INTRODUCTION TO
CLINICAL
PHARMACOLOGY

MARIE MONARD

INTRODUCTION TO
CLINICAL PHARMACOLOGY

MARILYN W. EDMUNDS, R.N., Ph.D.

Nursing Consultant in Pharmacology
Baltimore, Maryland

SECOND EDITION
With 203 illustrations

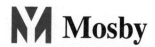

St. Louis Baltimore Berlin Boston Carlsbad Chicago London Madrid
Naples New York Philadelphia Sydney Tokyo Toronto

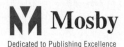

Editor: Robin Carter
Developmental Editor: Jeanne Allison
Project Manager: Patricia Tannian
Production Editors: Elizabeth C. Browning, Ann E. Rogers
Senior Book Designer: Gail Morey Hudson
Cover Designer: Teresa Breckwoldt
Illustrator and Cover Art: Mark Swindle
Manufacturing Supervisor: Kathy Grone

SECOND EDITION

Printed in the United States of America.
Composition by Carlisle Communications, Ltd.
Printing/binding by Custom Printing Company.

Mosby–Year Book, Inc.
11830 Westline Industrial Drive, St. Louis, Missouri 63146

Library of Congress Cataloging in Publication Data

Edmunds, Marilyn W.
    Introduction to clinical pharmacology / Marilyn W. Edmunds.—2nd
ed.
        p.   cm.
    Includes bibliographical references and index.
    ISBN 0-8016-7890-0
    1. Clinical pharmacology.   2. Nursing.   I. Title.
    [DNLM: 1. Pharmacology, Clinical—nurses' instruction.   2. Drug—
Therapy—nurses' instruction.   3. Drugs—administration & dosage—
nurses' instruction.   QV 38 E24i 1994]
RM301.28.E33   1995
615.5'8—dc20
DNLM/DLC
for Library of Congress   94-12193
                                                              CIP

94 95 96 97 98 / 9 8 7 6 5 4 3 2 1

Preface

Introduction to Clinical Pharmacology is a basic guide for nursing students beginning the study of pharmacology. With the second edition, the most current content is included, with discussions of contemporary medications, problems, regulations, and issues for nurses administering drugs. Many medications have been removed from the market, reflecting the Food and Drug Administration's reevaluation of effectiveness of medications. Many new medications have been included, in particular those that deal with HIV and hepatitis infections. Particular attention has been paid to pediatric and geriatric clients and the special care the nurse will need in administering medications to these individuals. A special section on cultural and ethnic variations in relation to taking medications is also included. Throughout the preparation of this text, making the content as clear and understandable as possible for today's nursing student was of great importance. Every effort has been made to incorporate in this edition the excellent suggestions of the nurses who used and evaluated the text.

The goals of *Introduction to Clinical Pharmacology* include the following:

▼ To focus on only the essential information that the nurse needs to know for safe administration of drugs.
▼ To present the material clearly and understandably.
▼ To feature a comprehensive unit on mathematics and calculations to enable students to review the mathematical skills required for medication administration.
▼ To use a consistent, practical format and extensive illustrations to help students develop a logical thinking process in the administration of drugs.
▼ To provide learning aids that help the student identify and learn what he or she needs to know.
▼ To use color to clarify concepts introduced in illustrations, mathematics, and conversions and to highlight what is most important for the student.

▼ To provide a comprehensive and useful *Instructor's Resource Manual* that helps the instructor teach pharmacology.

Organization

Pharmacology is a science: there are both right answers and wrong answers. Accuracy and precision are extremely important. In fact, nurses are legally responsible and accountable for how they administer medications. The science of medication administration for nurses is outlined in **Unit One: General Principles**. This unit stresses the nursing process, the importance of working with patients to assess medication needs and actions, and the differences among many types of medications; it also discusses establishing patient trust, teaching the patient or family about the medication and how to take it appropriately, and evaluating patient responses to medications.

Unit Two: Mathematics and Calculations also emphasizes precision—the precision required in dosage calculations. This unit includes review chapters on mathematical principles, equivalents, and drug dosage calculations.

Unit Three: Drug Groups briefly outlines essential information on 12 specific groups of medications.

Introduction to Clinical Pharmacology uses a **consistent, practical format** to help the student develop logical thinking skills in preparing and administering medications. Drugs are grouped by their therapeutic class within body system chapters, allowing students to learn quickly by making generalizations about similar drugs in a class. Each **drug class** is presented in a consistent format: its action, uses, adverse reactions, drug interactions, and a highlighted section "Nursing Implications and Patient Teaching." Content in this especially pertinent section is consistently divided into a **functional nursing process format:** assessment, planning, implementation, evaluation, and patient and family teaching. Headings throughout are in bold type so the student can find specific information easily and so that the organizing framework, which represents a useful, clinical approach to pharmacology, is reinforced by frequent repetition of these key headings.

New Features

▼ Geriatric considerations boxes have been added to reflect the special needs of this growing population.

▼ Similarly, pediatric considerations boxes are presented to address the special issues that exist with this age-group.

▼ Critical decision boxes have been added to highlight important aspects of medication administration and drug therapy.

▼ Critical thinking questions have been added to the end of each chapter to promote higher level thinking skills and to reinforce key concepts in the chapter.

▼ In addition, we have moved the key terms list to the beginning of each chapter to allow for a quick review of terminology so that the student is aware of what to look for in each chapter.

▼ Anatomy reviews have been added to chapter beginnings.

Faculty Input

As mentioned previously, our *focus* is on only the most essential information that nurses need to know. We have solicited input from experienced faculty members who reviewed the first edition of this book to ensure that the content is relevant, accurate, and current. The input from faculty members was invaluable for improving the readability and limiting the content throughout the book to only the most essential information.

We realize the importance of differentiating between what the student must learn from reading a pharmacology text and what kind of material to include strictly for reference. Because educators continually stressed the nursing students' need for both in a pharmacology textbook, we have retained the book's unique format that meets both of these needs: **narrative content** deals exclusively with major drug groups, whereas all the information related to specific drugs appears in **reference tables.** Using this approach, the student is not overwhelmed with extensive reading material but, at the same time, has ready access to generic names, trade names, forms, and dosages for individual drugs. We have marked trade name drugs available only in Canada with a ✦ for Canadian educators and students.

Readability

In discussing this book with those who regularly teach nursing students, we realized that pharmacology is a subject that is difficult to teach and to learn. We have made this text as *clear and readable* as possible to facilitate the instruction of pharmacology. Because of a combination of factors, many of today's students are not as well prepared as instructors would desire. Students from a variety of backgrounds add a welcome diversity to an educational program and, with it, a host of challenges in identifying and meeting the needs of today's student. We have used shorter sentences, simpler terminology, and shorter paragraphs to make the book less intimidating and more engaging to students.

Mathematics Review

A **comprehensive unit on mathematics and calculations** has been included to allow students to review the mathematic concepts necessary for understanding pharmacology. The content was also limited to what is most essential; numerous equivalencies and other mathematical reference features are included for student review or reference. Another feature of the mathematics unit is the use of **key point boxes** that break up the text and remind the student of basic mathematical principles or reinforce what has just been learned. This feature was included because of the difficulty many students have in learning and retaining basic mathematical skills. Color has been used specifically in these chapters to clarify and convey problem-solving concepts.

Numerous sample problems, which are solved in a logical step-by-step approach, provide students with concrete examples of how to work problems, in addition to giving them a systematic approach to solving the problems. Expanded problems for students to solve are included on **reproducible worksheets** and **quizzes** included in the *Instructor's Resource Manual.* These additional mathematical review tools can be used in a variety of ways: to assess students' current mathematical skills and abilities, to enable students to review mathematics at their own pace, and to test students in the classroom. A complete list of worksheets, quizzes, and tests is included in the front of the *Instructor's Resource Manual* for the educator's reference and class planning.

Illustrations

Over **70 two-color illustrations** have been created specifically for this book. We have included extensive illustrations of medication administration techniques; equipment; various forms and preparations; and sample forms relating to documentation, charting, or drug administration. The illustrations are clear, simple, and also attractive, and—perhaps most important—they employ color and various screens in a fresh and interesting way. Students who class-tested portions of the book consistently rated the illustrations as outstanding. Several anatomical drawings have been added to promote student understanding of the body systems.

Pedagogy

In addition to making the book readable, consistently and logically organized, and well illustrated, we have included **numerous pedagogical features** to further enhance learning. These include unit objectives and overviews, chapter objectives and overviews, key terms printed in color where they are first introduced and defined, chapter summaries, an alphabetical listing of the color key terms with page cross references at the beginning of each chapter, and critical thinking questions at the end of each chapter. Each of these

features has been built in to help the student identify and learn what is important. We believe that each of these features will make the student's learning experience and the instructor's teaching experience as positive as possible.

Ancillary Package

Our *Instructor's Resource Manual* is unique to the teaching of pharmacology. It includes unit objectives and overviews, chapter objectives and overviews, a list of key terms introduced and explained in each chapter, a chapter outline with related lecture content and reference material from the text, role plays, resources, and reproducible practice worksheets and quizzes.

In addition to the *Instructor's Resource Manual,* a separate *Student Learning Guide* is available either packaged with the text or for separate purchase. The student guide duplicates the worksheets included in the *Instructor's Resource Manual.* Also available to instructors are pharmacology transparency acetates to serve as visual aids to instruction. In addition, **Mosby's Pharmacology Update,** a biannual newsletter, is available to meet the special needs of nursing students and instructors by providing current and well-documented pharmacology information.

Conclusion

Nothing teaches the nurse more about pharmacology than actually giving medications to a patient. To develop mastery of this content, the nursing student should approach each encounter with a patient as an opportunity to learn. The nurse should accept it as a personal challenge to learn about each medication ordered for a patient under his or her care and to understand why the medication is given in that particular situation. Completing medication cards and personalizing the information to a specific patient are invaluable experiences in learning about medications. Because pharmacology is a rapidly changing and dynamic field, it is recommended that the student be exposed early on to supplemental drug information, such as package inserts or current drug handbooks. The student should be encouraged to develop the habit of seeking up-to-date and timely information to supplement this book and to provide specific details that cannot be covered in a textbook.

In working with patients, the nursing student will quickly learn that medication administration is one of the most challenging components of the nursing role. A nurse who develops the knowledge and skills needed to competently administer medications is highly visible and will gain the respect of both patients and colleagues in the health care system. Both the responsibilities and the personal rewards are great. The author and publisher sincerely hope this book helps the student to gain both. We welcome your suggestions or comments on *Introduction to Clinical Pharmacology*, second edition, so that we may continue to provide a clear and useful exposition of introductory pharmacology in future editions.

Acknowledgments

Writing a pharmacology text is like running a race that never ends. There are always new drugs arriving on the market and new information available about old products. The available information is endless, and it is a real challenge to try to acquire enough knowledge to be a safe practitioner.

I wish to acknowledge my personal stimulation from the many students who have asked challenging questions throughout my years as a teacher and the support of my professional colleagues. I am grateful for the help of the editorial, production, and design staff at Mosby–Year Book and specifically thank Jeanne Allison, Liz Browning, Robin Carter, Gail Hudson, Ann Rogers, and Patricia Tannian. I am also grateful to Mark Swindle for his highly original illustrations, including the cover illustration. I would also like to thank Sheila Rankin Zerr, R.N., M.Ed., Visiting Assistant Professor at the University of Victoria, British Columbia, for her careful research on Canadian drug legislation. As always, I owe a special debt of gratitude to my family, who is so important in my life and who supports me in all the things in which I get involved.

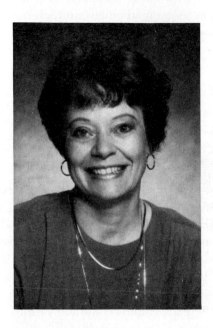

Marilyn Edmunds

Consultants

Pam Blake, RN, MSN
Indiana Vocational College
Valparaiso, Indiana

Julie Buntjer, RN, ADN
Willmar Technical College
Willmar, Minnesota

Rose Corder, RN, BSN, EMT-P
San Jacinto College of Nursing
Houston, Texas

Lola Cress, RN, MEd
Lawrence County Vocational School
Chesapeake, Ohio

Wanda Huffman, RN, BSN
Lawrence County Vocational School
Chesapeake, Ohio

Shirley P. Jones, RN, BS
Isabella Graham Hart School of Practical Nursing
Rochester, New York

Diana G. McLaughlin, RN, MS
Idaho State University
Pocatello, Idaho

Linda North, RN, MSN
Reid State Technical College
Evergreen, Alabama

Patricia B. Simmons, RN, MSN
Reid State Technical College
Evergreen, Alabama

Marilyn Fuqua Thompson, RN, MS
Lake Land College
Mattoon, Illinois

Richard E. Watters, RN, BSc, BEd
Nursing Consultant
Ottawa, Ontario

The author and publisher are especially grateful to the practical nursing students at Willmar Technical College, Willmar, Minnesota, for their willingness to class-test portions of the manuscript of the first edition and their many helpful comments.

Contents

Detailed Contents

xiii

INTRODUCTION TO
CLINICAL
PHARMACOLOGY

UNIT ONE

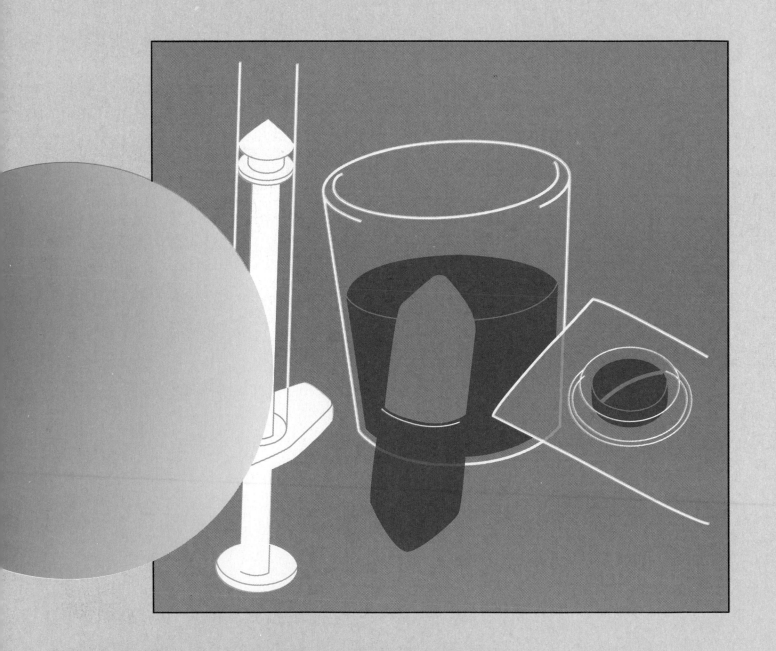

General Principles

OBJECTIVES

At the conclusion of this unit you should be able to:

1. Discuss the steps of the nursing process and how they are used in the administration of medications.

2. List the federal, state, and institutional regulations or policies that affect the nurse who administers medications.

3. Use basic terminology to describe the absorption, distribution, metabolism, and excretion of medications.

4. Evaluate whether responses to medications are therapeutic or nontherapeutic.

5. Describe the procedures for administration of enteral, parenteral, and percutaneous medications.

6. Outline the nurse's responsibility in giving medications.

OVERVIEW

The first four chapters of this book describe the basic nursing actions that will be used in the text. Chapter 1 explores the nursing process and shows how assessment, planning, implementation, and evaluation are used in administering medications. The goal is to give the nurse a clear idea of the special responsibility involved in giving medications.

Chapter 2 focuses on the legal rules and the basic federal laws that have shaped federal policy about drugs. A clear picture of how the federal regulations differ from other regulations is presented. State Nurse Practice Acts are discussed in detail, since they specify who has the authority to administer medications and how that authority must be obtained. Other state and institutional policies are discussed, relating to legal medication orders, ordering medications, and the use and supervision of controlled substances.

Chapter 3 discusses how drugs are used for medicinal purposes. The basic processes that all medications go through in the body are described, as well as the variables that affect a drug's action in the body.

Chapter 4 introduces information that applies to the following chapters. It covers the specific procedures for administering medications. The focus is on accuracy, accepting nursing responsibility, and maintaining asepsis as medications are given enterally (orally, nasogastrically, or rectally), parenterally (intradermally, subcutaneously, intramuscularly, or intravenously) or percutaneously (by application to the skin surface or through mucous membranes).

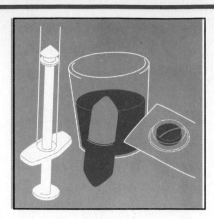

CHAPTER 1
The Nursing Process

Steps of the Nursing Process

Nursing actions are specific and deliberate, and are not performed in a random manner. A plan that organizes and coordinates the nurse's activities has developed over the years and is known as the nursing process. The nursing process consists of the following four major parts:

1. Assessment
2. Planning
3. Implementation
4. Evaluation

All of these steps are followed when giving medications to patients. The nursing process is illustrated in Fig. 1-1.

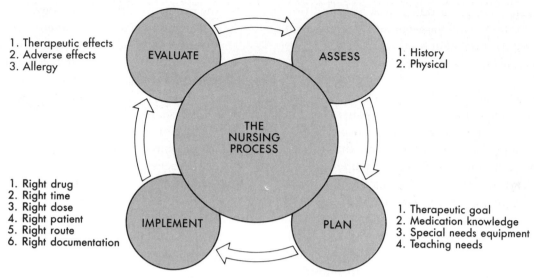

1. Therapeutic effects
2. Adverse effects
3. Allergy

EVALUATE

ASSESS

1. History
2. Physical

THE
NURSING
PROCESS

1. Right drug
2. Right time
3. Right dose
4. Right patient
5. Right route
6. Right documentation

IMPLEMENT

PLAN

1. Therapeutic goal
2. Medication knowledge
3. Special needs equipment
4. Teaching needs

Fig. 1-1   The nursing process.

ASSESSMENT

Assessment is a process that gathers information about the patient, the problem, and any factors that may influence the drug to be given. This step of the nursing process is especially important because it provides the beginning information, or **data base,** from which all other nursing process decisions will be made.

Assessment involves collecting information by taking the patient's history and evaluating the physical findings. When the patient is admitted to the hospital, she or he should be carefully questioned about present problems, past history of illnesses, surgery, and medications, and the response to previous drug therapy. This information is extremely important and helps the health care team members plan the patient's care. Information provided in the patient's history often directs the nurse and the physician to look for physical signs that may be present.

Information obtained through assessment is classified into two categories: subjective data and objective data. **Subjective data** are supplied by the patient or family, and may be felt or known only by the patient and may not be detected directly by anyone else. Examples of subjective information might include the following:

1. The chief complaint of the patient (in the patient's own words)
2. The detailed history of the course of the present illness

3. Past medical history
4. The family history of diseases
5. Social profile
6. Review of complaints and problems found in different body systems

Some patient complaints are more subjective than others. For example, if a patient complains of pain in the abdomen, the nurse must accept the patient's word that the pain is present. The nurse cannot see, hear, or feel the patient's abdominal pain. A patient may state that he or she has difficulty breathing. Although the nurse may observe the patient breathing more rapidly, the degree of difficulty experienced by the patient is not obvious. This is the patient's internal feeling; the nurse cannot actually document this. Information is considered to be subjective if the nurse has no documentation or evidence to support the patient's statement or if the perception cannot be discerned by anyone other than the patient. Information about the patient obtained in the history may be considered subjective until there are medical records or laboratory findings to document the existence of the problem.

Objective data are obtained from documentation that patients may bring with them, such as old electrocardiograms or x-ray scans, or from information obtained during the physical examination. Vital signs (respiratory rate, pulse, blood pressure, weight, height, temperature), physical findings discovered during **inspection** (looking closely), **palpation** (feeling), **percussion** (detecting differences in sound produced by vibration), and **auscultation** (listening with the stethoscope), and recent findings from laboratory tests and diagnostic procedures all provide objective evidence.

It is especially important to obtain subjective and objective assessment data when the patient is first examined or on admission to the hospital. This provides initial or baseline information that can be used to determine the severity of the patient's problems. Assessment is performed throughout the course of the disease to determine whether the patient is responding appropriately to the treatment.

The nurse may not always be responsible for collecting the subjective and objective data; however, the nurse is always responsible for learning this information from the chart, the physician, the family, or other health care team members, and using the information to plan nursing care.

Factors to consider in assessing the patient

Although the information in the patient's history and physical examination helps the nurse understand the patient and plan nursing care, certain information is especially important in planning drug therapy. The nursing assessment at the time of the patient's admission to the hospital should give special attention to the drug history. Information should be obtained from the patient (primary source), but occasionally a patient's relatives, old medical records, ECGs, or laboratory reports may provide the information (secondary sources). Literature about particular diseases, medications, or problems might also provide helpful information (tertiary sources).

When asking about the patient's drug history, the nurse makes assessments in the following areas:
1. Symptoms, signs, or diagnosed diseases that document the patient's need for medication (such as high blood sugar levels, high blood pressure, or pain).
2. Current (and sometimes past) use of all medications and drugs.
   a. All prescription medications (patients often forget to mention birth control pills in this category).
   b. Over-the-counter medications (such as aspirin, vitamins, laxatives, cold and sinus preparations, and antacids).
   c. Street drugs used for recreational purposes (such as marijuana or cocaine).

3. Any problems with drug therapy.
   a. Allergies: what is the patient's response to a medicine to which the patient believes he or she is allergic? Does it represent a true allergy? An adverse effect? A common side effect?
   b. Diseases that may contraindicate or limit prescription of some medications (such as sickle cell anemia, G6-PD deficiency, migraine headaches, or angina).

Assessment of the individual is not just conducted at the beginning of treatment or hospitalization. Assessment of changes in patient status that may influence drug therapy must be performed constantly during the course of the hospital stay.

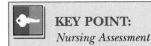

KEY POINT:
Nursing Assessment

Assessment includes collecting relevant information.

PLANNING

Based on the data collected, goals are established and care plans are developed. Plans have two participants: the nurse and the patient. Patient goals help the patient learn about the medication and how to use it properly. Nursing goals help the nurse plan what equipment or procedures are needed to give the medication. Using the information about the patient's history, medical and psychosocial problems, risk factors, and severity of problems, both types of plans can be constructed. The patient-oriented care plan should include any medications that will be given on either a short-term or long-term basis. For example, goals may be established for applying ointments or medicated patches, or for demonstrating patient-administered aerosol nebulizer treatments. Nursing goals may include developing the site rotation of injections, or educating the patient about specific side effects of medications that should be anticipated and reported.

Factors to consider in planning to give a medication

Planning to give a medication involves the following four steps:
1. Determine the therapeutic goal for each medi-

cation to be administered (for example, what is this drug to accomplish?).

2. Review specific information about the medication.
   a. Anticipated action of the drug.
   b. Side effects that may develop.
   c. Recommendations for dosage, route, and frequency.
   d. Contraindications to the drug (in what situations the drug must *not* be given).
   e. Drug interactions (what is the influence of another drug given at the same time?).
3. Anticipate special storage or administration procedures, techniques, or equipment needs.
4. Develop a teaching plan for the patient.
   a. What the patient needs to know about the medication's action and side effects.
   b. What the patient needs to know about the administration of the medication.
   c. What the patient needs to report to the nurse or physician about the medication and/or the patient's response.

The most important step in planning is to collect and use information about the patient and the medication. This step requires knowledge of drug agents and exercise of professional judgment.

Once the medication is ordered, the nurse must verify the accuracy of the order. This is usually done by comparing the medication card or Kardex order with the physician's original order in the chart. This step must be performed each time the medication is given. In this way, errors caused in recopying the order onto the medication card can be avoided.

The nurse must also compare the information known about the drug and the specific drug order to determine whether the drug and the dosage ordered seem correct. The nurse should also know enough about the patient's problem to understand why the medication is being given. No part of the order or the reason for giving the medication should be unclear. Any questions about the appropriateness or the safety of the medication for that patient should be answered before the medication is administered. The nurse must use professional judgment in carrying out the medication order. If the nurse decides (1) that any part of the order is incorrect or unclear, (2) the patient's condition would be worsened by the medication, (3) the physician may not have all the information needed about the patient in planning the therapy, or (4) there has been a change in the

patient's condition so that the medication should not be given, the medication should be withheld until the physician can be contacted. If the physician cannot be contacted or does not change the order under question, the nurse should notify the head nurse and nursing supervisor immediately. Most institutions have clear policies about who to contact, how to report this problem, and what to do next.

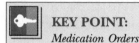

KEY POINT:
Medication Orders

Clarify and understand each part of the medication order.

Again, the planning phase gives the nurse time to do the following:

1. Obtain any special equipment needed to administer the medication (such as IV infusion pumps, TB syringes, or nebulizers).
2. Review administration procedures or techniques (such as Z-track injection technique, IV push policy).
3. Determine in advance what information the patient will need.

This information can be recorded on the nursing care plan or in the Kardex file so that other team members are included in the plan.

IMPLEMENTATION

Implementation is the performance of the nursing care plan by administering a helpful medication (therapeutic agent). This phase of the nursing process requires that the nurse understand all of the information about each patient and about the drug ordered as therapy. It is the nurse's responsibility to understand why each medication is ordered, to know detailed information about the drug itself, and to know how to safely administer it. For example, the nurse who adds an antibiotic solution to an intravenous line should have knowledge of the proper equipment, aseptic technique, rate of flow, interactions with the chemicals already in the tubing, and flushing of the line following therapy. Or perhaps the nurse may take the patient's pulse before giving digitalis to determine whether the medication may be given safely.

Implementation also implies that the nurse is

aware of any changes in the patient's status that may make it unwise to give the medication. For example, if the patient receiving antibiotics complains of an itchy rash on the chest and arms, the nurse will withhold the antibiotic and notify the patient's physician.

THE RIGHT DRUG. Many drug names are complicated and difficult to read. Many drug names are very similar. It is important to carefully check the spelling and concentration of each medication *before* the medication is administered. For example, digitoxin and digoxin are both cardiotonic drugs, but they are quite different in dosage and duration of action. Sometimes confusion arises when a medication is ordered by a trade name (such as Valium), but the pharmacy sends up a medication with the generic name (diazepam). The nurse must not assume that the correct medication has been sent without checking a reliable book or calling the pharmacy.

The drug may be delivered in a unit dose system or in an individually prepared prescription, or the medication may be taken from a unit stock. Regardless of the delivery method, the nurse must read the drug label at least three times:

1. Before removing the drug from the unit dose cart or shelf
2. Before preparing or measuring the prescribed dose of medication
3. Before replacing the medication on the shelf or just before opening the medication at the time of administration

THE RIGHT TIME. The drug order should specify when the medication is to be given. Hospitals have policies that determine which hours medications will be given when they are ordered (such as "every 4 hours" or "qid"). The nurse must be familiar with hospital policy and use only standard abbreviations in administering and recording medication therapy. To be effective, many drugs must be given on a rigid schedule day and night to keep the level of medication constant in the blood. Other medications may be given only during the day.

Medication administration often has to be planned around other patient activities. For example, if a patient is taking an anticoagulant to thin the blood and prolong the clotting time (to decrease the risk of blood clots), the medication must be given at the same time every day and a blood test to monitor the clotting time should also be taken at the same time every day. Patients with infections should have specimens cultured before starting antibiotic therapy. Patients under-

going evaluation of thyroid function should have blood tests done before having gallbladder x-ray scans, which confuse or make inaccurate thyroid function study results.

Medications are usually given when there is the maximum chance for absorption and the least risk for side effects. This may mean some medications should be given when the patient's stomach is empty; others need to be taken with food. Some medications require that the patient not eat certain foods (for example, imipramine has special dietary restrictions). Others are incompatible with alcohol (for example, metronidazole [Flagyl] causes severe vomiting if the patient takes any alcohol while taking the drug). When a patient is taking several medications, the patient must be observed for drug interactions. For example, some medications reduce the absorption of birth control pills, thus placing the patient unknowingly at risk for pregnancy.

Finally, one-time-only or emergency medications are especially important to check. The nurse must be certain that no one else has already administered the medication and that the appropriate time interval has elapsed for the administration of the drug. Narcotics are often given irregularly as "stat" or "prn" medications. Their administration should be promptly noted on the patient's chart so that it is clear whether or not the patient has been given the medication.

The box below summarizes the important considerations in giving the medication at the right time.

Factors to Consider in Administering Medication at the Right Time

Understand and follow the institution's policies regarding designated times for regularly scheduled drugs.

Follow drug treatment guidelines to maximize drug absorption and reduce chances for drug incompatibilities.

Give medications as ordered to enhance constant blood levels.

Coordinate drug therapy with other diagnostic and laboratory testing plans.

Be especially cautious in giving prn or stat medications to avoid risk of overdosing.

THE RIGHT DOSE. Medication dosages are usually intended for the "average" patient. A patient who is emaciated (bony and shrunken from severe weight loss as a result of illness), small, or obese may require variation in dosages. Pediatric patients often have dosages based on their body weight. Geriatric or elderly patients may be unusually sensitive to the action of many medications. If patients have coexisting diseases or reduced liver or kidney function, this may further complicate the dosage requirements. Patients who are nauseated and vomiting may be unable to take oral medications. Although the physician may order the correct dosage of the medication, changes in the patient's status may require that the dosage be altered.

Obtaining the correct dosage of a medication also requires that the nurse use the proper equipment (for example, insulin measured in an insulin syringe), the proper drug form (oral or rectal, water or oil base, scored or coated capsules), and the proper concentration (0.25 mg or 2.5 mg), and that accurate calculations are used to determine the drug dosage. Most institutions have specific policies that require two nurses to check any medication dosage that must be calculated, particularly medications such as narcotics, heparin, insulin, or intravenous medications.

THE RIGHT PATIENT. Although it seems like common sense to make certain the right patient gets the medication, errors may occur on a busy hospital unit. Four groups of patients are most at risk for error: the pediatric patient, the geriatric patient, the non–English-speaking patient, and the very confused or critically ill patient. The common factor these four groups share is their decreased ability to identify themselves accurately to the nurse. They also may not understand what the nurse is asking or what is being given to them. The identification bracelets on some patients may have been removed for tests or when blood was drawn for testing. Children especially enjoy hiding, changing beds, answering to another name, and so on. Each patient should be asked his or her name *as the nurse checks the identification bracelet.* Medications should *never* be administered to a patient without an identification bracelet.

THE RIGHT ROUTE. The drug order should clearly specify the route of drug administration. The nurse must never substitute one route for another without consulting the physician and having the order changed. There is great variation in the rate of absorption of medications administered by various routes.

The oral route is usually the preferred route of administration if the patient is oriented. In some cases, faster and higher blood concentrations are needed, and the medication may be given intravenously or subcutaneously. There may be special precautions for medications administered through these routes (such as rate of administration or dosage). Some injections should be given subcutaneously rather than intramuscularly. This requires proper technique by the nurse. Some medications are very painful if given intramuscularly, and intravenous administration would be more appropriate.

When breathing nebulizers are ordered, the nurse needs to find out whether the nebulizer is to be used through the nose or the mouth. The nurse must teach the patient the appropriate way to use the nebulizer so that the medication reaches the intended place. The same principle applies to the use of eye drops, ear drops, ointments, lotions, shampoos, and rectal and vaginal medications.

THE RIGHT DOCUMENTATION. A notation of the drug's administration should be made on the patient's chart as soon as possible after the drug is given. For emergencies and medications used only occasionally, this is very important. Institutional policy may require that the chart notation of intramuscular medications also include the site of the injection and any complaints made by the patient at the time of administration. The chart notation should identify the drug given, the dosage, and the time it is actually given (not the time it is supposed to be given). Progress notes should include any comments describing the patient's response to the medications. Any complaints or adverse effects should be noted in the chart and reported to the head nurse and the physician. The nurse should never record on the chart medications that were not given or before they are given.

It is clear that if all these principles are followed, the nurse must never give medication prepared by another nurse. Even when nurses are very busy, when emergencies occur, or when they are interrupted, the nurse cannot assume that all the "rights" are followed unless the person who prepares the medication is the one who gives the medication. Occasionally a physician will ask the nurse to prepare the medication for the physician to give. The nurse may then prepare the medication, but should go with the physician to see that the medication is given as ordered. It should be clearly documented that the physician gave the medication.

Following institutional policy, using common sense, and remembering the high standards that nurses should have will reduce the chance for medication error. Should an error be made, honesty in discussing the problem and prompt action to correct any damage are especially important in protecting the patient from harm.

KEY POINT:

The Six Rights of Medication Administration:

- Drug
- Time
- Dose
- Patient
- Route
- Documentation

EVALUATION

Evaluation is the process of looking at the results produced when the plan is implemented. When related to medications, evaluation requires the nurse to consider the patient's response to the drug, noting both expected and unexpected findings. When antipyretic medications (drugs that reduce fever) are given, the nurse should take the patient's temperature to determine whether the medication has been effective. When antidysrhythmic agents are given to make the patient's heartbeat more regular, taking the pulse will help determine the patient's response to the medication.

Evaluation of previous therapy is frequently part of the assessment process for continued drug therapy. Thus the nursing process may be viewed as a circular process (see Fig. 1-1, p. 3). For example, taking the patient's temperature is part of the evaluation phase of the nursing process, but it may also become an assessment that the patient's temperature is still elevated, requiring more medication or additional nursing actions.

Factors to consider in evaluating response to medication

Once medication has been administered to the patient, the nurse must closely observe the patient to see the response to the medication. The nurse checks for two types of responses to drug therapy: therapeutic effects and adverse effects.

Therapeutic effects are seen when the drug produces the intended reaction. If the nurse understands why the medication is being given or the therapeutic goal of the medication, the nurse will be able to decide whether or not that goal is being met. For example, if the patient has a fever and aspirin is given, the nurse should see a lower temperature when the temperature is taken in 1 to 2 hours.

Adverse or side effects are seen when the patient fails to respond to the medication in the anticipated manner or develops other signs or symptoms that create problems. For example, a patient with pneumonia may be given penicillin. Although the pneumonia infection may be controlled by the antibiotic, presence of a rash may indicate that the patient has developed an allergy to the medicine, and the penicillin must be stopped. A patient receiving an anticoagulant must be closely observed for signs of bleeding or bruising, which would indicate overdosage or overresponse to the medication. Sometimes side effects such as nausea or vomiting may be eliminated by decreasing the dosage or by giving the medication with food. Grading the severity of the side effects will help the physician determine whether the medication should be continued or stopped.

Because the nurse is the health care provider who is most often with the patient, the nurse is in an important and unique position to examine the patient's response to drug therapy. The careful and repeated assessment of the patient and the documentation of the findings are especially important in the care of the hospitalized patient.

KEY POINT:

Evaluating Response to Medication

It is important to evaluate the therapeutic response and any adverse side effects or allergic responses.

CRITICAL DECISION:

Points in Administering Drugs

- **Assessing the patient and clearly understanding why the patient is receiving a particular medication**
- **Preparing the medication to be administered (i.e., checking labels, preparing injections, observing proper asepsis techniques with needles and syringes)**
- **Accurately calculating dosages**
- **Administering the medication (proper injection techniques, aids to help swallowing, topical methods)**
- **Documenting medications given**
- **Monitoring the patient's reaction and evaluating the patient's response**
- **Educating the patient regarding his or her medications and medication regimen**

SUMMARY

The nursing process is an organized guide that helps the nurse provide good care to the patient and avoid making mistakes. Performing a patient assessment, planning medications, implementing the correct procedures and techniques, and evaluating the patient's response become automatic as the nurse gains greater skill and experience. For new nurses, the nursing process provides a predictable and safe direction to follow when learning many new and important skills.

 ## CRITICAL THINKING QUESTIONS

1. Identify each of the following as either *objective* (*O*) or *subjective* (*S*) information:
   _____ **a.** The patient complains of pain in the abdomen.
   _____ **b.** The nurse takes the patient's blood pressure and determines that it is too high.
   _____ **c.** The nurse counts respirations and concludes that the patient is short of breath.
   _____ **d.** After palpating the patient's abdomen, the nurse reports that it is tender to touch.
   _____ **e.** The patient complains of being "too fat."
   _____ **f.** Four-year-old Sean's thermometer registers a temperature of 102° F.
   _____ **g.** After weighing Mr. Tracy this morning, the nurse reports that he has gained 2 pounds in 6 days.
   _____ **h.** Ms. Jackson says that almost every day she has trouble breathing or "catching" her breath.
   _____ **i.** A 50-year-old female patients asks for aspirin, saying she's getting "hot flashes."
   _____ **j.** Mr. Clark tells the nurse, "My heart is really pounding!"

2. You are assigned to give medications to eight different patients this morning. Write a paragraph describing the step-by-step procedure you would use to ensure that you are observing the six rights of drug administration.

3. Describe four things a nurse might do for a patient taking morphine that would fall under the category of *assessment*.

4. What's the difference between *planning* and *evaluation* in drug administration? Are they sometimes the same thing? Give examples of each.

5. What's the difference between *palpation* and *percussion*? Describe the performance of each, illustrating the differences.

6. Match the following abbreviations with their correct meanings:
_____ OD	a. twice a day
_____ q2h	b. one dose if necessary
_____ bid	c. drops
_____ D	d. give
_____ sos	e. right eye
_____ gr	f. lozenge
_____ gtt	g. mouth
_____ AS	h. every 2 hours
_____ troch	i. four times a day
_____ qid	j. left ear
_____ os	k. grain

7. Why does the nurse have to keep repeating assessment of the patient receiving medications?

8. Identify three areas of assessment necessary in completing a patient's drug history.

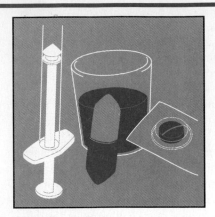

CHAPTER 2
Legal Aspects Affecting the Administration of Medications

OBJECTIVES

At the conclusion of the chapter you should be able to:

1. List major federal legislation about drugs and drug use.
2. Explain what is meant by "scheduled drugs" and give examples of drugs in the different schedules.
3. Compare regulations by state and institution that affect administration of medications by nurses.
4. Identify the traditional parts of a patient's chart and the information given in each part.
5. Describe the information contained in the patient Kardex file.
6. Explain the nurse's responsibility for controlled substances.
7. List the information required in a medication order or prescription.
8. Define and give examples of the four different types of medication orders.

KEY TERMS

controlled substances, p. 11
legal responsibility, p. 15
nurse practice act, p. 14
over-the-counter (OTC) medications, p. 11
physical dependence, p. 11
prescription medications, p. 11
problem-oriented medical record (POMR), p. 16
professional responsibility, p. 14
psychologic dependence, p. 11

Pharmacology and Regulations

Nurses who give medications come under the authority of regulations at the following three levels:

1. *Federal legislation,* which describes conditions under which certain medications may be given
2. *State legislation and regulations,* which describe who may prescribe, dispense, and administer medications, and under what conditions
3. *Individual hospital or agency regulations,* which establish further guidelines and policy regarding medication administration and reporting

FEDERAL LEGISLATION

Legislation passed by Congress generally tries to make medications as safe as possible for patients to take and makes certain that the medication does what it claims to do (effectiveness). Congressional legislation created the Food and Drug Administration (FDA) to oversee the testing and marketing of new drugs. A great deal of legislation is also directed at controlling potentially dangerous drugs and trying to limit drug abuse. Table 2-1 summarizes major federal drug legislation.

Federal legislation has created the following three categories of drugs in the United States:

1. **Controlled substances,** which include major pain killers (narcotics) and some sedatives or tranquilizers
2. **Prescription medications,** such as antibiotics and oral birth control pills
3. **Over-the-counter (OTC) medications,** which may be purchased without prescription

Controlled substances

Controlled substances are the most heavily regulated drugs because of their high potential for abuse. The Controlled Substances Act of 1970 classified these medications into five "schedules." The degree of control, the recordkeeping required, the order forms, and other regulations vary with regard to these five classifications.

Table 2-2 describes the five drug schedules, with examples of medications included in each category.

Physical dependence refers to the physiologic need for a medication to relieve shaking, pain, or other symptoms. **Psychologic dependence,** on the other hand, refers to a feeling of anxiety, stress, or tension felt if the patient does not have the medication. One type of dependency often leads to the other; they are often found together in the same individual.

Federal and state laws make the possession of controlled substances a crime, except in specifically exempted cases defined clearly by the law. The professional practice acts within each state define which health professionals may dispense and prescribe controlled substances. Medications are usually dispensed by pharmacists; the responsibility for prescribing is reserved for physicians, dentists, and sometimes osteopaths. In about half the states, nurse practitioners, nurse anesthetists, physician's assistants, and/or nurse-midwives may also have prescribing privileges. Professional and licensed practical nurses may give controlled substances only under the direction of a health professional who is licensed to dispense or prescribe these drugs.

Nurses may not have controlled substances in their possession unless:

1. The nurse is giving them to the patient for whom they are ordered.
2. The nurse is the individual designated responsible for the control of the supply of medications of a ward or department.
3. The nurse is the patient for whom a physician has prescribed the medication.

There are specific state and institutional regula-

Table 2-1	Summary of major federal drug legislation	
Title of legislation	**Year**	**Description of legislation**
Harrison Narcotic Act	1914	Limits the indiscriminate use of addictive drugs. Regulated the importation, manufacture, sale, and use of opium, cocaine, and their compounds and derivatives. Amended many times and finally repealed and replaced in 1970.
Federal Food, Drug and Cosmetic Act	1938	Authorized the Food and Drug Administration of the Department of Health and Human Services to determine the safety of drugs before marketing to determine labeling specifications, and to assure that advertising claims are met.
Durham-Humphrey Amendment	1952	Restricts the number of prescriptions that can be refilled.
Kefauver-Harris Act	1962	Provides greater control and surveillance of clinical testing and distribution of investigational drugs. Product must be proven to be both safe and effective before it may be released for sale.
Comprehensive Drug Abuse Prevention and Control Act (Controlled Substances Act)	1970	Composite law that repealed almost 50 other laws. Designed to improve the administration and regulation of manufacturing, distributing, and dispensing of controlled drugs. Drug Enforcement Administration (DEA) created to enforce Controlled Substances Act, gather intelligence, train investigators, and conduct research on potentially dangerous drugs and drug abuse.

Table 2-2   Controlled substance schedule

Schedule	Potential for abuse	Comments and examples
I	High	No currently accepted medical use in the United States. Lack of accepted safety for use under medical supervision. *Examples:* hashish, heroin, lysergic acid diethylamide (LSD), marijuana, peyote, STP.
II	High	Abuse potential that may lead to severe psychologic or physical dependence. *Examples:* amphetamines, meperidine, methadone, methaqualone, morphine, pentobarbital, oxycodone (Percodan), secobarbital.
III	High, but less than I or II	Abuse potential that may lead to moderate or low physical dependence or high psychologic dependence. *Examples:* glutethimide (Doriden), aspirin with codeine (Empirin with codeine), aspirin with butalbital and caffeine (Fiorinal), methyprylon (Noludar), paregoric, acetaminophen with codeine (Tylenol with codeine).
IV	Low compared with III	Abuse potential that may lead to limited physical or psychologic dependence. *Examples:* chloral hydrate, flurazepam (Dalmane), meprobamate (Equanil), chlordiazepoxide (Librium), paraldehyde, phenobarbital, chlorazepate (Tranxene), diazepam (Valium).
V	Low compared with IV	Abuse potential of limited physical or psychologic dependence. *Examples:* diphenoxylate with atropine sulfate (Lomotil), guaifenesin with codeine sulfate (Robitussin A-C), terpin hydrate with codeine.

tions that cover the ordering, receiving, storing, and recording of use of controlled substances. All schedule medications must be counted every 8 hours. Every pill or ampule must be accounted for. Institutional policy determines which nurses will be involved in the legal transferring of responsibility from shift to shift and how medications will be counted and checked. All controlled substances ordered for patients but not used must be returned to the pharmacy when the patient is discharged.

In a time when drug abuse is so common, the nurse assuming the responsibility for the controlled substances must remain alert. Abuse is not limited to patients. Some health care professionals may be unable to resist a large supply of medication and will seek to disguise or hide their use of patients' medication. For example, if a pattern develops of personnel frequently dropping or spilling medications, or if records show that patients are receiving large or frequent doses of medications on certain shifts but the patients get no relief from pain, suspicion might be raised that the medication is being taken by the nurse. Most states have as part of the state profes-

sional nursing organization "impaired nursing committees" to help nurses who have drug abuse or other problems that affect their ability to carry out their professional duties.

Regulations about drug administration and controlled substances are under close inspection at all levels of regulation, and breaking the rules is considered serious. Illegal behavior will result in the loss of the nurse's license to practice. Violation of the Controlled Substances Act or failure to comply with its regulations is punishable by a fine, imprisonment, or both.

Prescription drugs

The federal government has also designated that many drugs are sufficiently dangerous that their use must be carefully supervised by a knowledgeable health professional (physician, dentist, or nurse practitioner). This control is maintained through use of a written prescription or order before the drug may be given. Prescription drugs represent the largest category of drugs and account for most of the medications the nurse will be giving to hospitalized patients.

Prescription drugs are tested before they are put on the market. They must meet certain standards for safety and effectiveness. However, even though a good deal of information is known about the medication, each patient may display a slightly different reaction. The nurse must be alert and watch for signs of the expected response to the drug, as well as adverse reactions that may develop. The patient often receives several medications at the same time, and drug interactions may make evaluation of the patient response more complex.

The Omnibus Reconciliation Acts of 1989, 1990, and 1991 placed further controls on drugs for patients on Medicare. Drug utilization review is required.

Over-the-counter medications

Many medications have been classified by the Food and Drug Administration as available without prescription and may be readily purchased at a drug store or pharmacy. These medications are generally available in a very low dosage, and their use presents little hazard to the individual. Warning labels and special packaging help make them relatively safe for the average consumer. These medications represent standard therapy for many common human miseries: colds, allergies, headaches, burns, constipation, and upset stomach. Their use often represents the first line of treatment for patients before they seek medical treatment from a physician or other health practitioner.

Although over-the-counter medications are freely available, they are not without risk. Some medications produce more adverse effects than others. Education about the use of over-the-counter medications is especially important.

Many medications given in the hospital setting also are from this category and are given for minor problems that hospitalized patients sometimes have. Although these medications do not require a prescription for purchase, a physician's order is required before they may be administered in the hospital.

KEY POINT:

Federal regulations

The nurse should identify federal regulations that pertain to the administration of medication.

CANADIAN DRUG LEGISLATION

The Canadian Health Protection Branch of the Department of National Health and Welfare corresponds to the United States Food and Drug Administration of the Department of Health and Human Services. This branch is responsible for the administration and enforcement of federal legislation for the Food and Drug Act, the Proprietary or Patent Medicine Act, and the Narcotic Control Act. These acts, together with provincial acts and regulations that govern the sale of poisons and drugs and those that govern the health professions, are designed to protect the Canadian consumer from health hazards, deceptive advertising of drugs, cosmetics, and devices, and adulteration of food and drugs.

The Canadian Food and Drug Act divides drugs into various categories. Regulations covering the various categories or schedules of drugs differ, making it important to have a clear identification system. Table 2-3 illustrates the three major classifications of drugs under the Food and Drug Act: nonprescription drugs, prescription drugs, and restricted drugs.

The regulations within the Canadian Food and Drug Act allow the government to withdraw from the market drugs found to be unduly toxic. New drugs introduced to the market must have shown effectiveness and safety in human clinical studies to the satisfaction of the manufacturer and the government.*

The Proprietary or Patent Medicine Act provides for a class of products that may be sold to the general public by anyone. The drug formula is not found in the official compendia or printed on the label. The formula for all such secret nonpharmacopoeial medicines must be registered and approved for licensing under the Proprietary or Patent Medicine Act. The nurse needs to be aware of this act in the case of possible drug interactions and the dangers of such interactions.

The Canadian Narcotic Control Act governs the possession, sale, manufacture, production, and distribution of narcotics in Canada. Only authorized persons can be in possession of a narcotic. All persons authorized to be in possession of a narcotic must keep a record of the name and quantity of all narcotics

---

*For more specific information, the nurse can obtain a copy of Health Protection and Drug Laws from Supply and Services Canada, Canadian Government Publishing Centre, Ottawa, Canada, K1A 0S9.

Table 2-3	Canadian drug classification	
Classification	Description	Specific substances
NONPRESCRIPTION DRUGS		
Proprietary medicines	Drugs that may be widely purchased for self-treatment of symptoms of minor self-limiting diseases; identified by a six-digit code preceded by letters GP	Cough drops, medicated shampoos, minor pain relievers
Over-the-counter drugs	Drugs available through a pharmacy and used on advice of a health professional for control of symptoms of minor self-limiting diseases; identified by a six-digit code preceded by letters DIN	Laxatives, cough syrups, cold remedies, sinus preparations, certain vitamins
PRESCRIPTION DRUGS		
Schedule F	Over 200 drugs that may not be used except after professional consultation; identified by symbol Pr on label	Hormones, antibiotics, tranquilizers
Schedule G	Drugs that affect central nervous system (e.g., stimulants, sedatives); identified by symbol C on label	Amphetamines, barbiturates
Narcotics	Drugs used primarily for relief of pain, but also possessing significant psychotropic activity; identified by letter N on label	Cannabis (marijuana), cocaine, codeine, morphine, opium, phencyclidine
RESTRICTED DRUGS		
Schedule H	Drugs with no recognized medical use and significant danger of physiologic and psychologic side effects; available only to institutions for research	Lysergic acid diethylamide (LSD), N_2N-diethyltryptamine (DET), N,N-dimethyltryptamine (DMT), 2,5-dimethoxy-4-methyl-amphetamine (STP; DOM)

From Clark JB, Queener SF, Karb VB: *Pharmacological basis of nursing practice*, ed 2, St Louis, 1990, Mosby.

dispensed and they must ensure the safekeeping of all narcotics. The law governing this act is enforced by the Royal Canadian Mounted Police. A nurse is in violation of this Act if he or she is guilty of illegal possession of narcotics.

Over-the-counter drugs are regulated in Canada by the Canadian Food and Drug Act. These medications can be purchased without prescription but have regulations controlling packaging, labeling, and dispensing. The nurse needs to be aware of the risks these medications present, and assess for possible adverse effects and interactions with other drug therapies. There are differences in over-the-counter drugs that are available in Canada and those available in the United States. It is important for the nurse to assess over-the-counter drug habits when taking a patient's health history.

STATE LEGISLATION AND INSTITUTIONAL POLICY

Although many regulations about the administration of medications come from federal legislation, the details about who may administer medications are determined by each state. This authority is spelled out for nurses in each state's nurse practice act. This legislation varies from state to state and has changed over the years to reflect the increased responsibility many nurses have for administering medications.

The ability to administer medications is clearly specified for licensed practical nurses, registered nurses, and nurse practitioners in the state **nurse practice act.** This is a privilege granted to those individuals who can document their educational preparation and show the willingness to accept **professional responsibility** for drug administration. It also involves accepting **legal responsibility** for judgment and actions while performing professional duties. Because of the variability of practice in different states, it is mandatory that each nurse learn what is legally authorized with regard to medications, and ensure that the rules are clearly followed. Because people in our society tend to relocate so frequently, it is particularly important for nurses to know what is in the nurse practice act as they move from state to state and accept different nursing positions and responsibilities.

State regulations often list minimum standards of practice. Therefore institutional policies and guidelines are often more specific or restrictive than state nurse practice acts. Institutional employers usually provide:

1. Written policy statements regarding:
   a. Educational preparation of nurses administering medications
   b. Institutional policies nurses must follow
2. Orientation to particular policies, procedures, and recordkeeping requirements

Acceptance of employment in an institution, in turn, implies the nurse's willingness to obey established policies or procedures and to participate in their revision and modification as needed.

KEY POINT:

State nurse practice act

It is important to understand how your state nurse practice act describes your drug administration responsibilities.

Some requirements the nurse must meet to administer medications are very formal. It may be an institution's policy to give a nurse with a current nursing license the authority to administer medications. Although the nurse has the authority, this action is valid only when the nurse has a medication order signed by an authorized prescriber.

Some of the other requirements to administer medications are less formal and rely on the professional judgment and knowledge of the nurse. The institution expects the nurse to carry out the steps of the nursing process and, in fact, holds the nurse responsible for consequences resulting from the assessment, planning, implementation, and evaluation of the patient as the nurse gives the medication.

Thus, the nursing process is not just a "nice" thing that might be thought about when giving medications. It is a professional and, implicitly, a legal requirement to use this process. *The nurse must understand the patient:* symptoms, diagnosis, and why the medication is to be given. The nurse must also know other information about the patient's past medical history, allergies, risk factors, and reaction to medications or any information that contraindicates (forbids) the medication being ordered. *The nurse must be knowledgeable about the medication itself:* the dosage, the route of administration, the expected response, and adverse reactions. Knowledge about other medications is also mandatory, so the nurse must watch for possible drug interactions. *The nurse must understand the procedure:* how, when, and where the medication is to be given, and equipment or special techniques needed. The nurse must monitor the patient's response after the medication is given, document the administration, and report promptly to the physician any unexpected results. And finally, the nurse must take every opportunity to teach the patient and the family the major information needed for continued and safe administration of this medication.

Patient charts

The patient's chart is a legal record. It is the major source of information about the patient and the activities in which the patient participates while in the hospital. It provides a central place where all members of the health care team communicate about the patient. The physician describes the patient's condition on admission and determines the plans to identify and/or resolve the patient's problems. The nurse records the assessment of the patient's condition, the implementation of basic nursing procedures, the patient's response, and the progress in meeting the diagnostic and therapeutic plans.

The chart belongs to the hospital. It is not the property of the patient, the nurse, or the physician. It is the legal record of the patient's stay in the hospital. It is kept after the patient has been discharged, and is often used for billing, insurance, and auditing activities; in medical or nursing research; and to provide foundational information if the patient should be admitted again. In cases of court action or lawsuits, the chart may be used by lawyers as evidence. It is especially important that meaningful and accurate information be recorded by the nurse in a legible and complete manner.

Increasingly, health care facilities are computerizing client records, including medication records. The nurse is responsible for checking that the transcription of the medication order is correct by comparing it with the original order.

Every institution develops its own particular forms and order for the patient's chart. Institutional policy will clearly define what information is to be placed in each section. Although there is variety, certain traditional parts of the chart are usually found. These parts are summarized in the box below.

Many hospitals use the chart format developed by Lawrence Weed in 1969, called the **problem-oriented medical record (POMR)**. The POMR uses a list of

KEY POINT:
The patient's chart

It is important to understand different parts of the patient's chart.

numbered patient problems as an index to the chart. The way the individual notes are written in the chart also helps make information easy to find.

Figs. 2-1 to 2-8 illustrate the various parts of the chart.

Parts of the POMR Patient Chart

Summary sheet

The summary sheet is the standard hospital information form that gives basic information about the patient: name, address, date of birth, sex, marital status, nearest relative, employer, insurance carrier or payment arrangements, religion, date and time of admission, admission diagnoses, and attending physician. It may also contain information about allergies, past diagnoses or admissions, and the patient's occupation. A summary of surgeries, diagnoses, and the date and time of discharge may also be added when the patient leaves.

History and physical examination

On admission, a comprehensive history and a physical examination are completed by the physician. The nurse admitting the patient may also conduct a nursing history and a physical examination to supplement the physician's report. All findings are listed and the problem list is constructed from this information.

Problem list

The problem list contains all the symptoms, signs, problems, and diagnoses that have been identified. New problems are added as indicated. The list is numbered and dates are given for when each problem began and when it was detected. All further entries in the chart that relate to a given problem would use the problem number.

Physician's orders

All procedures and treatments are ordered on the physician's order form. These orders include general care (activity level, diet, vital signs), diagnostic and laboratory tests (blood work, x-ray scans), and medications and treatments (hot packs, dressings, physical therapy).

Progress notes

The progress notes section contains observations made by health care workers about the patient. Physician and nurses' notes are written in a SOAP format: **S**ubjective information, **O**bjective findings, **A**ssessment of problem, and **P**lan of care. (Some hospitals put physicians' and nurses' notes into separate sections.)

Graphic record

The graphic record section contains forms for recording vital signs, fluid intake and output, and treatments. In some hospitals, medications are also recorded in this section. In other hospitals, medications are kept in a separate medication Kardex and are not part of the chart until the patient is discharged.

Laboratory tests

All laboratory test results are recorded either on a single sheet as they return to the unit as separate entries, or as sequential entries or summaries updated by computers. (If a patient is critically ill, charts may be developed to show all laboratory tests so any changes can be easily seen.) These are often called "flow charts." ECGs, EEGs, x-ray scans, or other test results may be placed here, or there may be another section for other diagnostic reports.

Consultations

When other specialists are asked to evaluate the patient, the summary of their findings and recommendations is placed in this section.

GENERAL HOSPITAL

Patient ID Number: 437-56-5268 **Admitting date:** Sept. 16, 19••

NAME: YOUNG, Edward SEX: M MOTHER'S BIRTH NAME: Wilson

BIRTHDATE: 6-16-•• AGE: 47   TELEPHONE: 301-555-5555

ADDRESS: 1234 Flamingo Path   Ellicott City, Maryland 21043

ATTENDING PHYSICIAN: J. Smarts   SERVICE: Medical 4 East

ADMITTING DIAGNOSIS: Peptic ulcer

INSURANCE: Blue Cross-Blue Shield High Option

Fig. 2-1   Example of a summary sheet for chart.

GENERAL HOSPITAL

Problem Number	Date Onset	Date Recorded	Description	Status Active Inactive

Fig. 2-2   Example of a problem list.

History and Physical Examination Form (Page 3 - History)

HISTORY

Date:_____ Time:_____
Examiner:_____

Chief Complaint:_____

History of present illness:_____
_____
_____
_____
_____
_____
_____

PAST HISTORY
PERSONAL HISTORY

Occupation_____
Drugs (include alcohol and cigarettes)
_____
_____

Allergies_____
Steroids_____
Bleeding tendency_____
Transfusions_____ Reactions?_____

PAST MEDICAL-SURGICAL PROBLEMS
Hospitalization_____
Surgery_____
Chronic medical illness_____

FAMILY HISTORY
Diabetes_____
Cancer_____
Hypertension or heart disease_____
Other_____
_____
_____

History and Physical Examination Form (Page 2 - Circle appropriate responses)

Circle appropriate res

GENERAL
Weight change NO YES
Fatigue   NO YES
Fever   NO YES
HEAD AND NECK
     Normal Abnormal_____
EYES
     Normal Abnormal_____
EARS/NOSE/THROAT
     Normal Abnormal_____
MOUTH
     Normal Abnormal_____
LUNGS
     Normal Abnormal_____
BREASTS
     Normal Abnormal_____
HEART
     Normal Abnormal_____
GASTROINTESTINAL
     Normal Abnormal_____
URINARY
     Normal Abnormal_____
GENITAL
     Normal Abnormal_____
BONES, JOINTS, AND MUS
     Normal Abnormal_____
BLOOD/LYMPHATIC
     Normal Abnormal_____
NEUROLOGIC
     Normal Abnormal_____
PSYCHOLOGIC
     Normal Abnormal_____

History and Physical Examination Form (Page 1 - Physical exam)

Temp_____ (R___O___
Pulse_____/min___

Circle appropriate response
SKIN
     Normal Abnormal_____
HEAD AND NECK
     Normal Abnormal_____
EYES
     Normal Abnormal_____
     Fundi- Normal Abnorm
NOSE
     Normal Abnormal_____
EARS
     Normal Abnormal_____
MOUTH/THROAT
     Normal Abnormal_____
THYROID
     Normal Abnormal_____
LYMPH NODES
     Normal Abnormal_____
CHEST - BREASTS
     Normal Abnormal_____
BREATH SOUNDS
     Normal Abnormal_____
HEART
     Size   Normal Abnorm
     Rhythm   Normal Abnorm
     Sounds   Normal Abnorm
ABDOMEN
     Size and Shape   Normal Abnormal_____
     Palp organs   Normal Abnormal_____
     Tenderness   Normal Abnormal_____
     Masses   Normal Abnormal_____
     Bowel Sounds   Normal Abnormal_____

ASSESSMENT _____
_____
_____
_____

Fig. 2-3   Example of a history and physical examination form.

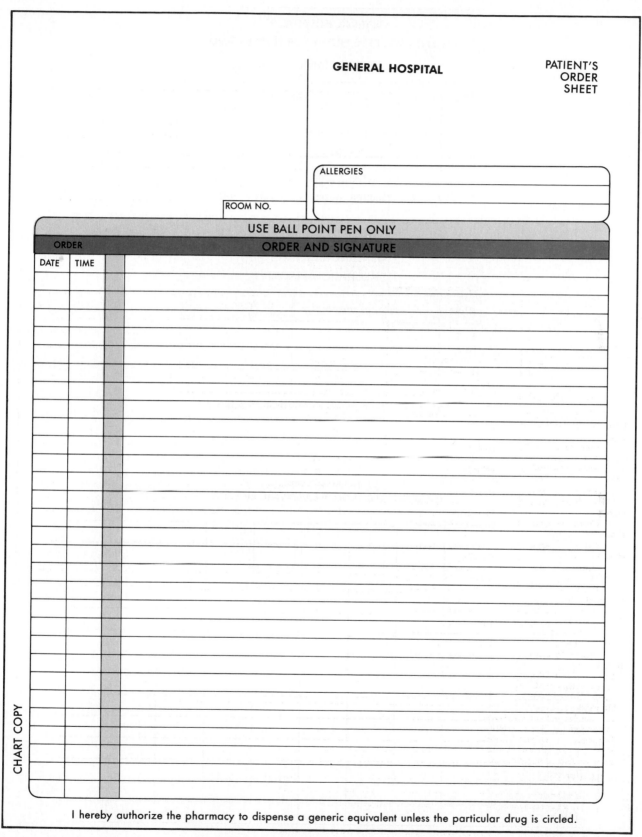

Fig. 2-4   Example of a physician's order sheet.

GENERAL HOSPITAL

PATIENT PROGRESS NOTES FOR NURSES AND PHYSICIANS

Date	Time	Comments

Fig. 2-5   Example of patient progress notes.

GENERAL HOSPITAL

CONSULTATION REPORT

Date	Consultation record of	Service

Fig. 2-6   Example of a consultation report.

GENERAL HOSPITAL
GRAPHIC RECORD OF LABORATORY TESTS

DATES									
WBC									
Neutrophil									
Eosinophil									
Basophil									
RBC									
HBG									
Hct									
Uric acid									
Glucose									
Sodium									
Potassium									
Chloride									
BUN									

Fig. 2-7   Example of a record of laboratory tests.

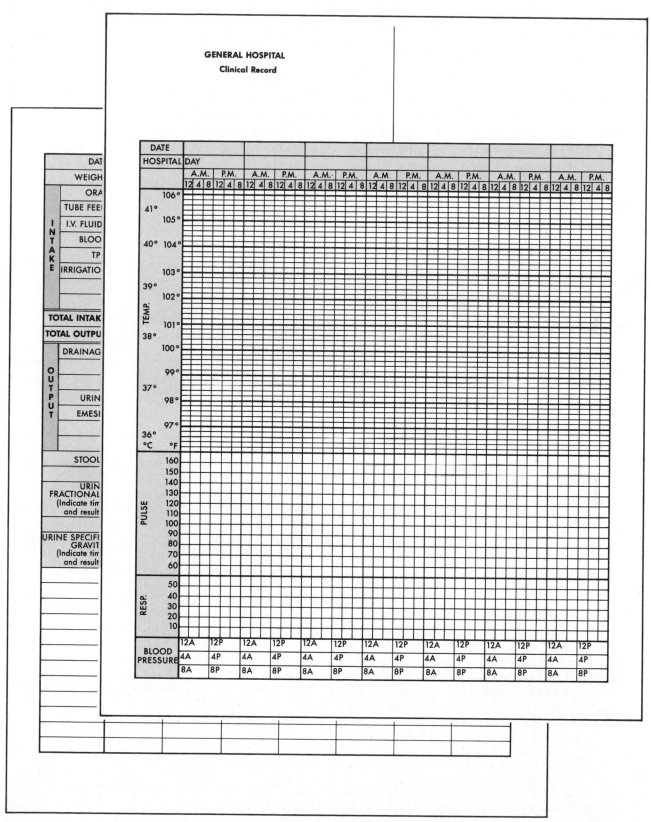

Fig. 2-8   Example of a clinical record.

Kardex

The Kardex is a flip-file card system that contains important information from the patient summary form and the physician's orders. It is regularly updated and changed to reflect current orders. This format keeps important information about the patient readily available for all team members. All tests, medications, and treatment orders are listed here, along with the nursing care plan (Fig. 2-9). All medication cards (Fig. 2-10) may be compared with the order written in the Kardex to verify the accuracy of the orders. If a unit dose system is used, individual medication cards are not needed because all medications are listed in the Kardex or medication profile sheet (Fig. 2-11). The Kardex card is discarded when the patient is discharged. It is not a legal document and serves no further purpose.

Drug distribution systems

Each institution has its own procedure for ordering and administering medications. Although institutional formats may vary, there are three commonly used drug distribution systems:

1. The floor or ward stock system
2. The individual prescription order system
3. The unit dose system

These three different systems are described in the box below.

Common Drug Distribution Systems

Floor or ward stock system

In the floor or ward stock system, all frequently used medications (except potentially dangerous or controlled substances) are stocked in large containers at the nursing station. This system is usually used in small hospitals, institutions with no pharmacist, or where there are no direct charges to patients for the medications (such as most government hospitals). Medication is taken from each container as needed for each patient.

Advantages: Few inpatient prescription orders; minimal return of medications; and ready availability of medications.

Disadvantages: Increased potential for medication errors; potential for unnoticed drug deterioration; potential for use of medication by hospital personnel; potential for increased number of expired drugs that may be difficult to detect; storage and space problems; lack of review of medication order by pharmacist.

Individual prescription order system

In the individual prescription order system, medication orders are sent to the pharmacy, which issues an individual box or bottle for each drug. The container may hold a 3- to 5-day supply of the drug. Medications are stored in a cabinet at the nursing station. Medications are arranged either alphabetically by drug name or according to the patient's room number. Medication is taken from each container by the nurse as needed and distributed to the patient.

Advantages: Review of prescription by both pharmacist and nurse before administration; less chance for deterioration of the drug or for drug misuse; smaller total drug inventories needed; medication frequently available for stat or prn usage; easy charging and billing mechanisms.

Disadvantages: Frequent need to return or discard unused medications; complex ordering, preparing, administering, controlling and recording systems required.

Unit dose system

Single-unit packages of drugs are dispensed to fill each dosage requirement as ordered. Each package is clearly labeled and is often dispensed by the pharmacy into drawers assigned to individual patients in a special medication cart or an individual patient drug cabinet near the patient's room (this is known as a "nurse service" format). Every 24 hours the pharmacist refills this cart or cabinet with all the medications required for the patient for 1 day. This is the safest and most economical method of drug distribution in use today.

Advantages: Little nursing time is required for preparation of medications; better use of pharmacist skills and knowledge, since the pharmacist has greater information about the patient and is able to evaluate each order for contraindications or drug interactions; errors are reduced, since no drug calculations by the nurse are required; little waste or misuse of medication, because only small doses are dispensed; credit can be given for unused drugs because medication packages have not been opened.

Disadvantages: Nurses must administer a medication prepared by someone else, occasionally leading to an error; may lead to delays in starting medications if no stock is on hospital unit; requires presence of pharmacist(s) at hospital, which may be unavailable or very expensive in some areas.

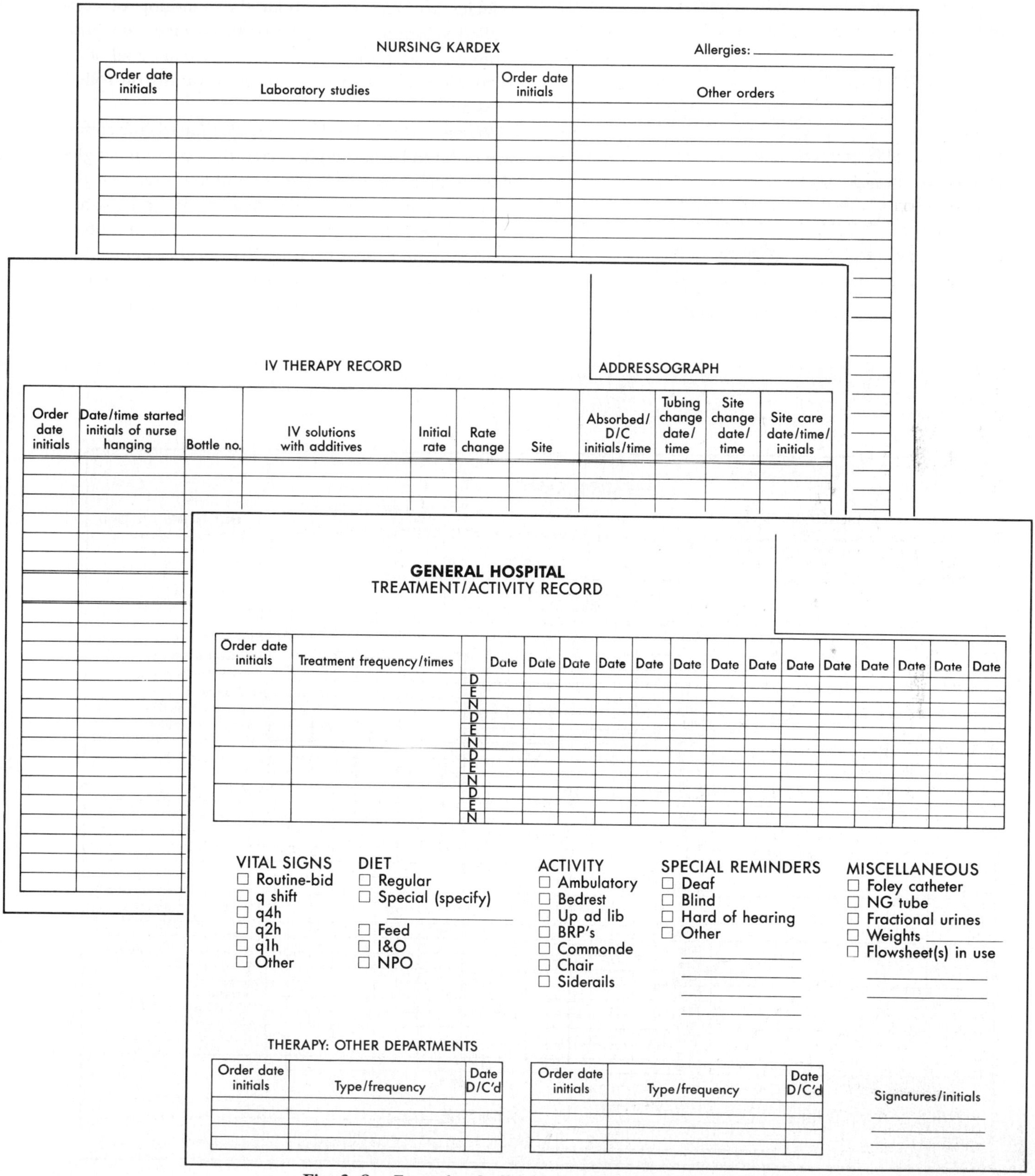

NURSING KARDEX   Allergies: _____

Order date initials	Laboratory studies	Order date initials	Other orders

IV THERAPY RECORD   ADDRESSOGRAPH

Order date initials	Date/time started initials of nurse hanging	Bottle no.	IV solutions with additives	Initial rate	Rate change	Site	Absorbed/ D/C initials/time	Tubing change date/ time	Site change date/ time	Site care date/time/ initials

GENERAL HOSPITAL
TREATMENT/ACTIVITY RECORD

Order date initials	Treatment frequency/times		Date	Date	Date	Date	Date	Date	Date	Date	Date	Date	Date	Date	Date	Date
		D E N														
		D E N														
		D E N														
		D E N														

VITAL SIGNS
☐ Routine-bid
☐ q shift
☐ q4h
☐ q2h
☐ q1h
☐ Other

DIET
☐ Regular
☐ Special (specify)
_____
☐ Feed
☐ I&O
☐ NPO

ACTIVITY
☐ Ambulatory
☐ Bedrest
☐ Up ad lib
☐ BRP's
☐ Commonde
☐ Chair
☐ Siderails

SPECIAL REMINDERS
☐ Deaf
☐ Blind
☐ Hard of hearing
☐ Other
_____
_____
_____

MISCELLANEOUS
☐ Foley catheter
☐ NG tube
☐ Fractional urines
☐ Weights _____
☐ Flowsheet(s) in use

THERAPY: OTHER DEPARTMENTS

Order date initials	Type/frequency	Date D/C'd

Order date initials	Type/frequency	Date D/C'd

Signatures/initials
_____
_____
_____

Fig. 2-9 Example of a Kardex treatment/activity record.

Name ______ Room ______

Drug ______

Dosage ______

Time ______

Date ______ Initials ______

Fig. 2-10 Example of a medication card.

Narcotic control systems

Both federal and state laws as well as institutional policies are very clear about the handling of controlled substances in the hospital. Formats vary little from institution to institution. The primary goal of all regulations is to verify and account for all controlled substances.

When controlled substances, particularly narcotics, are ordered from the pharmacy, they come in single-dose units or prefilled syringes and are attached to a special inventory sheet. The nurse receiving the order must inspect the medication and return to the pharmacy a signed record stating that all the medication ordered was received and that it was in acceptable condition. As each medication is used, it must be

MEDICATION KARDEX

PRN MEDICATIONS

Order date initials	Expir. date	Medication dose/frequency/route	Doses given
			Date
			Time
			Initials
			Date
			Time
			Initials
			Date
			Time
			Initials
			Date
			Time
			Initials
			Date
			Time
			Initials
			Date
			Time
			Initials
			Date
			Time
			Initials
			Date
			Time
			Initials
			Date
			Time
			Initials
			Date
			Time
			Initials
			Date
			Time
			Initials

IM Injection Site Code
1. Rt. posterior gluteal
2. Lt. posterior gluteal
3. Rt. anterior gluteal
4. Lt. anterior gluteal
5. Rt. anterolateral thigh
6. Lt. anterolateral thigh
7. Rt. deltoid
8. Lt. deltoid

Indicate the number of the site used with each IM dose given.

Record site with time.

Signatures/Initials

ALLERGIES ______ DIAGNOSIS ______

ROOM NO. ______ NAME ______ DOCTOR ______ AGE ______

Fig. 2-11 Example of a medication Kardex.

accounted for on the inventory sheet by the nurse administering the medication.

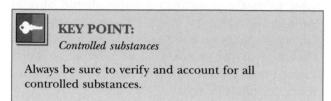

> ### 🔑 KEY POINT:
> *Controlled substances*
>
> Always be sure to verify and account for all controlled substances.

The use of controlled substances is carefully monitored on the hospital unit. Medication is stored in a special locked cabinet. The key to this cabinet is carried by the head nurse or by a medication nurse. These individuals assume legal responsibility for the appropriate use and recording of all the controlled substance medications during that shift, whether or not they give all the medications.

When a controlled substance is ordered for a patient, the nurse responsible for administering the medication first checks the order and verifies the dosage and the last time the medication was given before obtaining the key to the cabinet. The inventory record is completed before the drug is removed from the cabinet. The record indicates the patient's name, date, drug, dosage, and the signature of the nurse administering the medication. If a smaller dose is ordered than that provided (so that some medication must be discarded), or if the medication is accidentally dropped, contaminated, spilled, or otherwise made unusable and unreturnable, two nurses must sign the inventory record and describe what happened. The medication administration should be noted in the patient's chart, as well as subsequent evaluations of the patient's response to the medication.

At the end of each shift the responsibility for all controlled substances and the key to the controlled substances cabinet are transferred to another nurse from the new shift. The contents of the locked cabinet are counted together by a nurse from each shift. The numbers of each ampule, tablet, and prefilled syringe must match the numbers listed on the inventory report form. All medications used during the shift should be signed out by the nurse. Sealed packages are kept sealed. Opened packages of medications must be individually inspected and counted. Prefilled syringes in particular should be examined to make sure they all have the same color, the same fluid levels, and the same amounts of air within them. Both nurses must sign the inventory report saying that the

	GENERAL HOSPITAL				
	NARCOTIC INVENTORY FORM				
MEDICATION:	Demerol prefilled tubex			Dosage: 100 mg	
Number	Date	Time	Patient's name	Room	Nurse
10					
9					
8					
7					

Fig. 2-12   Example of a narcotic inventory form.

records and inventory are accurate at that time (Fig. 2-12).

Occasionally the inventory and the report do not agree. Any discrepancies in the number of remaining doses and the inventory report must be analyzed and explained. All nurses having access to the key must be asked about medication they have given to see if someone forgot to record any medication. Patient charts might also be checked to see if medication was administered that was not signed for on the inventory report. If errors in the report cannot be found, both the pharmacy and the nursing service office must be notified. If the inaccuracy is large, the hospital administrator and security police are usually also contacted.

The nurse with the key assumes a great deal of responsibility in overseeing the controlled substances on the hospital unit. This nurse is usually a mature individual, often the head nurse or a nurse who has been with the hospital for some time, who has demonstrated trustworthiness. It is the duty of this nurse to give the key only to nurses authorized to administer the controlled substances. Keys are never given to physicians or to other health care workers. (Occasionally a physician will want to give the medication, but the nurse should obtain the medication and sign the inventory report.) This nurse should be in a position to evaluate activity relating to controlled substances on a daily basis, so that if patterns develop, deviations from normal are easily seen. A hospital unit that has many patients returning from surgery will have a high frequency of narcotic use during the immediate postoperative period, and this should taper off within 2 to 3 days. Patients who require large or frequent doses

GENERAL HOSPITAL

Patient's name _____

Room number _____

PHARMACY MEDICATION ORDER FORM

Date	Medication order per physician
1	
2	
3	
4	

Fig. 2-13. Example of a pharmacy medication order form.

or prolonged narcotic use should draw attention. Nurses who habitually "drop," "spill," or give smaller doses of medications than normal should also be evaluated thoughtfully to see if there is a problem. Any activity that causes concern relating to controlled substances should be noted by the head nurse. Sometimes patterns do not become evident until examined over a period of months.

The drug order

Both state law and institutional policy make it clear that all medications administered in hospitals must be ordered by licensed health providers acting within their areas of professional training. This generally

DEA # _____

ROBERT S. GOODWIN, M.D.
BONNIE BOCK, R.N., A.N.P.
MARILYN EDMUNDS, R.N., A.N.P.-C.
STEVENS FOREST PROFESSIONAL CENTER
OAKLAND MILLS VILLAGE CENTER
9650 SANTIAGO ROAD
COLUMBIA, MD 21045

Name _____

Address _____ Date _____

℞

☐ Label

Refill _____ times PRN NR

_____ M.D.

To insure brand name dispensing, prescriber must write 'Dispense As Written' on the prescription.

Fig. 2-14. Example of a prescription pad order form.

restricts prescriptive authority (the ability to write an order or prescription for medication) to physicians, dentists, and in some states nurse practitioners, nurse midwives, and physician's assistants.

Prescriptions for hospitalized patients are written on the order form in the chart. Sometimes the order is on a tear-off sheet that can be sent directly to the pharmacy to obtain the medication. Other times, the order must be rewritten or transcribed by the nurse or unit secretary to a special pharmacy order form (Fig. 2-13).

Prescriptions for patients leaving the hospital are written on regular prescription pads and taken to a pharmacy or drug store to obtain the medication (Fig. 2-14).

Whether the prescription is for hospitalized or nonhospitalized patients, the order contains the same information: the patient's full name, date, name of drug, route of administration, dosage, frequency, duration, and signature of prescriber. Additional details about administration may also be written: "Take with meals," "Avoid milk products with this drug," "Do not refill," "Please label." Frequently, pharmacies will also want the patient's age and address on the prescription. This information may help the pharmacist ensure appropriate drug dosage for the patient (if it is a child or older adult), or verify the patient's identity.

In emergencies or when the physician is not in the hospital, the nurse will occasionally be given either a verbal order or an order over the telephone by the physician. All institutions have policies regarding non-written orders. Usually the nurse taking the order is responsible for writing the order on the order form in the chart, including both the name of the nurse and the name of the doctor. This order must then be cosigned by the physician, usually within 24 hours, for the order to be valid.

Medication orders may usually be classified into one of four types of orders:

1. The standing order
2. The single order
3. The emergency or "stat" order
4. The prn order

The institution's policy will clearly define each of these types of orders and the format for implementation of each. The general definition of each type of order and examples of each are presented in Table 2-4. Table 2-5 lists common abbreviations used in pharmacology, which the nurse must memorize.

KEY POINT:
Institutional regulations

The nurse should identify specific institutional regulations regarding the administration of medications.

Table 2-4 Types of medication orders	
Description	**Example**
STANDING ORDER	
Indicates that the drug is to be administered until discontinued, or for a certain number of doses; hospital policy dictates that most standing orders expire after a certain number of days and that a renewal order must be written by the physician before the drug may be continued	"Amoxicillin trihydrate 500 mg PO × 10 days." "Ibuprofen 600 mg PO q6h."
STAT ORDER	
One-time order to be given immediately	"Lidocaine 50 mg IV push stat."
SINGLE ORDER	
One-time order to be given at specified time	"Meperidine 100 mg IM 8 AM preoperatively."
PRN ORDER	
Given as needed based on nurse's judgment of safety and patient need	"Docusate calcium 100 mg PO hs prn constipation."

Table 2-5 Common abbreviations used in pharmacology

Abbreviation	Definition	Abbreviation	Definition
aa	equal parts	O	pint
ac	before meals	OD	everyday
AD	right ear	OD	right eye
ad	up to	OH	every hour
ad lib	as desired	Ol	oil
AM	before noon	ON	every night
aq	water	OS	left eye
aq dest	distilled water	os	mouth
AS	left ear	OU	both or each eye
AU	each or both ears	oz	ounce
bid	twice a day	pc	after meals
bin	twice a night	pil	pill
BT	bedtime	PM	after noon
c	with	PO	per os, by mouth
cap	capsule	PR	per rectum
comp	compound	prn	as required
D	give	q	every
d	day	qd	every day
dil	dilute	qh	every hour
div	divide	q2h	every 2 hours
dos	dose	qid	four times daily
dr	dram	qs	as much as required
elix	elixir	repetat	repeated
ext	extract	Rx	take
fl	fluid	S	mark
ft	make	s	without
gm	gram	SC	subcutaneous
gr	grain	Sig	write on label
gt (gtt)	drop(s)	SOS	one dose if necessary
h	hour	ss	one half
hs	at bedtime or hour of sleep	stat	immediately
IM	intramuscular	tab	tablet
IV	intravenous	tal	such
M	mix	tid	three times daily
m	minim	tin	three times a night
m et n	morning and night	tr	tincture
mist	mixture	ung	ointment
m m dict	as directed	ʒ	dram
noct/n	night	℥	ounce
non	not to be		

SUMMARY

The nurse's authority to administer medications has grown gradually out of a complex and interlocking system of federal, state, and institutional policies. These policies describe not only general procedures and regulations, but very specific responsibilities of the nurse who administers medications. The nurse is also legally responsible for exercising professional judgment and responsibility in carrying out these tasks.

CRITICAL THINKING QUESTIONS

1. Identify three levels of regulations the nurse must adhere to in giving medicines.
2. What is the major focus of federal legislation on drugs? state legislation? agency regulations?
3. Identify three categories of "scheduled" drugs and define the sort of drugs that fit into each schedule.
4. On a blank sheet of paper, draw and fill out a sample patient medication card.
5. On another sheet of paper, block off sections and give them headings similar to the appropriate parts of a patient's chart. Within each section, write a brief description of the kind of information each normally contains.
6. Research the Nurse Practice Act in your state. Discuss at least three of your findings with the rest of the class.
7. Interview nurses in your practice setting to discover institutional policy regarding drug administration. Share your findings with the class. If you're in a hospital setting, do some agency regulations apply more frequently to specific types of floor nurses?
8. Explain the difference between a drug order form, a prescription, and a verbal order. How should the nurse respond to each?
9. Identify the difference between standing, stat, single, and prn orders.
10. Assume that it is your responsibility to take inventory of the narcotic box at the end of your shift. What should you do if you discover that an injectable narcotic is missing (i.e., the count does not match the written inventory report)?

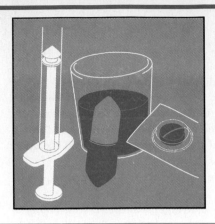

CHAPTER 3
Basic Concepts in Pharmacology

OBJECTIVES

At the conclusion of the chapter you should be able to:

1. Define the key words used in pharmacology and drug administration.
2. Explain the differences in the chemical, generic, official, and brand names of medicines.
3. Describe the four basic physiologic processes affecting all medications.
4. List the basic principles of drug action.
5. Identify specific considerations in giving medications to pediatric or elderly patients and those from various cultures.

KEY TERMS

absorption, p. 32
additive effect, p. 36
adverse reactions, p. 34
agonists, p. 31
anaphylactic reaction, p. 35
antagonistic effect, p. 36
antagonists, p. 32
biotransformation, p. 33
chemical name, p. 31
desired action, p. 34
displacement, p. 36
distribution, p. 32
drug interaction, p. 35
enteral route, p. 32
excretion, p. 33
generic name, p. 31
half-life, p. 34
idiosyncratic response, p. 35
official name, p. 31
parenteral route, p. 32
partial agonists, p. 32
percutaneous route, p. 32
receptor site, p. 31
side effects, p. 34
solubility, p. 32
synergistic effect, p. 36
trade name, p. 31

Drug Names

Medicines have several different names that may make it confusing when first learning to work with drugs. It is very important to know the various names of a medicine so that mistakes are not made in drug administration. Sometimes a medication is ordered by one name and the pharmacist labels it with another name. It is important to know whether the medicine is the same or a different drug. For example, Valium (trade name) is the same as diazepam (generic name).

 Key Words Used in Pharmacology and Drug Administration

Drug comes from the Dutch word "droog," which means "dry." For centuries, most drugs used for treating people came from dried plants.

Medicines are those drugs used in the prevention or treatment of diseases.

Pharmacology deals with the study of drugs and the action of drugs on living organisms. It comes from the Greek word *pharmakon*, which means "drugs," and *logos*, which means "science."

Therapeutic regimen refers to the combination of treatment methods planned by the physician for treatment of disease. This combination may include plans for special diets; use of hot packs, whirlpools, or ultraviolet lights; counseling, biofeedback, psychotherapy; as well as drug therapy.

The most commonly used name is the **generic,** or nonproprietary, name. This is the name manufacturers use for a drug, and it is the same in any country. It is usually a name given to a drug before there is an official name, or when the drug has been around for so many years and is commonly made by many manufacturers. An example would be digitalis or tetracycline. Generic names are assigned by the American Pharmaceutical Association, the American Medical Association, and the United States Adopted Names Council. Generic names are not capitalized when written.

Another common drug name is the **trade,** or brand, **name.** This name is followed by the symbol ®, which indicates that the name is registered to a specific manufacturer or owner and no one else can use it.

This is the name the drug is marketed under and is often descriptive, easy to spell, or catchy sounding so that physicians will remember it easily and will be more likely to order it. The first letter of the trade name is capitalized. Examples of trade names are Dimetapp, Lanoxin, or Pen-Vee K.

Chemical names are often the most difficult to remember because they use the chemical composition of the drug. These names are usually hyphenated, long, and describe the atomic or molecular structure. An example would be ethyl-1-methyl-4-phenylisonipecotate hydrochloride, the chemical name for meperidine (Demerol).

The final type of name is the **official name,** which is the name given by the Federal Drug Administration (FDA). Sometimes this name is similar to the brand or chemical name. The first letter of the official name is also capitalized. An example would be Ethacrynic acid.

Principles of Drug Action

DRUG ATTACHMENT

Drugs participate in chemical reactions that change the physiologic activity of the body. They do this most commonly when the medication bonds chemically at a specific site in the body called a **receptor site** (Fig. 3-1). The chemical reactions are possible only when the receptor site and the chemical can fit together like pieces of a jigsaw puzzle or a key fitting into a lock. If the chemical fits the receptor site well, the chemical response is generally good. We call these drugs **agonists.** Some drugs compete with other chemicals that are already bonded to a receptor site and replace them, producing a different action.

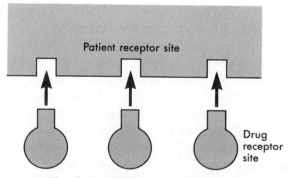

Fig. 3-1   Drug receptor sites.

Some drugs attach at the receptor site, but then produce no new chemical reaction. These drugs are called **antagonists.** Other drugs attach, but produce only a small chemical response and may even prevent other reactions from occurring. These drugs are called **partial agonists.** The box below summarizes the various types of receptor site activity.

> **KEY POINT:**
> *Drug receptor sites*
>
> **Agonist:** Chemical fits receptor site well; chemical response is usually good.
> **Antagonist:** Drug attaches at drug receptor site, but then remains chemically inactive; no chemical drug response is produced.
> **Partial agonist:** Drug attaches at drug receptor site, but only a slight chemical action is produced.

BASIC DRUG PROCESSES

All drugs go through four basic processes in the body. Each drug has different characteristics of absorption, distribution, metabolism, and excretion. To understand how a drug works, the nurse must understand each of these processes for the drug being administered.

The process of absorption

Absorption involves the way a drug enters the body and passes into the body fluids and tissues. Absorption takes place through processes of diffusion, filtration, or osmosis. The rate of absorption depends on three factors: solubility of the drug, route of administration, and degree of blood flow through the tissue where the medication is found. These mechanisms of absorption are more fully described in the box on p. 33.

All medication must be dissolved in body fluid before it can enter body tissues. The ability of the medication to dissolve is called **solubility.** Sometimes the medication must be dissolved quickly; sometimes it should be dissolved slowly. Solubility of the drug is often controlled by the form of the medication: solutions are more soluble than capsules. Enteric-coated capsules are covered with a substance that causes them to be absorbed slowly. An injection with an oil base may be given to delay absorption from the tissue. When the patient takes water with a tablet, it not only helps in swallowing, but helps dissolve the medication and increase its solubility.

The route of administration also influences absorp-tion. Medication routes are **enteral** (directly into gastrointestinal tract through oral, nasogastric tube, or rectal administration); **parenteral** (directly into dermal, subcutaneous, or intramuscular tissue, or into the bloodstream through intravenous injections); or **percutaneous** (through topical [skin], sublingual [under the tongue], or inhalation [breathing] administration).

In areas where the blood flow through tissues is very high, medication will be rapidly absorbed. Examples of this include placing a nitroglycerin tablet under the tongue right next to blood vessels or spraying steroids into the nose and lungs through a nebulizer. Medications injected intravenously into the bloodstream have the fastest action. Oral or rectal medications usually take much longer because they need to dissolve and diffuse across the gastric mucosa and then be transported to the body tissues.

The process of distribution

Once the medication is absorbed, it must travel throughout the body. The term **distribution** refers to the ways that drugs move from circulating body fluids to the sites of action in the body. The drug is usually carried by the bloodstream and lymphatic system throughout the whole body. The organs that have the greatest blood supply receive the medication faster, and areas of skin and fat receive the medication more slowly. Some drugs cannot pass through some cell barriers, such as the placenta or the blood-brain barrier. Thus, the distribution is selective for some types of drugs.

The chemical properties of a drug also influence how the drug is distributed. Some chemicals bind together with proteins, such as albumin (found in the blood plasma), which serve as carriers for drugs that are not easily dissolved. Thus, a drug may be a complex (more than one part), with part of its chemicals locked to the protein and part of its chemicals free to diffuse into the tissues. The ratio of bound chemical to free chemical remains the same in the blood. As more of the free chemical diffuses into the tissues, more of the bound chemical becomes unlocked, and thus available to diffuse.

Some medications are attracted to tissues other than the target receptor sites. For example, medications that dissolve easily in lipid (fat) prefer adipose or fat tissue, and stores of the medication may accumulate in these areas. As the medication circulating in the body binds at the receptor site, more medication will gradually be given up by the fat cells. Thus, a

Mechanisms Involved in Absorption

Diffusion

Diffusion is the tendency of the molecules of a substance (gaseous, liquid, or solid) to move from a region of high concentration to one of lower concentration.

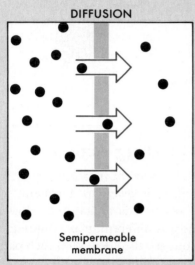

Filtration

Filtration is the passage of a substance through a filter or through a material that prevents passage of certain molecules.

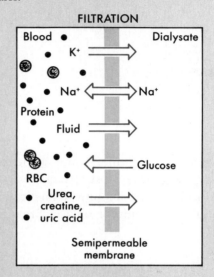

Osmosis

Osmosis is the diffusion of fluid through a semipermeable membrane, the principal flow being from the less dense solution to the more dense solution.

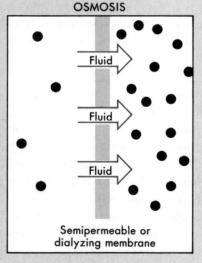

---

lipid-soluble medication may remain in the body for a long time.

The process of metabolism

Once the medication is absorbed and distributed in the body, the body's enzymes use it in chemical reactions through the process of metabolism. The medication is gradually broken down, primarily in the liver, through complex chemical reactions until it becomes chemically inactive. This process is called **biotransformation.** A great deal of medication is actu-

ally inactivated by the liver before it can be distributed to other portions of the body.

The process of excretion

All inactive chemicals, chemical by-products, and waste (often referred to as metabolites) are eventually discarded from the body through the process of **excretion.** Fibrous or insoluble waste is usually excreted through the gastrointestinal tract as feces. Chemicals that are more easily dissolved may be filtered out as they pass through the kidneys, and are

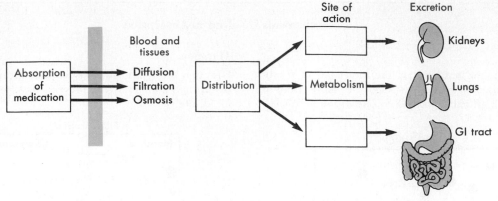

Fig. 3-2 Processes of absorption.

then excreted in the urine. Some chemicals are exhaled from the lungs or lost through evaporation from the skin. Very small amounts of medication may also escape in tears, saliva, or milk of breastfeeding mothers.

• • •

These four major processes are fundamental to understanding how medications are used in the body. The major processes are illustrated in Fig. 3-2.

Half-life

Some chemicals are quickly excreted from the body. Other drugs remain for a long time. A standard method of expressing how long it takes to metabolize and excrete a drug is the **half-life,** or the time it takes to eliminate 50% of the drug from the body. Because these rates are usually the same for most individuals, the half-life helps determine the dosage and frequency needed for the administration of different drugs. If a drug has a long half-life, it may need to be administered only once a day. If a person takes too much medication with a long half-life, it may cause a serious situation, because the action lasts for such a long time. If the half-life of a drug is short, such as for many antibiotics, the person must take frequent doses to maintain an effective level in the blood. If the liver or the kidneys of an individual do not function correctly, medications may not be properly metabolized or excreted, thus causing higher dosages of medication to circulate for a longer time and producing symptoms of overdosage. Therefore, it is important to monitor kidney and liver function through renal and hepatic tests, and to alert the physician if there are any problems.

Basics of Drug Action

When a drug is given to a patient, a predictable chemical reaction is anticipated. However, because each patient is different, many unpredictable chemical reactions are also seen. With each patient, giving a medication is somewhat of a therapeutic experiment and the patient must be monitored closely to determine the effects of the medication.

The expected response of the medication is called the **desired action.** This is when the medication produces the action the physician intended and the therapeutic goal is achieved (for example, Demerol relieves pain).

Because the medication also has the potential for influencing many body systems at the same time, the action of the medication is often not specific. Other reactions may be produced, which are called side effects or adverse reactions. **Side effects** are usually regarded as mild but annoying responses to the medication. **Adverse reactions,** or adverse effects, usually imply more severe symptoms or problems that develop because of the drug. Because substantial testing is required for each drug before it can be placed on the market, most side effects and adverse reactions are predictable. Some side effects, such as drowsiness, may go away after the patient takes the medication for a while. Some side effects, such as nausea, may be eliminated if the dosage is reduced. Some side effects are such a problem that the medication must be changed or discontinued. An example of this might be hyperactivity or inability to sleep. Certainly if adverse effects such as bleeding or liver damage develop, the medication must be stopped.

Occasionally a patient may experience a reaction to a drug that is not anticipated. Strange, unique, or unpredicted responses are called **idiosyncratic responses.** These reactions often are caused by underlying enzyme deficiencies from genetic or hormonal variation. They often produce either an unanticipated result, such as pain or bleeding, or an overresponse to the drug. These types of reactions are usually rare.

A second type of unanticipated reaction is that produced by hypersensitivity or allergy. Some medications and some individuals are more likely to be associated with allergic reactions than others. Allergic reactions usually occur when an individual has been exposed to a drug and his or her body has developed antibodies to it. When the body is reexposed to the drug, the antigen-antibody reaction produces hives, rash, itching, or swelling of the skin. These mild allergic reactions are extremely common and the nurse should always question patients about them. Patients with an allergy to one medication may be more likely to develop an allergy to another medication, and individuals commonly develop a reaction to

medications that they have taken previously without problem.

Occasionally the allergic reaction is so severe that the patient has difficulty breathing and may even have cardiovascular collapse. This life-threatening allergic response is called an **anaphylactic reaction.** A patient who has had a mild reaction to a medication is much more likely to develop the more severe anaphylactic reaction if the medication is given again. These individuals should always be warned about their allergy so they will not take the drug again, and they should wear a Medic-Alert badge or carry identification regarding their allergy.

Patients commonly report allergy to medication that does not represent a true allergy, but only a common side effect. It is important to clarify the nature of the response to the drug if a patient claims an allergy to a particular medication. If a patient experiences nausea or stomach pain when taking aspirin, that is a side effect, but not an allergy.

The common responses to medications are summarized in the box below.

Common Responses to Medications

Desired effect

When the desired effect takes place, the therapeutic goal is achieved. The drug does what it is supposed to do. An example would be temperature reduction after taking aspirin.

Side effect

Side effects are mild but annoying responses to medication. An example would be gastric burning caused by aspirin.

Adverse effects

Adverse effects are more severe symptoms or problems that arise because of the medication. An example would be that the patient might develop severe gastric bleeding from an ulcer caused by aspirin.

Idiosyncratic response

Idiosyncratic responses are strange, unique, or unpredicted reactions. An example would be blood in the urine caused by aspirin. This is rare.

Allergic response

An allergic response is an antigen-antibody reaction. The body develops hives, rashes, itching, or swelling of the skin. A rash or shortness of breath is occasionally seen in patients allergic to aspirin.

Anaphylactic response

An anaphylactic response is a severe form of allergic reaction that is life threatening. The patient develops severe shortness of breath, may stop breathing, or may have cardiac collapse.

DRUG INTERACTIONS

When one drug alters the action of another drug, a **drug interaction** is present. Some medications are given together because the drug interactions are helpful. For example, probenecid is given with penicillin to increase the absorption of penicillin in treat-

ing venereal disease. Other drug interactions produce adverse effects. For example, some antibiotics make birth control pills less effective, thus placing a woman at risk for pregnancy.

Several types of effects are seen with drug interactions (see box on p. 36). If two drugs given together

Common Drug Interactions

Additive

An additive effect takes place when two drugs are given together and double the effect is produced.

Antagonistic

An antagonistic effect takes place when one drug interferes with the action of another drug.

Displacement

A displacement effect takes place when one drug replaces another at the drug receptor site, increasing the effect of the first drug.

Incompatibility

Incompatibility occurs when two drugs mixed together in a syringe produce a chemical reaction so they cannot be given.

Interference

Interference occurs when one drug promotes the rapid excretion of another, thus reducing the activity of the first.

Synergistic

A synergistic effect takes place when the effect of two drugs taken at the same time is greater than the sum of each drug given alone.

---

double the effect produced, an **additive effect** is seen. If one drug interferes with the action of another drug, it is described as an **antagonistic effect.** At times, one drug may replace another drug at a receptor site, increasing the effect of the first drug. This is called **displacement.** Sometimes drugs are chemically incompatible. Attempts to mix them together in a syringe result in a chemical reaction such that the drugs cannot be given. Interference is sometimes seen when one drug promotes the rapid excretion of another drug, thus reducing its activity. Finally, if the effect of two drugs taken at the same time is greater than the sum of each drug given alone, the drugs have a **synergistic effect.**

PATIENT VARIABLES THAT MAY AFFECT DRUG ACTION

Extensive research is conducted on all drugs before they are marketed. A great deal of information is known about every medication and certain parameters have been established. These drug parameters include the therapeutic response, side effects, adverse effects, and probable interactions with other drugs. This information is listed by the manufacturer on a slip of paper inserted into the product container.

Just as medications vary, there are variations among individuals that influence the absorption, distribution, metabolism, and excretion of the medications also. General variables that influence drug activity often help the nurse anticipate individual response to medication. Some of these patient variables are summarized in the box on p. 37.

Special considerations in the pediatric patient

The changes that occur as the child progresses from birth to adolescence have profound influences on drug action and effect. Some changes are obvious, but subtle changes in the response to drugs occur throughout the growth and developmental cycle.

Clear-cut variations in drug effects on neonates are the result of the infants' small body mass, low body fat content, high body water volume, and enhanced membrane (i.e., skin, blood-brain barrier) permeability. Immediately after birth there are several factors that influence drug absorption: lack of gastric acid, absence of intestinal flora and enzyme function, and increased gastrointestinal transit time. The drug inactivation systems are immature, and incomplete development of the renal excretion system also contributes to modification of drug effects in neonates.

In the older infant and young child, the decrease in total body water, increase in body mass, decrease in membrane permeability, and changes in body fat produce less obvious alterations in drug response. The infant has a high metabolic rate and a rapid turnover of body water, which result in a proportionately higher fluid, calorie, and drug dosage requirement per kilogram of body weight than that of the adolescent. Maturation of drug metabolizing systems and the development of urinary elimination mechanisms also result in changes in drug response.

Patient Variables Influencing Drug Action

Body weight

An *overweight* individual requires a larger dosage. An *underweight* individual requires a smaller dosage.

Age

Infants and *children* require smaller dosages, since they have smaller fat and total water content, immature enzyme systems, reduced kidney function, and variation in circulating blood proteins.

Elderly individuals may require smaller dosages because of changes in cellular composition and functioning throughout the body (especially in the liver and kidney), the presence of several disease processes, and the necessity for many medications.

Illness

The type of pathologic process influences body processes. *Nephrotic syndrome, dehydration, malabsorption or malnutrition* may cause changes in blood volume and protein composition. *Kidney disease* produces changes in blood and electrolyte concentration. *Liver disease* leads to decreased metabolism of drugs. *Hyperthyroidism* may produce higher metabolic rate which increases drug metabolism. A patient in *shock* may have reduced circulation with delays in drug distribution in tissues.

Cumulative drug effects

A drug may reach a higher level than needed because it is administered too often, the dosage is too high, or other drugs or chemicals (such as alcohol) that increase the effect of the drug are taken at the same time. The drug may accumulate in a high concentration and produce side effects.

Psychologic overlay

The patient's attitude about drug acceptability and effectiveness is important. *Placebos,* an inert or ineffective substance, may be given to some individuals and will be as effective as if the real medication were given. Other patients develop *tolerance,* or a need for an increased dosage over time to produce the same effects.

Dependence

An individual may develop both a physical and a psychologic need for a drug, usually a controlled substance. This may also be termed *addiction* or *habituation.*

The growth spurt, increase in adrenal steroids, and rise in sex hormones (i.e., estrogen in girls, androgens in both sexes) that precede puberty affect drug response in the pubescent child and adolescent. Increase in male muscle mass, increase in female body fat, and stabilization of basal body temperature in both sexes also affect adolescent drug response.

These facts are important to consider in evaluating a child's sensitivity to medication. For example, infants and children require a total daily digoxin dose that is approximately twice that of an adult on a basis of the ratio of drug to dose. This increased requirement of digoxin has been attributed to a greater affinity of the child's developing myocardial digoxin receptors for digitalis derivatives. Variations in development of drug receptors may make the neonate very sensitive to anesthetics such as curare, but resistant to other anesthetics such as succinylcholine.

Special considerations in the geriatric patient

At the other end of the age spectrum, elderly patients also react differently to drugs. Medications are absorbed, metabolized, and excreted more slowly and less completely in the elderly. Impaired circulation can delay the transport of injected drugs to the tissues they affect. Drugs also can be deposited in fat cells, which have a greater attraction for the drug chemicals than do active cells. Because elderly persons have a higher proportion of fat cells to active cells than do younger persons, they are especially vulnerable to a cumulative effect. Decreases in kidney and liver function and changes in the chemical binding of proteins in the older person's body fluids alter the body's ability to detoxify and eliminate harmful drug chemicals and utilize those that are helpful. All of these factors contribute to the accumulation and extended duration of action of drugs taken by an elderly person.

Because chronic illnesses typically affect persons in the later stages of life, daily medications may be a way of life for many older adults. These drugs are helpful, but also present a very real hazard to the elderly. Ninety percent of older people experience adverse reactions to drugs, and 20% of these reactions require hospitalization. As many as 30,000 people may die each year as a result of adverse drug reactions.

Many times drug interactions cause problems for the elderly patient. Patients may see several specialists, and the medications prescribed by each, when taken together, may have negative consequences for the patient.

All medications are potentially hazardous, but the medications most dangerous to the elderly patient are tranquilizers, sedatives, and other drugs that alter the mind and change perception. Diuretics and cardiac drugs such as digitalis also pose special dangers and must be given with caution and careful monitoring of the patient's response. Because liver and kidney function are decreased in elderly patients, they don't metabolize medication as quickly as younger persons, and are much more susceptible to side effects and toxicity with normal adult dosages. Monitoring of laboratory values for kidney and liver function should be done routinely, and vigilant assessment for side effects and signs of toxicity is vitally important. If a problem is found, it should be discussed with the physician immediately. Symptoms of toxic reactions and adverse side effects of drugs include diminished level of mental function, increased fatigue, restlessness, irritability, depression, weakness, dizziness, headache, and disorientation. It is important to recognize that these symptoms may be caused by drugs and should not simply be dismissed as "typical" of elderly persons.

Elderly persons must be taught how to take prescription medications and the danger of taking nonprescription drugs. Failure of the elderly to follow their medication regimens can be caused by a number of personal and environmental factors. The cost of the drug, difficulty in getting it from a pharmacy, poor memory and motivation to take it regularly, depression, and feelings of being overwhelmed by the responsibility of self-medication all contribute to noncompliance. In some cases arthritis or other disabling physical disease may make getting up or struggling with bottle caps a problem. Poor eyesight may cause a problem in drawing up insulin or reading dosages accurately. Many elderly patients also diagnose each other's ailments and exchange medication, thus causing severe difficulties in monitoring effects.

Cultural influences related to medications

Over the years, cultural diversity has widened among the citizens of the United States. There are many differences between the values and practices of the dominant white, middle-class Americans and the minority groups that are increasingly found in the health care system. Effective nursing care, whatever the setting, is dependent on an ability to assess these differences and to adapt or accommodate nursing strategies to these differences.

Some racial or ethnic group differences are obvious. These commonly relate to attitudes and practices related to birth, death, and general health care; susceptibility to specific diseases; responses to suffering, pain, and loss; standards of personal hygiene and need for privacy; acceptance of male and female children and tolerance of their behavior; rate of growth and development of children; and adjustment to life changes. The words and concepts used to communicate feelings and behaviors related to health practices and remedies for sickness are quite different in each cultural subgroup and relate directly to the accepted values of the group.

In the United States, health care workers have traditionally been influenced by Western medical science and have been taught the values and beliefs of the white, middle-class society. Many of the minority groups that health care workers deal with do not necessarily share these values and beliefs. Thus, problems in communication, priorities, and solutions develop.

Many cultural health beliefs are based on "folk medicine," passed down through the generations within a culture. Many cultures have their own "healers" in the form of a medicine man, shaman, or *curandera*. Those within the culture often seek the advice of this person before going to a scientific health professional. Beliefs in the various cures that the cultural healer suggests are difficult to overcome. Respect for the person's cultural beliefs in all areas is necessary on the part of the nurse for her advice and teaching to be meaningful.

Culture guides behavior into acceptable ways for the people in a specific group. It is learned by each new generation through both formal and informal life experiences. Cultural practices often arise because of a group's social and physical environment and adapt over time. As subcultures live within a dominant culture, their ideas and values change, and they may gradually be assimilated into the more dominant group. Subcultures develop through ethnicity, when the group has a common heritage; or through race, when the group members share specific physical characteristics. The role of the male and the female, how much privacy or personal space is needed, the meaning of food and nutrition, and relative economic freedom all influence the subculture of the minority group. Indeed, much has been written about the culture of poverty and its effects on health care.

Whether a patient will be willing to take the medication provided by the nurse depends on what meaning the medication has to the patient and the beliefs the patient has about its helpfulness or harm. So the nurse must learn more about the patient's culture if he or she is to be effective.

Cultural assessment involves talking with the patient about differences in values, religion, dietary practices, family lines of authority, family life patterns, and beliefs and practices related to health and illness. A great deal of research has documented this information for subcultures within the United States. If the nurse works with minority groups on a regular basis, this is important information to have mastered in providing care to the clients.

Attempt to accommodate the cultural dietary practices of patients as much as possible. Do not force a patient to participate in care that conflicts with the patient's values. If the patient is forced to accept the care, it may even be harmful because resulting feelings of guilt and alienation from a religious or cultural group are likely to threaten the patient's well-being.

SUMMARY

As the nurse prepares to administer medication, he or she must be aware of the pharmacologic parameters of each drug. The information gained through assessment of the individual and the nurse's knowledge about the expected patient response, side effects, adverse effects, and drug interactions become the foundation for the planning, implementation, and evaluation of the patient's response to the medication.

 CRITICAL THINKING QUESTIONS

1. Complete the following chart, identifying the appropriate names for each drug:

Generic Name	Chemical Name	Official Name	Brand Name
phenobarbital	___	___	___
metronidazole	___	___	___
___	___	___	Keflex
albuterol	___	___	___
___	___	___	Valium

2. Sometimes the brand name of a drug is more expensive than a generic version of the same drug. Can you always substitute a generic drug for a brand name version? Explain.

3. To get an idea of the range of chemical reactions that can be involved with a single drug, take the following steps:

A. Pick a drug from the index of this text and look up and describe each action or reaction below, as it applies to the drug you've chosen to investigate:
 - additive effect
 - adverse reaction
 - anaphylactic reaction
 - antagonistic effect
 - desired action
 - drug interaction
 - idiosyncratic response
 - side effect
 - synergistic effect

B. What did you learn about the differences in these effects or reactions? For instance, what is the difference between a side effect, adverse reaction, and idiosyncratic response?

C. Now, if time permits, repeat this exercise with another drug of your choice.

4. In the second column of the table below, define the following physiologic processes (listed in the first column). Choose a drug. In the third column, describe how that drug is absorbed, distributed, metabolized, and excreted.

Drug: _____

Process	Definition	Action
Absorption		
Distribution		
Metabolism		
Excretion		

5. Define the following and give examples, using the index and a little help from Unit Three:
 - Agonist
 - Antagonist
 - Partial agonist

6. Using Unit Three as your resource, work with a partner to find examples of each of the different types of drug interactions:
 - Additive
 - Antagonistic
 - Displacement
 - Incompatibility
 - Interference
 - Synergistic

7. Four-year-old Jesse has never been in the hospital before. His mother spent the night with him last night and stayed with him for most of today. Now he's been crying

quite a bit ever since his mother left to pick up her other two children from school. She has told you she'll be back after her husband gets home from work. That means she won't be here for another hour yet, and it's time for Jesse to take his pills—and without Mom! Identify some strategies you might use to help Jesse take his medication.

8. Mrs. Anderson, 87, says she cannot take her capsules because they are too large and get stuck in her throat. She looks a little panicky as you approach her with her medicine cup. She tries to stay calm, though, and asks you if she can either chew the capsules or sprinkle their contents onto her food. "If I can't," she says, "then I'm just not going to take them, honey. I just can't!" What can you do?

9. Ms. Kim, an elderly Korean woman, has been brought in by her grandson, who speaks English perfectly. Now, however, it's time for her first dose of presurgery medication, but her grandson is nowhere to be seen. When you approach Ms. Kim with the medication, she smiles but shakes her head no. "No," she says, shaking her head emphatically. "No pill." When you try to explain her dosage regimen to her, you quickly discern that Ms. Kim does not seem to understand English—and you don't understand Korean. Is Ms. Kim saying no because she expects another route of medication? Because she hasn't been told about it? Or does she have an allergy you aren't aware of? Is she distrustful of the medication? Is it against her religion? What should you do?

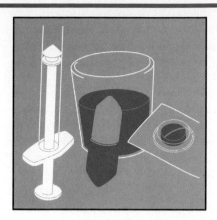

CHAPTER **4**

Preparing and Administering Medications

OBJECTIVES

At the conclusion of the chapter you should be able to:

1. Compare and contrast dosage forms for medications administered by the enteral route.
2. Outline the techniques for giving medications enterally, parenterally, and percutaneously.
3. Identify anatomic landmarks used for giving parenteral medications.
4. Outline recommendations for the prevention of HIV transmission.

KEY TERMS

This chapter provides an overview of basic principles of medication administration. Section One discusses all medications taken by the enteral route: oral, nasogastric, or rectal. Section Two describes the procedures for giving medications parenterally. Section Three describes the methods for giving medications percutaneously.

SECTION ONE: ENTERAL MEDICATIONS

Objectives

At the conclusion of this section you should be able to:
1. Compare and contrast the different dosage forms of oral medications.
2. Use common terms to describe oral medications and the equipment used to administer them.
3. Outline the procedure for administering oral, nasogastric, or rectal medications.

Overview

Enteral medications are administered directly into the gastrointestinal tract through the oral, nasogastric, or rectal routes.

The most common route of administration of medications is through the mouth, or orally. The order is often written, "give PO," meaning per os or by mouth. Advantages of oral preparations are as follows:
1. They are convenient for the nurse to give and for the patient to swallow.
2. Most medications are available in this form.
3. It is relatively inexpensive to make oral preparations.
4. If a patient takes too much of an oral medication, the drug could be removed by gastric lavage or by having the patient vomit.

The major disadvantages of oral preparations are as follows:
1. They cannot be administered to very nauseated, vomiting, or unconscious patients.
2. Some substances lose their effectiveness if mixed with gastric secretions.
3. The onset of action may vary because of changes in absorption in the gastrointestinal tract.

There are many different forms of oral medications. Each form is desired for a particular purpose (for example, to increase absorption, delay absorption, reduce gastric irritation). The term **pill** is often used by patients to describe capsules or tablets. Tablets and capsules are very common and are made up of several different chemicals. Tablets may be covered with a special coating that resists the acidic pH of the stomach, but will dissolve in the alkaline pH of the intestine.

The box on p. 43 summarizes the various oral dosage forms and their characteristics.

The Oral Route

The basic procedure in administration of medication is the same, regardless of type or route of administration. General principles that underlie all procedures include accuracy, acceptance of responsibility, and **asepsis** (prevention of infection). The legal policies and regulations, along with the nursing process and knowledge about the medication, are all used in administering medications. The steps involved in administering medications by the various routes should be followed exactly as outlined in the following sections. Following these steps each time medications are administered will reduce the possibility of medication error.

KEY POINT:
General principles that underlie all procedures

- Accuracy
- Acceptance of responsibility
- Asepsis

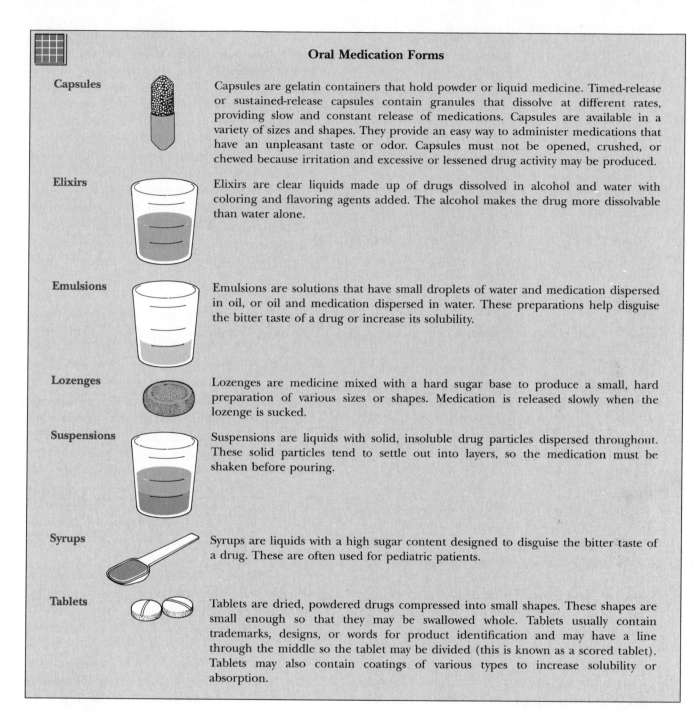

Oral Medication Forms

Capsules

Capsules are gelatin containers that hold powder or liquid medicine. Timed-release or sustained-release capsules contain granules that dissolve at different rates, providing slow and constant release of medications. Capsules are available in a variety of sizes and shapes. They provide an easy way to administer medications that have an unpleasant taste or odor. Capsules must not be opened, crushed, or chewed because irritation and excessive or lessened drug activity may be produced.

Elixirs

Elixirs are clear liquids made up of drugs dissolved in alcohol and water with coloring and flavoring agents added. The alcohol makes the drug more dissolvable than water alone.

Emulsions

Emulsions are solutions that have small droplets of water and medication dispersed in oil, or oil and medication dispersed in water. These preparations help disguise the bitter taste of a drug or increase its solubility.

Lozenges

Lozenges are medicine mixed with a hard sugar base to produce a small, hard preparation of various sizes or shapes. Medication is released slowly when the lozenge is sucked.

Suspensions

Suspensions are liquids with solid, insoluble drug particles dispersed throughout. These solid particles tend to settle out into layers, so the medication must be shaken before pouring.

Syrups

Syrups are liquids with a high sugar content designed to disguise the bitter taste of a drug. These are often used for pediatric patients.

Tablets

Tablets are dried, powdered drugs compressed into small shapes. These shapes are small enough so that they may be swallowed whole. Tablets usually contain trademarks, designs, or words for product identification and may have a line through the middle so the tablet may be divided (this is known as a scored tablet). Tablets may also contain coatings of various types to increase solubility or absorption.

ADDITIONAL GUIDELINES

Solid-form oral medications

1. Do not crush tablets or break capsules without checking with the pharmacist. Many medications have special coatings that are essential to the proper absorption of the medication.
2. If a patient has difficulty swallowing the medication, have him or her take a few sips of water before placing the medication in the back of the mouth, then follow with more water. Patients should keep their heads forward while swallowing, as they do when they eat. It is generally not helpful to move the head backward.
3. If the patient is unable to swallow the medication as ordered, discuss this problem with the physician.

4. Always give the most important tablets, such as heart medications and antibiotics, first. Other medications might even be withheld until you talk with the doctor, if the patient has great difficulty taking them.

Liquid-form oral medications

1. Liquids often must be shaken before they are poured. Although it seems like a commonsense idea, always check to make certain the lid is tightly closed before shaking the bottle.
2. Remove the lid from the bottle and place the lid upside down (flat part down) on a flat surface. This protects the inside of the lid from contamination.
3. When pouring liquids from a bottle into a medication cup, hold the bottle so the label is in your hand. This will prevent medication from running down onto the label and making it unreadable.
4. Hold the medication cup at eye level to read the proper dosage. Often the medication is not level, but is higher on the sides than in the middle. Read the level at the lowest point in the medication cup.
5. The medication could also be drawn up from the bottle or medication cup with a syringe or a medicine dropper. These methods are particularly helpful in improving accuracy when a small dosage is ordered and are frequently used when giving medications to infants or small children. The syringe or medicine dropper is placed halfway back in the baby's mouth, between the cheek and gums, and slowly emptied, giving the baby time to swallow it. The medication in the syringe or medicine dropper could also be emptied into a nipple on which the baby is sucking.
6. Wipe any excess medication from the bottle top and replace lid promptly to avoid contamination.
7. Do not dilute a liquid medication unless ordered to do so by the physician.

Nasogastric Administration

The **nasogastric tube** is another route for enteral medication. Patients who cannot swallow or who are weak or nauseated may be able to take medications through this tube, which leads directly to the stomach. Some individuals find the nasogastric tube so irritating to the nose that the medication must be given parenterally. The procedure for giving nasogastric medications is similar to that given for oral medications, but with the following precautions:

1. Liquid medications may be ordered for patients who have disorders of the esophagus, are comatose, or have problems swallowing. Some tablets may be crushed, mixed with 30 ml of water, and administered by way of the nasogastric tube.
2. Because many of the patients receiving medications by nasogastric tube are seriously ill or comatose, it is especially important to be accurate in all phases of administering the medication. The patient may not be able to assist you in identifying any irregularity. Question any irregularity.
3. Make certain that the nasogastric tube is in the stomach. Aspirate stomach contents with a syringe, or inject 5 or 10 ml air into the tube and listen for a gurgling sound in the abdominal area caused by the air. This may be heard by placing a stethoscope over the stomach. The nurse might also listen for breath sounds, indicating that the tubing might be in the lung, by holding the tubing to the ear. Medication must not be injected if there is any question about the placement of the nasogastric tube. Usually the tube is left in place once inserted.
4. The procedure for administering nasogastric medications is very similar to steps 1, 2, and 4 of administering oral medications (see pp. 46-47). The major difference is that the medication is put into the tube rather than having the patient swallow it. If nasogastric suction is attached to the tubing, detach it and clamp the suction tube. Clamp the nasogastric tube and attach a bulb syringe. Next, pour the medication into the syringe, unclamp the tube, and let the medication run in by gravity. Add water, usually at least 50 ml, to flush the tubing. Reclamp the tube. The tube should remain clamped for at least 30 minutes before the suction tube is reattached so that the medication has time to be absorbed. This procedure is illustrated in Fig. 4-1.

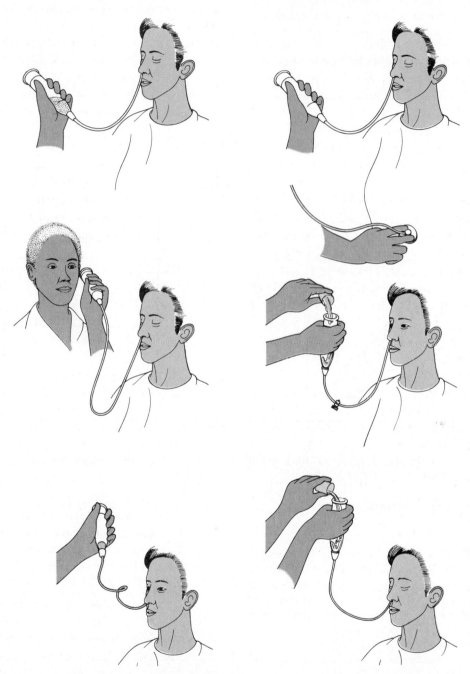

Fig. 4-1   Administration of medication by nasogastric tube. Make certain the nasogastric tube is in place by, **A**, aspirating stomach contents; **B**, listening for gurgling sound in stomach with stethoscope; or **C**, listening for breath sounds. **D**, Put the medication into tubing and, **E**, let it run in by gravity. **F**, After the medication is almost out of the tubing, add water to flush the tubing.

Step one: getting ready

1. Check the medication order on the Kardex. Check the accuracy of the order as written and the time to be given. Clarify any information now known about the patient or the medication such as allergies.

2. Wash your hands. This is essential to avoid contaminating the medication. Although it seems an obvious step, it is often neglected by busy nurses.

3. Assemble the medication equipment. In addition to the medication order or card, obtain the medication tray, souffle or medication cups, medication cart, glass, water or juice, and straw if needed (see *a* through *f*). Unlock medication cart if necessary.

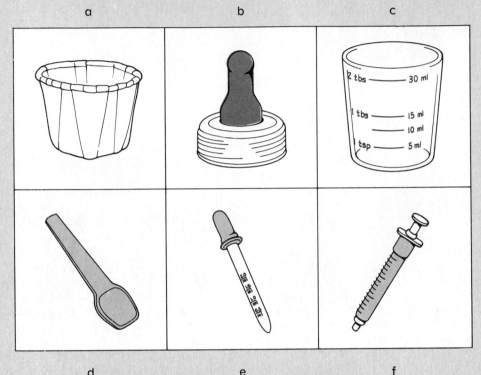

a, Soufflé cup; *b*, nipple; *c*, graduated medication cup; *d*, medication spoon; *e*, medication dropper; *f*, syringe for administering oral liquids.

Step two: preparing the medication

1. Read the order on the medication card or Kardex, and obtain the correct medication from the cabinet or cart. Medications may come in a cardboard or plastic container, a bottle, or an individually wrapped package.

2. Compare medication card with label on container. First check for the right patient, drug, route, dosage, and time of administration.

3. Open the container and pour the correct number of tablets or capsules into the medication cup. Do not touch the medication with your hands, but pour the medication directly into the bottle lid or the cup. Return any extra medication to the container (see *g* through *i*). To avoid errors, hold the medication cup at eye level when pouring liquids (see *j*).

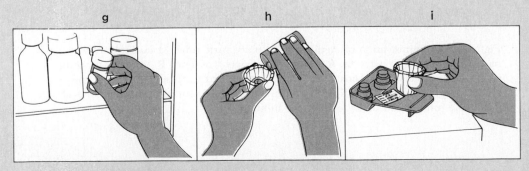

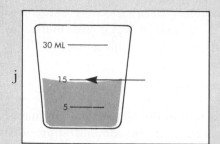

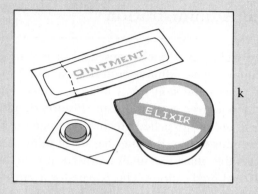

If the unit dose system or nurse service is used, the medication will come in a labeled package. It is not removed from the wrapping until the nurse is at the patient's bedside (see *k*).

4. Compare the information on the medication card to the label on the container. This is the second check for accuracy.
5. Close the box or replace the lid on the container, and check the information for the third time with the medication card.

Step three: administering the medication

1. Go the patient's bedside. Help the patient get into an upright position if possible. Ask patient his or her name at the same time you are checking the patient's identification bracelet and bed tab. Never give medication without positively identifying the patient. Confused or critically ill patients may answer to any name.
2. Explain what you are giving and answer any of the patient's questions. Give any special instructions or teach the patient about the medication as indicated. Make any special assessments required. If the patient makes any comment about the medication looking different from usual, having just taken the medication, or not having had that medication before, recheck the medication order.

Step four: concluding

1. Throw away the medication cup. Clean the medication tray or cart. Wash your hands.
2. Note on the chart the time that the medication was given and sign your name or initials. Record accurately that the medication was given as ordered. Also record if the drug was refused or omitted.

Medication lids are always replaced immediately after use. Medication that requires special storage (such as refrigeration) should be replaced immediately.

6. Put the medication container back on the shelf.
7. Place the cup containing the medication next to the medication card on the tray.
8. Repeat this process for each medication ordered for the patient. All of the tablets for one patient may be placed in the same medication cup.

3. Give the patient a glass of water or juice and have the patient place medication in the back of the mouth, take a sip of water, and swallow. Most medication dissolves better and causes less stomach discomfort when it is taken with adequate liquid.
4. Remain at the bedside until the medication is swallowed. Do not leave medication at the bedside for the patient to take later. You are responsible for making certain the medication is given when ordered.

3. Check the patient again later and note any particular responses or adverse effects that should be recorded on the chart and reported.

Rectal Administration

When a patient is severely nauseated or is vomiting, medication may be administered rectally, thus bypassing the mouth and stomach. Unlike an enema, when medication is given rectally, the medication should be absorbed and not expelled. Accurate dosage through rectal administration is somewhat more difficult and unpredictable than the small, accurate preparations used in oral medications. This is true for a variety of reasons:

1. Some required medications are not available in suppository or enema form.
2. Sometimes the patient has diarrhea and cannot retain the medication.
3. Sometimes other rectal problems may make this route less desirable.
4. If the patient has a lot of fecal material already present, the medication may not be well absorbed.

The procedure for administering rectal medications is described in Procedure 4-2. You will note that steps 1, 2, and 4 again are similar to those for administering oral medications.

SUMMARY

This section of the chapter has emphasized the nursing procedure in the administration of enteral medications. Specific steps are outlined for giving medications orally, by nasogastric tube, and rectally. Specific precautions are also presented for administering medications by the different routes.

KEY POINT
Safe medication administration equation

Legal regulations
+ Nursing process
+ Knowledge about pharmacology
Safe medication administration

SECTION TWO: PARENTERAL MEDICATIONS

Objectives

At the conclusion of this section you should be able to:

1. List universal precautions for prevention of HIV transmission.
2. Describe different preparations used for giving parenteral medications.
3. Compare and contrast types of equipment used for giving parenteral medications.
4. Identify anatomic landmarks for parenteral injections.
5. Outline the procedure for administering intradermal, subcutaneous, intramuscular, and intravenous medications.

Universal Precautions

In 1987, in an effort to protect health care workers from exposure to HIV, hepatitis B virus, and other blood-borne pathogens, the Centers for Disease Control and Prevention (CDC) issued recommendations for universal precautions. They recommend that health care workers use gloves, gowns, masks, and protective eyewear when exposure to blood or body fluids is likely and to consider that all patients might be infected.

In 1988 an update from the CDC clarified the specific body fluids affected by universal precautions (see box on pp. 51–52). Epidemiologic evidence has implicated only blood, semen, vaginal secretions, and possibly breast milk in transmissions. Universal precautions also apply to a variety of other bodily functions (see box on pp. 51–52), although the risk is unknown.

Universal precautions recommend the use of puncture-resistant containers for disposing of all needles and sharps. Needles should not be recapped, since most needlestick injuries occur at this time.

Procedure 4-2
Administering Rectal Medications

Step one: getting ready

1. Check the medication order on the Kardex. Check the accuracy of the order as written and the time to be given. Clarify any information now known about the patient or the medication.
2. Wash hands. This is essential to avoid contaminating the medication.
3. Assemble all the necessary equipment. In addition to the medication order or card, obtain the medication tray, souffle or medication cups, medication cart, lubricant, and rubber glove.

Step two: preparing the medication

1. Read the order on the medication card and obtain the correct medication from the cabinet, refrigerator, or cart. Medication may come in a bottle, in a plastic container, or as a suppository individually wrapped in foil.
2. Compare the medication card with the label on the container. First check for the right patient, drug, route, dosage, and time of administration.
3. Obtain the proper amount of liquid, disposable medicated enema, or suppository. Suppositories should be firm or they cannot be properly inserted. If the suppository has melted, it may be hardened by being put in a small container of ice for a few minutes.

    If the unit dose system or nurse service is used, the medication comes in a labeled package. It is not removed from the wrapping until the nurse is at the patient's bedside.
4. Compare the information on the medication card to the label on the container. This is the second check for accuracy.
5. Replace the medication container and check the information on it for the third time with the medication card.

    Medication such as suppositories requiring special storage (refrigeration) should be replaced immediately.
6. Place the cup containing the medication next to the medication card on the tray. Suppositories should be given promptly to avoid melting.

Step three: administering the medication

1. Explain what you are giving and answer any of the patient's questions. Give any special instructions, such as not expelling the medication, and teach the patient about the medication as indicated. Make any special assessments required.

2. Go to the patient's bedside. Help the patient turn over on the side with one leg bent over the other in a Sims' position. Protect the patient's modesty as much as possible by closing the drapes and draping the patient.
3. Ask the patient his or her name at the same time you are checking the patient's identification bracelet and bed tag. Never give medication without positively identifying the patient.
4. Put on the glove. Remove the suppository from the foil packet and place a small amount of water-soluble lubricant on the tip of the suppository and on the inserting finger. Tell the patient that you are ready to begin. Hold the suppository at the anal sphincter for a few seconds, and tell the patient to take a deep breath and to bear down slightly. This will relax the sphincter so you may push the suppository into the rectum about 1 inch. Use fourth finger (which is smaller) for children. The patient should remain on the side for about 20 minutes. With children you may have to hold their buttocks together to prevent them expelling the suppository (see *a* through *d*).

    If you are giving the patient medication by disposable enema, the procedure is the same except that the lubricated tip is inserted into the rectum and the 50 to 150 ml of medication is slowly squeezed from the disposable container (see *e* through *g*).

Step four: concluding

1. Dispose of the foil packet or plastic containers and the gloves. Clean the medication tray or cart.
2. Leave patients with tissues to wipe themselves if needed.
3. Wash your hands.
4. Note on the chart the time that medication was given and sign your name or initials. Record accurately that the medication was given as ordered.
5. Check the patient again later and note any particular responses or adverse effects that should be recorded on the chart and reported. Medicated enemas may be given for severe asthma, to relieve constipation, or to instill steroids used to treat bowel disorders. The nurse should always look for and report any response to the medicated enema.

Continued.

Procedure 4-2
Administering rectal medications—cont'd

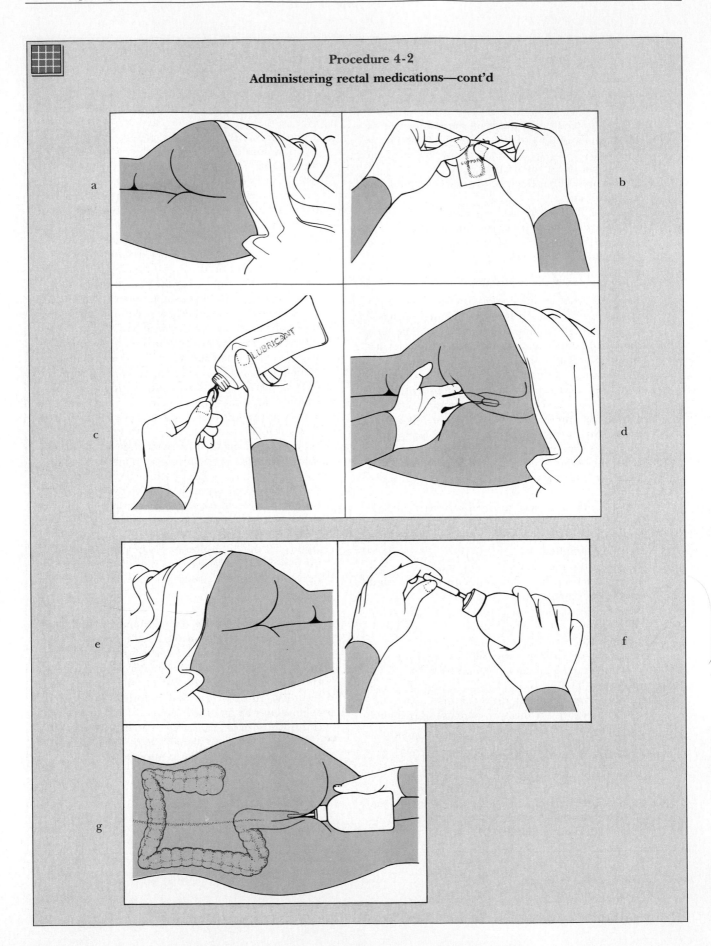

Summary of Universal Precautions: Prevention of Transmission of Human Immunodeficiency Virus, Hepatitis B Virus, and Other Blood-Borne Pathogens in Health Care Settings

Under universal precautions, blood and certain body fluids of all patients are considered potentially infectious for human immunodeficiency virus (HIV), hepatitis B virus (HBV), and other blood-borne pathogens. Blood is the single most important source of transmission of HIV and HBV and other blood-borne pathogens in health care settings. Infection control efforts for HIV, HBV, and other blood-borne pathogens must focus on preventing exposures to blood as well as on delivery of HBV immunization.

Epidemiologic evidence has implicated only blood, semen, vaginal secretions, and possibly breast milk in transmissions. Although the risk is unknown, universal precautions also apply to tissues and the following fluids: cerebrospinal fluid, synovial fluid, pleural fluid, peritoneal fluid, and amniotic fluid. Universal precautions do not apply to feces, nasal secretions, sputum, saliva (except in situations where contamination with blood is likely, such as dental settings), sweat, tears, urine, and vomitus unless they contain visible blood. The risk of transmission of HIV and HBV from these materials is extremely low to nonexistent.

Health care workers are at risk for exposure to blood from patients and must consider all patients as potentially infected with blood-borne pathogens. Health care workers must, therefore, adhere rigorously to infection control precautions for all patients.

Precautions to prevent transmission of HIV
General precautions

- Consider all patients potentially infected.
- Wear gloves when touching blood, body fluids containing blood, and body fluids to which universal precautions apply; for handling items or surfaces soiled with blood or applicable fluids; and for performing venipuncture and other vascular access procedures. Change gloves after each contact with a patient.
- Use protective barriers (i.e., wear masks, protective eyewear or face shields, and gowns or aprons) when performing procedures that may produce blood or body fluid droplets or splashes.
- Wash hands and skin surfaces immediately and thoroughly with warm soap and water if contaminated with blood or other body fluid to which universal precautions apply; wash between patients and after removal of gloves even when they are intact.

- Take precautions to prevent injuries from needles, scalpels, and other sharp instruments during procedures, when cleaning instruments, during disposal, or when handling. To prevent needlestick injuries, needles should not be recapped, purposely bent or broken by hand, removed from disposable syringes, or otherwise manipulated. After they are used, disposable syringes and needles, scalpel blades, and other sharp items should be placed in puncture-resistant containers for disposal.
- Use mouthpieces, resuscitation bags, or other ventilation devices when mouth-to-mouth resuscitation is likely to be performed in emergency situations.

Special considerations

- Health care workers who have exudative lesions or weeping dermatitis should refrain from all direct patient care and from handling patient care equipment until the condition resolves.
- Pregnant health care workers are not known to be at greater risk of contracting HIV infection than health care workers who are not pregnant; however, if a health care worker is infected with HIV during pregnancy, the infant is at risk of infection from perinatal transmission. Because of this risk, pregnant health care workers should be especially familiar with and strictly adhere to precautions to minimize the risk of HIV transmission.

Precautions for invasive procedures

(Here an invasive procedure is defined as any surgical entry into tissues, cavities, or organs, or repair of major traumatic injuries.) General blood and body fluid precautions listed earlier, combined with the precautions listed below, should be the minimal precautions for all such invasive procedures.

- All health care workers who participate in invasive procedures must routinely use appropriate barrier procedures to prevent skin and mucous membrane contact with all patients' blood and other body fluids to which universal precautions apply.
- Gloves and surgical masks must be worn for all invasive procedures.
- Protective eyewear or face shields should be worn for all procedures that commonly result in generation of droplets, or splashing of blood, body fluids containing blood, or other applicable body fluids.

Continued.

Summary of Universal Precautions: Prevention of Transmission of Human Immunodeficiency Virus, Hepatitis B Virus, and Other Blood-Borne Pathogens in Health Care Settings—Cont'd

■ Gowns or aprons made of materials providing an effective barrier should be worn during an invasive procedure likely to result in the splashing of blood or other pertinent body fluids.

■ All health care workers who perform or assist in vaginal or cesarean delivery should wear gloves and gowns when handling the placenta or the infant until blood and amniotic fluid have been removed from the infant's skin. Gloves should be worn until postdelivery care of the umbilical cord.

■ If a glove is torn or a needlestick or other injury occurs, the glove should be removed and a new glove used as promptly as patient safety permits; the needle or instrument involved in the incident should also be removed from the sterile field.

Data from Centers for Disease Control: Recommendations for prevention of HIV transmission in health care settings, *MMWR* 36(suppl 25), 1987; Update: Universal precautions for prevention of transmission of human immunodeficiency virus, hepatitis B virus, and other bloodborne pathogens in health care settings, *MMWR* 37(24), 1988; and *MMWR* 38(suppl 6): 9-18, 1989.

Needles may be cut from the syringe in a special disposal or immediately discarded intact into a well-marked "hazardous material" plastic canister. Research indicates that the frequency of needlestick injury is probably underestimated, and that efforts to prevent needle capping should continue.

Parenteral Administration

The **parenteral route** of medication administration commonly refers to intradermal, subcutaneous, intramuscular, or intravenous injections. Drugs are administered parenterally for the following reasons:

1. When the patient cannot take an oral medication
2. When medication must be given quickly
3. When the medication might be destroyed by the gastric enzymes
4. When medication must be given at a controlled rate
5. When the medication preparation is not available in an enteral form

For example, vomiting or unconscious patients may receive intramuscular or intravenous antibiotics; intravenous medication may be given in a life-threatening emergency; or a patient may receive continuous intravenous medication to control heart dysrhythmias.

Intramuscular (IM) and subcutaneous (SC or SQ) injections require some time for the medication to reach the bloodstream, so the onset of action may be slower than if given intravenously (IV). If an individual is filled with fluid (edema), has large quantities of fat, or has poor circulation (particularly if in shock), the rate of absorption may be unusually long for IM or SQ injections.

IV injections or infusions may be needed when medication must go directly into the bloodstream because the action of these methods is rapid. IV medications usually are effective for only a short time, requiring frequent doses. Overdosage errors of IV medications can be very serious. Also, the cost is generally greater for IV medication, even though the total dose may be smaller than if the medication were given orally.

Although all medication administration should be 100% accurate, the nurse administering parenteral medication has a special responsibility for careful and accurate administration because any errors in technique or dosage may have far-reaching consequences. Once injected, the medication cannot be withdrawn. Accurate drug dosage must be ensured to prevent overdosage. Accurate site of injection is mandatory to avoid pain and damage to tissues, nerves, or blood vessels. Aseptic technique must be followed to reduce chances of infection. A slow and gradual rate of injection is important for most drugs. This will reduce pain, prevent overdosage, and decrease adverse reactions, such as respiratory collapse or heart dysrhythmias.

Basic Equipment

SYRINGES

Syringes, or instruments for injecting fluids, are available in 1, 3, 5, 10, 20, and 50 ml sizes and in plastic or glass. Plastic syringes are commonly used once and thrown away. This makes them convenient in packaging and disposal, but they are more expensive than glass, cannot be used with some medications, and dosage lines or calibration may be more difficult to read. Reusable glass syringes are more economical, but they may break, may become loose with constant usage, and must be cleaned, packaged, and sterilized.

Syringes are made up of three main parts (Fig. 4-2). The **tip** is the portion that holds the needle. The needle screws onto the tip or fits tightly so it does not fall off. The **barrel** is the container for the medication. The calibrations are printed numbers on the barrel, and they indicate the volume of medication in either minims (m), milliliters (ml), units (U), or cubic centimeters (cc) (Fig. 4-3). The **plunger** is the inner portion that fits into the barrel. The medication is forced out through the needle when the plunger is pushed into the barrel.

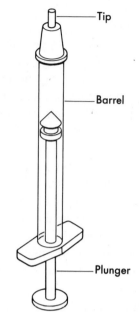

Fig. 4-2   Parts of a syringe.

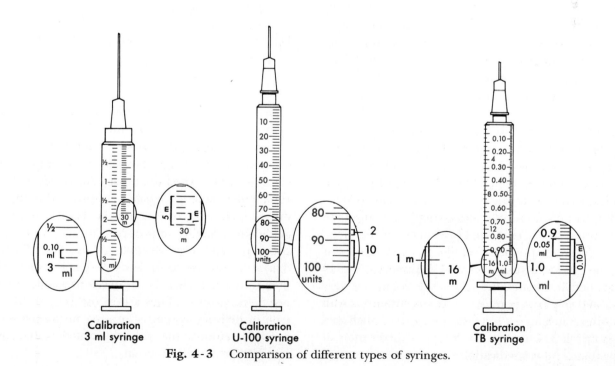

Fig. 4-3   Comparison of different types of syringes.

NEEDLES

The needle must be selected according to the needs of the medication. The **needle** is made up of the hub or bottom part, which attaches to the syringe; the shaft, which is the hollow part through which the medication passes; and the beveled tip, which pierces the skin (Fig. 4-4). The longer the bevel of the needle, the more easily the needle enters the skin. The diameter of the needle is called the gauge. The larger the number of the gauge, the smaller the hole (for example, a 25 gauge needle is smaller than a 16 gauge needle). Thick solutions require larger diameters for injection. The needle gauge is written on the needle hub and on the package.

Needles also come in varying lengths, from ⅜ inch to 3 inches. Generally the smaller the needle (larger the gauge), the shorter the needle. The smallest needles are used for intradermal or subcutaneous injections because they do not extend very far into the skin.

There are also several special intravenous needles that are used when a needle is to be left in place in the vein for a prolonged period of time. Short, small needles with plastic "wings" are used in infants and children, in the smaller veins of the hands in elderly patients, or in adults who are moving around. These needles are referred to as scalp vein, butterfly, or wing-tipped needles, and all have small pieces of plastic on either side of the needle that can be pinched together during needle insertion and then flattened against the skin and anchored with tape. These needles have a small, capped plastic tube attached to the needle that can be used to withdraw blood specimens or inject medication such as heparin. Other special needles include plastic needles or intracatheters that use a stainless steel needle for insertion and leave in place a plastic tube in the vein after the metal needle is withdrawn. Because there is no metal tip left inside the vein, there is less chance for the catheter to puncture the surrounding tissue and less irritation to the vein wall itself (Fig. 4-5).

The sizes of the needle and syringe to be used are determined by the viscosity or thickness of the medication and the amount or volume to be injected. For example, blood is very thick and requires a 15 to 19 gauge needle. Sometimes when the volume is very small and the dosage must be very accurate (as with heparin or insulin), a small gauge needle (such as a 27 gauge) is essential to avoid loss of medication. If more than 3 ml of medication is to be given intramus-

Table 4-1	Suggested guide for selecting syringe and needles		
Route	Gauge	Length (inches)	Volume to be injected
Intradermal	25 to 27 G	⅜ to ½	0.01 to 0.1 ml
Subcutaneous	25 to 27 G	½ to 1	0.5 to 2 ml
Intramuscular	20 to 22 G	1 to 2	0.5 to 2 ml
Intravenous	15 to 22 G	½ to 2	Unlimited

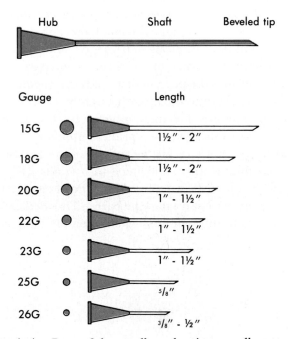

Fig. 4-4   Parts of the needle and various needle gauges.

cularly, the medication should be divided and given in two injections to avoid injecting large pools of medication, which would be irritating to the tissues. The hub of the syringe should be ¼ to ½ inch above the skin surface when the medication is injected. This allows the needle to be easily grasped and removed if the patient jerks or the needle breaks. A general guide for selecting appropriate syringe and needle sizes is presented in Table 4-1. A "needleless" syringe that uses pressure to force small droplets of medication into tissue has been developed, and various needleless infusion lines are in use (Fig. 4-6). This type of delivery system is growing in popularity because it removes the risks associated with reusing needles and needle disposal.

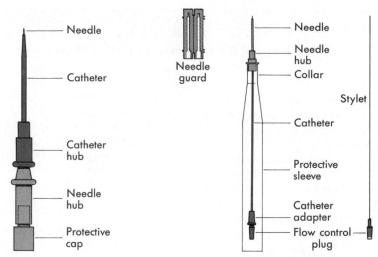

Fig. 4-5   Over-the-needle catheters. Puncture the vein with a metal large-bore needle. Thread a 4- to 6-inch small-gauge plastic catheter inside and up into the vein before removing the metal needle. Use this type of needle when intravenous therapy must continue for several days.

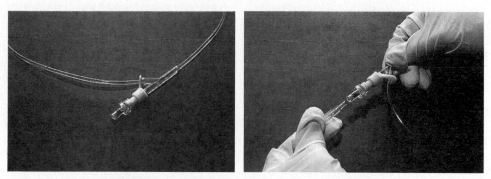

Fig. 4-6   Needleless device using valvelike system.

Basic Procedure for Preparing and Administering Parenteral Medications

The basic procedure for preparing and administering parenteral medications is similar to that for oral medications (pp. 46-47). You will note in the following procedure that there is greater emphasis on sterile technique in giving parenteral medications, because the risk for infection is high. There is also a need to correctly determine the proper site for the injection.

The type of parenteral injection and the medication itself often require special equipment or injection techniques. Accurate selection of the syringe and needle and the packaging of the medication help determine the specific steps to follow in drawing up the medication.

FORMS OF PARENTERAL MEDICATIONS

All equipment and medication used in parenteral injections should be clearly labeled. All packages should be closely inspected to make certain the

Procedure 4-3
Preparing and Administering Parenteral Medications

Step one: getting ready

1. Check the medication order on the Kardex. Check the accuracy of the order as written and the time to be given. Clarify any information now known about the patient or the medication.
2. Wash your hands. This is essential to avoid contaminating the medication and equipment. Although it seems an obvious step, it is often neglected by busy nurses.
3. Assemble all the necessary equipment. In addition to the medication order or card, obtain the medication tray, the proper size needles and syringes, alcohol swabs, tubes, and medication cart. Make certain the equipment is sterile. The expiration date on the plastic or paper wrapping should indicate when the equipment must be discarded or resterilized.

Step two: preparing the medication

1. Read the order on the medication card and obtain the correct medication from cabinet or cart. The medication may come in ampule, vial, Mix-o-vial, or infusion set.
2. Compare the medication card with the label on the container. First check for the right patient, drug, route, dosage, and time of administration.
3. Attach the needle to the syringe, keeping the needle covered with a cap.
4. Ready the medication for withdrawal by opening the ampule, if necessary.
5. Compare the information on the medication card to the label on the container. This is the second check for accuracy.
6. Insert the needle into the medication container and fill the syringe with the proper amount of medication. (See the discussion regarding drawing up medications from different dosage forms on pp. 57-59.) If any air bubbles are present, tap barrel of syringe so air moves into needle and can be removed. Check the information for the third time with the medication card.
   Do not mix more than one medication in a syringe without checking to see if the medications are compatible.
7. Put the unused medication containers away.
8. Change the needle for a new sterile needle if medication has been withdrawn through a rubber stopper or used with a multidose vial.
9. Place the syringe and alcohol swabs next to the medication card on the tray.

Step three: administering the medication

1. Go to the patient's bedside. Help the patient get into the proper position for the injection. The patient may need to turn over, roll onto the side, or remove the gown. Ask the patient his or her name at the same time you are checking the patient's identification bracelet and bed tag. Never give medication without positively identifying the patient. Confused or very ill patients may answer to any name. Put on gloves.
2. Explain what you are giving and answer any of the patient's questions. Give any special instructions or teach the patient about the medication as indicated. Make any special assessments required. Assess previous sites of injections for signs of necrosis, infection, or swelling. Examine the site to be injected. If the patient makes any comments about the medication being different than usual, having just taken the medication, or not having had that medication before, recheck the medication order.
3. Using an alcohol wipe, carefully rub the skin for several seconds to cleanse it. Following the specific procedure for intradermal, subcutaneous, or intramuscular injection (described in detail on pp. 60-69), insert the needle firmly, pull back slightly on the plunger to aspirate for blood, and inject the medication. To aspirate is to look for blood, indicating that the needle has been accidentally placed in a blood vessel, artery, or vein. If blood comes into the syringe when the plunger is pulled back, remove, prepare new medication for administration, and select another site for injection.
4. Assist the patient to a comfortable position.

Step four: concluding

1. Dispose of the alcohol wipe. Return to the nursing station and dispose of the syringe and needle according to hospital procedure. Do not attempt to put the cap back on the needles, because you may accidentally poke yourself. Most hospitals have the policy that any accidental scratching or injection of a used syringe should be reported according to a designated procedure because of the risk of AIDS or hepatitis. Clean the medication tray or cart. Wash hands.
2. Note on the chart the time the medication was given, and sign your name or initials. Record accurately that the medication was given as ordered or was refused.
3. Check the patient again later and note any particular responses or adverse effects that should be recorded and reported. Particularly note any complaints of pain, numbness, or tingling at the injection site.

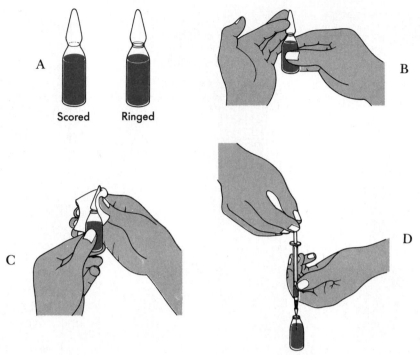

Fig. 4-7 **A**, Examples of scored and ringed ampules. **B**, Shake medication from the top to the bottom portion of the ampule by flicking the top lightly with your finger. **C**, Wrap a gauze pad around the neck of the ampule and use a snapping motion to break off top of ampule along prescored line at neck. Always break away from your body. **D**, Insert the needle into the ampule and draw up the medication.

contents are sterile. Any equipment that appears old or crumpled or that has holes in the packaging should be thrown away. Any medication with a questionable seal or with changes in color or appearance should be returned to the pharmacy. Dates should be checked to make certain the sterilization date has not expired.

Parenteral medications are supplied in a variety of different containers. Ampules, vials, Mix-o-vials, and prefilled tubes are the most common dosage forms.

Ampules contain one dose of medicine in a small, breakable glass container. The narrow neck of the ampule may need to be filed with a small ampule file, or may have a line (score) or ring around it indicating a weakened area where the top can be broken. All the medicine can be shaken into the bottom of the ampule by flicking the top lightly with your fingers. Grasp the top above the scored or ringed area with an alcohol wipe or gauze pad and pull down sharply on the glass top. The top should easily fall off, allowing insertion of the needle into the ampule to draw up the medicine (Fig. 4-7).

Small single- or multiple-dose glass containers of medication are called **vials.** The top of the glass container is covered first with a rubber diaphragm and then with a small aluminum lid. A tightly fitting metal band holds the rubber diaphragm in place. First the metal lid is removed, then the rubber diaphragm is cleansed with an alcohol wipe, and the needle is inserted through the rubber diaphragm into the medication. An amount of air equal to the amount of solution to be withdrawn is inserted to ease the withdrawal of the medication (Fig. 4-8). The vial may contain a solution or it may contain a powder to which sterile water or normal saline must be added just before administration.

Needles should always be inserted with the bevel up, so the nurse may inspect the needle as it goes into the rubber stopper. The needle is always changed before administering the medication to the patient because forcing the needle through the rubber stopper may dull it or create sharp irregular edges called "burrs" that would produce pain when inserted into the patient.

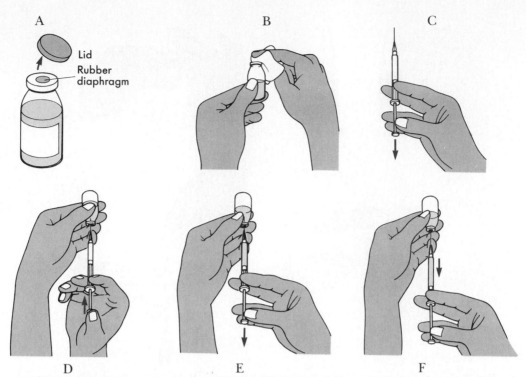

Fig. 4-8 **A**, Example of a vial. **B**, Remove the metal lid and cleanse the diaphragm with an alcohol wipe. **C**, Pull into the syringe an amount of air equal to the amount of solution to be withdrawn. **D**, Insert the needle with the bevel up, and inject the air into the space above the solution. **E**, Withdraw the medication. **F**, Move the needle downward to allow needle to continue to fill.

Occasionally two medications may be ordered that may be given in the same syringe. Two compatible medications are often ordered to be given together as a preoperative medication before surgery (for example, meperidine [Demerol] and promethazine HCl [Phenergan]). Another example is the common practice of ordering two types of insulin (for example, regular and NPH) to be given together. Many antibiotics, on the other hand, must be given in separate syringes because chemically they harden, separate into layers, or become inactive if mixed together. It is important when mixing medications in one syringe to remember the following:

1. The compatibility of the two medications must be known.
2. Air must be injected into both bottles before any medication is withdrawn (to avoid sucking medication down into another bottle).
3. The medication with the shorter action or weaker dosage must be withdrawn first. (This idea can be understood if we use insulin as an example: regular insulin acts more quickly than NPH insulin. If regular insulin is put into the syringe first and a small amount accidentally drops into the NPH insulin when it is being added, the patient will not be affected. However, if NPH insulin accidentally contaminates the regular insulin bottle, it could change the time at which the patient experiences the onset of the action of the insulin.)
4. New guidelines for drawing up nonanimal insulins state that insulin may now be shaken before being drawn up. This reverses previous precautions.
5. When two different types of insulin are mixed in one syringe, they should be injected within 5 minutes of drawing. If this is not possible, the nurse or patient should wait at least 30 minutes before injecting.

Some medications come as a powder and must have solution added immediately before use. Normal saline solution or sterile water may be drawn into a 1 or

A   B   C   D

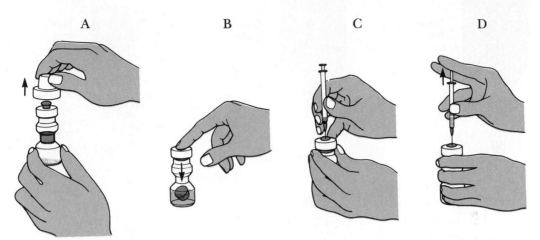

Fig. 4-9 **A,** Remove the protective sterile cap from the Mix-o-vial. **B,** Push the rubber plunger on the top compartment; this will force the rubber stopper into the bottom compartment and let the solution dissolve the powder. The solution is mixed by gently rolling the container. **C,** The needle is inserted through the top rubber diaphragm into the solution. **D,** The required dose is withdrawn into the syringe.

2 ml syringe and added to the powder. Some of these medications come in a two-compartment vial called a **Mix-o-vial.** The top compartment contains a sterile solution, the bottom compartment contains the medication powder. The two areas are separated by a rubber stopper. Pressure on the rubber plunger of the top compartment forces the rubber stopper below to fall into the bottom compartment, letting in the solution to dissolve the powder. The solution is gently rolled (not shaken) to dissolve the powder completely. A needle may then be inserted to withdraw the solution (Fig. 4-9).

Any multiple-dose vial or newly mixed (reconstituted) powder-solution must be clearly labeled when it is first opened. The date, time, and concentration should be included, as well as the expiration time of the medication. The nurse who opened or mixed the medication should also initial the label.

Some narcotics and emergency drugs (such as adrenalin) may come in prefilled syringes or tubes. These medication tubes may be quickly slipped into a plastic or metal "Tubex" holder, screwed into place, needle added, and administered (Fig. 4-12). Prefilled tubes are particularly helpful when time is important (such as during a cardiac arrest) or when the dosage of medication rarely varies. Plastic holders may be soaked in a bleach solution for cleaning.

Medications or solutions to be given intravenously come in large plastic or glass containers of from 250 to 1000 ml. The opening to the glass container is plugged with a hard rubber stopper, a thin rubber diaphragm, and a metal cover. The metal cover and diaphragm are removed just before inserting the infusion tube that connects the bottle to the tube through a small hole in the hard rubber stopper. In many products, there is also a second small hole in the rubber stopper that allows air to enter the container to replace the amount of medication being infused. The plastic container comes sealed in another plastic bag, which is not opened until the infusion is to begin. Air may enter the plastic bag either at the bag opening, or farther down on the infusion tubing (Fig. 4-10).

Some medications (such as antibiotics) are ordered every few hours. This medication would come from the pharmacy already mixed or as a solution to be injected into a smaller bottle, usually containing 50 to 250 ml of fluid, and hung with new tubing that is "piggybacked" or "secondary" to an infusion that is already running. The existing solution is clamped off while the piggyback medication is administered, usually over 20 to 60 minutes, and then the original solution is restarted (Fig. 4-11).

After studying the general procedure for administering parenteral medications, the nurse should examine specific techniques necessary for administration of intradermal, subcutaneous, intramuscular, and intravenous medications. The equipment, sites of injection, and technique must be completely understood.

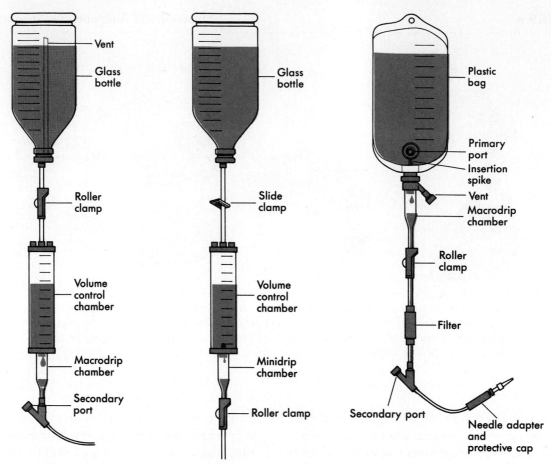

Fig. 4-10 Intravenous bottle or bag and tubing.

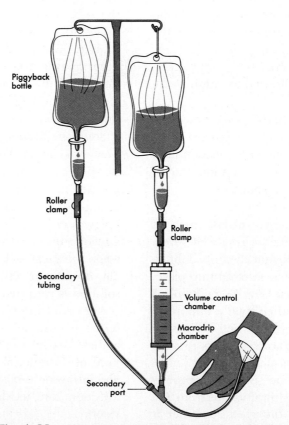

Fig. 4-11 Intravenous setup with piggyback bottle.

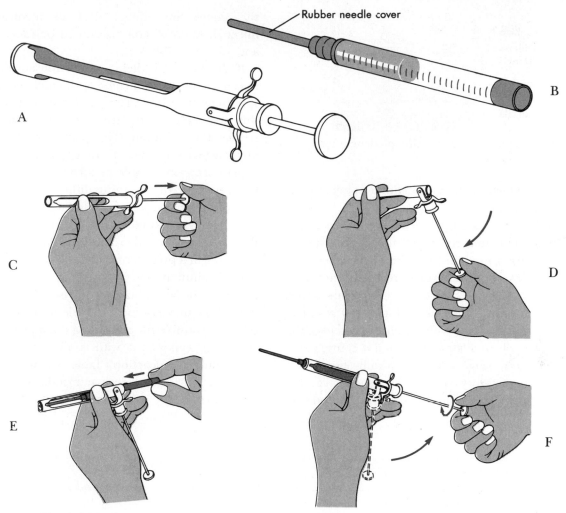

Fig. 4-12   Examples of **A**, a reusable plastic or stainless steel cartridge holder and, **B**, a disposable prefilled medication cartridge. **C**, Plunger of cartridge holder is pulled back. **D**, Barrel is opened at the hinge, and, **E**, the medication cartridge is inserted into the holder. **F**, Pull the plunger up and twist the end of the plunger to secure.

ADMINISTERING INTRADERMAL MEDICATIONS

Intradermal injections are used to determine whether someone has an allergy (allergy sensitivity testing), for vaccination, and for allergy desensitization. They are also used for injection of local anesthetics before wart removal, superficial suturing, and minor procedures. The medication is injected into the dermal layer of the skin, the superficial layer of skin just below the epidermis (Fig. 4-13). Injections are made into the inner aspect of the forearm, the scapular area of the back, and the upper chest if they are free from hair. Usually just a small volume is injected, producing a small bump like a mosquito bite, called a bleb. The blood supply to this area of the skin is less than in other areas, resulting in very slow absorption from the intradermal layer. Once the medication has been injected, the skin should not be restricted or compressed by clothing.

Equipment and technique

Usually 0.01 to 0.1 ml is injected, so a needle that is both small (25 gauge) and short (⅜ inch) is used. The needle should be inserted firmly at a 15-degree angle. The bevel of the needle should be pointing upward. The medication is injected and the needle is swiftly removed. The small bleb should be seen on the

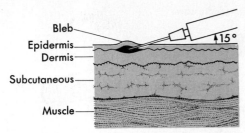

Fig. 4-13 Anatomy of skin showing placement for intradermal injections.

skin at the point where the medication was injected in the intradermal layer.

If the injection was given for allergy or sensitivity testing, it is important to record the concentration of the medication used and the site of the injection. Many reactions to intradermal injections are not apparent for several hours or even days after injection. It is sometimes helpful to draw a circle around the injection site with a pen to help identify the site accurately at a later date when it is inspected for any reaction (Fig. 4-14). Clinically significant reactions to sensitivity testing are shown if the patient develops a wheal or elevated area around the

site where the diluted dose of medication was injected. Areas of swelling should be noted at 5, 10, and 15 mm (Table 4-2).

If the patient is being tested for an allergy, the injection site may become reddened, swollen, and very itchy (pruritic). The patient should not scratch this area and should use cool wet compresses to reduce the irritation. The patient should call the physician or go to an emergency room if he or she experiences any symptoms affecting other body systems, particularly breathing difficulties such as shortness of breath, puffiness of the face, or hives.

Reactions to intradermal allergy injections or sensitivity testing for tuberculosis (PPD test) must be evaluated at a predetermined time after the injection. Each institution has a policy on how the patient reaction will be evaluated and recorded. When testing is done on an outpatient basis, a reliable patient is often responsible for examining the injection site and returning a postcard with a picture most clearly resembling the reaction. Table 4-2 illustrates common reactions to intradermal injections and how they are described.

Table 4-2   Description of intradermal skin reactions

Observation of skin	Recording symbols		Reaction
	–	(0)	No reaction
	+	(1+)	Redness or erythema of skin
	+ +	(2+)	Redness and solid elevated lesions (or papules) up to 5 mm in diameter
	+ + +	(3+)	Redness, papules, and vesicles (fluid-filled elevated lesions) up to 5 mm
	+ + + +	(4+)	Generalized blister larger than 5 mm

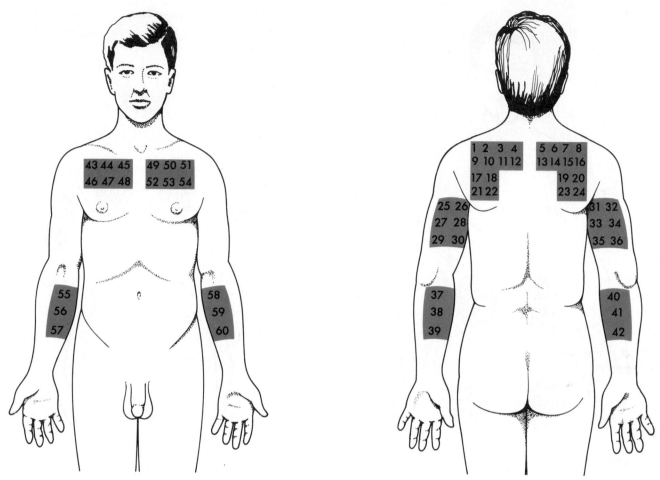

Fig. 4-14   Sites used in intradermal skin testing for allergy.

ADMINISTERING SUBCUTANEOUS MEDICATIONS

Subcutaneous injections involve placing no more than 2 ml of fluid into the loose connective tissue between the dermis of the skin and the muscle layer (Fig. 4-15). Because there is normally less blood supplied to this area than to muscle, any medication injected here will be slowly, but completely, absorbed. This produces a relatively slow onset of medication action, but a long drug action.

Medications injected into the subcutaneous tissue are usually very strong, but concentrated into small doses. For example, insulin and heparin are the most frequently given subcutaneous injections. Because these medications are often given daily for a long time in patients with chronic illnesses, special care must be taken not to irritate the skin tissue with repeated injections in the same area.

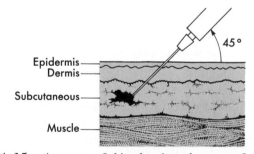

Fig. 4-15   Anatomy of skin showing placement for subcutaneous injections.

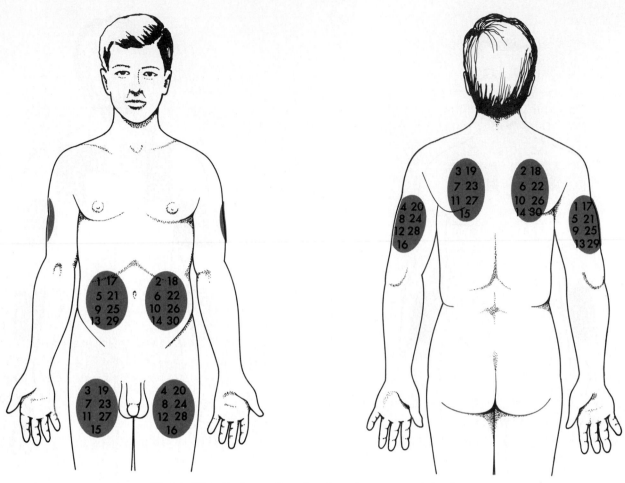

Fig. 4-16   Body rotation sites for subcutaneous injections.

Equipment

In preparing the subcutaneous injection, only a small syringe and needle are needed. Usually a 25 or 27 gauge needle is used, and one that is no longer than ⅝ inch in length.

The sites used for subcutaneous injection depend on whether the nurse or the patient is giving the injection. Commonly the nurse will give subcutaneous injections in the upper arms, upper back, or scapular region. The nurse often begins teaching the patient about chronic or long-term administration of subcutaneous medications while the patient is in the hospital and can practice the technique under the nurse's supervision. The patient will be able to inject himself or herself most easily in the upper arms, anterior thighs, and abdomen. A rotation plan for injection sites should be established and posted with

the patient's medications or by the patient's bedside. Fig. 4-16 front view shows areas usually used for self-administration. The back view shows less commonly used areas that may be used by the nurse. Recording of medication administration should include the site used.

Recent recommendations for diabetics have advised them to use the abdominal wall exclusively for insulin injections. Because it may be hard for patients to remember where they last injected the insulin, a "tape-dot" method has been developed. Using the face of a clock, patients inject themselves at 3, 6, 9, and then 12 o'clock. After each injection they put a small dot of tape over the injection site. When they get around to the 3 again, they move ½ inch to the side, and start their new series of dots. Thus, the sites are rotated in an organized fashion.

Technique

The technique for subcutaneous injection is identical to that for other parenteral medications with the following three exceptions:

1. Because the dosages are so small and so potent, it is important to draw up the prescribed dose of medication and then add 1 to 2 minims of air. This will force all the medication into the tissue when it is injected and not leave any drops in the needle. It is especially important that the medication is precisely administered, especially in children where small variations in dosage might have a large effect.

2. In injecting the medication, grasp the skin and hold it flat with one hand, inserting the needle firmly at a 45-degree angle with the other hand. In areas of the scapula or abdomen, it is often easier to grasp the skin with your hand, pull it up into a small roll, and insert the needle quickly at a 90-degree angle. Slowly inject the agent while watching for a small wheal or blister to appear.

3. Although it is the policy to always aspirate for blood by pulling back on the plunger and checking the syringe for any blood, you must not aspirate when you are injecting heparin. The increased vacuum on the tissues would lead to damage and bruising when the heparin is injected.

ADMINISTERING INTRAMUSCULAR MEDICATIONS

The intramuscular route is by far the most common for parenteral injections. Many antibiotics, preoperative sedatives, and narcotics are administered intramuscularly. In **intramuscular injections** the medication is deposited deep into the muscle mass, past the dermis and subcutaneous tissue (Fig. 4-17) where the rich blood supply allows for rapid and complete absorption. The muscles also contain large blood vessels and nerves, making it important to correctly place the needle to avoid damage to these structures.

Equipment

The syringe chosen needs to be big enough to hold the volume of medicine injected. Generally 0.5 to 2 ml is injected intramuscularly, although infants and children rarely receive more than 1 ml. On rare occasions when more than 3 ml of medicine is or-

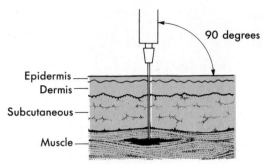

Fig. 4-17   Anatomy of skin showing placement for intramuscular injections.

dered, it should be given in two doses rather than in one syringe. The needle length should also be chosen to allow deeper placement of the needle. Usually 1 or 1½ inch needles are used. Very obese patients may require a longer needle; very thin or emaciated patients may require a shorter needle. The gauge of the needle should be chosen on the basis of the type of medication and how liquid it is. Usually 20 to 22 gauge needles are used.

Sites for injection

There are five muscles commonly used for intramuscular injections: the deltoid, dorsogluteal, rectus femoris, vastus lateralis, and ventrogluteal muscles. Each site has advantages and disadvantages and must be correctly identified for safe administration. These sites have been selected because they are away from major blood vessels and nerves, and are therefore safer to use. The box on p. 66 summarizes the five sites for intramuscular injections and how to identify them. Also see the accompanying illustrations (Figs. 4-18 through 4-22).

Technique

The technique for administration of intramuscular injections is the same as that for other parenteral medications, except for several additional items:

1. Carefully select the site and expose the landmarks before picking up the syringe. Have all equipment ready once the site is identified. This is especially true for children, who will not hold still for a prolonged time after the site is identified.

2. Insert the needle firmly, usually at a 90-degree

Text continued on p. 69.

Sites for Intramuscular Injections

Deltoid muscle

The deltoid muscle is easily reached and frequently used as an injection site. No more than 2 ml may be injected here (less in children), and the substance should not be irritating but quickly absorbed. An imaginary line should be drawn across the armpit at the level of the axilla and the lower edge of the acromion, the sharp point of the shoulder. Two more imaginary lines should be drawn down on either side, one third and two thirds of the way around the outer lateral aspect of the arm. This creates a small rectangle in which medication can be safely given.

Dorsogluteal muscle

The dorsogluteal muscle is a common injection site for adults because it is free from nerves and major blood vessels. However, it is not developed enough to be used for children under 3 years of age. The patient must lie prone (on stomach) on a flat surface and point the toes inward to relax the muscles. An imaginary cross should be drawn from the anus laterally, and from the posterior superior iliac spine down the leg. The injection should be given in the upper, outer quadrant of the cross (see Fig. 4-19). Hold the syringe perpendicular to the flat surface and inject the medication.

Rectus femoris muscle

The rectus femoris muscle lies medial to (toward the middle of the body) the vastus lateralis muscle, but does not cross the midline of the anterior thigh. It is used in both children and adults, especially for self-injection, but it must be carefully located because it lies close to the sciatic nerve and major blood vessels. Injections here may be painful if the muscle is not well developed.

Vastus lateralis muscle

The vastus lateralis muscle is located on the anterior lateral thigh away from blood vessels and nerves. It can absorb a large volume of medication. This is the preferred site for IM injections in infants; it is also a good site for healthy, ambulatory adults. The muscle mass here tends to shrink or become smaller in elderly or very ill patients and may be inadequate. The muscle extends from one handbreadth below the greater trochanter to one handbreadth above the knee.

Ventrogluteal muscle

The ventrogluteal muscle is a large muscle mass and is free of major nerves and blood vessels. Whether the site may be used for children depends on the extent of muscle development. The patient should lie on the side with the upper leg flexed, or the patient should lie prone (on stomach) and point the toes inward to relax the muscles. The palm of the nurse's hand should be placed on the lateral portion of the greater trochanter, the index finger on the anterior superior iliac spine, and the middle finger extended to the iliac crest. The injection should be made into the center of the "V" formed between the index and middle fingers, with the needle directed slightly upward toward the crest of the ilium.

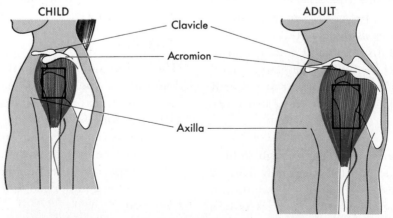

Fig. 4-18   Sites for intramuscular injections in deltoid muscle.

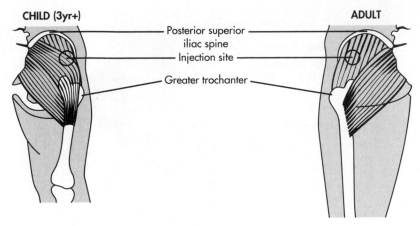

Fig. 4-19   Sites for intramuscular injections in dorsogluteal muscle.

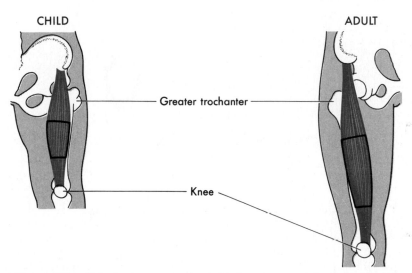

Fig. 4-20   Sites for intramuscular injections in rectus femoris muscle.

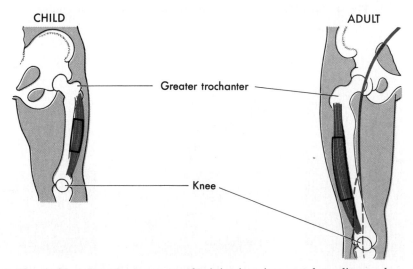

Fig. 4-21   Sites for intramuscular injections in vastus lateralis muscle.

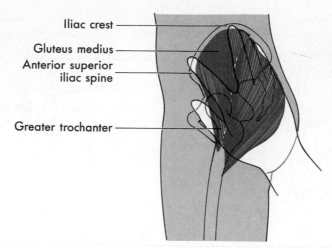

Fig. 4-22 Sites for intramuscular injections in ventrogluteal muscle.

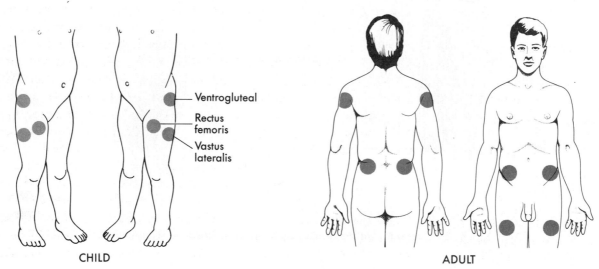

Fig. 4-23 Master rotation sites for intramuscular injections.

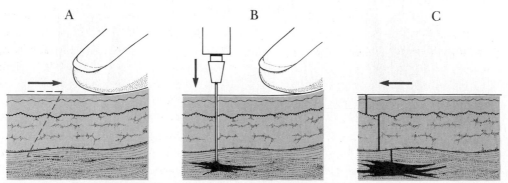

Fig. 4-24 Z-track injection technique. **A,** Pull the tissue laterally. **B,** Insert the needle straight down into the muscle, and inject the medication. **C,** Release the tissue as the needle is withdrawn; this allows the skin to slide over the injection track and seal the medication inside.

angle. After removing the needle, apply gentle pressure to the site with a dry cotton pad (use of an alcohol swab may cause burning). Massaging the area may increase pain if a large amount of medication has been injected. Because bleeding often occurs after IM injections, a small bandage may be necessary. Rotate the site of injections as shown in Fig. 4-23.

3. Some medications are irritating or may stain the skin (iron is an example). Use the "Z-track technique" of injection (Fig. 4-24) for these medications. The Z-track technique uses the skin itself as a door to seal in the medication and prevent it from leaking back out. The dorsogluteal site is used whenever possible because of the muscle mass involved. Use a long needle and add 0.5 ml of air to the syringe after drawing up the medication to ensure that all medication is injected from the needle. Stretch or pull the skin approximately 1 inch to one side. Insert the needle, aspirate, inject the medication slowly, and wait approximately 5 seconds. Remove the needle and let the skin slide back to its normal position. Do not massage the injection site. Avoid pressure on the area from clothing, although walking helps increase absorption.

ADMINISTERING INTRAVENOUS MEDICATIONS

The **intravenous** (IV) **route** is used when medication needs to enter the bloodstream directly. Sometimes large doses of medication must be given, either every few hours or over a long period of time. Because IV medication has not been exposed to other enzymes or tissues before reaching the bloodstream, the rate of absorption and the onset of action are increased. In addition, some medications cannot be given orally, and may be very painful or irritating if given intramuscularly. In emergencies medication may be injected directly into a vein, but usually the IV medication is given on a scheduled basis or infused slowly through IV tubing or an infusion line that is already in the vein.

If a patient must have numerous medications injected daily, both the patient and the nurse generally prefer IV administration. Some patients do not like to be "tied down" by the tubing and feel some general discomfort and irritation from the needle and the medication. Nurses must use greater skill to adminis-

ter medication intravenously than with other routes, and must be especially diligent to prevent infection at the needle site. In addition, because the effect of the medication is immediate, drug overdosages, errors in calculation, or failure to control the rate of administration may produce serious problems for the patient. Thus, the nurse has an increased responsibility for implementing and evaluating the medication given.

Equipment

IV solutions come in large volume, plastic or glass containers, ranging from 250 to 1000 ml. Medications in vials, ampules, or prefilled syringes marked specifically "For IV use" may be added to these containers. Many hospitals receive solutions from the pharmacy with the medications already added.

Some hospitals have "IV teams," who can be called to insert the IV needle and start the initial medications. More frequently, the nurse has the responsibility for performing the venipuncture and starting the infusion. All hospitals have clear policies about what nurses may do in starting infusions. Most of these policies have been updated to protect the nurse from accidental exposure to the human immunodeficiency virus (HIV), which may be spread by direct contact with blood and other body fluids and may lead to the development of acquired immune deficiency syndrome (AIDS). It is mandatory that nurses review these policies before attempting to start an IV, for their own protection and the protection of others. Policies clearly define when gloves should be worn and how to dispose of the equipment contaminated with the patient's blood.

Sites for IV insertion

IVs are generally inserted into the smallest veins and as close to the hands as possible. Arteries are never used. As more infusion sites are needed, the needle is inserted farther and farther up the vein, closer to the patient's heart. This principle allows one vein to be used multiple times (Fig. 4-25). The metacarpal, dorsal, basilic, and cephalic veins are commonly used in adults. Veins in the lower extremities, over sharp bony areas or joints, or in areas of recent injury or surgery should be avoided. Veins commonly used in infants and children include the scalp vein in the temporal area, the dorsum of the foot, and the back of the hand (Fig. 4-26). Elderly or emaciated individuals generally have such fragile skin that needles will not stay in the veins of the hand.

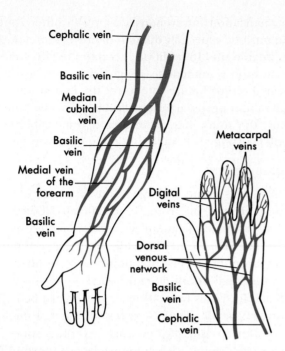

Fig. 4-25 Intravenous sites used in the hand and forearm of adults.

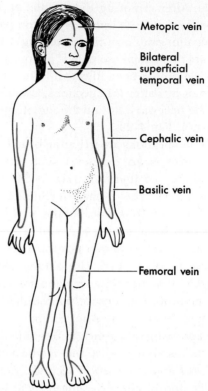

Fig. 4-26 Intravenous sites used in children.

Venipuncture and IV infusion

The procedures for venipuncture and starting an intravenous infusion are somewhat different from those with other routes of administration. Procedure 4-4 summarizes the steps involved in venipuncture and IV infusion.

Modifications in technique for specific situations

1. *Adding medication by syringe to an infusion.* IV medications are commonly added by syringe to an already running IV infusion. This is done by using the medication portal available on the IV tubing. The nurse should wear gloves while carrying out this procedure. The tubing should be clamped above the self-sealing IV portal of the infusion tubing. The portal should be cleaned with an alcohol swab, and a syringe containing the medication should be inserted through the portal. A short needle should be used to avoid accidentally pushing the needle all the way through the tubing. The plunger on the syringe should be drawn back until blood is seen in the tubing above the needle at the skin insertion site. This verifies that the needle is in the vein. The medication should then be slowly injected into the IV line, according to the prescribed rate of infusion for that medication. Once all the medication is injected, the needle is withdrawn and the tubing is unclamped. Any blood or fluid is cleaned up and the rate of infusion is readjusted. The gloves are then removed and the hands are washed.

   All gloves, needles, swabs, and equipment must be taken to the nurses' station or to the dirty utility room for disposal according to hospital policy. The hands are washed again.

2. *Adding medication to a plastic bag or an intravenous bottle.* The top of the plastic bag or the intravenous

Procedure 4-4
Preparing and Administering Intravenous Medications

Step one: getting ready

1. Check the medication order on the Kardex. Check the accuracy of the order as written and the time to be given. Clarify any information now known about the patient or the medication. Complete any calculations needed for dosage, flow rate, and length of infusion.
2. Wash your hands. This is essential to avoid contaminating the medication and equipment. Although it seems an obvious step, it is often neglected by busy nurses.
3. Assemble all the medication equipment. In addition to the medication order or card, obtain the medication tray, proper size needles, tubing, tape, IV infusion poles, alcohol swabs, and medication cart. Make certain that the equipment is sterile. The expiration date on the plastic or paper wrapping should indicate when the equipment must be discarded or resterilized.

Step two: preparing the medication

1. Read the order on the medication card, and obtain the correct medication from the cabinet or cart. Medications may come in an ampule, a vial, a Mix-o-vial, or an infusion set.
2. Compare the medication card with the label on the container. First check for the right patient, drug, route, dosage, and time of administration.
3. Attach the needle to the syringe, keeping the needle covered with a cap.
4. Ready the medication for withdrawal by opening the ampule, if necessary.
5. Compare the information on the medication card to the label on the container. This is the second check for accuracy.
6. Insert the needle into the medication container and fill the syringe with the proper amount of medication. (See the discussion regarding drawing up medications from different dosage forms on pp. 57-59.) Check the information for the third time with the medication card. Dilute the medication in the proper volume and type of solution. Always follow the manufacturer's recommendations. Do not mix medications with blood or albumin. Do not administer any solution that is hazy or cloudy or that has a precipitate or any particles in it. Once mixed, label the container with the medication, date, time, and your initials. IV infusions are generally usable for 24 hours. Any solution not used during that time should be returned to the pharmacy. Some medications require special precautions: shading from sunshine or infusion over a certain time period. Make certain that the infusion is completely infused and that the tubing is cleared before other medication is added.

7. Put the unused medication containers away.
8. If using an IV bottle, remove the metal covering over the IV bottle top. Cleanse the top of the rubber diaphragm on top of the IV bottle or plastic IV bag with an alcohol wipe. Insert the needle with an unused syringe through the rubber diaphragm or medication port into the IV container and withdraw air, creating a vacuum inside the IV container. Now insert the needle with the syringe containing the medication and inject the contents into the IV container through one of the medication ports.
9. Place the syringe and alcohol preps next to the medication card on the tray. Bring other needed equipment to the bedside.

Step three: inserting the needle into the vein

1. Go to the patient's bedside. Help the patient get into the proper position to receive the infusion. The patient may need to turn over, roll onto one side, or remove the gown. Ask the patient his or her name at the same time you are checking the patient's identification bracelet and bed tag. Never give medication without positively identifying the patient.
2. Explain what you are giving and answer any of the patient's questions. Give any special instructions or teach the patient about the medication as indicated. Make any special assessments required. Assess previous sites of injections for signs of necrosis, infection, or swelling. Examine the site to be injected. If the patient makes any comments about the medication being different from usual, having just taken the medication, or not having had that medication before, recheck the medication order.
3. Before performing the venipuncture, tear strips of adhesive tape for anchoring the needle. Open up the infusion set, insert the tubing into the IV container, allow the solution to run into the tubing, and then clamp it shut. Hang the container on the IV pole.
4. Put on gloves. Use correct barrier procedures, as determined by hospital policy, to protect yourself from HIV infection.
5. Apply a tourniquet 2 to 3 inches above the proposed insertion site. Use a slip knot to allow quick release of the tourniquet (Fig. 4-27).
6. Identify the vein to be used and palpate it with fingers of left hand.
7. Using an alcohol wipe, carefully rub the skin for a few seconds to cleanse. Wipe firmly in a circular pattern, moving inside to outside. Let the skin air dry.

Continued.

8. Grasp the needle in your dominant hand, stretch the skin with the other hand, and stabilize the vein. With the needle bevel up at an angle less than 45 degrees, insert the needle into the skin about ½ inch below the point of entry into the vein. Then decrease the angle to 15 degrees and slowly push the needle into and along the vein. Blood will flow down into the tubing when the needle is in the vein.

9. Connect the tubing to the needle, release the tourniquet, and cleanse the area to remove any blood that may have gotten on the skin or tubing. Remove the gloves.

10. Anchor the tubing with adhesive tape. Mark on the tape the time that the needle was inserted and your initials (Fig. 4-28).

11. Immobilize the arm or hand by taking it to an infusion board.

12. Adjust the rate of infusion. An infusion pump may be used to monitor the flow rate and to alert the nurse with an alarm if a problem develops (Fig. 4-29). There are many types of pumps to control infusion rate. The nurse is responsible for checking the equipment's functioning and accuracy.

13. Assist the patient to a comfortable position.

Step four: concluding

1. Dispose of the alcohol wipes and gloves according to the hospital procedure. Clean the medication tray or cart and put away the equipment.

2. Note on the chart the time the medication was given and sign your name or initials.

3. Check the patient again later and note any particular responses or adverse effects that should be recorded and reported. Particularly note any complaints of pain, burning, or stinging at the needle insertion site. Note the infusion rate.

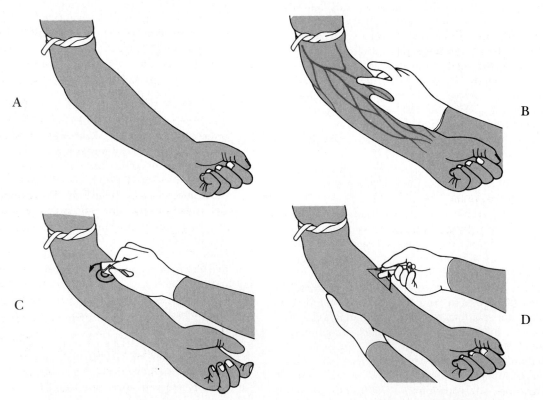

Fig. 4-27   Insertion of needle for venipuncture. **A**, Select site and apply a tourniquet. **B**, Palpate vein to be used for infusion. **C**, Wipe skin with an alcohol swab, moving in a circular pattern. **D**, With the bevel up and the syringe at a 45-degree angle, the needle is inserted through the skin and into the vein. Slowly reduce the angle and thread the needle up into the vein once blood is seen in the syringe. Remove tourniquet and apply adhesive dressing.

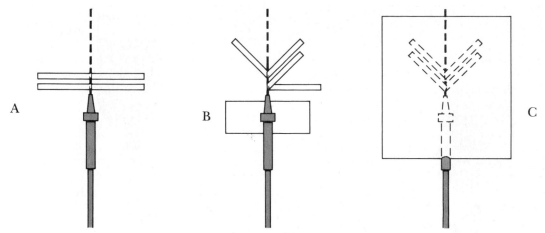

Fig. 4-28   Taping of intravenous tubing after insertion. **A,** Place two small adhesive strips under the needle or the catheter with the adhesive side up. **B,** Cross adhesive tapes and fasten them securely to the skin on both sides. **C,** Place a large piece of tape over the tubing and skin to stabilize the needle. Mark the date and time of insertion and your initials or name.

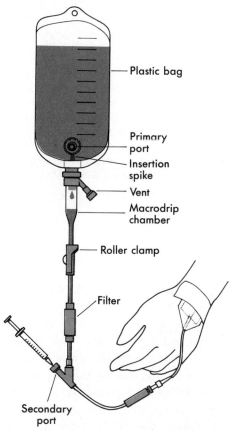

— Plastic bag

— Primary port
— Insertion spike
— Vent
— Macrodrip chamber

— Roller clamp

— Filter

Secondary port

Fig. 4-29   Adding IV push medication to an IV line. Close the IV tubing with a roller clamp. Insert the syringe with the medication into the secondary port. Inject the medication slowly. Release the IV tubing at the roller clamp and allow the infusion to resume.

glass bottle has an air portal, a tubing portal, and an injection portal (Fig. 4-30). Identify the proper portal and cleanse it with an alcohol wipe. Allow the portal top to air dry. Fill the syringe with medication and inject the medication slowly with a small needle through the medication portal into the bag or glass container. Slow administration will allow air to escape from the container while the medication is being injected. Label the bottle or bag with the date, time, dosage, and medication added, and sign your initials.

3. *Adding medication to a volume control.* Draw up the medication in a syringe. Fill the volume chamber with the specified amount of intravenous solution and clamp the tubing between the intravenous bottle or bag and the volume control chamber. Cleanse the medication portal on the volume control chamber with an alcohol wipe and slowly inject the medication into the chamber. Adjust the rate of flow, allowing for infusion of the fluid in the tubing and the volume control chamber within the specified time limit (Fig. 4-31). Label the container with the date, time, dosage, and medication added, and sign your initials.

4. *Adding a medication by **piggyback infusion.*** While an infusion is running to keep a vein open, it may be clamped off and a second IV infusion added to allow administration of medication. In this case, rather than injecting medication directly into the

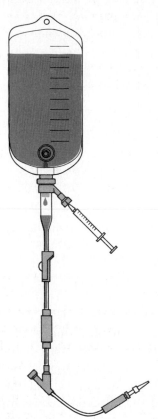

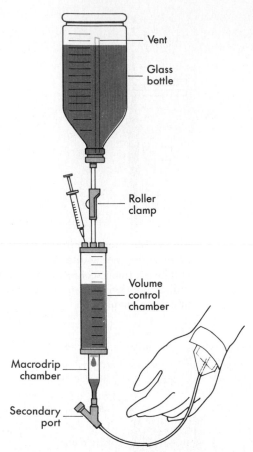

Fig. 4-30 Adding medication to an IV plastic bag or glass bottle. Close the IV tubing with a roller clamp. Clean medication port with alcohol swab. Add the medication to the primary port of bag or the medication vent on the rubber stopper of the IV bag. Air must be let out of the container to equal that of the medication being injected or the medication will leak back out. Gently rotate container to mix the medication in the solution. Release the roller clamp and start the infusion.

Fig. 4-31 Adding medication to a volume-control chamber. Remove the IV bottle from the pole and squeeze all the liquid from the volume-control chamber back into the bottle. Close the IV tubing with the roller clamp. Rehang the IV bottle on the pole. Add the medication in the syringe to the volume-control chamber through the medication portal. Reopen the roller clamp and slowly infuse the medication.

medication portal, the medication is added to a second, small IV bottle, which is inserted into the medication portal with a small needle. If this second, or piggyback, IV container is hung slightly higher than the first IV and the tubing to the first container is clamped off, the medication from the smaller bottle will be infused (refer back to Fig. 4-12, p. 61). Usually antibiotics are given in this manner. The smaller IV bottle should be completely labeled with the time, date, medication, and dosage and the nurse's initials. The order will specify the time in which the piggyback infusion should be completed. Once the smaller volume is

infused, the setup is removed and the clamp reopened to the original bottle.

5. *Administration of medication when there is no IV but only a heparin lock.* Wear disposable gloves and use an alcohol wipe to cleanse the top of the rubber diaphragm at the end of the heparin lock. Pull back the plunger to aspirate blood into the tubing and then slowly inject the medication into the tubing. Follow this by inserting another syringe with 1 to 2 ml of normal saline to flush the tubing of medication. Some institutions will also use 1 ml of heparin to help keep the tubing open. The nurse must carefully follow the hospital's policy.

Clean up any spilled blood or fluid, remove the gloves, and dispose of the equipment properly. Figs. 4-32 and 4-33 illustrate the taping of a heparin lock and the addition of medication.

Intravenous infusion rates

Since so many factors influence the gravity flow, a solution may not necessarily continue to run at the speed originally set. Therefore, intravenous infusions must be monitored frequently to verify that the fluid is flowing at the intended rate. The IV flask or bag should be marked with tape to indicate the rate so that the nurse can tell at a glance whether the correct amount has been infused. The flow should be calculated when the solution is originally hung, then rechecked at least hourly. To calculate the flow rate, the number of drops delivered per milliliter must be ascertained. This number varies with equipment and is usually printed on the solution set packaging. A formula that can be used to calculate the drop rate follows:

$$\frac{\text{gtt/ml of given set}}{60 \text{ (min in hour)}} \times \text{total hourly volume} = \text{gtt/min}$$

A variety of infusion pumps is available to assist in intravenous fluid delivery. These devices allow more accurate administration of fluids and medications than is possible with routine gravity-flow setups. Some pumps have flow rates calibrated in terms of milliliters/hour and are referred to as volumetric pumps (Figs. 4-34 to 4-36). Others are calibrated in drops/minute and are referred to as infusion controllers. It is important to read the manufacturer's directions carefully before using any infusion pump or controller because there are many variations in available models. Use of these devices does not eliminate the need for frequent monitoring of the infusion and the patient.

Small pumps weighing about half a pound are now available as portable infusion systems for continuous drug treatment of certain patients with type 1 diabetes or cancer. The systems currently in use generally consist of a battery, a programmable electronic "brain," an electric motor and a pump, and a syringe, all of which are detachable as a unit from the small needle kept in place either in subcutaneous abdominal or thigh tissue (for diabetes) or by Silastic catheter inserted into an artery supplying the malignant tumor. Some systems are designed to be worn externally over clothing, stored in a pocket, or suspended from a belt or a neck chain (Figs. 4-37 and 4-38). Others are implanted within a subcutaneous pocket in the lower abdomen or elsewhere. The starting dosage levels and six other parameters of therapy are currently programmed initially by the physician. Demand systems may soon be available, since there is much experimental research in this area.

Innovative delivery systems

Implanted capsules of a progestin hormone, called the Norplant method, are being used for contraception. Implantation takes 5 minutes and is immediately effective with contraceptive effects lasting 5 to 7 years.

General nursing actions for a patient with an IV infusion

A patient receiving an intravenous infusion should be checked hourly, and the rate of infusion should be closely monitored. It is possible to slow infusions, but an infusion rate should never be increased to "catch up" if the rate was accidentally slowed. Many patients with bad hearts, poor circulation, or kidney failure could be overwhelmed by too much fluid. Intake and output records should be closely monitored. The patient should maintain an hourly output of 30 ml or more of urine. Any decrease in this level should be reported to the physician.

When one IV infusion has been completed and another should be started, the rate should be turned down very low to keep the vein open, but not stopped. Using aseptic technique, the old infusion container should be clamped off, the old container exchanged for a new container, and the drip chamber filled halfway before the tubing is unclamped and the rate recalculated.

If the completed infusion is to be discontinued, the nurse should explain to the patient what is to happen, then clamp the tubing, loosen the adhesive tape, and put on gloves. Holding a gauze pad in the nondominant hand, apply gentle pressure on the venipuncture site as the needle is carefully withdrawn with the dominant hand. The needle should be inspected to make sure it is intact. The area should be cleaned with an alcohol wipe and elevated if possible, and direct pressure should be applied to stop any bleeding at the site. Check for bleeding after 1 to 2 minutes, then apply an antibiotic ointment and a clean pressure dressing. Dispose of all contaminated equipment in the authorized way.

Text continued on p. 78.

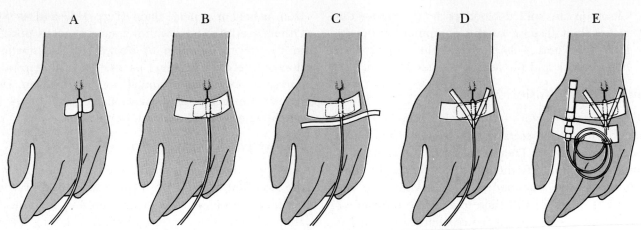

Fig. 4-32   Taping of a butterfly needle with a heparin lock. **A,** Hold the two plastic wings together and insert the butterfly needle into the vein. **B,** Flatten the plastic wings out and place a strip of tape over them. **C,** Place the tape just below the wing and under the IV tubing, adhesive side up. **D,** Cross the tape over the wing-tips to anchor into place. **E,** Coil IV tubing with the heparin lock and tape it into place.

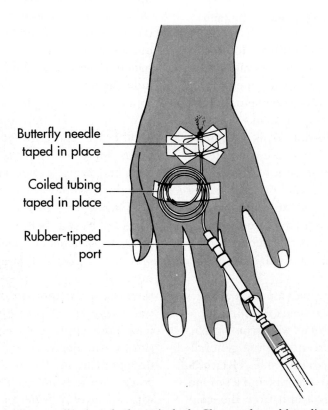

Butterfly needle taped in place

Coiled tubing taped in place

Rubber-tipped port

Fig. 4-33   Adding medications by heparin lock. Cleanse the rubber diaphragm on the end of the tubing with an alcohol wipe and allow it to air dry. Slowly inject the medication by inserting the needle through the diaphragm. Withdraw the needle and cleanse the diaphragm again with an alcohol wipe. Insert the needle of a syringe containing saline, and flush the reservoir with 1 to 2 ml of sterile saline. Remove syringe and needle and cleanse diaphragm with alcohol wipe.

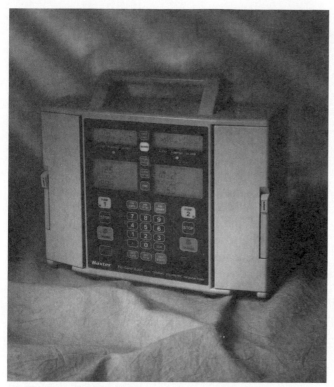

Fig. 4-34 Flo-gard 6301 Dual Channel Volumetric Infusion Pump. (Courtesy of Baxter Healthcare Corp.)

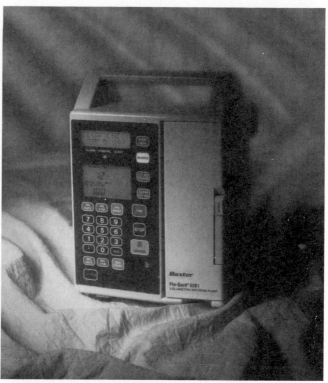

Fig. 4-35 Flo-gard 6201 Volumetric Infusion Pump. (Courtesy of Baxter Healthcare Corp.)

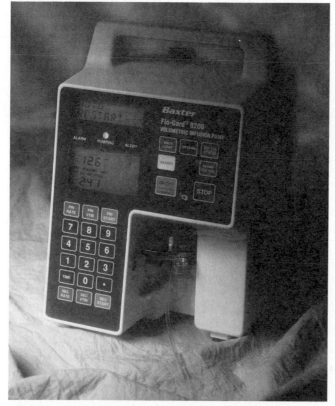

Fig. 4-36 Flo-gard 8200 Volumetric Infusion Pump. (Courtesy of Baxter Healthcare Corp.)

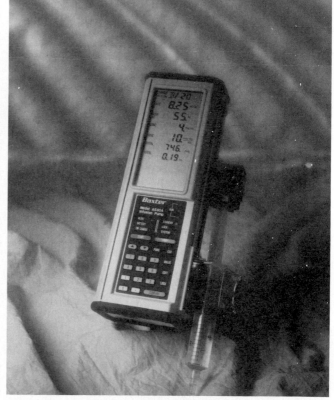

Fig. 4-37 AS40A Auto Syringe Infusion Pump. (Courtesy of Baxter Healthcare Corp.)

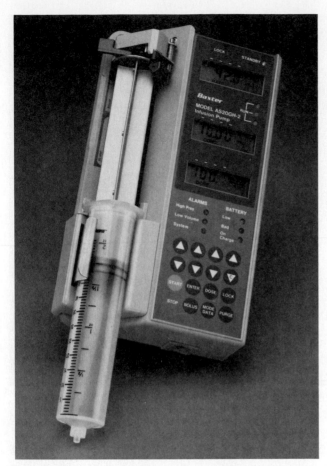

Fig. 4-38 Auto Syringe Model AS20GH-2 Infusion Pump. (Courtesy of Baxter Healthcare Corp.)

In evaluating the patient receiving an infusion, there are six primary areas of concern:

1. *Failure to infuse properly.* Occasionally the tubing may become kinked or may be under the patient, preventing proper infusion. At other times the needle may become lodged against the wall of the vein, and slightly pulling back on it and reanchoring the needle will start it again. Sometimes the rate of infusion is so slow that a small clot may form at the end of the needle, obstructing the flow. Sometimes the IV bottle needs to be elevated to keep adequate pressure for infusion, or blood pressure cuffs or tight gowns restricting fluid flow need to be removed. Starting at the bottle and moving down, check every part of the infusion setup for problems. If the IV bottle is placed below the needle site, gravity should cause blood to run back into the tubing if the needle is in place and not obstructed. If

blood fails to return to the tubing, the nurse may suspect that the needle is out of place or blocked.

2. *Infiltration.* Another common complication occurs when the needle becomes dislodged from the vein, allowing infusion or infiltration of medication and fluid into the tissues. This produces pain, swelling of the area, and redness. When some kinds of medication accidentally leak into tissue, they can irritate and damage the tissue. Whenever IV infiltration is discovered, the infusion site must be carefully inspected for signs of injury. The infusion should be discontinued and the physician contacted, especially if necrosis, sloughing, blistering, or unusual swelling is seen. Warm, moist compresses should be applied to the area. Sometimes other drugs are injected to counteract the medication that accidentally infused into the tissue.

3. *Air in the tubing.* Air infused into a patient is potentially dangerous, producing a bubble of air in the bloodstream. If air is seen in the tubing, the tubing should immediately be clamped below the air bubble, and, using aseptic technique, the air should be withdrawn through a syringe and needle inserted at the piggyback portal, or at the hub of the needle. All air, fluid, and blood in the syringe should then be discarded. Small amounts of air probably will not harm the patient. Should a larger amount of air actually enter the patient through the tubing, the patient should be placed with the head down and turned on the left side, and the physician notified. The patient should be given oxygen if he or she complains of shortness of breath.

4. *Signs of infection.* Redness, swelling, warmth, and burning along the course of the vein are signs of infection or phlebitis and are often produced or aggravated by irritating medication. They are commonly seen with medications such as potassium, antibiotics, or anticancer drugs, but may occur with any infusion. The IV should be stopped, the physician notified, and warm, moist compresses applied to the area.

A contaminated infusion that causes a systemic infection is rare. If the patient suddenly develops chills, fever, nausea, vomiting, and headache, the infusion should be immediately stopped, the patient closely monitored, and the physician contacted. The solution should be

Table 4-3 Common problems with intravenous infusions	
Problem	**Nursing action to follow**
Failure to infuse properly	Check for kinked tubing, needle against vein wall, or small clot at needle end; the IV pole may be too low, or the needle may be out of the vein. Check for damage done from tissue infusion. Stop infusion and restart it if required.
IV infiltration	Check to see if any tissue was damaged. Notify physician of any necrosis or sloughing. Apply wet compresses to the area to reduce pain. Stop infusion and restart it if required.
Air in tubing	Clamp tubing and remove the air with a syringe. If air was infused into the patient, put the patient in the head down position, lying on left side, and notify the physician.
Signs of infection	Check for local and systemic symptoms. Stop infusion, restart with a fresh setup, and notify physician. Treat symptomatically. Save the solution for testing.
Allergic reactions	Stop infusion and notify the physician.
Circulatory	Watch for problems of pulmonary edema: shortness of breath, poor color, weight gain, restlessness, edema. Notify the physician. Watch for problems of pulmonary emboli: poor color, shortness of breath, chest pain, coughing up blood. Notify the physician.

saved so that cultures may be taken.

5. *Allergic reactions.* Some products create an allergic response in the patient. Antibiotics often cause shortness of breath, temperature elevation, or rash. Reactions to blood or blood products are also common, producing shaking chills, hematuria, and temperature elevations. The medication infusion should be stopped and the physician notified.

6. *Circulatory problems.* Problems in systemic circulation are produced primarily in two forms: circulating particles or excess fluid volume.

   a. *Pulmonary embolism.* When particles of medication or pieces of a blood clot break loose and travel in the patient's bloodstream, they may stop in the lungs, causing shortness of breath as blood flow is blocked. Poor color, chest pain, restlessness, and coughing up blood may also be signs of pulmonary emboli. Infusion bottles and the IV lines should be kept clean, medications should be adequately dissolved, and filters should be used routinely in the IV lines. Embolism is usually an emergency and the physician should always be notified promptly.

   b. *Pulmonary edema.* Elderly patients, emaciated patients, infants, and children are particularly sensitive to the amount of fluid infused. These individuals often have heart, lung, or kidney problems that may decrease their ability to handle extra fluid. Circulatory overload may develop when fluids are infused too rapidly, or when the volume is too great. Signs of circulatory overload include:

    Dyspnea
    Weakness
    Lethargy
    Reduced urine output
    Edema
    Swelling of extremities
    Dependent edema
    Weak, rapid pulse
    Shallow, rapid respirations

In some individuals, the excess fluid accumulates primarily in the lungs, producing coughing, troubled breathing, crackles in the lung sounds, and frothy sputum. The infusion should be slowed and the physician notified if these symptoms develop.

Table 4-3 summarizes the problems that may occur with an IV infusion and the appropriate nursing actions to take.

SUMMARY

This section has stressed the procedures involved in administering parenteral medications, including the equipment, anatomic sites, and aseptic technique involved. The nurse should follow the standard institutional procedure to ensure safe administration of parenteral medications and protection of staff from personal risk of infection.

SECTION THREE: PERCUTANEOUS MEDICATIONS

Objectives

At the conclusion of this section you should be able to:

1. Describe the different forms of medications administered percutaneously.
2. Compare and contrast the procedures used to administer topical and mucous membranes medications.
3. Outline the procedures commonly used to apply topical products to skin, eyes, ears, nose, and respiratory tract.

Administration of Percutaneous Medications

The application of medication for absorption through the mucous membranes or skin is called **percutaneous administration**. The medication generally acts locally to cleanse, soften, disinfect, or lubricate the skin rather than to produce broad systemic effects. However, there are exceptions, such as nitroglycerin, which is given for its effect on the whole body.

It is hard to predict how topical medications will be absorbed. They often have a short duration of action and require frequent applications. Some medications must be properly inhaled, spread, or shampooed to be effective. In addition, many of these medications are greasy or messy to apply and leave stains on clothing and bedding.

The amount of medication absorbed through the skin or mucous membranes depends on several factors:

1. The size of the area covered by medication
2. The concentration or strength of the drug
3. The length of time the medication stays in contact with the skin

The general condition of the skin itself also makes a difference. Important factors include:

1. The amount of skin irritation and breakdown
2. The thickness of the skin involved
3. The general hydration, nutrition, and tone of the skin

Methods of percutaneous administration include:

1. Putting solutions onto the mucous membranes of the ear, eye, nose, mouth, or vagina
2. Applying topical creams, powders, ointments, or lotions
3. Inhaling aerosolized liquids or gases to carry medication to the nasal passages, sinuses, and lungs

The nurse should follow the same procedures outlined for other routes of administration when applying medications to the skin or mucous membranes. The nurse must also strictly follow the rules of safety. The general procedure for administering percutaneous medication is outlined in Procedure 4-5. However, the site of administration and the form of medication may require minor adjustments in the technique.

TOPICAL PRODUCTS

Topical medications are applied directly to the area of skin requiring treatment. The most common forms of topical medications include creams, lotions, and ointments, although there are many others. Each form of topical application has particular advantages and characteristics (see box on p. 81).

Administering topical medications

1. Always clean the skin before applying medication. This not only reduces the chances of infection, but removes any residue of medication previously applied and prevents the buildup of medication in that area. Water-based and alcohol-based products may be removed with soap and water alone. Oil-based products may be removed with cottonseed oil and gauze. Coal tar products may be removed with corn oil and gauze.
2. Gloves are worn to protect the nurse. Many skin lesions contain infectious material that could be spread to the nurse during the treatment process. Also, many medications may be absorbed through the skin of the person applying the medications.
3. Lotions are shaken until they are a uniform color throughout and are then applied by dabbing the medication onto the skin with a cotton ball or

Common Forms of Topical Medications

Astringents

Astringents are alcohol-based medications used for cleaning oily skin, and for cooling and soothing skin. They have a drying effect.

Creams

Creams are semisolid emulsions (mixture of two liquids) that contain medicine and a water-soluble base. They are rubbed into the skin.

Disks or patches

A disk or a transdermal patch is a semipermeable membrane pad containing medication that is attached to the skin with adhesive. The pad is left in place for 24 hours, providing gradual release of medication into the skin. The dosage depends on the concentration of the medication and the area of skin covered.

Lotions

Lotions are aqueous (watery) preparations that contain suspended materials. They cleanse or soothe the skin, or act as a drawing agent or astringent. Lotions should be shaken thoroughly and applied sparingly by patting on the skin, not rubbing.

Ointments

Ointments are semisolid preparations of medicines in an oily base, such as petrolatum or lanolin. Ointments provide good skin contact and are not easily removed. They are used sparingly, sometimes according to an application guide, and are often covered with dressings.

Powders

Powders are finely ground medication particles in a talc base. They are used for their drying, cooling, or protective effects.

Shampoos

Shampoos are medication in an aqueous or alcohol base that is poured onto the hair, allowed to stand, and then rubbed into hair and scalp before being rinsed. They are designed to treat problems of hair and scalp.

Soaps

Medicated soaps may be used to cleanse the skin and to moisten dry skin. Some soaps also leave a residue that helps reduce bacteria and oil.

Solutions

Medicated solutions of chemicals mixed with water or normal saline are used as washes or baths, or are applied to wet dressings for wrapping the skin. Chemicals used commonly include boric acid, Burow's solution, potassium permanganate, and silver nitrate. The mixing directions must be closely followed. Many of these solutions stain the skin and clothing.

---

gauze. Lotions are not rubbed into the skin.

4. Ointments and creams should be applied with a tongue depressor or a cotton-tipped applicator. Medication is scooped out or squeezed onto the applicator and then applied to skin with a firm stroke. If the area is to be covered with a dressing, the ointment may be applied directly to the gauze with the tongue depressor and then the gauze is applied to the skin. Creams are generally rubbed into the area, whereas ointments are just spread thinly and evenly over the skin. More is not better; this is an error that both patients and nurses commonly make with ointments.

5. Squeeze excess medication from wet dressings so they are not dripping. Directions should be closely followed. Dressings should be anchored with hypoallergenic tape or the physician may specify that the patient should have wraps, ace bandages, gauze pads, plastic wrap, or gloves covering the area. These coverings increase the sticking and absorption of the medication. They may also reduce staining and greasiness on clothes and bedding, but may limit the patient's ability to move.

6. Many patients with skin lesions worry about their appearance. The treatment process and application of dressings also may draw attention to unattractive areas or disfigurement. These patients need to be cared for in privacy and given opportunities to express their feelings about the problem and treatment. Opportunities to build up the patient's self-esteem should be sought.

7. Many treatments for skin problems extend beyond the time that patients are in the hospital. Take every opportunity to teach the patient how to

Procedure 4-5
Preparing and Administering Percutaneous Medications

Step one: getting ready

1. Check the medication order on the Kardex. Check the accuracy of the order as written and the time to be given. Clarify any information now known about the patient or the medication.
2. Wash your hands. This is essential to avoid contaminating the medication. Although it seems an obvious step, it is often neglected by busy nurses.
3. Assemble all the medication equipment. In addition to the medication order or card, obtain the medication tray; medication jars, tubes, or boxes; medication cart; gloves; plastic wrap; and tongue blades.

Step two: preparing the medication

1. Read the order on the medication card, and obtain the correct medication from the cabinet or cart. Medications may come in bottles, disks, patches, tubes, drops, sprays, and jars. Medication containers are commonly taken to the bedside for administration.
2. Compare the medication card with the label on the container. First check for the right patient, drug, route, dosage, and time of administration.
3. Place the medication next to the medication card on the tray.

Step three: administering the medication

1. Go the patient's bedside. Help the patient get into a position appropriate for the medication being given. Ask the patient his or her name at the same time you are checking the patient's identification bracelet and bed tag. Never give medication without positively identifying the patient. Confused or very ill patients may answer to any name.
2. Explain what you are giving and answer any of the patient's questions. Give any special instructions or teach the patient about the medication as indicated. Make any special assessments required. If the patient makes any comments about the medication looking different from usual, having just taken the medication, or not having had that medication before, recheck the medication order.
3. Cleanse the site of previous medication if necessary. Examine for signs of irritation, infection, or swelling.
4. Compare the information on the medication card to the label on the container. This is the second check for accuracy.
5. Put on gloves.
6. Before beginning administration check the information for the third time with the medication card.
7. Follow the specific procedure for applying the solution, powder, ointment, or shampoo. Cover the area with a plastic wrap or a dressing as ordered to increase absorption.

Step four: concluding

1. Discard all used dressings and gloves in the dirty utility room.
2. Note on the chart the time the medication was given and sign your name or initials. Record accurately that the medication was given as ordered.
3. Check the patient again later and note any particular responses or adverse effects that should be recorded and reported.

administer the medication and apply the dressings. If possible, have the patient administer the medication and apply any dressings under the nurse's supervision.

8. Medicated ointment is an increasingly common method of administering nitroglycerin to patients with chest pain from angina. When properly applied, nitroglycerin ointment (Nitrol or Nitro-Bid) can provide continuous release of medication to help prevent anginal attacks and is especially helpful at night.

To apply nitroglycerin ointment, cleanse the skin gently with an alcohol wipe. Individuals may use the chest, upper arm, or flank areas. An area without hair should be used. Adhesive tape applied to the skin and removed quickly should help remove small hairs. Shaving may cause skin irritation and should not be done. The physician will order nitroglycerin ointment to be applied by specifying the number of inches. A measuring applicator is provided with the medication (Fig. 4-39). The measuring applicator is laid on top of

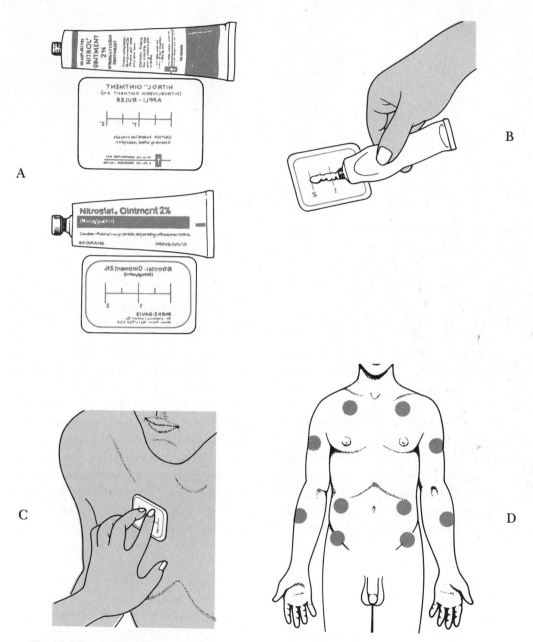

Fig. 4-39 **A,** Nitroglycerin ointment and special application papers. Note that the papers are printed backward. **B,** The correct amount of ointment is squeezed onto paper, and, **C,** it is applied to the patient's skin, **D,** in one of the sites shown. Clear plastic wrap is applied over the paper to increase absorption.

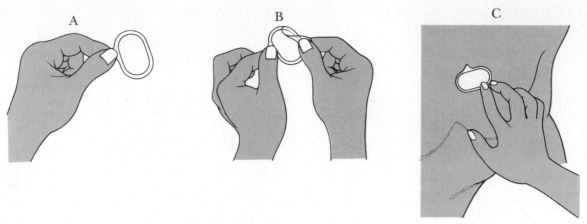

Fig. 4-40 **A,** Nitroglycerin patch. **B,** Remove the plastic backing, being careful not to touch inside. **C,** Place the exposed side on the patient's skin and press it into place.

the skin where the medication is to be applied and the correct number of inches is squeezed onto the applicator paper as a small ribbon of medication. The measuring applicator is then turned over onto the skin, ointment side down, and left in place. The area is not rubbed. The paper is covered with a plastic wrap and is taped in place. It must be changed every 3 to 4 hours.

9. Disks or patches are another method of providing continuous medication through the skin and are becoming more common as a means to provide nitroglycerin, some female hormones, and medications for motion sickness. Some antismoking programs also use nicotine patches. The principles for administration are similar to that for applying nitroglycerin ointment.

The medication comes packed over a semipermeable membrane and an adhesive patch. A site is chosen for application, according to a standard rotation pattern. The patch is carefully picked up and the clear plastic backing is removed from the patch, exposing the medication (Fig. 4-40). The medicated side is then pressed firmly onto the skin. The outer edge of the patch is adhesive and will hold the patch tightly to the skin. Patches are changed daily, unless they become partially dislodged and require replacement. Transderm Nitro and Nitro-Dur may be worn while showering; all other medicated patches should be applied after bathing.

ADMINISTERING MEDICATIONS TO MUCOUS MEMBRANES

The mucous membranes represent the other major route of percutaneous medication administration. In general, medication is easily absorbed across mucous membranes and it is easy to obtain therapeutic dosages. However, all mucous membranes do not have the same sensitivity to medication or the same capacity to absorb chemicals. The blood supply under the mucous membranes also varies. These different characteristics may be used advantageously. For example, putting medication in an oily base will slow its absorption and might help deliver antibiotics, whereas an aqueous medication would be quickly absorbed and its action quickly gone.

There are seven places where medications are commonly applied to mucous membranes: under the tongue (**sublingual administration**), against the cheek (**buccal administration**), in the eye, nose, or ear, or inhaled into the lung through an aerosol. Vaginal suppositories, creams, or douches also represent treatment through mucosal membranes. The medications might come as tablets, drops, ointments, creams, suppositories, or metered-dose inhalers.

The administration procedure for medications to mucous membranes follows the general format previously outlined. Different mucous membranes require minor adjustments in technique, which are summarized in the box on p. 85.

Procedure 4-6
Administering Medications to Mucous Membranes

Buccal area of cheek

The patient holds the medication between the cheek and molar teeth, where it is rapidly absorbed into the bloodstream and reaches the systemic circulation without being metabolized by the liver. This area is used for nitroglycerin tablets to relieve chest pain (Fig. 4-41).

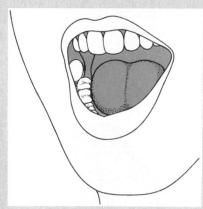

Fig. 4-41   Buccal medication administration.

Ear

Localized infection or inflammation of the ear is treated by dropping a small amount of a sterile medicated solution into the ear. Very low dosages of medication are required, and the medication must indicate it is for otic (ear) usage. The medication should be at room temperature. The patient should lie on the side with the affected ear up. Shake the medication well and draw the medication up into the dropper. In infants, gently pull the earlobe downward; in adults and children, gently pull the earlobe up and back. This will straighten the external canal so that the medication may be dropped into canal. Do not touch the dropper to the ear. The patient is to remain on that side for 5 minutes to allow the medication to coat the surface of the inner canal. A cotton ball may also be inserted if ordered. Repeat in the other ear if indicated (Fig. 4-42).

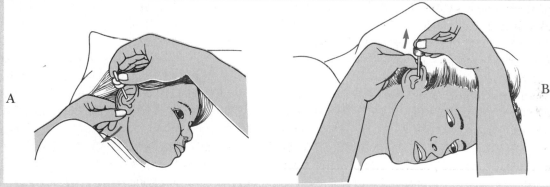

Fig. 4-42   Administering ear drops in a child and an adult. **A,** Pull earlobe downward in a child and, **B,** pull upward in an adult.

Continued.

Additional guidelines

1. All medications applied to mucous membranes must be administered aseptically. The nurse's hands must be washed before preparing medications. Gloves should be used to protect the nurse from suspected or confirmed infections. Universal precautions recommended by the Centers for Disease Control and Prevention (CDC) should be followed each time a medication is administered.

Eye and ear drops must be instilled carefully to prevent contamination of the droppers or the spread of the infection from one eye or ear to the other. Equipment and dressings used during medication administration must be disposed of properly.

2. Accurate documentation of medication administration should be made as soon as the medication

Procedure 4-6
Administering Medications to Mucous Membranes—cont'd

Eye

Sterile drops or ointments in very low dosage and specifically labeled for ophthalmic (eye) use may be applied to the eye. Gloves are used during the procedure. The eye may be cleaned with normal saline and cotton balls to remove exudate or previous medication. Wipe from the nasal side out. The medication should be at room temperature. Infants may need to be restrained. Have the patient look up, and pull out the lower lid to show the conjunctival sac (Fig. 4-43). Never touch the eye with the dropper or the ointment tip. Drop the medication or squeeze the ointment into the conjunctival sac, not onto the eye itself. Using a cotton ball, apply gentle pressure to the inner corner of the eyelid on the bone for 1 to 2 minutes to ensure adequate concentration of medication and prevent medication from draining rapidly into the nose. The patient should move the eyes around with eyelids closed to spread the ointment over the surface of the eye. Sterile dressings may be ordered to cover the eye at conclusion of treatment.

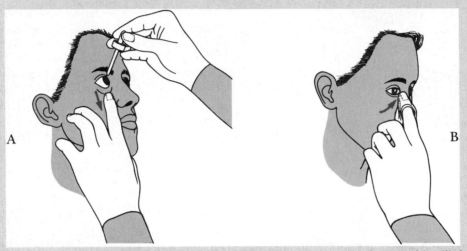

Fig. 4-43   Administering eye drops. **A,** While wearing gloves, pull the lower lid down and instill drops into the conjunctival sac while the patient looks upward. **B,** Apply gentle pressure with a tissue to the inner corner of the eyelid for 1 to 2 minutes to keep the medication in eye.

Continued.

is given. Medications involving site rotation should be carefully recorded. When medications are given for angina, the nurse must return within a few minutes to assess the patient's response to medication. Further medication may need to be given or the physician may need to be called.

3. Administration of medications presents an excellent teaching opportunity. The nurse should take advantage of it each time medication is given and teach the patient about the medication's actions, the important points to follow in administration of the medication, and the problems to report. When the medication is to be taken at home, the patient should begin self-administration under the supervision of the nurse as soon as possible. This will provide additional opportunities for the nurse to assess the patient's learning needs and to answer questions.

SUMMARY

Percutaneous medication involves applying medication to the skin and the mucous membranes through a variety of procedures and preparations. The basic techniques in percutaneous administration do not usually require the accuracy and precision of parenteral or oral medications. However, the nurse's responsibility in medication administration remains significant.

Procedure 4-6
Administering Medications to Mucous Membranes—cont'd

Nose

Nasal solutions act locally to treat minor congestion or infection. The patient should gently blow the nose and then lie down with the head hanging back over the side of the bed. The medication should be drawn up in the dropper, held just over one nostril, and then the required number of nose drops is administered. The patient should turn the head slightly, and the procedure is repeated for the other nostril. Infants may need to be restrained. If a nasal spray is used, the patient sits upright, one nostril is blocked, and the tip of the nasal spray is inserted into the nostril. As the patient takes a deep breath, a puff of spray is squeezed into the nostril. Less medication is required with the spray, and the medication is rapidly absorbed into the vascular areas of the nose for prompt action (Fig. 4-44).

Respiratory mucosa

Medication may be carried through the mouth or nose and down into the respiratory tract through use of aerosol nebulizers, Spinhalers, or metered-dose inhalers. These techniques require special equipment that must be kept very clean, and that breaks the medication up into very small particles, which can be carried with air down into the lungs where the desired action takes place.

Aerosols

Aerosols use a special nebulizer mouthpiece, and medications are diluted according to a special concentration. Oxygen is used to deliver the medication. The patient sits upright, places the nebulizer mouthpiece loosely in the mouth, and breathes in and out slowly and deeply while the oxygen is directed through the nebulizer until the medication is gone. The equipment must be cleaned after it is used.

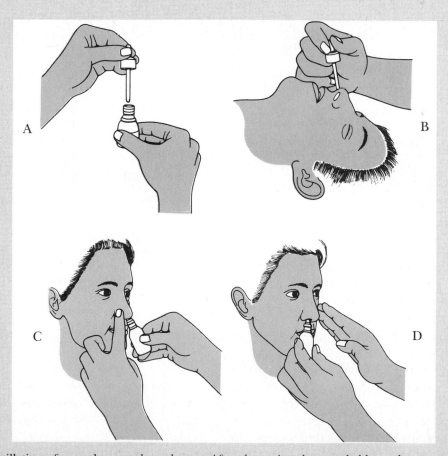

Fig. 4-44   Instillation of nose drops and nasal spray. After the patient has gently blown the nose and has placed the head backward, **A**, draw the nose drops and, **B**, carefully squeeze the drops into each nostril, taking care not to touch the dropper to the skin. For nasal spray, shake the solution and, **C**, cover one nostril and insert the tip into the other nostril. **D**, Squeeze a puff into the nostril while the patient inhales deeply.

Continued.

Procedure 4-6
Administering Medications to Mucous Membranes—cont'd

Metered-dose inhalers

Metered-dose inhalers are used to deliver specific amounts of corticosteroids or bronchodilators to nasal or lung tissue. These small canisters are pressurized with gas, which propels the medication out and breaks it up into small particles that can be carried deep down in the lungs as the patient takes a deep breath. The medication is carried directly to the site of action with very little systemic effect. The onset of action is rapid. Some medications are designed to be administered through the mouth, some through the nose. It is important to read the directions completely. The medication should be shaken before use. Instruct patient to sit upright, hold the nebulizer in the hand 1 to 2 inches in front of the mouth or at the opening of the nose. The patient should exhale, then squeeze the canister in its holder (Fig. 4-45) as the next inspiration begins. This will carry medication down into the lungs. The patient should hold the breath as long as possible before exhaling to allow the medication to settle before administering in other nostril or taking another puff. It is important to time the squeezing of the nebulizer to ensure that medication travels in with the next breath and is not just squirted on the back of the throat or nose. The nebulizer must be cleaned with water after each use. It is important that the patient keep an adequate supply of medication on hand. See Fig. 4-46 for determining medication level in canister.

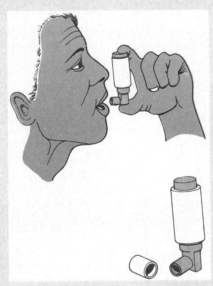

Fig. 4-45 Using a metered-dose inhaler. The patient should open the mouth and hold the mouthpiece up to but not touching the mouth. The patient should take a deep breath and blow out all air. At the same time as the next breath, the patient should squeeze the canister from the top, producing a small spray of medication that will travel to the lungs.

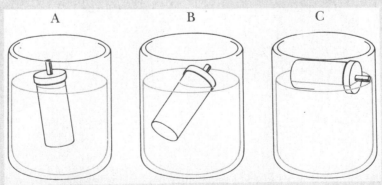

Fig. 4-46 Checking a metered-dose canister for medication by placing it in a glass of water. **A,** Canister is full. **B,** Canister is partially filled. **C,** Canister is nearly empty.

Procedure 4-6
Administering Medications to Mucous Membranes—cont'd

Sublingual mucosa

The patient places the tablet under the tongue, where it dissolves and is rapidly absorbed through the blood vessels and enters the systemic circulation. This site is used for nitroglycerin tablets to relieve chest pain (Fig. 4-47).

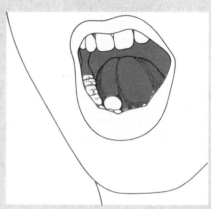

Fig. 4-47   Sublingual medication administration.

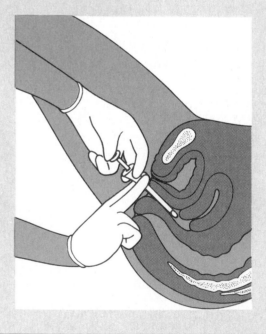

Vaginal

Medication to treat local infections or irritation may be applied vaginally through creams, jellies, tablets, foams, suppositories, or irrigations (douches). Room temperature suppositories are inserted into the vagina with a gloved hand, much like a rectal suppository is inserted. Creams, jellies, tablets, and foams are inserted with a special applicator that comes with the medication. With the patient lying down, the vaginal applicator is inserted as far into the vaginal canal as possible and the plunger is pushed, depositing the medication. The patient is instructed to remain lying down for 10 to 15 minutes so all the medication can melt and coat the vaginal walls. The patient may need a perineal pad to catch any drainage or prevent staining. Gloves must be carefully discarded according to hospital regulations.

Some medicated solutions are used to wash the internal vaginal area when infection and irritation are present. These solutions are administered as douches. The patient may be on a bedpan or reclining in a bathtub. A douche bag containing a medicated solution is hung on an IV pole or shower head, about 12 inches above the patient's hips. The tubing is clamped shut. The vulva is gently washed by slowly unclamping the tubing, and then the douche nozzle is inserted into the vaginal canal 3 to 4 inches and pointed downward towards the patient's tail bone (coccyx) (Fig. 4-48). The labia are held shut while the solution is gently introduced. As much solution as possible is allowed to fill the vaginal canal before the labia are opened and the solution flows out. The nozzle should be rotated gently, to allow the solution to reach and wash all areas. When all the solution has been used, the nozzle is withdrawn and all the equipment is cleaned and put away and the gloves are discarded.

Fig. 4-48   Vaginal medication administration.

CRITICAL THINKING QUESTIONS

1. With a partner, use a jar of vitamins or aspirins or a small bottle of juice, a small paper cup, and a notecard (for the Kardex) to practice pouring and administering tablets and liquids. Prepare to demonstrate each step as your partner explains, and vice versa, to the rest of the class. As you practice, keep in mind *all* the steps laid out in the procedures descriptions in the text—it's not as easy as it sounds to remember everything and to do it all in the right order as well!

2. Test yourself on the administration of rectal medications by sectioning a sheet of paper off into four blocks. Label these blocks as follows: "Getting Ready," "Preparing the Medication," "Administering the Medication," and "Concluding the Process." Now fill in as many steps within each phase of administration as you can remember. Without checking your work against the book, exchange lists with a partner and fill in steps you know of that he or she has left out. Now answer these two questions:

- Did your partner's list include anything that you left out of yours? What?
- Did your partner add anything to your list that you hadn't thought of?
- Now check your own work against the text. How many steps in this apparently "simple" procedure did you leave out altogether?

3. Write these three headings across the top of a sheet of paper: "Dose form," "Description," and "Indications." Now put the oral dose forms listed below in column 1, skipping at least 3 spaces between.

buccal forms	elixirs	emulsions
capsules	lozenges	pills
suspensions	syrups	tablets

Now distinguish these forms from one another by completing your table. How are they distinct not only in form but in indications?

4. Describe techniques and considerations unique to nasogastric medication administration.

5. You have just entered the medication room where Lisa, a fellow nurse, has just finished pouring capsules for Mr. Johnson, when she is called away in an emergency. As she rushes past you, she calls back, asking you to please give Mr. Johnson his medication. She points to the cup as she slips out the door. What should you do?

6. You've been responsible for Mrs. Davis' care for 2 days now, counting today. When you enter her room with her medication tray, she seems groggy and confused; she probably just woke up, you think. You greet her, set down the tray, but then discover that she no longer has her identification band on. Still, it's time for her pills, you know her well, she answers to her name, and you don't want to have to delay her medication. Is it okay to go ahead and give it to her for now and then find out what happened to her ID? Explain your answer.

7. Describe universal precautions for preventing the transmission of HIV.

8. What is the purpose of the Z-track injection technique? Describe how it's given.

9. Point out the differences in site, absorption, and technique among each of the following parenteral routes: intradermal, subcutaneous, intramuscular, and intravenous.

10. How do you get rid of bubbles in a filled syringe? Why should you bother?

11. List as many forms of percutaneous medications as you can. Now check your work in the text; add whatever you left out. Identify *unique* steps in the administration of each.

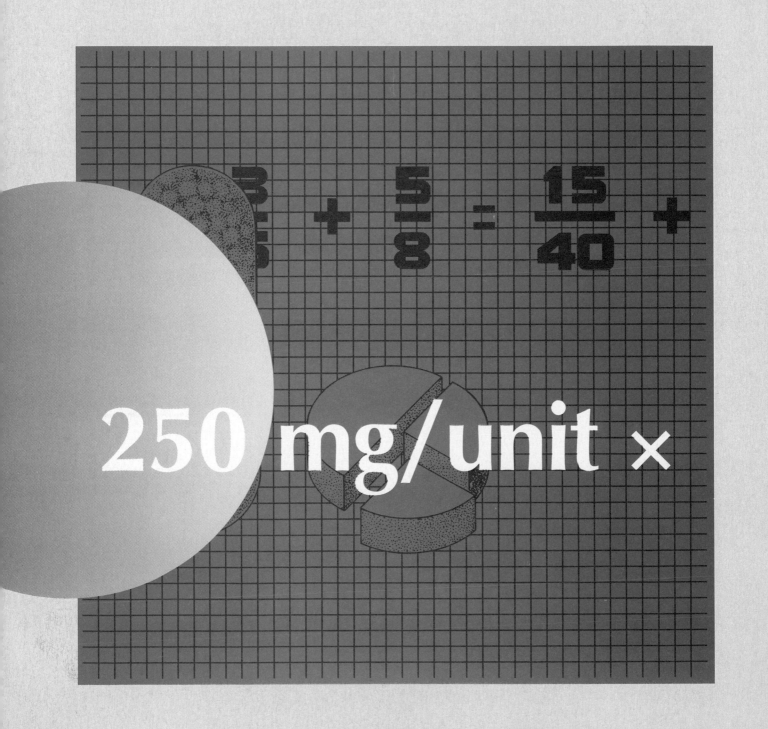

Mathematics and Calculations

OBJECTIVES

At the conclusion of the unit you should be able to:

1. Work basic mathematical calculations involving fractions, decimal fractions, percentages, ratio, and proportions.

2. Convert numbers between apothecary, household, and metric equivalents.

3. Convert temperature readings between centigrade and Fahrenheit scales.

4. Accurately perform mathematical calculations used in computing drug dosages.

OVERVIEW

This unit is divided into three major chapters: Chapter 5 contains a general review of mathematical principles. Chapter 6 presents mathematical equivalents in pharmacology. Chapter 7 applies basic mathematical principles to the calculation of medication dosages. Key concepts and tasks are described, and illustrations and examples provided for each area.

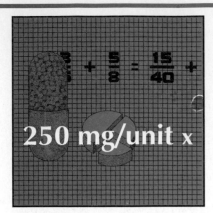

CHAPTER 5

Review of Mathematical Principles

OBJECTIVES

At the conclusion of the chapter you should be able to:

1. Work basic multiplication and division problems.
2. Interpret Roman numerals correctly.
3. Apply basic rules in calculations using fractions, decimal fractions, percentages, ratios, and proportions.

KEY TERMS

common denominator, p. 97
complex fraction, p. 97
denominator, p. 95
fraction, p. 95
improper fraction, p. 96
mixed number, p. 96
numerator, p. 95
percent, p. 100
proper fraction, p. 96
proportion, p. 100
ratio, p. 100
Roman numeral system, p. 95

Overview

The ability to accurately and quickly calculate basic mathematical problems rests on the nurse having a good foundation of basic math. Although most nurses feel comfortable with subtraction and addition, most students profit from a review of basic concepts in multiplication and division to increase their speed. By memorizing and drilling these basic facts you will have confidence and speed in completing the calculations ahead. These number relationships form important building blocks for tasks the nurse must master.

Multiplication and Division

Included in the box below is a basic grid for multiplication and division. To multiply a number in the top row by a number in the left-hand column, draw a straight line from each number to where they intersect.

Multiplication and Division Grid

1	2	3	4	5	6	7	8	9	10	11	12
2	4	6	8	10	12	14	16	18	20	22	24
3	6	9	12	15	18	21	24	27	30	33	36
4	8	12	16	20	24	28	32	36	40	44	48
5	10	15	20	25	30	35	40	45	50	55	60
6	12	18	24	30	36	42	48	54	60	66	72
7	14	21	28	35	42	49	56	63	70	77	84
8	16	24	32	40	48	56	64	72	80	88	96
9	18	27	36	45	54	63	72	81	90	99	108
10	20	30	40	50	60	70	80	90	100	110	120
11	22	33	44	55	66	77	88	99	110	121	132
12	24	36	48	60	72	84	96	108	120	132	144

For example: What is 7×8? Follow across to the right from number 7 on the left; follow down from number 8 on the top. The two lines intersect at 56. Therefore, $7 \times 8 = 56$.

If you want to review a division fact, find the number on the left-hand side of the chart that is the same as the divisor. Follow the number to the right until you come to the exact number or the number closest to that being divided. Follow the number up to the top to learn the number of times the larger number may be divided by the number on the left.

For example: How many times will 9 go into 81? Find 9 in the column on the left. Follow the line across until you come to 81. Follow the column up from 81 to 9. Therefore, 81 divided by $9 = 9$. If you were seeking to learn how many times 9 would go into 84, 9 would still be the closest number, but there would be a remainder of 3.

KEY POINT:
Multiplication hint

Zero times any number is zero!

Roman Numerals

The numbers commonly used today in expressing quantity and value are called Arabic numerals. Examples of Arabic numerals are 1, 2, 3, etc. Another number system in common use is the **Roman numeral system.** Roman numerals from the values of 1 to 100 are commonly used as units of the apothecaries' system of weights and measures in writing prescriptions. They may also be used to express dates in copyrights and in formal manuscripts. Seven numerals make up the basic building blocks of the Roman numeral system (see the box below).

After memorizing the seven Roman numerals and their values, it is important to learn four rules in using Roman numerals (see the box on p. 96).

Roman Numerals and Their Values

I = 1	C = 100
V = 5	D = 500
X = 10	M = 1000
L = 50	

Fractions

A good understanding of fractions is important to the nurse because all units of the apothecaries' system are written as common fractions for all amounts less than one. Fractions also form the foundation in dosage calculations when medication is in a different available dose form than that ordered.

BASIC PRINCIPLES

A **fraction** is one or more equal parts of a unit. It is written as two numbers separated by a line, such as $\frac{1}{2}$ or $\frac{3}{4}$. The parts of the fraction are called the terms. The two terms of a fraction are the **numerator** and the **denominator.** The numerator is the top number (the number above the line). The denominator is the bottom number (the number below the line). In $\frac{1}{2}$, 1 is the numerator and 2 is the denominator.

The denominator tells into how many equal parts

Rules in using Roman numerals

1. Whenever a Roman numeral is repeated, or when a smaller numeral *follows* a larger one, the values are added together.
   For example:

   II = 2 (1 + 1 = 2)

   LVII = 57 (50 + 5 + 1 + 1 = 57)

   CXIII = 113 (100 + 10 + 1 + 1 + 1 = 113)

2. Whenever a smaller Roman numeral *comes before* a larger Roman numeral, subtract the smaller value.
   For example:

   IV = 4 (5 − 1 = 4)

   CD = 400 (500 − 100 = 400)

3. Numerals are never repeated more than three times in a sequence.
   For example:

   III = 3

   IV = 4

4. Whenever a smaller Roman numeral comes between two larger Roman numerals, subtract the smaller number from the numeral following it.
   For example:

   XIX = 19 (10 + [10 − 1] = 19)

   LIV = 54 (50 + [5 − 1] = 54)

In expressing dosages in the apothecaries' system, lowercase rather than capital Roman numerals are used. A dot is always placed over the Roman numeral i whenever lowercase numbers are used. For example, iii or vi is the proper form rather than III or VI.

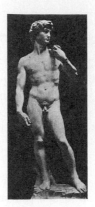

N
U
—
D
E

Fractions may be raised to higher terms by multiplying both terms of the fraction by the same number.

For example, to raise $\frac{3}{4}$ to a higher term, multiply both the numerator and the denominator by 2, converting it to $\frac{6}{8}$; $\frac{3}{4}$ and $\frac{6}{8}$ have the same value.

$$\frac{3}{4} \times \frac{2}{2} = \frac{6}{8}$$

Fractions are reduced to lower terms by dividing both the numerator and denominator by the same number. For example, to lower $\frac{3}{9}$ to a lower term, divide both the numerator and the denominator by 3, converting it to $\frac{1}{3}$; $\frac{3}{9}$ and $\frac{1}{3}$ have the same value.

$$\frac{3}{9} \div \frac{3}{3} = \frac{1}{3}$$

Proper fractions are part of a whole number, or any number less than a whole number (1, 3, and 5 are examples of whole numbers). The number $\frac{3}{4}$ is a proper fraction because it is less than 1; its numerator is less than its denominator.

Improper fractions have a numerator the same as or larger than the denominator. The number $\frac{6}{4}$ is an improper fraction because the numerator (6) is larger than the denominator (4).

In using fractions in calculations, the numerator and the denominator must be of the same unit of measure. For example, if the numerator is in grains, the denominator must be in grains.

A **mixed number** is a whole number and a proper fraction. Examples of mixed numbers include: $4\frac{1}{3}$, $3\frac{3}{4}$, $5\frac{16}{35}$.

It is often necessary to change an improper fraction to a mixed number or to change a mixed number to an improper fraction when doing certain

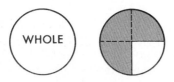

the whole has been divided. The numerator tells how many of the parts are being used.

It is important not to confuse these two parts of the fraction. One way to remember which part belongs where is to think of the word NUDE. The N is on top; the D is on the bottom, like this:

calculations. To change an improper fraction to a mixed number, divide the denominator into the numerator. The result (quotient) is the whole number. The remainder is placed over the denominator of the improper fraction.

For example: $\frac{17}{3}$ is an improper fraction. To convert $\frac{17}{3}$ to a mixed number:

1. Divide the denominator (3) into the numerator (17):

$$
\begin{array}{r}
5 \leftarrow \text{quotient} \\
3\overline{)17} \\
-15 \\
\hline
2 \leftarrow \text{remainder}
\end{array}
$$

2. Move the remainder (2) over the denominator (3)

3. Put the quotient (5) in front of the fraction:

$$5\frac{2}{3}$$

To change the mixed number $5\frac{2}{3}$ to an improper fraction, multiply the denominator of the fraction (3) by the whole number (5), add the numerator (2), and place the sum over the denominator.

For example:

$$
\begin{array}{r}
3 \times 5 = 15 \\
+\ 2 \\
\hline
17 \leftarrow \text{sum}
\end{array}
$$

The sum (17) goes over the denominator of the fraction: $\frac{17}{3}$ is the improper fraction.

A **complex fraction** has a fraction in either its numerator, its denominator, or both. For example $\frac{1/5}{50}$ or $\frac{30}{2/3}$ or $3\frac{1/2}{1/8}$ are examples of complex fractions. Complex fractions may be changed to whole numbers, proper or improper fractions by dividing the number or fraction above the line by the number or fraction below the line.

For example, change $\frac{\frac{1}{2}}{100}$ to a proper fraction as follows:

$$\frac{\frac{1}{2}}{100} = \frac{1}{2} \div 100$$

$$
\boxed{
\begin{aligned}
&= \frac{1}{2} \div \frac{100}{1} \\
&= \frac{1}{2} \times \frac{1}{100}
\end{aligned}
}
$$

To divide by $\frac{100}{1}$, simply invert or reverse the numerator (100) and the denominator (1) and multiply by the result, or by $\frac{1}{100}$

$$= \frac{1}{2 \times 100}$$

$$= \frac{1}{200}$$

Adding fractions

If fractions have the same denominator, simply add the numerators, and put the sum above the common denominator:

For example:

$$\frac{1}{11} + \frac{3}{11} = \frac{4}{11} \quad \begin{array}{l}\text{(sum of 1 + 3)} \\ \text{(same denominator)}\end{array}$$

Also:

$$\frac{2}{12} + \frac{3}{12} + \frac{6}{12} = \frac{11}{12} \quad \begin{array}{l}\text{(sum of 2 + 3 + 6)} \\ \text{(same denominator)}\end{array}$$

If the fractions have different denominators, they must be converted to a number that each denominator has in common, or a **common denominator.** You can always find a common denominator by multiplying the two denominators by one another. Sometimes, however, both numbers will go into a smaller number. For example: $\frac{1}{12} + \frac{3}{8} + \frac{3}{4} = ?$ What is the smallest common denominator?

1. The smallest whole number all these denominators (12, 8, and 4) have in common is 24; 24, then, is the lowest common denominator.

2. Divide the lowest common denominator by the denominator of each fraction and multiply both terms of the fraction by the quotient. This is often easier to see if we write the problem vertically:

$$
\begin{aligned}
\frac{1}{12} &= \frac{?}{24} \\
+\ \frac{3}{8} &= \frac{?}{24} \\
+\ \frac{3}{4} &= \frac{?}{24}
\end{aligned}
$$

3. Next, divide 12, 8, and 4 into 24 and multiply the numerator and denominator by the answer (quotient):

$$
\begin{aligned}
\frac{1}{12} \times \frac{2}{2} &= \frac{2}{24} \\
+\ \frac{3}{8} \times \frac{3}{3} &= \frac{9}{24} \\
+\ \frac{3}{4} \times \frac{6}{6} &= \frac{18}{24}
\end{aligned}
$$

4. Then add the numerators and bring down the denominator:

$$\frac{2}{24} + \frac{9}{24} + \frac{18}{24} = \frac{29}{24}$$

5. Reduce to lowest terms:

$$\frac{29}{24} = 1\frac{5}{24}$$

Subtracting fractions

If fractions have the same denominator, subtract the smaller numerator from the larger numerator. Leave the denominator the same, and then reduce to the lowest terms, if necessary.

For example:

$$\frac{5}{10} - \frac{1}{10} = \frac{4}{10} = \frac{2}{5}$$

If fractions do not have the same denominator, change the fractions so they have the smallest common denominator, subtract the numerators, and leave the denominator the same.

For example:

$$\frac{15}{28} - \frac{3}{14} =$$

Since 28 is a multiple of 14 ($14 \times 2 = 28$), 28 is a common denominator of 28 and 14. Divide the smallest common denominator by the denominator of each fraction, and multiply the numerator and denominator of the fraction by the quotient.

$$\frac{15}{28} = \frac{15}{28} \text{ (no change necessary)}$$

$$- \frac{3}{14} \times \frac{2}{2} = \frac{6}{28} \text{ } (28 \div 14 = 2)$$

Subtract the numerators and leave the denominators the same.

$$\frac{15}{28} - \frac{6}{28} = \frac{9}{28}$$

Multiplying fractions

When multiplying fractions, reduce all terms to their smallest form to simplify the calculation. For example, $\frac{12}{24}$ is the same as $\frac{1}{2}$, but $\frac{12}{24}$ is more difficult to work with. To reduce to the lowest terms, divide the same number into both the numerator and the denominator (i.e., $\frac{2}{10}$ can be divided by 2; $\frac{2}{10}$, therefore, $= \frac{1}{5}$; $\frac{9}{36}$ can be divided by 9; $\frac{9}{36}$, therefore, $= \frac{1}{4}$).

When the fractions are in their simplest form, multiply the numerators together, and then multiply the denominators together.

KEY POINT:

Multiplying fractions

Because 3 is a whole number it is the same as $\frac{3}{1}$. The 1 can be added as a denominator if it makes it easier to understand.

For example:

$$\frac{1}{20} \times \frac{5}{3} \times 3 =$$

By reducing, this can be simplified as follows:

$$\frac{1}{20} \times \frac{5}{3} \times \frac{3}{1} =$$

$$\frac{1 \times 5 \times 3}{20 \times 3 \times 1} =$$

$$\frac{15}{60} = \frac{1}{4}$$

If the number is a mixed number (a whole number and a fraction), change it to an improper fraction before solving.

For example:

$$2\frac{1}{2} \times \frac{2}{3} \times 6 = \frac{5}{2} \times \frac{2}{3} \times \frac{6}{1}$$

$$= \frac{5}{\cancel{2}} \times \frac{\cancel{2}}{\cancel{3}} \times \frac{\cancel{6}}{1}$$

$$= \frac{10}{1}$$

$$= 10$$

Dividing fractions

To divide a fraction by a fraction, invert (or turn upside down) the divisor and then multiply.

For example:

$$\frac{4}{6} \div \frac{2}{6} = ?$$

Invert the divisor.

$$\frac{4}{6} \times \frac{6}{2} = ?$$

Simplify, then multiply the numerators and then the denominators.

$$\frac{\cancel{4}}{\cancel{6}} \times \frac{\cancel{6}}{\cancel{2}} = 2$$

Decimal Fractions

A decimal fraction has a denominator of 10 or a multiple of 10. Instead of writing the denominator, a decimal point is added to the numerator.

For example:

$$\frac{1}{4} = \frac{25}{100} = 0.25$$

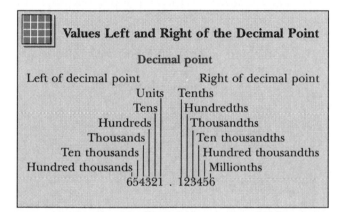

Values Left and Right of the Decimal Point

Decimal point

Left of decimal point   Right of decimal point

Units   Tenths
Tens| |Hundredths
Hundreds|| ||Thousandths
Thousands||| |||Ten thousandths
Ten thousands|||| ||||Hundred thousandths
Hundred thousands||||| |||||Millionths

654321 . 123456

All numbers left of the decimal point represent whole numbers. Numbers to the right represent fractions. Zeros may be placed to the right of the decimal without changing the value of the whole number (i.e., 45 is the same as 45.0 or 45.00).

Decimals increase in value from right to left; they decrease in value from left to right. Decimals increase in value in multiples of 10. Each column in a decimal has its own value, according to where it lies from the decimal point (see the box above).

ADDING AND SUBTRACTING DECIMAL FRACTIONS

Place the numbers so that the decimal points fall in a straight line. Keep the columns straight. Add zeroes to the right if necessary. Then add or subtract as you would for whole numbers. The decimal point goes in the answer just below the decimal points in the problem.

For example: add 0.0678 and 1.082

```
    0.0678
 + 1.0820      (add one zero)
   1.1498
```

The decimal point is in line with the other decimal

points. Subtract 3.053 from 6.046:

```
   6.046
 - 3.053
   2.993
```

MULTIPLYING AND DIVIDING DECIMAL FRACTIONS

To multiply decimal fractions, multiply the two numbers and count off from right to left as many decimal places in the product (answer) as there were in the multiplier and multiplicand.

For example:

```
   44.61     Multiplicand (has 2 decimal places)
 ×  2.3      Multiplier (has 1 decimal place)
  13383
  89220
 102.603×    Count off 3 places right to left
             and insert decimal point.
```

To divide by a decimal fraction, first move the decimal point in the divisor (the number you are dividing with) enough places right to make it a whole number. Then move the decimal point in the dividend (the number you are dividing) as many places as it was moved in the divisor. Place the decimal point in the quotient (answer) directly above that in the dividend.

For example: divide 32.80 by 8.2

8.2)‾3‾2‾.‾8‾0   8.2 is the divisor; 32.80 is the dividend

Move the decimal point in the divisor to the right to make it a whole number, then move it the same number of places in the dividend.

8⌣2.)‾3‾2⌣8‾.‾0

Solve the problem:

```
        4.0
 82.)‾3‾2‾8‾.‾0‾0
      328.00
          0
```

A short cut may be taken when multiplying or dividing by 10, 100, or 1000.

To multiply a decimal fraction by 10, 100, or 1000, move the decimal place as many places to the right as there are zeros in the multiplier.

For example:

$$0.0006 \times 1000 = ?$$

In 1000 there are three zeros, so

$$0.0006 \times 1000 =$$

$$0⌣000.6 = 0000.6 = 0.6$$

To divide a decimal fraction by 10, 100, or 1000, move the decimal place as many places to the left as there are zeros in the divisor.

For example:

$$0.5 \div 100 = ?$$

100 has two zeros, so

$$0.5 \div 100 = 0.00{\scriptstyle\smile}5 = 0.005$$

Ratios

A **ratio** is a way of expressing the relationship of one number to another number, or of expressing a part of a whole number. The relationship is expressed by separating the numbers with a colon (:). The colon means division. The expression 1:2 means there is one part to two parts. Ratios are commonly used to express concentrations of a drug in a solution.

For example, a ratio written as 1:20 means 1 part to 20 parts. A ratio may also be written as a fraction (i.e., 1:10 is the same as 1/10).

Percents

The term **percent** or the symbol % means parts per hundred. Thus, the percentage may also be expressed as a fraction or as a decimal fraction.

For example:

30% means 30 parts per hundred or 30/100

70% means 70 parts per hundred or 70/100

Percents should also be reduced to their lowest common denominator, when appropriate:

For example:

20% is 20/100 or 1/5

40% is 40/100 or 2/5

To change a fraction to a percent, divide the numerator by the denominator and multiply the results (quotient) by 100 and add a percent sign (%).

For example:

To change $\frac{8}{10}$ to a percent:

$$8 \div 10 = 0.8$$
$$0.8 \times 100 = 80\%$$

To change $\frac{2}{5}$ to a percent:

$$2 \div 5 = 0.4$$
$$0.4 \times 100 = 40\%$$

To change a ratio to a percent, the ratio is first expressed as a fraction. The first number or term of the ratio becomes the numerator and the second number or term becomes the denominator (i.e., 1:200 becomes 1/200).

The fraction is then changed to a percent as shown:

$$1{:}200 = \frac{1}{200}$$
$$1 \div 200 = 0.005$$
$$0.005 \times 100 = 0.5\%$$

To change a percent to a ratio, the percent becomes the numerator and is placed over the denominator of 100.

For example, to change 20% and 50% to ratios:

$$20\% \text{ is } \frac{20}{100} = \frac{1}{5} \text{ or } 1{:}5$$
$$50\% \text{ is } \frac{50}{100} = \frac{1}{2} \text{ or } 1{:}2$$

A percent may easily be expressed as a decimal, a fraction, or as a ratio.

For example:

$$20\% = 0.20 = \frac{20}{100} = \frac{1}{5} = 1{:}5$$

It is very easy to change between decimals, fractions, percents, and ratios. The rules that summarize these changes are presented in the box on p. 101.

Proportions

A **proportion** is a way of expressing a relationship of equality between two ratios. In other words, the first ratio listed is equal to the second ratio listed. The two ratios are separated by a double colon (::), which means, "as." The numbers of each end of the relationship are the extremes, and the two numbers in the middle are the means. ***The product of the extremes equals the product of the means.*** This means that if one of the terms is not known, it may be calculated. The unknown term is defined by an x.

For example:

$$5{:}500 :: 2{:}x$$

(when x is the unknown) means

"The relationship of 5 to 500 is the same as the relationship of 2 to x."

```
        ┌─extremes─┐
        │ ┌means┐  │
        5:500 :: 2:x
```

Rules for Changing Between Percents, Decimals, Fractions, and Ratios

To change a fraction to a ratio, write the two numbers with a colon between them instead of the dividing line.

Example: $\frac{1}{5} = 1:5$

To change a fraction to a decimal fraction, divide the numerator by the denominator.

Example: $\frac{1}{5} = 0.20$

To change a fraction to a percent, divide the numerator by the denominator (use as many decimal places as needed); then move the decimal point two places to the right and add the percent sign.

Example: $\frac{1}{5} = 0.20 = 20\%$

To change a percent to a decimal fraction, move the decimal point two places to the left and omit the percent sign.

Example: $10\% = 0.10$

To change a percent to a fraction, drop the percent sign, write the number as the numerator, with 100 as the denominator, and reduce to the lowest terms.

Example: $10\% = \frac{10}{100} = \frac{1}{10}$

To change a percent to a ratio, drop the percent sign, use the number as the first term, 100 as the second term, and reduce to the lowest terms; or change to a fraction and then use a colon instead of the dividing line.

Example: $10\% = 10:100 = 1:10$ or

$10\% = \frac{1}{10} = 1:10$

To change a decimal fraction to a percent, move the decimal point two places to the right (multiply by 100) and add the percent sign.

Example: $0.20 = 20\%$

To change a decimal fraction to a common fraction, omit the decimal point and place the number over the appropriate denominator of 10, 100, or 1000, and reduce to the lowest terms.

Example: $0.20 = \frac{20}{100} = \frac{1}{5}$

To change a decimal fraction to a ratio, write the number as the first term; then put 10, 100, or 1000 as the second term; finally, reduce to the lowest terms.

Example: $0.20 = 20:100$ or $1:5$

To change a ratio to a fraction, write the numbers with a dividing line instead of a colon.

Example: $1:20 = \frac{1}{20}$

To change a ratio to a decimal fraction, divide the first term by the second term.

Example: $1:20 = 0.05$

To change a ratio to a percent, divide the first term by the second term, move the decimal point two places to the right in the answer, and add a percent sign.

Example: $1:20 = 0.05 = 5\%$

---

5 and x are the extremes; 500 and 2 are the means.

Proportions may be written as fractions. To find x, express the proportion as a relationship, and solve:

$$\frac{5}{500} = \frac{2}{x}$$
$$2 \times 500 = 1000$$
$$5x = 1000$$
$$x = \frac{1000}{5}$$
$$x = 200$$

In addition to being equal, proportions must also be written in the same system in both ratios (e.g.,

minims is to grains as minims is to grains; ml is to grams as ml is to grams).

For example:

15 (m) : 60 (gr) :: 13 (m) : x (gr)   Correctly written
15 (m) : 60 (m) :: 13 (m) : x (gr)   Incorrectly written

The calculation of ratios provides one of the major foundations in drug dosage calculations. Often the nurse knows the desired concentration of a drug and needs to calculate how much to give of a medication on hand. The nurse is able to figure how much medication to give by using the principles of proportion.

SUMMARY

The nurse must understand and be able to use basic math principles to administer drugs. These basic math principles include the use of multiplication, division, and Roman numerals, and the calculation of fractions, decimal fractions, percentages, ratios, and proportions.

CRITICAL THINKING QUESTIONS

1. Match the following mathematical expressions or components (marked in bold) on the left with their appropriate labels in the right-hand column:

a. 2/3	_____	ratio
b. 25/4	_____	denominator
c. 5 1/8	_____	improper fraction
d. $\frac{\mathbf{1}}{}$	_____	mixed number
e. **3**	_____	numerator
f. 3:4	_____	percent
g. 75%	_____	proper fraction
h. $\frac{1}{4} + \frac{2}{5} = \frac{13}{\mathbf{20}}$	_____	common denominator

2. Review multiplication and division by doing the following problems:
   $7 \times 11 =$ $9 \div 3 =$ $8 \times 7 =$
   $(252)(41) =$ $98 \times 7 =$ $360 \div 3 =$
3. Calculate the following division problems.
   $516 \div 7 =$ $637 \div 4 =$ $7849 \div 60 =$
4. Change the following Roman numerals into Arabic, and the Arabic numerals into Roman numerals.
   CDVIII =
   XXXIV =
   LXXVII =
   MCMXIII =
   93 =
   562 =
   1934 =
   2597 =
5. Find the common denominators and add or subtract. Reduce, if necessary.
   a. $\frac{1}{4} + \frac{2}{5} =$ b. $\frac{4}{25} + \frac{3}{25} =$
   c. $\frac{1}{4} + \frac{2}{3} =$ d. $\frac{3}{4} - \frac{4}{7} =$
6. Subtract the following:
   a. $\frac{5}{6} - \frac{7}{9} =$ b. $\frac{4}{25} - \frac{3}{20} =$
   c. $5\,\frac{3}{8} - 2\,\frac{3}{4} =$ d. $7\,\frac{1}{3} - 4\,\frac{2}{5} =$
7. Multiply the following fractions and reduce to lowest terms.
   a. $\frac{2}{7} \times \frac{3}{5} =$ b. $\frac{4}{11} \times \frac{3}{8} =$
   c. $\frac{5}{12} \times \frac{2}{3} \times \frac{1}{2} =$ d. $\frac{3}{4} \times \frac{4}{5} \times \frac{2}{3} =$
8. Divide the following fractions:
   a. $\frac{5}{9} \div \frac{2}{3} =$ b. $\frac{3}{4} \div \frac{3}{5} =$
   c. $5\frac{1}{2} \div 2\frac{3}{4} =$ d. $7\frac{1}{5} \div 4\frac{2}{5} =$
9. Change the following decimals to fractions:
   a. .591 = b. 1.34 = c. 2.547 =
10. Convert to common fractions or mixed numbers in lowest terms:
    a. 1.56 = b. 5.27 = c. 3.375 =
11. Find:
    a. $11.019 + 52.70 + 7.141 =$ b. $97.30 - 9.071 =$
    c. $1.59 \times 2.301 \times 1.977 =$ d. $121.4 \div 8.12 =$
12. Change to a percent:
    a. .65 = b. $5\frac{3}{7} =$ c. $\frac{4}{9} =$
13. Change to decimal fractions:
    a. 23% = b. 116% = c. $\frac{2}{7}\% =$
14. Express as decimals:
    a. $7\frac{3}{8} =$ b. 321% = c. 52% =
15. Express as percents:
    a. 2.47 = b. 1.55 = c. $2\frac{2}{3} =$
16. Express as ratios:
    a. $\frac{1}{6}$ to $\frac{1}{5}$ b. 2 feet to 6 inches c. 100 mph
17. Calculate the following:
    a. $\frac{3.5}{6.7} = \frac{x}{8.9}$ b. $\frac{2}{3} \times \frac{x}{.49}$ c. 0.3:1 : : 0.5:x

Answers

1. f, e, b, c, d, g, a, h
2. 77; 3; 56; 10,332; 686; 120
3. 73 R5; 159 R1; 130 R49
4. 408; 34; 77; 1913; XCIII; DLXII; MCMXXXIV; MMDXCVII
5. a. $\frac{13}{20}$ b. $\frac{31}{100}$ c. $\frac{11}{12}$ d. $\frac{5}{28}$
6. a. $\frac{1}{18}$ b. $\frac{1}{100}$ c. $2\frac{5}{8}$ d. $2\frac{14}{15}$
7. a. $\frac{6}{35}$ b. $\frac{3}{22}$ c. $\frac{5}{36}$ d. $\frac{2}{5}$
8. a. $\frac{5}{6}$ b. $1\frac{1}{4}$ c. 2 d. $1\frac{7}{11}$

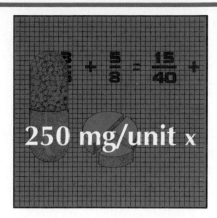

CHAPTER 6

Mathematical Equivalents Used in Pharmacology

OBJECTIVES

At the conclusion of this chapter you should be able to:

1. Use the apothecaries' system to convert from one measure to another.
2. Use the metric system to convert from one measure to another.
3. State the values of common household measures and their equivalents.
4. Compare the units used in the apothecaries', metric, and household measures systems.
5. Use common abbreviations and symbols to interpret and solve medication problems.

KEY TERMS

apothecaries' system, p. 103
Celsius, p. 107
Fahrenheit, p. 107
gram, p. 104
liter, p. 104
meter, p. 104
metric system, p. 103

Overview

Three established systems of weights and measures are used to compute and prepare medications. Perhaps the most commonly known system is that of general household measures. This system is adequate when more accurate measures are either not available or not needed, and is used primarily in the home. The English have used the **apothecaries' system** for many centuries. It relies on different units for solid and liquid measures. The **metric system** was developed in France and is based on the decimal system, with measures expressed in increments of tens, hundreds, and thousands. The metric and apothecaries' systems are commonly used by physicians and pharmacists as medication is ordered and prepared. The metric system is used the most frequently.

The nurse must be able to use all three systems of measures to calculate medication dosages accurately. Some nurses may be apprehensive about learning these new systems because they seem foreign or different to them. However, once the basic words and values are memorized, the nurse should be able to solve problems confidently.

Apothecaries' System

The apothecaries' system uses the basic units of grain (for solids) and minim (for liquids). Whole numbers and fractions are used in this system. The whole numbers are written as lower case Roman numerals, such as iv and x; decimals are not used. A few Arabic symbols are used to express dram (℥) and ounce (℥) and fractions. When ½ is desired, a special abbreviation from Latin, ss, may be used. In the apothecaries' system, the unit abbreviation comes before the quantity (i.e., gr ½ [grains one-half] or m xxx [minims thirty]). If no abbreviation is used, the quantity comes before the unit (i.e., ½ grain or 30 minims).

The apothecaries' system makes a clear distinction between solid and liquid measures. One minim (a liquid measure) equals 1 grain (a solid measure). Although there are many units of measure in the system, only a few are commonly used. These common measures are listed in the box below.

The Apothecaries' System

Liquid measures

60 minims (m) = 1 fluid dram (℥)
8 fluid drams = 1 fluid ounce (fl oz or ℥)
16 fl ounces = 1 pint (pt or 0)
2 pints = 1 quart (qt)
4 quarts = 1 gallon (gal)
480 minims = 1 ounce (oz)

Solid measures

60 grains = 1 dram (℥)
8 drams = 1 ounce (oz or ℥)
480 grains = 1 ounce (oz)
12 ounces = 1 pound (lb)*

*Generally not used. 16 oz = 1 lb is commonly used from the avoirdupois table.

Metric System

The metric system relies on a decimal system; it is built on multiples of 10. The metric system uses **meter**

The Metric System

Measures of length (meter)

1 meter (m) = 100 centimeters (cm) = 1000 millimeters (mm)
1 centimeter (cm) = 0.01 meter (m)
1 millimeter (mm) = 0.001 meter (m)

Measures of volume (liter)

1 decaliter (ml) = 10 liters (L)
1 liter (L) = 10 deciliters (dl) = 1000 milliliters (ml) or 1000 cubic centimeters (cc)

Measures of weight (gram)

1 kilogram (kg) = 1000 grams (gm)
1 gram (gm) = 1000 milligrams (mg)
1 milligram (mg) = 1000 micrograms (μg)

for the unit of length, **liter** for the unit of volume, and **gram** for the unit of weight.

The most common measures used in the metric system are listed in the box above.

KEY POINT:

Common metric equivalents

Milliliters, cubic centimeters, and grams are approximately equivalent; 1 ml or 1 cc weighs approximately 1 gm.

1 ml = 1 cc = 1 gm, whereas 1 kg = 2.2 lb.

Relying on what you know about the decimal system, you can change measures within the same system:

To change milligrams to micrograms, move the decimal point three places to the right.

000×000.07   000000.07

To change micrograms to milligrams, move decimal point three places to the left.

000.000×07   000.00007

To change grams to milligrams, move the decimal point three places to the right (multiply by 1000).

1×000.067   1000.067

To change milligrams to grams, move the decimal point three places to the left (divide by 1000).

1.345×0789   1.3450789

KEY POINT:

Metric system prefixes

Prefixes of the metric system indicate the multiples or fractions of the unit:

  milli = one-thousandth
  centi = one-hundredth
  deci = one-tenth
  deca = ten
  hecto = hundred
  kilo = thousand

Metric and Apothecaries' Equivalents

Most problems are easier to solve when metric system numbers are involved. Most nurses find it helpful to change all the units in the apothecary system to the metric system in drug calculations.

Units in the apothecaries' and metric systems are not quite equivalent or equal, but they are close enough that they are commonly used. In calculating the changes from one system to another, fractions sometimes make a difference. There are actually 64 mg in 1 grain and 16 grains in 1 gm, but 60 and 15 are much easier to work with and they are often employed in making calculations.

Rounding a number up or dropping to a lower number is often significant. When you are working with small portions, such as minims, it is important to be precise. Do not give vague equivalents or round off calculations for dosages in milliliters, dosages for

infants or children, dosages of cardiovascular or cancer drugs, or tablets, capsules, or medications for diagnostic tests. Additionally, dosages for heparin or other anticoagulants and insulin must be calculated precisely.

Rather than memorizing all the different units in the apothecaries' and metric systems, the nurse should do the following:

1. Master the most familiar units system.
2. Learn equivalents in the two systems.
3. Know where information may rapidly be found to help in calculating less common unit dosages.

Most hospital units, clinics, and offices have some basic pharmacologic text with information on conversion from one system to another. This information should always be consulted when the nurse is unclear about a mathematical calculation.

There are a number of common equivalent values for the two systems of measurement that the nurse should memorize. Basic rules for conversion are based on the assumption that the nurse has mastered these basic relationships. Study the following chart and memorize the information presented. This information is reprinted on the inside front cover of this book for easy reference.

There are a few basic rules that may be followed to convert measurements from one system to another. These rules are presented in the first box on p. 106. Remember that 1 minim weighs 1 grain. If you are using measures from two different systems, always convert the numbers to one system, and then to grains, using whichever system is easiest to convert.

Sometimes as you work with new number systems it is difficult to keep things in proper perspective. The answer you arrive at through calculation may appear

Approximate Equivalents in the Apothecaries' and Metric Systems*

Apothecaries' system		Metric system
1 gallon (gal)	=	4000 ml or 4000 cc or 4 liters
1 qt or 32 oz	=	1000 ml or 1000 cc or 1 liter
1 pt or 16 oz 2 cups	=	500 ml or 500 cc or 500 gm
1 oz, 8 drams	=	30 to 32 ml or 30 to 32 cc or 30 to 32 gm
1 dram, 60 to 64 grains, or 60 to 64 minims	=	4 to 5 ml or 4 to 5 cc or 4 to 5 gm
15 to 16 grains, 15 to 16 minims	=	1 ml or 1 cc or 1 gm
2.2 lb	=	1000 gm or 1 kg
1 grain	=	60 or 64 mg or 0.06 gm
1/60 grain	=	1 mg

*15 rather than 16 grains is often used in calculations; 60 is often used in place of 64. These account for the variances seen in the table.

Rules for Converting from One System to Another

To convert grains to grams, divide by 15 or 16.
To convert grains to milligrams, multiply by 60 or 64.
To convert grams to grains, multiply by 15 or 16.
To convert grams to milligrams, move the decimal point three places to the right.
To convert milligrams to grains, divide by 60 or 64.
To convert milligrams to grams, move the decimal point three places to left.
To convert milliliters to minims, multiply by 15 or 16.
To convert minims to milliliters, divide by 15 or 16.

Common Household Measures

60 drops (gtt)	=	1 teaspoonful (t or tsp)
3 to 4 teaspoonsful	=	1 tablespoonful (T or Tbs)
2 tablespoonsful	=	1 ounce (oz)
6 to 8 teaspoonsful	=	1 ounce (oz)
6 ounces	=	1 teacupful
8 ounces	=	1 glass

Common Equivalents for Metric Measures

1 meter = 39.37 inches = 3.28 feet = 1.09 yards
1 centimeter = 0.39 inch
1 millimeter = 0.04 inch
1 kilometer = 0.62 mile
1 liter = 1.06 liquid quarts
1 gram = 0.04 ounce
1 kilogram = 2.2 pounds
1 inch = 25.4 millimeters
1 foot = 0.3 meter
1 yard = 0.91 meter
1 mile = 1.61 kilometers
1 ounce = 28.35 grams
1 pound = 0.45 kilogram

abnormally small or tremendously large. As you gain experience, common sense will help you determine whether or not your answer is correct. As you begin to change numbers from one system to another, you will soon learn shortcuts to help you in the mathematical calculations. For example, converting between grams and grains often produces large fractions that are difficult to reduce. It is often easier to change the grams to milligrams and then carry out the calculation.

Household Measures

The final system of measures that nurses need to be able to use involves common household measures. These measures are often used when dosages do not need to be exact.

The basic units of measure in the household system involve drops, teaspoons, tablespoons, and ounces. Their values are presented in the box at top, right. Although teaspoons and tablespoons found in the home come in varying sizes, these measures refer to the official measuring spoons one would use in baking or cooking. These measurements are not precise enough to substitute in hospital calculations.

Household measures may be converted to either the apothecaries' system or to the metric system. The drop is the unit in the household system equivalent to the minim and the grain. Remember, household measures are *very rough equivalents*. Thus it is possible to accept calculations using household measures when the amounts are very small. As the size of the dosage or volume increases, there is less and less accuracy in the dosage calculated. For example, 60

KEY POINT:
Converting household measures

The key relationship to understand in converting household measures to other systems is that 1 minim equals 1 drop and weighs 1 grain.

gtts equals one teaspoonful. But it would be foolish to calculate 240 gtts to get one tablespoonful. It is better to refer to a standard table of equivalents rather than calculating the dosage.

In comparing various measurement systems, several obvious differences appear. These differences are seen in Table 6-1.

Examples of common conversions between household measures, apothecaries' system measures, and metric system measures are shown in Table 6-2.

At times it may be difficult to keep these measures in perspective. Other common equivalents with more familiar measures may help you understand the relative size and weight of some of these measures. These are included in the box above.

Table 6-1   Comparison of metric, apothecaries', and household systems

Apothecaries'	Metric	Household
UNITS OF MEASURE		
grain, minim, dram, ounce	milligram, gram, milliliter, cubic centimeter, liter	drops, teaspoons, tablespoons, ounces, glasses
STRUCTURE		
Ancient English system including familiar household measures; some measures not commonly used in this system	Built on decimal system (French) so logic of change from one unit to another is clear	Commonly used for small amounts when dosages need not be exact
FORMAT		
Roman numerals and common fractions are used; abbreviations or symbols are given before the amount number	Arabic numbers and decimal fractions are used; the amount is given before the abbreviation	Arabic numbers are used; the amount number is given before the abbreviation

Converting Temperature Readings

For years nurses have used the Fahrenheit (F) scale to take temperatures. In the last 20 years institutions have placed increasing emphasis on the centigrade, or Celsius, scale (C) for hospital use. Although electronic thermometers with digital readouts are used in some hospitals, nurses may use either Fahrenheit or Celsius thermometers on occasion.

Thermometers used in many hospitals come in either Fahrenheit or Celsius scale. Oral thermometers come with either a long flat tip or oblong or stubby tips. The oblong or stubby tips may also be used for rectal or axillary temperatures.

On the Fahrenheit scale, 212° is the boiling point and 32° is the freezing point. Outdoor temperature thermometers generally include these points. The Fahrenheit thermometer is used for medical measurement ranges from 95° to 105°, with individual divisions representing 0.2°. Because body temperature generally does not vary more than a few degrees, this smaller range is sufficient to measure the normal body range of 97.6° to 99.4° F and any common variations from normal.

The Celsius scale has a boiling point of 100° and a freezing point of 0°. The Celsius thermometer also has a restricted range for medical use, with each division on the scale representing 0.1°. The normal body range as measured on the Celsius scale varies from 36.5° to 37.5° C.

Table 6-2   Conversions between household, apothecaries', and metric systems

Household measure		Apothecaries' system		Metric system
1 teaspoonful	=	1 dram or 60 minims	=	4 or 5 ml
1 tablespoonful	=	3 or 4 drams	=	15 or 16 ml
2 tablespoonsful	=	8 drams or 1 ounce	=	30 or 32 ml
1 teacupful	=	6 ounces	=	180 ml
1 glassful	=	8 ounces	=	240 ml

Since both Fahrenheit and Celsius scales are commonly used in hospitals, the nurse must understand how to accurately read each thermometer, correctly note changes from normal, and convert from one system to another. If a nurse needs to give an antipyretic medication to help reduce an elevated temperature, the nurse must clearly understand the variations from normal in either system.

The formulas for converting from one scale to another are very simple. Because the normal range of temperatures varies so little in individuals, even a little experience converting temperatures will aid the nurse in rapidly understanding this process.

Thus, the formula for converting Fahrenheit to Celsius is:

$$(°F - 32) \times \frac{5}{9} = °C$$

KEY POINT:

Converting temperatures

The key relationships to understand in converting temperatures are:
   One degree on the Fahrenheit scale equals ⅝ of one degree on the Celsius scale.
   One degree on the Celsius scale equals ⅝ of one degree on the Fahrenheit scale.

For example:

$$102° \text{ F is } ?° \text{ C?}$$

$$(102 - 32) \times \frac{5}{9} = 70 \times \frac{5}{9} = 38.9° \text{ C}$$

The formula for converting Celsius to Fahrenheit is:

$$(°C \times \frac{9}{5}) + 32 = °F$$

For example:

$$40° \text{ C is } ?° \text{ F}$$

$$(40 \times \frac{9}{5}) + 32 = 72 + 32 = 104° \text{ F}$$

SUMMARY

This section has summarized all the basic rules regarding the measurement systems used to calculate drug dosages and interpret thermometer readings. This is an especially important section to master, because many of the physician's orders will use a variety of the basic scales for weights and measures in the apothecaries', metric, and household systems. Common equivalents in the three systems and procedures for converting from one system to another are valuable to memorize. The nurse must be able to use these different measurement systems accurately and appropriately. It is important for the nurse to be able to complete these calculations with confidence.

 CRITICAL THINKING QUESTIONS

1. 50 cc = __10__ dram = _____ oz
2. 160 cc = _5.33_ oz = _43_ dram = _500_ pt
3. 7 cc = _1.4_ dram = _____ tsp
4. 3 oz = _____ teacupful = _____ dm
5. Change 7 kilograms to pounds. _15.4_
6. Change 9 kg to lb.
7. Change 8 L to liquid quarts.
8. Change 80 gm to oz.
9. Change 9 liquid quarts to L.
10. Change 3 lb to kg.
11. If 150 ml solution contains 75 gm of alcohol, how many grams of alcohol are there in 25 ml of solution?
12. It takes 7 gm of a substance to make 35 ml of solution. How many ml of solution can be made with 42 gm of the substance?
13. Your patient weighs 137 lb. What is her weight in kilograms?
14. A certain medication comes in a 16-fl-oz bottle with four bottles to a package. The same medication is also sold in a package containing two 1-liter bottles. Which contains more medicine, the four-pack or the two 1-liter bottles?

#2 — 160 ÷ 30 = 5.33
8 drams = 1 oz
5.33 × 8 = 42.64 → 43 drams
16 drams = 1 pt
16 × 5 = 80 pt
16 ÷

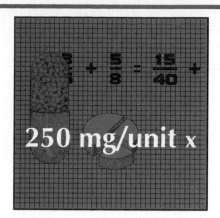

Calculating Drug Dosages

Overview

How medications are ordered will differ among physicians, drugs, and institutions. Some institutions require physicians to order generic products or only those drugs stocked by the pharmacy. Some drugs are traditionally ordered in units of one measurement system (for example, atropine usually comes in metric units [such as 0.6 mg], whereas other drugs come in apothecary units [such as morphine sulfate, which comes as ¼ grain.]) Physicians' patterns in ordering drugs develop from their experiences in medical school and in the clinical institutions where they have worked. Some physicians are highly influenced by pharmaceutical salespeople. Thus there are many reasons why medication orders appear in a variety of forms, and the nurse must be prepared to understand them all.

Calculation Methods

Calculating dosages involves the following three steps:

1. Determine whether the drug dosage desired (what is written in the physician's order) comes in the same measurement system as the drug dosage available. If they are not in the same measurement system, convert between the two systems.
2. Simplify by reducing to the lowest terms whenever possible.
3. Calculate the dosage quantity to be administered. This may be done by using fractions, ratios, or proportions.

FRACTION METHOD

When using fractions to compute drug dosages, write an equation consisting of two fractions. First set up a fraction showing the number of units to be given over x, the unknown number of tablets or milliliters. For example, if the physician's order states "ibuprofen 600 mg," you would put $\frac{600 \text{ mg}}{x}$. On the other side of the equation, write a fraction showing the drug dosage as listed on the medication bottle over the number of tablets or milliliters. The ibuprofen bottle label states "200 mg per tablet," so the second fraction would be $\frac{200 \text{ mg}}{1}$. The fractions then read:

$$\frac{600 \text{ mg}}{x \text{ tab}} = \frac{200 \text{ mg}}{1 \text{ tab}}$$

You will note that the same units of measure are in both numerators and the same measures are in both denominators. Now, solve for x:

$$\frac{600 \text{ mg}}{x \text{ tab}} = \frac{200 \text{ mg}}{1 \text{ tab}}$$

$$\frac{600}{x} = \frac{200}{1}$$

$$200x = 600$$

$$x = 3 \text{ tablets}$$

RATIO METHOD

In using the ratio method, first write the amount of the drug to be given and the quantity of the dosage (x) as a ratio. Using the example above this would be 600 mg : x tab. Next, complete the equation by forming a second ratio consisting of the number of units of the drug in the dosage form and the quantity of that dosage form, as taken from the bottle. Again,

using the example above, the second ratio would be 200 mg : 1 tablet. Solving for x determines the dosage.

$$200 \text{ mg} : 1 \text{ tab} :: 600 \text{ mg} : x \text{ tab}$$

Multiply the means (inside); divide by the extremes (outside).

$$600 \times 1 = 600$$

$$200x \overline{)600} \atop 600 ^{3}$$

This, again, gives us 3 tablets.

DESIRED OVER AVAILABLE METHOD

A third method for drug dosage calculation combines the conversion of ordered units into available units and the computation of drug dosage into one step. The equation for doing this is:

$$\frac{\text{DESIRED}}{\text{Units}} \times \frac{\text{Conversion}}{\text{Factor}} \times \frac{\frac{\text{Quantity}}{\text{(Caps, tabs, etc)}}}{\frac{\text{Quantity}}{\text{AVAILABLE}}} = x \text{ (Quantity to give)}$$

If a physician orders 10 grains of a drug and the drug is available only in 300 mg tablets, the dose may be easily calculated with this formula.

Substitute 10 gr (DESIRED) for the first element of the equation. Then use the conversion fraction $\frac{60 \text{ mg}}{1 \text{ gr}}$ as the second portion of the formula. The third element of the equation shows the quantity of dosage form (capsule or tablet) for the dosage AVAILABLE. One tablet contains 300 mg. The completed equation then is:

$$10 \text{ gr} \times \frac{60 \text{ mg}}{1 \text{ gr}} \times \frac{1 \text{ tab}}{300 \text{ mg}} = x =$$

$$10 \times \frac{60}{1} \times \frac{1}{300} = \frac{600}{300} = 2 \text{ tablets}$$

Solving for x, you find that the patient should receive two 300 mg tablets.

As you can see, all three methods of drug calculation (fractions, ratios, or proportions) use the same information and much of the same format in solving the problems. With minor variations, they do the same thing. Some methods will seem to make more sense to you or be easier for you to follow. As we move throughout the calculation sections, use the method for drug calculation that makes the most sense to you. Return here for review if you have difficulty.

Calculating Dosages

ORAL MEDICATIONS

Although there are many forms of oral products, oral medications usually come in capsules, tablets, or liquids. Medications dispensed via the unit-dose system are packaged by the pharmacist according to the dosage ordered. The nurse usually does not have to calculate the medication dosage, but does check the accuracy of the preparation.

When medication is ordered individually or through an open-stock system, the nurse usually calculates the proper drug dosage. These drug calculations are required when:

1. The drug available is in a smaller dose than that ordered.
2. The drug available is in a larger dose than that ordered.
3. The drug available is in a different unit of measure than that ordered.

CAPSULES AND TABLETS

Capsules cannot be broken or divided. This makes calculating the drug dosage more difficult. More than one capsule may be given to provide an accurate dosage; a part of one capsule cannot. Manufacturers of drugs provide capsules in different dosages to help in arriving at the proper dosage. If your calculations specify that you should give a fraction of a capsule, give an additional capsule if the fraction is ½ or more; do not give an additional capsule if the fraction is less than ½. (For example, if you find the calculations work out to 2¾, give three capsules; if it is 2¼, give two.)

Some tablets may be easily divided if they are "scored" (Fig. 7-1, *A*). Examples of unscored tablets include coated tablets (Fig. 7-1, *B*) and layered tablets (Fig. 7-1, *C*). If a tablet is not scored, it should *not* be broken or cut apart. Sometimes tablets may be cut to fill a smaller drug dosage order, or combined to fill a larger drug dosage order.

The medication order usually states the dosage of grams, grains, or milligrams to give. Therefore, the nurse understands the dosage DESIRED. The order also specifies how often the medication is to be given, such as twice a day (bid) or four times a day (qid). It may or may not specify for how many days the medication is to be given. If the order does not

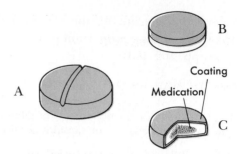

Fig. 7-1 **A,** scored, and **B** and **C,** unscored tablets. The tablet in **B** is layered, and the tablet in **C** is coated.

indicate a specific length of time (i.e., give for 5 days), the drug is given on a continuous basis, unless the institution has a specific policy limiting the length of time a drug may be given without reordering. (Antibiotics and narcotics usually have an automatic stop date after a certain period of time.) Therefore, the nurse may also need to calculate how much medication to order, depending on the length of time the patient will receive the medication. The nurse needs to know how much medication is NEEDED.

For example, the order reads: diazepam (Valium) 10 mg PO stat and 2 mg bid × 10 days. The medication DESIRED is diazepam 10 mg and diazepam 2 mg. The nurse must know the dosage AVAILABLE of the medication. A check with the pharmacy reveals that diazepam comes in 2 mg, 5 mg, and 10 mg tablets.

The nurse NEEDS one 10 mg diazepam tablet and enough 2 mg tablets for 10 days, or enough 2 mg tablets to fill the whole order (bid means twice a day). Thus, the nurse needs to order:

One 10 mg tablet plus
One 2 mg tablet × 2 times a day × 10 days =

$1 \times 2 \times 10 = 20$ 2 mg tablets plus 1 10 mg tablet

or because five 2 mg tablets are the same as one 10 mg tablet, the nurse may order:

Five 2 mg tablets plus one 2 mg tablet ×
2 times a day × 10 days =

$5 + (1 \times 2 \times 10) = 25$ tablets

 KEY POINT:
Parentheses in math problem

When parentheses are used in a math problem, it means to do all the calculations inside the parentheses first, then complete the rest of the problem.

The formula to calculate the number of capsules or tablets to order is a basic proportion problem (review proportions, pp. 102-103):

$$\underset{\text{DESIRED}}{\text{Dose}} : \underset{\text{AVAILABLE}}{\text{Dose}} :: \underset{\substack{\text{capsules}\\\text{per dose}}}{\text{Tablets or}} :$$

$$\underset{\text{(tablets or capsules)}}{\text{Drug form}} = \underset{\text{or capsules per dose}}{\text{Numbers of tablets}}$$

For example, the order reads "sulfadiazine 1.0 gm q6h × 3 days." Sulfadiazine comes in 300 or 500 mg tablets.

DESIRED: 1.0 gm

AVAILABLE: 500 mg = 0.5 gm (converted from mg to gm)

$$\frac{1.0 \text{ gm}}{0.5 \text{ gm}} = 2 \text{ tablets}$$

Therefore, give two 500 mg tablets every 6 hours for 3 days. Two tablets given four times a day for 3 days equals 24 tablets total. In simple terms this means:

$$\frac{\text{(Dose DESIRED)}}{\text{(Dose AVAILABLE)}} \times \underset{\text{or capsule}}{\text{Tablet}} = \underset{\text{or capsules per dose}}{\text{Number of tablets}}$$

To illustrate, let's try a few examples. Order: ASA gr x stat and prn for temperature elevation. ASA is labeled as 0.3 gm/tab.

KEY POINT:
Dosage formula hint

To help you remember the usual formula, remember DESIRED over AVAILABLE, D/A, or "D.A." A District Attorney (D.A.) often helps solve the mystery. You are helping to solve the mystery of the dosage needed.

KEY POINT:
Steps to completing dosage formula

1. First change dosages to the same unit of measurement
2. Reduce to the simplest terms
3. Calculate the dosage, using fractions, ratios, or proportions
4. Use common sense to check your answer

$$\frac{\text{(Dose DESIRED)}}{\text{(Dose AVAILABLE)}} \frac{\text{gr } x}{0.3 \text{ gm}}$$

$$\left(\text{gr } 16 = 1 \text{ gm, so } \frac{\text{gr } x}{16} = 0.6 \text{ gm}\right)$$

$$\frac{\text{D}}{\text{A}} = \frac{0.6 \text{ gm}}{0.3 \text{ gm}} \times 1 = 2 \text{ tablets}$$

Order: methocarbamol 1.5 gm qd. The medication comes in 750 mg tablets.

$$\frac{\text{(Dose DESIRED)}}{\text{(Dose AVAILABLE)}} \frac{1.5 \text{ gm}}{750 \text{ mg}} \times 1 = ?$$

$$(1.5 \text{ gm} = 1500 \text{ mg})$$

$$\frac{\text{D}}{\text{A}} = \frac{1500 \text{ mg}}{750 \text{ mg}} \times 1 = 2 \text{ tablets}$$

LIQUIDS

The process and formulas used to calculate dosages of liquids are the same as those used to compute dosages of capsules or tablets. Only the unit of measure is different.

To review:

$$\frac{\text{(Dose DESIRED)}}{\text{(Dose AVAILABLE)}} \times \underset{\text{(minims, ml, drams)}}{\text{Drug form}} =$$
$$\underset{\text{per dose}}{\text{Amount of liquid}}$$

Order: phenobarbital elixir 0.2 gm hs. The drug is available in 20 mg/5 ml.

$$\frac{\text{(Dose DESIRED)}}{\text{(Dose AVAILABLE)}} \frac{0.2 \text{ gm}}{20 \text{ mg/5 ml}} = \frac{200 \text{ mg}}{20 \text{ mg/5 ml}}$$

$$20 \text{ mg} : 5 \text{ ml} :: 200 \text{ mg} : x \text{ ml} = 50 \text{ ml/dose}$$

PARENTERAL MEDICATIONS

When medication is to be injected, it comes in three different forms:

1. A prefilled syringe labeled with a certain dosage in a certain volume (e.g., meperidine [Demerol] 100 mg in 1 ml).
2. A single- or multiple-dose ampule labeled with a certain dosage in a certain volume (e.g., epinephrine [Adrenalin] 1:1000 in 0.1 ml).
3. A vial with a powder or crystals that must be mixed or reconstituted with sterile water or normal saline solution. The drug may be measured in grains, grams, milligrams, or units. The amount of solution to be added varies and must be calculated according to the instructions with the vial. Medications given intradermally or subcutaneously generally involve very small

amounts of solution, whereas IV preparations may involve 50 ml or more of solution.

Again, proportion is the standard method for calculating this dosage:

Drug AVAILABLE : Dilution :: Drug DESIRED : *x*

KEY POINT:

Dosage solution formula

$$\frac{\text{Dose DESIRED}}{\text{Dose AVAILABLE}} \times \frac{\text{Dilution or}}{\text{amount of solution}} =$$

Amount of solution per dose

To illustrate, let's try a few examples:

Order: digoxin 0.2 mg IM. Drug is available as 0.5 mg/ml.

$$\frac{\text{(Dose DESIRED)}}{\text{(Dose AVAILABLE)}} \frac{0.2 \text{ mg}}{0.5 \text{ mg}} \times 1 \text{ ml} =$$

$$\frac{2}{5} \times 1 \text{ ml} = 0.4 \text{ ml or 6 minims}$$

Order: KCl 24 mEq stat PO. Solution labeled potassium chloride contains 20 mEq/10 ml.

$$\frac{\text{(Dose DESIRED)}}{\text{(Dose AVAILABLE)}} \frac{24 \text{ mEq}}{20 \text{ mEq}} \times 10 \text{ ml} = \frac{6}{5} = 12 \text{ ml}$$

Order: Cedilanid-D 0.6 mg IM qd. Drug is available in 0.8 mg/4 ml ampules.

$$\frac{\text{(Dose DESIRED)}}{\text{(Dose AVAILABLE)}} \frac{0.6 \text{ mg}}{0.8 \text{ mg}} \times 4 \text{ ml} =$$

$$\frac{3}{4} \times 4 \text{ ml} = 3 \text{ ml (0.6 mg)}$$

Again! Do not forget your common sense! If the answer tells you to inject 20 ml, you know you have made a mistake!

Many chemicals are very fragile. Heat, light, and time cause the medication to change or deteriorate. To avoid these problems, some medications come as powders or crystals, making them more stable. When the medication is ordered, liquid must be added to the drug to dissolve the medication in the solution (reconstitute the drug). The medication must then be given within a few hours or it will decay.

Some chemicals come in a single-dose vial. When the medication is ordered, usually 1 to 2 ml of liquid is added, the solution is gently shaken to dissolve it, and the whole amount is drawn into a syringe and injected. This is very common for some antibiotics.

At other times, an ampule will contain several doses of the powdered medication. The instructions for adding the liquid (diluent) must be followed carefully. Some multiple-dose vials for steroids contain the diluent in the top part of the bottle, separated from the powder in the bottom part of the container. Pushing on the top part forces the liquid down into the bottom part, dissolving the medication. The instructions will usually be found on the package, on the ampule label, or on the package insert in the box, and they must be followed exactly. If instructions are not included, it is common to dissolve the drug in enough diluent so that the dose ordered may be given in no more than 0.5 to 1 ml.

Once powders have been dissolved in liquid or reconstituted, the bottle must be carefully labeled so that further doses may be accurately given from it. It is especially important to note the date and time the powder was dissolved, as well as the concentration of the reconstituted medication.

If instructions are not given for diluting the medication, a modification of the familiar proportion formula may be used:

Dose desired : 1 ml :: Total drug available : *x*

Look at the relationships in the above formula.

The dose desired to the known amount of liquid is compared to the total amount of the drug to an unknown amount of liquid.

Multiply the means, divide by the extremes. (NOTE: In this formula, the dose AVAILABLE is on the top of the formula, the dose DESIRED is on the bottom. Think clearly as you establish your problems. Keep the logic of the proportions clear. DESIRED doesn't always go over AVAILABLE!)

KEY POINT:

Dosage formula

$$\frac{\text{Total drug AVAILABLE}}{\text{Dose DESIRED}} \times 1 \text{ ml} =$$

Amount diluent required to add to vial
powder so that dose ordered equals 1 ml

For example, order: cephalothin (Keflin) 500 mg q6h IM. It comes in a multiple-dose vial containing 3 gm of powder. Prepare it so that 500 mg equals 1 ml. Convert 3 gm to 3000 mg.

500 mg : 1 ml :: 3000 mg : x =
           6 ml diluent to add to obtain 1 ml = 500 mg/ml

or

$$\frac{\text{(Dose AVAILABLE)}}{\text{(Dose DESIRED)}} \frac{3000 \text{ mg}}{500 \text{ mg}} \times 1 \text{ ml} = 6 \text{ ml to add}$$

Order: give 500,000 U penicillin IM. Dilute 1,000,000 U penicillin so that 500,000 U equals 1 ml.

1,000,000 U : x :: 500,000 U : 1 ml = 2 ml diluent

or

$$\frac{\text{(Dose AVAILABLE)}}{\text{(Dose DESIRED)}} \frac{1,000,000 \text{ U}}{500,000 \text{ U}} \times 1 \text{ ml} =$$
                                        2 ml diluent added

Order: Give cephalosporin 200 mg in 1 ml IM. The drug comes in 1 gm units of powder. What is the amount of diluent to add?

$$\frac{\text{(Dose AVAILABLE)}}{\text{(Dose DESIRED)}} \frac{1 \text{ gm}}{200 \text{ mg}} = \frac{1000 \text{ mg}}{200 \text{ mg}} \times 1 \text{ ml} =$$
                                        5 ml diluent

HYPODERMIC TABLETS

Some narcotics come as sterile tablets. A tablet is put into a syringe, 1 to 2 ml of diluent is drawn into the syringe, and the medication is dissolved by gently turning the syringe. Rather than breaking the tablet, the proper amount is calculated and any extra solution is discarded before the medication is injected. The usual dilution is 1 ml. The standard formula is used:

Amount available : 1 ml :: Amount desired : x ml

For example, the order reads: give morphine gr ⅙. The available tablets are gr ¼.

$$\frac{\text{(Dose DESIRED)}}{\text{(Dose AVAILABLE)}} \frac{\text{gr } 1/6}{\text{gr } 1/4} \times 1 \text{ ml} = \frac{1}{6} \times \frac{4}{1} \times 1 \text{ ml}$$
$$= \frac{2}{3} \text{ ml or 11 minims}$$

INSULIN

Insulin is a parenteral medication that replaces insulin not being produced by the patient. Great accuracy is important in preparing and administering insulin, because the quantity given is very small and even

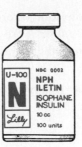

Fig. 7-2   U-100 vial.

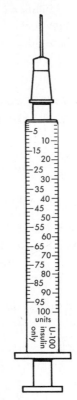

Fig. 7-3   U-100 syringe.

minor variations in dosage may produce adverse symptoms in the patient.

Calculating and preparing insulin dosage is unique in the following three ways:

1. There are many kinds of insulin, but they all come in a standardized measure called a *unit*. Insulin is available in 10 ml vials and in two strengths (concentrations): U-100 (100 units per 1 ml solution) (Fig. 7-2) and U-500 (500 units per 1 ml solution). U-500 is five times stronger (more concentrated) than U-100. This preparation is rarely used.

2. Insulin should be drawn up in a special insulin syringe that is calibrated in units (Fig. 7-3). If an

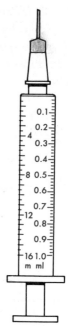

Fig. 7-4   Tuberculin syringe.

insulin syringe is not available, a tuberculin syringe that is calibrated in minims may be used (Fig. 7-4).

3. The insulin order, the insulin bottle, and the insulin as drawn up should always be rechecked by another nurse for maximum accuracy. Small errors can cause big problems.

Let's try some examples:

Order: 48 U Lente insulin U-100 (insulin zinc suspension) 1 hour before breakfast.

$$\frac{\text{(Dose DESIRED)}}{\text{(Dose AVAILABLE)}} \quad \frac{48 \text{ U}}{100 \text{ U}} \times 1 = 48 \text{ U}$$

It is easy to see then, that if the insulin and the syringe are both U-100, all you have to do is draw up the number of units ordered.

When the order calls for two different types of insulin, both may be given at the same time in the same syringe. One will be short-acting (regular) insulin and the other will be an intermediate or longer-acting type (NPH or zinc suspension). Draw up the regular insulin first, then the longer acting. Give both in the same syringe.

For example, order: 20 U regular (Iletin) insulin U-100 and 30 U NPH (isophane insulin suspension) U-100 before breakfast. Using a U-100 syringe, draw

up 20 U regular insulin; then draw up 30 U NPH insulin to equal 50 U in the syringe.

Sometimes U-100 syringes are not available and a tuberculin (TB) syringe must be used. The number of minims that will equal the units ordered must be calculated. The formula for determining insulin dosage when a TB syringe is used is as follows:

$$\frac{\text{(Insulin DESIRED)}}{\text{(Insulin AVAILABLE)}} \times 16 \text{ minims} =$$

Number of minims to administer

Order: 80 U of regular (Iletin) U-100 insulin, to be given in a TB syringe:

$$\frac{\text{(Dose DESIRED)}}{\text{(Dose AVAILABLE)}} \quad \frac{80 \text{ U}}{100 \text{ U}} \times 16 = \frac{64}{5} =$$

12.8 minims

> **NOTE:** You *must* use 16 minims—not 15 minims/ml—for these very accurate calculations.

INTRAVENOUS INFUSIONS

Flow rates

Regulating the intravenous infusion rate is a common nursing task. The completeness of physicians' orders for intravenous infusions varies widely. Some physicians are more specific in their instructions than others. A complete order specifies not only the type of solution and the volume to be infused (usually 500 or 1000 ml), but the length of time that the medication should be given. More commonly, the nurse is left to calculate the flow rate, or how fast the infusion will be completed.

There are three mathematical procedures that the nurse must be familiar with regarding intravenous infusions:

1. Calculating the flow rate for IV fluid administration
2. Making modifications in flow rates for infants
3. Calculating total administration time for IV fluid

To *calculate the flow rate for IV fluid administration,* two concepts must be understood: the flow rate and the drop factor. The rate at which IV fluids are given is the **flow rate,** and this is measured in drops per minute. The **drop factor** is the number of drops per milliliter of liquid and is determined by the size of the drops. The drop factor is different for different manufacturers of IV infusion equipment, and it must be checked by reading it on the infusion set itself. Regular infusion sets generally range between 10 and 15 drops per milliliter. Infusion sets have different drop factors for use with blood infusion sets (usually 10 to 12 drops per milliliter) because the drops are larger, whereas pediatric setups use very small drops called microdrops (often with 50 or 60 microdrops per milliliter).

 KEY POINT:
IV fluid administration

- The flow rate for infusions can be calculated.
- The drop factor for infusions depends on the type of equipment, and must be read from the setup label.

Once the nurse has learned the drop factor for the equipment being used, the flow rate may be calculated by using the following formula:

Drop factor × Milliliters per minute =
$$\text{Flow rate (drops/minute)}$$

Order: IV infusion to run at a slow rate to keep vein open. The rate is to be at 2 ml/minute. The IV infusion set delivers 10 drops/ml. The goal is to determine the flow rate in drops/minute.

$$10 \text{ (drop factor)} \times 2 \text{ ml/min} = 20 \text{ drops/minute}$$

Order: 1000 ml NS to be administered in 5 hours. The drop factor is 15.
Use:

$$\frac{\text{Total of fluid to give}}{\text{Total time (minutes)}} \times \text{Drop factor} = \text{Flow rate (drops/minute)}$$

$$\frac{1000 \text{ ml}}{300 \text{ min}} \times 15 = \frac{15000 \text{ ml}}{300 \text{ min}} = 50 \text{ drops/minute}$$

Flow rates for infants and children

Infants and small children are very sensitive to extra amounts or volumes of fluids. Smaller total amounts of IV fluids are often given, and the infusions are given in very small drops to avoid quickly overloading the infant's circulation. This is a built-in safety mechanism to try to prevent fluid overloading resulting from accidental delivery of too much fluid.

The drop factor must be determined from the

infusion setup. Usually 60 microdrops per ml is the drop factor for infants. For calculating the flow rates in infants, the same formula is used, but the microdrop drop factor must be substituted into the formula for the adult drop factor.

$$\frac{\text{Total of fluid to give}}{\text{Total time (minutes)}} \times \text{Drop factor} = \frac{\text{Flow rate}}{\text{(drops/minute)}}$$

For example, give 50 ml of D_5W IV in 4 hours. The drop factor is 60 microdrops/ml.

$$\frac{50 \text{ ml}}{240 \text{ min}} \times 60 = \frac{300}{24} = 12.5 \text{ microdrops/minute}$$

Total infusion time

Sometimes physicians order how fast they want infusions to run. To plan nursing care of the patient and to anticipate when new IV bottles may be needed, the nurse needs to calculate the total time the infusion will run.

Calculating the total administration time for IV fluid depends on calculating the total number of drops to be infused. Using this information, plus the drop factor, the total infusion time can be easily determined by using the following formula:

$$\frac{\text{Total drops to be infused}}{\text{Flow rate (drops/min)} \times 60} = \frac{\text{Total infusion time}}{\text{(hours or minutes)}}$$

For example, if the physician orders 1000 ml 5% dextrose in water (D_5W) to be given at 50 drops per minute with a drop factor of 10 drops/ml:

1. *Determine the total number of drops ordered.* The total number of drops to be infused comes from the physician's order for the amount of fluid (i.e., 1000 ml) × the drop factor (read from the infusion setup).
2. *Determine the number of minutes that the IV is to flow.* The number of drops per minute (50) is multiplied by 60 to give the number of drops infused in 1 hour (3000). This figure is then divided into the total number of drops. This will give the number of minutes for the total infusion. For example:

$$1000 \text{ ml} \times 10 \text{ drops/ml} = 10,000 \text{ drops}$$

$$\frac{10,000 \text{ drops}}{3,000 \text{ drops/hr}} = 3.33 \text{ hr or 3 hours, 20 minutes}$$

Other factors influencing flow rates

There are many other factors that influence the flow rate of an infusion. The nurse has no control over many of them, such as the age, size, and condition of the patient, the size of the vein, the type of fluid, and the need for the fluid. Other factors, such as the size of the needle, the needle's position in the vein, the height of the IV pole, the condition of the filter, the air in the air vent, and movement of the patient, may be changed or altered to assist in infusion of IV fluids. If the fluid does not infuse at the calculated rate, the IV should be carefully checked from the IV bottle to the site of the needle's insertion.

Calculating Dosages for Infants and Children

Drug dosages are calculated to give the maximum blood and tissue concentration of a medication without causing overdosage or adverse effects. Because infants are very sensitive to medications, and because infants and children are so much smaller than adults, almost all dosages given to infants and children are less than those given to adults. Most pharmaceutical companies list the recommended dosages for a child or infant. If it is not listed in the instructional material with the medication, the nurse should question whether the medication may be safely given to a child.

Although children's dosages were frequently calculated in the past, there remain only a few medications that require the nurse to calculate how much to give a child. Over the years several general rules have developed to calculate these special reduced dosages for infants and children.

One of the most popular methods for determining the dosage for children is based on the child's body weight and is known as **Clark's rule.** Again, ratios and proportions may be used to calculate the new value. If we assume that a normal adult weighs 150 lb and we know the adult dosage, then if we know the child's weight we can calculate the child's dosage:

Adult weight : Adult dosage :: Child's weight :

x Child's dosage

For example, if the adult dose of Demerol is 100 mg, what is the dose for a 50 lb child?

$$\frac{\text{Weight of child}}{\text{Weight of adult}} \times \text{Adult dose} = \text{Child's dose}$$

so

$$\frac{50}{150} \times 100 \text{ mg} = \frac{100}{3} = 33 \text{ mg}$$

Other formulas substitute kilograms for pounds in calculating the weights. The formula remains the same.

Clark's rule is by far the most popular method of assessing children's dosages. If no other formula is specified, use Clark's rule to determine a child's dosage.

Two other popular methods for calculating pediatric dosages involve the child's age. **Young's rule** is used for children ages 2 to 12; **Fried's rule** is used for infants and children under age 2. Obviously all children of the same age are not the same size. When the pediatric patient is approximately the "normal" size for his or her age, these rules may be used. If the child is unusually large or small for his or her age, it is better to use a weight calculation.

Young's rule for children from 2 to 12 years of age states:

$$\frac{\text{Child's age}}{\text{Child's age} + 12} \times \text{Adult dose} = \text{Child's dose}$$

Fried's rule for children under 2 years states:

$$\frac{\text{Infant's age in months}}{150} \times \text{Adult dose} = \text{Infant's dose}$$

For example, using Young's rule, if the adult dose of aminophylline is 0.5 gm, what is the dose for a child who is 8 years old?

$$\frac{8 \times 0.5 \text{ gm}}{8 + 12} = \frac{4}{20} = 0.20 \text{ gm}$$

Using Fried's rule, if the adult dose of Staphcillin is 1 gm (1000 mg), what is the dose for a child who is 3 months old?

$$\frac{3 \text{ months} \times 1000 \text{ mg}}{150} = \frac{3000 \text{ mg}}{150} = 20 \text{ mg}$$

Medications that require very careful dosage use the **body surface area (BSA)** of the child, which is the most accurate method for determining pediatric dosages. The reason for using the body surface area is that children have a greater surface area than adults in relation to their weight. For these drugs, charts are used to calculate the body surface area in square meters. These are constructed from height and weight figures. The surface area-to-weight ratio varies inversely (opposite) to length. Thus infants would have more surface area proportionally because they weigh less and are shorter than children. These charts may be used only if the child has normal height for weight. Even with the use of standardized charts, the calculated dosages are more accurate for children than for very young infants. An example of a **nomo-**

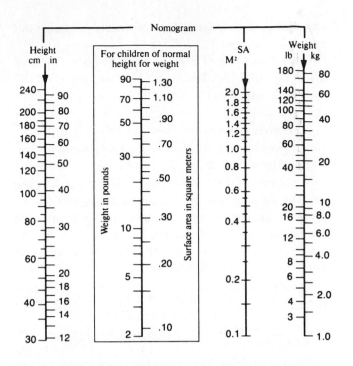

Fig. 7-5   Nomogram for body surface area of a child.
From Behrman RE, Vaughn VC, editors: *Nelson's textbook of pediatrics*, ed 12, Philadelphia, 1983, WB Saunders.

gram, or a chart used to calculate body weight, is shown in Fig. 7-5.

The total body surface area value is determined, and is put into the following formula:

$$\frac{\text{Surface area of the child in square meters}}{\text{Surface area of an adult in square meters (1.73 m}^2)} \times \text{Usual adult dose} = \text{Child's dose}$$

A straight edge is placed from the patient's height in the left column to his or her weight in the right column and the intersection on the body surface area column indicates the patient's body surface area.

Use the nomogram to solve these two sample problems, using the body surface area to calculate pediatric dosages (use 1.73 m^2 as the accepted adult body surface area):

1. If the adult dose of kanamycin is 0.5 gm, what is the pediatric dose for a 10-month-old child who weighs 22 pounds and is 29 inches long?

2. If the adult dose of sulfisoxazole (Gantrisin) is 500 mg, what is the pediatric dose for an 8-year-old child who weighs 48 pounds and is 47 inches tall?

SUMMARY

This chapter presented concepts and examples that illustrate common calculations that nurses are required to perform in administering medications. Mastery of this information is important for accuracy and speed. The foundation of multiplication facts, fractions, decimals, ratios, and proportions, added to the principles of metric, household, and apothecaries' systems come together in the practical application of dosage calculations. This chapter should be reviewed if you have difficulty with dosage calculations or need to review material that you have not worked with for some time.

 CRITICAL THINKING QUESTIONS

1. Convert the following using the metric and apothecaries' systems where applicable:
   a. 0.065 gm = _____ gr
   b. m vi = _____ cc = _____ ml
   c. 4 gm = _____ mg
   d. 35 mg = _____ gm
   e. gr 3/4 = _____ mg = _____ gm
   f. 45 cc = _____ ml

2. Your patient's drug order reads "3600 ml PO q24h." How many glassfuls would the patient have to drink?
3. The drug order is for 0.6 gm PO. The drug of choice is only available in 240 mg capsules. How many capsules would you give?
4. An IV infusion of tetracycline 4 mg/ml is ordered; tetracycline 500 mg/100 ml is available. The drop factor is 10 drops/ml. What is the flow rate? How much medication is received per minute?
5. Change 36° C to degrees F.
6. Give 250 ml IV over 24 hours. The drop factor is 60 microdrops. What should the flow rate be?
7. The adult dose of a given drug is 0.8 mg. What would be the dose for a 40-lb child?
8. Penicillin 500,000 U q8h is ordered. Drug is available as penicillin 1,000,000 U per 5 ml. How many ml would be given?
9. If a solution contains gr 1/40 of drug/ml, how many minims would you give for gr 1/160?
10. The physician orders 0.0015 gm OD of a drug. The drug is available in tablets labeled 2.5, 1.5, and 10 mg. Which would you order and how many would you give for each dose?

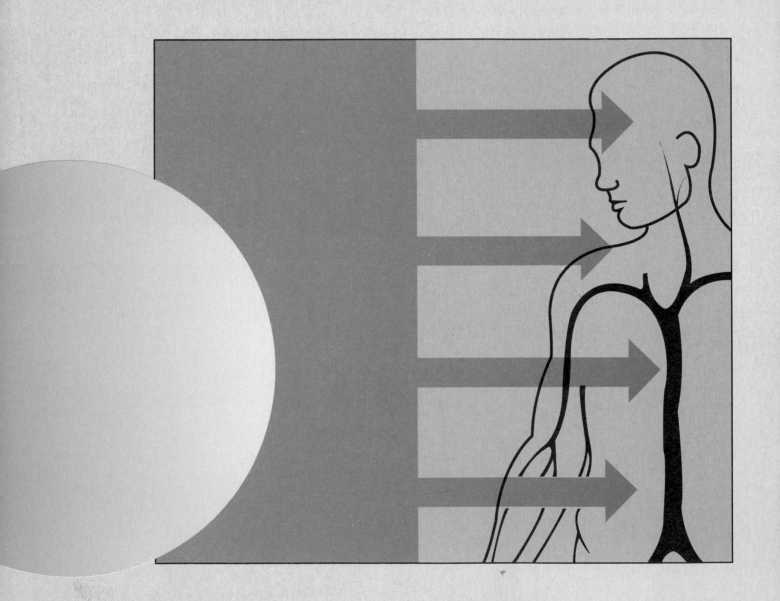

Drug Groups

OBJECTIVES

At the conclusion of this unit you should be able to:

1. List the actions and uses for the major drug groups.
2. Identify common adverse reactions associated with the major drug groups.
3. Describe the most common drug interactions among the major drug groups.
4. Apply the nursing process to information about the major drug groups.
5. Develop specific teaching plans for patients taking medications from the major drug groups.

OVERVIEW

The following chapters present brief discussions of the major drug groups, emphasizing the most important information the nurse must know about these medications. These chapters are designed to answer basic questions, highlight major areas of concern and knowledge, and help the nurse prepare to give the medications listed in each group. Special attention is given to the teaching requirements for all medications. The nurse assumes major responsibility for administering the drugs and for teaching the patients about the medications. These chapters provide the initial information necessary for safely carrying out these tasks.

We have marked trade name drugs available only in Canada with a ♣ for Canadian educators and students.

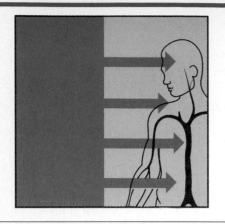

CHAPTER 8

Allergy and Respiratory Medications

OBJECTIVES

At the conclusion of this chapter you should be able to:

1. Identify major antihistamines used to treat respiratory problems.
2. Describe the action of antitussive medications.
3. List medications used to treat and prevent asthma attacks.
4. Describe the major actions and the adverse reactions of the two main categories of bronchodilators.
5. Identify at least six medications commonly used as decongestants.
6. Describe the mechanism of action for expectorants.
7. List the major contraindications to the use of nasal steroids.

KEY TERMS

OVERVIEW

This chapter discusses medications that affect the respiratory system. Section One, antihistamines, describes medications used to treat respiratory problems caused by allergies. Section Two discusses antitussives, or medications used to control coughing. Section Three describes medications used for **prophylaxis** (prevention) of asthma attacks. Sympathomimetics and xanthine derivatives are presented in Section Four, bronchodilators. Sections Five and Six cover decongestants and expectorants. The final section discusses nasal steroids used to treat respiratory problems.

Respiratory System

The respiratory system is composed of the lungs and the respiratory passages (Fig. 8-1). The structures of the oral and nasal cavity, sinuses, pharynx, larynx, trachea, and bronchus provide the conduit for air to move into the lungs. The lungs themselves are divided into lobes. The respiratory system functions to exchange gases (oxygen and carbon dioxide) between the blood and the air and regulates blood pH.

During inspiration the diaphragm drops, accompanied by the contraction of the intercostal muscles, which raises the ribs and increases the chamber size in the chest and creates a negative pressure. The negative pressure causes air to rush into the lungs through the respiratory passages. With exhalation the muscles relax, the pressure increases in the chest, and air is passively forced out of the lungs.

Abnormality may be present within any of the respiratory passages or structures, as well as the lung itself. Strictures or obstructions caused by infection or mucus, collapse of the bronchioles caused by asthma, or infective masses or tumors are common examples of problems requiring medication. The upper airways are often the site of allergic reactions and bacterial and viral infections.

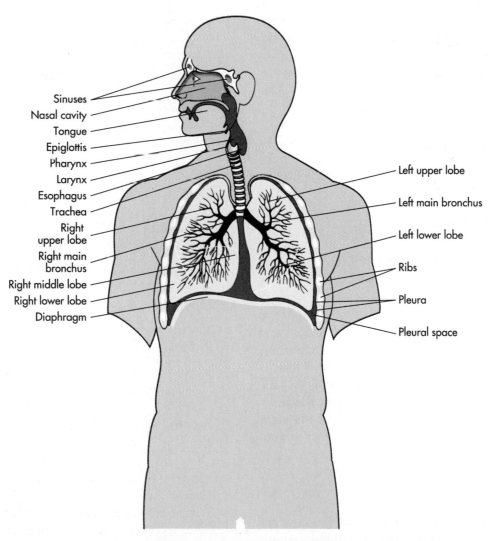

Fig. 8-1   The respiratory system.

SECTION ONE: ANTIHISTAMINES

Objectives

At the conclusion of this section you should be able to:

1. Describe the action of antihistamines in treating respiratory symptoms caused by allergy.
2. List major uses for antihistamine agents.
3. Identify three adverse effects of antihistamines.
4. Develop a teaching plan for a patient taking an antihistamine for an acute problem.

OVERVIEW

Histamine is the chemical produced by the body that is responsible for the inflammatory response. The mast cells found near capillaries and the white blood cell basophils contain large quantities of histamine. When the body is injured, the histamine is released, and it causes the smooth muscle and vascular system to increase blood flow by dilating the capillaries. This also makes the skin turn red. Fluid escapes from the capillaries into the tissues, producing swelling.

Histamines and other chemicals are released in varying degrees after an injury or an allergic stimulation. **Antihistamines** relieve the effects of histamine on body organs and structures.

ACTION

Antihistamines block the action of histamine by competing with it for the H_1 receptor sites on the effector structures (i.e., vascular and nonvascular smooth muscles, salivary glands, and respiratory mucosal glands). This serves to limit the vasodilation and increased capillary permeability, and to reduce the edema caused by histamine. Antihistamines also inhibit the release of acetylcholine, exerting an anticholinergic (drying) effect, particularly in the bronchioles and gastrointestinal system. Antihistamines also have a sedative effect on the central nervous system (CNS).

USES

Antihistamines are used to treat allergic perennial or **seasonal rhinitis** and other types of rhinitis (runny nose). They are used to relieve symptoms of allergic disorders (particularly urticaria [hives], angioneurotic edema, serum sickness, reactions to blood or plasma) and as an adjunctive therapy in anaphylactic reactions. They are used in combination cold remedies to decrease mucus secretion and at bedtime for sedation.

There are six main groups of antihistamines, with various characteristics and actions. These groups and some specific drugs within each group are summarized in the box below.

Major Antihistamine Groups

Alkylamines

Brompheniramine
Chlorpheniramine
Dexchlorpheniramine
Triprolidine

Ethanolamines

Carbinoxamine
Clemastine
Diphenhydramine

Ethylenediamines

Pyrilamine
Tripelennamine

Phenothiazines

Methdilazine
Promethazine
Trimeprazine

Piperidines

Azatadine
Cyproheptadine
Phenindamine

Miscellaneous

Astemizole
Loratadine
Terfenadine

ADVERSE REACTIONS

Potential adverse reactions to monitor in the patient receiving antihistamine medications include hypertension, hypotension, tachycardia, blurred vision, confusion, dizziness, drowsiness, excitation, insomnia, paradoxical excitation, restlessness, sedation, tinnitus (ringing in the ears), anorexia, constipation, diarrhea, dry mouth, nausea, vomiting, difficult or painful urination, impotence, urinary retention or frequency, photosensitization, rash, urticaria, nasal congestion, thickening of bronchial secretions. *Antihistamine overdosage is potentially fatal, particularly in children. The symptoms of overdosage occur when the CNS is being stimulated and depressed at the same time.*

DRUG INTERACTIONS

The sedative effect commonly associated with antihistamines is increased when other CNS depressants (such as hypnotics, sedatives, tranquilizers, depressant analgesics, and alcohol) are used along with the antihistamine. Antihistamines also add to the effect of anticholinergic drugs, and they can intensify the anticholinergic side effects of monoamine oxidase (MAO) inhibitors as well as tricyclic antidepressants. When antihistamines are used concurrently with **ototoxic** drugs (that is, drugs that may damage hearing, such as large doses of aspirin or other salicylates, streptomycin), the ototoxic effects may be masked. Antihistamines can decrease the effect of corticosteroids and many hormones. They may also interfere with the effects of anticholinesterase drugs. Astemizole is contraindicated for concurrent use with ketoconazole, itraconazole, and erythromycin because of its potential for severe cardiovascular side effects.

 ## NURSING IMPLICATIONS AND PATIENT TEACHING

▼ Assessment

The nurse should obtain a complete health history, including the presence of hypersensitivity, other drug use, presence of asthma, glaucoma, peptic ulcer, prostatic hypertrophy, bladder neck obstruction, respiratory or cardiac disease, and the possibility of pregnancy. A patient with thyroid disease or migraine headaches may be unable to take antihistamines because of the tachycardia (rapid heartbeat) pro-

duced. These conditions are contraindications or precautions to the use of antihistamines.

The patient may have a history of allergic reactions with allergic nasal congestion (usually seasonal in onset), runny nose, or cough related to a cold or allergy. The nurse may observe symptoms of rhinitis: sneezing, nasal discharge, and inflamed nasal mucosa. The patient may also have edema, skin lesions, dermatographism, conjunctivitis, eczema, insect bites, or contact dermatitis. The nasal mucosa may be swollen, boggy, and pale, and there may be nasal obstruction or a clear watery discharge. Increased sinus pressure may be found when palpating the frontal or maxillary sinuses.

The use of antihistamines in young children may cause hallucinations, convulsions, and even death. Elderly patients are also extremely sensitive to these preparations. Some products may produce **teratogenic effects** (deformities) in a fetus. Antihistamines should be used with caution in children with a family history of sleep apnea or sudden infant death syndrome (SIDS), or in children with symptoms of Reye's syndrome.

▼ Planning

The sedative effect is common to most antihistamines, except for new products such as terfenadine and astemizole. The sedation caused by antihistamines makes operating heavy machinery or driving particularly hazardous.

Most antihistamines are administered orally. Many are available in over-the-counter preparations, although the forms with the highest dosage are available only by prescription. Most manufacturers have at least one preparation that can be obtained by prescription, so that people with Medicare-Medicaid benefits are able to obtain these drugs with their cards.

▼ Implementation

Antihistamines should be taken only when needed. The type and dosage should be chosen according to the desired effect and the individual being treated. For example, ethanolamine derivatives have a high incidence of causing drowsiness, and they probably should not be used by people who perform activities that require alertness. Some preparations produce less drowsiness, but may not be as effective in resolving symptoms.

If tolerance to one type of antihistamine develops,

Table 8-1 Antihistamines

Generic name	Trade name	Comments and dosage
ALKYLAMINES		Alkylamines are effective at low dosages and are practical for daytime use; they may cause both CNS stimulation (excitation) and depression (drowsiness); the individual response is variable.
Brompheniramine	Bromphen Dimetane	Dimetane tablets and elixir are the only alkylamine products available without a prescription. *Adults:* 4 to 8 mg PO tid or qid; sustained-release tablets: 8 to 12 mg PO q8 to 12h. *Children over 6 years:* 4 mg PO tid or qid. *Children under 6 years:* 0.5 mg/kg/day PO.
Chlorpheniramine Dexchlorpheniramine	Chlor-Trimeton Polaramine ♣	Sustained-release forms are not for use in children under the age of 6; there is a low incidence of side effects. *Adults:* 2 to 4 mg PO tid or qid; sustained-release tablets: 8 to 12 mg PO q8 to 12h during the day or at bedtime. *Children:* 1 to 2 mg PO tid or qid.
Triprolidine	Actidil	*Adults and children over 12 years:* 2.5 mg q4 to 6h.
ETHANOLAMINES		Ethanolamines have the highest incidence of drowsiness but GI side effects are infrequent.
Carbinoxamine	Clistin	*Adults:* 4 to 8 mg q6 to 8h.
Diphenhydramine	Benadryl Caladryl Genahist Nordryl	It has anticholinergic, antitussive, antiemetic, and sedative properties, with high incidence of CNS depressant effects; drowsiness increases with use. *Adults:* 25 to 50 mg PO tid or qid. *Children over 20 pounds:* 12.5 to 25 mg PO tid or qid or 5 mg/kg/day PO.
ETHYLENEDIAMINES		
Pyrilamine	Pyrilamine Nisaval	High incidence of GI upset and moderate sedation, paradoxical excitation and hyperirritability. *Adults:* 25 to 100 mg PO bid to qid. *Children 6 to 12 years:* 12.5 to 25 mg PO bid to qid.
Tripelennamine	PBZ	There is a low incidence of side effects; the elixir is very palatable. *Adults:* 25 to 50 mg PO q4 to 6h, maximum 600 mg PO in 24 hours; sustained-release tablet: 100 mg in the AM and PM. *Children over 5 years:* 50 mg PO in the AM and PM; maximum 300 mg in 24 hours.
PHENOTHIAZINES		Phenothiazines have a strong CNS depressant effect (drowsiness). Phenothiazines may suppress the cough reflex or mask signs of intestinal obstruction, brain tumor, or overdosage from toxic drugs. See additional sections on phenothiazines.
Methdilazine	Tacaryl	Chew chewable tablets well. *Adults:* 8 mg PO bid to qid. *Children over 3 years:* 4 mg PO bid to qid.

Continued

switching to another type may restore responsiveness. Medications can be rotated to keep the symptoms under control.

The patient should not chew sustained-release tablets or capsules.

Gastrointestinal side effects can be minimized by administering oral doses with meals or milk. Antihistamines given orally are usually well absorbed; parenteral administration is rarely needed. When an IM preparation is used (such as diphenhydramine), it should be injected deep into the muscle to prevent tissue irritation. Antihistamines should not be given subcutaneously (SQ). IV administration of these agents should be done slowly, with the patient lying down. Long-term use of topical nasal antihistamines increases the risk of sensitization, often causing a **rebound effect** or an increase in symptoms.

See Table 8-1 for a summary of antihistamines.

Table 8-1   Antihistamines—cont'd

Generic name	Trade name	Comments and dosage
Promethazine	Phenergan Promethazine	High incidence of side effects, including severe drowsiness; potent drug with prolonged action; use cautiously in ambulatory patients. *Adults:* 25 mg PO or IM at bedtime; may also give 12.5 mg PO before meals and at bedtime if needed. *Children under 12 years:* 6.25 or 12.5 mg PO tid; may also give 12.5 mg IV or IM.
Trimeprazine	Temaril	Drowsiness decreases with continued use. *Adults:* 2.5 mg PO qid maximum 10 mg in 24 hours. *Children 3 to 12 years:* 2.5 mp PO at bedtime or tid if necessary. *Children 6 months to 3 years:* 1.25 mg PO at bedtime or tid if necessary; maximum of 5 mg PO in 24 hours.
PIPERIDINES		
Azatadine	Optimine	Not for use in children under 12 years of age; dosage should be individualized; drug has prolonged action. *Adults:* 1 to 2 mg PO bid.
Cyproheptadine	Periactin	Available by prescription only. *Adults:* 4 to 20 mg PO qd.
Phenindamine	Nolahist	*Adults and children 6 to 12 years:* 12.5 to 25 mg q4 to 6h.
MISCELLANEOUS		These new products reflect three different drug families. They reportedly produce less drowsiness, but they are not as effective in some individuals as other medications; they are relatively expensive.
Astemizole	Hismanal	*Adults and children over 12 years:* maintenance dose is 10 mg/day. Take on an empty stomach at least 2 hours after a meal. Do not eat for at least 1 hour after taking medications. Has severe drug interactions.
Loratadine	Claritin	*Adults and children over 12:* 1 tablet per day.
Terfenadine	Seldane	May also be used in some lower respiratory conditions such as histamine-induced bronchoconstriction in asthmatics and exercise-induced and hyperventilation-induced bronchospasm. *Adults and children over 12:* 30 to 60 mg bid. *Children under 12 years:* 15 to 30 mg bid.

▼ Evaluation

The therapeutic effect of antihistamines should cause the symptoms of allergy to decrease. The nurse should watch for the development of adverse reactions, which are common but are usually mild (see box, 128).

Elderly patients are more likely to develop extrapyramidal side effects such as dizziness, syncope, confusion, dyskinesia, and tremor (see box, p. 128).

Antihistamine use may cause the respiratory tract to dry and mucus to thicken. The patient must drink large amounts of fluid to thin the secretions and keep the tissues moist.

If any dermatologic reactions occur, the drug should be discontinued at once. The CNS depressant effects of antihistamines may be increased if the patient exceeds the recommended dosage.

▼ Patient and family teaching

The nurse should provide the patient and family with the following instructions:

1. The patient should take the medications as ordered and not exceed the recommended dosage.
2. Most antihistamines produce drowsiness, and the patient must avoid tasks, such as driving, in which alertness is required.
3. These drugs may cause dizziness, thickening of secretions, and upset stomach, which may require a physician's attention if reactions continue.
4. If the medication causes stomach upset, this can be decreased by taking medication with meals or milk.
5. A wide variation exists in the occurrence of side

Pediatric Considerations
ANTIHISTAMINES

Infants and young children are very susceptible to anticholinergic side/adverse effects.

Closely monitor pediatric patients with spastic paralysis or brain damage, since they generally have an increased reaction to these agents, requiring a dosage reduction.

Anticholinergics, especially high doses, may cause a paradoxical type reaction of increased nervousness, confusion, and/or hyperexcitability.

Children receiving these agents where hot weather prevails or environmental temperatures are high have an increased risk of developing a rapid body temperature increase (anticholinergic drugs suppress sweat gland activity).

Dosage adjustments are often necessary for infants. Down syndrome patients, and blonds since they generally have an increased response to this drug category. Flushing, increased temperature, irritability, and increased pulse and respiratory rate may occur.

Start with low doses and increase gradually, as needed and tolerated.

From McKenry LM, Salerno E.: *Mosby's pharmacology in nursing*, ed 18, St Louis, 1992, Mosby.

effects among antihistamines; even though a patient may experience many side effects from one agent, another antihistamine may produce few adverse reactions.

6. Tolerance may develop after use of an antihistamine, and another antihistamine should be tried for better control of symptoms if one product seems to become less effective over time.

Geriatric Considerations
ANTIHISTAMINES

The elderly are highly susceptible to anticholinergic side effects, especially constipation, dry mouth, and urinary retention (usually in males).

Memory impairment has been reported with continuous administration of these agents, especially in older patients.

When usual adult doses are administered, some elderly may have a paradoxical reaction: hyperexcitability, agitation, confusion, and/or sedation.

Anticholinergic dosing in the elderly should begin at the lowest dose with gradual increases, until maximum improvement is noted or intolerable side effects occur.

From McKenry LM, Salerno E: *Mosby's pharmacology in nursing*, ed 18, St Louis, 1992, Mosby.

7. The patient should discontinue the use of antihistamines for 48 hours before undergoing skin tests for allergies.
8. Many antihistamines can be purchased over the counter, whereas others require prescriptions; make certain the patient has a prescription if it is needed.
9. The patient should not take any other medications without the knowledge of the physician; it is especially important for the patient to avoid alcohol or sedative drugs while on this medication.
10. This medication must be kept out of the reach of children and others for whom it is not prescribed; overdosages may be very serious.

SECTION TWO: ANTITUSSIVES

Objectives

At the conclusion of this section you should be able to:

1. Describe the action of antitussive medications.
2. Identify major uses for antitussive medications.
3. List other drugs commonly combined with antitussive medications.
4. Identify several major adverse reactions associated with antitussive medications.
5. Indicate when a narcotic antitussive may be useful.
6. Construct a teaching plan for a patient taking an antitussive medication for a chronic problem.

OVERVIEW

Drugs used to relieve coughing are called **antitussives** These medications may either (1) act centrally on the cough center in the brain, (2) act peripherally by anesthetizing stretch receptors in the respiratory tract, or (3) act locally, primarily by soothing irritated areas in the throat. Products vary in their effectiveness. Antitussives are commonly combined with other drugs and are usually sold as nonprescription medications. Medications containing narcotics are controlled substances and are available only by prescription.

ACTION

The main action of an antitussive depends on whether a narcotic is included or not. Narcotic antitussives suppress the cough reflex by acting directly on the cough center in the medulla of the brain. Nonnarcotic antitussives reduce the cough reflex at its source by anesthetizing stretch receptors in respiratory passages, lungs, and pleura, and by decreasing their activity.

USES

Antitussives are used for the symptomatic relief of overactive or nonproductive coughs.

ADVERSE REACTIONS

Adverse reactions to antitussives include constipation, drowsiness, dry mouth, nausea, and postural hypotension.

DRUG INTERACTONS

Narcotic antitussives have an additive effect with other CNS depressants, and so the dosage should be reduced. Antitussives increase the analgesic effect of aspirin, which may be helpful.

 NURSING IMPLICATIONS & PATIENT TEACHING

▼ Assessment

The nurse should obtain a complete health history, including hypersensitivity to antitussives, presence of chronic pulmonary disease, possibility of pregnancy, and other drugs or alcohol that the patient is taking that may cause drug interactions. These conditions may be contraindications or precautions to the use of antitussives.

The patient may have a history of a nonproductive cough or an overactive cough, which may keep the patient awake at night or cause muscular pain.

▼ Planning

Do not use antitussives in patients with hypersensitivity to these drugs or those with chronic pulmonary disease. Narcotic antitussives may produce drug dependence. Some of these preparations are Schedule C-II controlled substances.

These preparations may cause drowsiness, so the patient should be cautioned to avoid tasks requiring alertness after taking the medication.

▼ Implementation

Antitussives come only in oral forms. They should be used only for short periods of time, since they can be addictive.

See Table 8-2 on page 130 for a summary of antitussives.

▼ Evaluation

The nurse should watch for therapeutic effects: resolution of cough, decrease in frequency and duration of coughing spells, and ability to sleep better at night. The nurse should monitor the patient for adverse reactions and drug tolerance.

▼ Patient and family teaching

The nurse should provide the patient and family with the following instructions:
1. The patient should take the medication as ordered and not alter the dosage or frequency.
2. Narcotics may cause drowsiness, and the patient must use caution when performing tasks requiring alertness.
3. Overuse of these medications may cause severe constipation and may also lead to addiction.
4. This drug will increase the effects of alcohol and other drugs that slow the nervous system; the patient should not take any other medications while taking this drug.
5. The patient may become nauseated during the first few minutes after taking the medication; this will resolve if the patient lies down.
6. The drug occasionally causes lightheadedness, dizziness, or fainting when getting up from a lying or sitting position; the patient should be cautioned to change positions slowly.
7. The patient should take the drug with food or milk to decrease stomach upset.
8. This medication must be kept out of the reach of children and others for whom it is not prescribed.

Table 8-2 Antitussives

Generic name	Trade name	Comments and dosage
NARCOTIC ANTITUSSIVES		
Codeine	Codeine sulfate Codeine phosphate	The average antitussive dose ranges from 10 to 20 mg q4 to 6h and is effective at this level; protect codeine from light; do not use in children under 12 years of age. *Adults:* 10 to 20 mg q4 to 6h. *Children:* 5 to 10 mg PO tid to qid.
Hydrocodone	Hycodan	*Adults:* 1 tablet q4 to 6h.
NONNARCOTIC ANTITUSSIVES		
Benzonatate	Tessalon Perles	Anesthetizes stretch receptors; do not chew drug, because local anesthesia of the mouth will develop. *Adults and children over 10 years:* 100 mg PO tid as needed; maximum of 600 mg in 24 hours.
Dextromethorphan	Benylin DM Formula 44 Robitussin Allerdyl ♣ Insomnal ♣	Centrally depresses the cough center. *Adults:* 10 to 20 mg PO q4h or 30 mg PO q6 to 8h; maximum of 120 mg daily. *Children 2 to 12 years:* 2.5 to 10 mg PO q4h or 15 mg PO q6 to 8h; maximum of 60 mg daily.
Diphenhydramine	Benylin cough Tusstat	Potent antihistamine; safe and effective antitussive. *Adults:* 25 mg PO q4h; maximum of 150 mg daily. *Children:* 6.25 to 12.5 mg PO q4h; maximum of 75 mg daily.

SECTION THREE: ASTHMA PROPHYLAXIS MEDICATION

Objectives

At the conclusion of this section you should be able to:
1. Describe the difference between asthma treatment and asthma prophylaxis (or prevention) therapy.
2. Identify the major asthma prevention drug.
3. Explain how cromolyn is administered.
4. Present key ideas to be included in teaching a patient about administering cromolyn.

OVERVIEW

Asthma is a condition in which there is increased cellular inflammation and mucus production, leading to bronchiolar collapse. The lumen (inside diameter of the bronchial tubes) becomes smaller as the patient attempts to breathe out. This traps air inside the lungs. The patient feels a lack of oxygen, and responds by breathing faster, trapping even more air inside the lungs. As some air is forced out through the small, mucus-lined passages, a musical respiratory sound called **wheezing** is heard.

Asthma is caused by a variety of factors, such as respiratory enzyme deficiencies, reaction to an allergy, or by hard exercise. Some individuals have a genetic tendency to develop asthma. It often develops in childhood. For some individuals it becomes a chronic condition. For others, it may be associated only with acute illnesses or self-limiting problems.

ACTION

The main action of the asthma medication cromolyn is indirect antiasthmatic activity by inhibiting the degranulation of sensitized mast cells. This drug inhibits the release of histamine and the slow-reacting substance of anaphylaxis (SRS-A) induced by inhaling specific antigens. It may provide some hyposensitization after long-term use by preventing the release of phospholipase A. This enzyme assists in the release of chemical mediators from nonsensitized mast cells.

USES

Cromolyn sodium and nedocromil sodium are used to manage bronchial asthma in selected patients. These drugs have no antihistaminic, antiinflammatory, or bronchodilator activity. Thus, they are effective only as a prophylactic agent and should not be used in an acute attack of asthma. They are used in some patients with food allergies to prevent GI and systemic reactions, in patients with allergic rhinitis, eczema and other forms of dermatitis, for patients with chronic urticaria, and those with postexercise bronchospasm.

ADVERSE REACTIONS

Adverse reactions to cromolyn or nedocromil include: dizziness, headache, vertigo, rash, nausea, dysuria, urinary frequency, bronchospasm, cough, nasal congestion, wheezing, anaphylaxis, tearing of eyes, and swollen parotid gland. Because these drugs are rapidly eliminated from the body, they are practically nontoxic except to those who have a hypersensitivity to the drug.

DRUG INTERACTIONS

No drug interactions with cromolyn or nedocromil have been currently reported.

 NURSING IMPLICATIONS & PATIENT TEACHING

▼ Assessment

The nurse should obtain a complete health history, including specific respiratory signs and symptoms, other medications, hypersensitivity, possibility of pregnancy, and presence of infection.

The patient may have a history of allergies, asthma, bronchitis, emphysema, recurrent acute or chronic attacks of wheezing, cough with or without mucoid sputum, dyspnea, fatigue, intolerance for exercise, and, in severe cases, cyanosis. Acute upper or lower respiratory tract infections may precede the onset of acute symptoms.

▼ Planning

Cromolyn is reported to be more effective in children than in adults.

Initiate administration of this drug when an acute

attack of asthma is over, the airway is clear, and the patient can breathe easily.

The amount of drug used by the lung depends on the proper use of the inhaler, the degree of bronchospasm present, and the amount of secretion in the tracheobronchial tree. Only about 5% to 10% of the inhaled drug reaches the lung.

▼ Implementation

Occasionally cough and bronchospasm may follow administration of cromolyn or nedocromil. Thus, some patients may not be able to continue using it even with concurrent administration of bronchodilators.

Caution should be used when decreasing the dosage or discontinuing the use of cromolyn or nedocromil; this can cause asthmatic symptoms to recur.

Cromolyn and nedocromil are not absorbed through the GI tract, so they are ineffective when taken orally. Cromolyn is available under the name Intal in 20 mg capsules for inhalation using an oral inhaler called a Spinhaler. A capsule is inserted in the Spinhaler and the patient sucks in hard on the inhaler, which then spins the medication into small particles that move down into the lung with the breath. The Spinhaler is washed after each use. For adults and children 5 years and over, use 20 mg doses inhaled at four *equal* intervals daily. The dosage can be decreased gradually to the minimum effective level, usually 20 mg three times daily.

The nurse should instruct the patient concerning proper use and care of the Spinhaler and have the patient return a demonstration of the procedure.

The cromolyn capsules should be protected from light, moisture, and heat.

Cromolyn and nedocromil are also available as aerosol solutions.

▼ Evaluation

Improvement in symptoms can be expected within 4 weeks of using cromolyn or nedocromil. The nurse should monitor for therapeutic effect: suppression of asthmatic attacks. Because the drug should be given when a patient's condition is stable, a visit should be scheduled 2 weeks after the initial administration, and at least once more within the first 4 weeks for evaluation of effectiveness of the preparation.

Supervise the patient carefully when reducing the dosage or discontinuing the drug. Reevaluate the drug regimen if no effect is achieved within 4 weeks.

▼ Patient and family teaching

The nurse should provide the patient and the family with the following instructions:

1. The patient should not swallow the capsules.
2. The capsules should be protected from light, heat, and moisture.
3. The airway should be cleared of as much mucus as possible before taking the drug.
4. The patient should avoid using this drug if they cannot take a deep breath and hold it, or if they feel they are having an asthma attack.
5. This drug must be administered *every* day at *regular* intervals.
6. If the patient is using a bronchodilator at the same time, it should be used first; then after several minutes the cromolyn may be taken.
7. Throat irritation, dryness of the mouth, and hoarseness may be prevented by rinsing and gargling after each dose.
8. To deliver the appropriate dosage, the patient must use the Spinhaler correctly and keep it clean.
9. Suddenly stopping the medication can make the patient have an acute attack of asthma.
10. The physician should be notified if symptoms do not improve or if they get worse.
11. The patient should avoid breathing out moisture into the inhaler. Because the drug is a powder, moisture may cause the particles to clump and may interfere with the correct dosage.

SECTION FOUR: BRONCHODILATORS

Objectives

At the conclusion of this section you should be able to:

1. Identify the two major groups of drugs used in bronchodilation.
2. Describe indications for the use of bronchodilators.
3. Compare the actions and adverse effects of sympathomimetic and xanthine derivatives.
4. List common drug interactions that occur with bronchodilators.

OVERVIEW

Many respiratory diseases produce a narrowing or collapse of the bronchial airways. This bronchoconstriction or **bronchospasm** narrows the lumen of the bronchi, decreasing the amount of air taken into the lungs or pushed out of the lungs with each breath. This causes the patient to cough, have difficulty breathing, and have feelings of chest tightness.

Two types of **bronchodilators** may be given to open the bronchi and allow air to pass more freely: the sympathomimetics and the xanthine derivatives. The **sympathomimetics** are beta-adrenergic agents and they dilate the bronchi. They are also known as adrenergic stimulants. The **xanthines** act directly to relax the smooth muscle cells of the bronchi, thereby dilating or opening up the bronchi. These groups will be discussed in detail.

SYMPATHOMIMETICS

ACTION

The main action of sympathomimetic bronchodilators is to relax the smooth muscle cells of the bronchi by stimulating beta$_2$-adrenergic receptors. They also stimulate alpha receptors, which produces a vasoconstriction response throughout the body (systemically), especially contraction in the blood vessels of the bronchial mucosa. This results in reduced mucosal and submucosal edema. Sympathomimetic bronchodilators also stimulate beta$_1$ receptors, which results in an increased rate and force of the heart's contractions. The sympathomimetic drugs vary in their selectivity for alpha and beta receptors. Some act solely on beta$_2$ receptors, and others have beta$_1$ and beta$_2$ effects. If the drug action is specific to beta$_2$ receptors, there are fewer side effects.

USES

Sympathomimetic bronchodilators are used for symptomatic treatment of bronchospasm occurring in acute and chronic asthma, bronchitis, and emphysema.

ADVERSE REACTIONS

Adverse reactions to sympathomimetic bronchodilators include dysrhythmias, hypotension, increased heart rate, anorexia, anxiety, headache, insomnia, nausea, pallor, perspiration, polyuria, restlessness, vomiting, weakness, and urinary hesitancy and retention. Overdosage will result in exaggeration of the adverse reactions.

DRUG INTERACTIONS

Thyroid drugs, tricyclic antidepressants (MAO inhibitors), some antihistamines, and amphetamines increase the effects of sympathomimetic drugs. Two or more sympathomimetic drugs taken together may cause the symptoms to become worse. Patients on digitalis or diuretics may experience dysrhythmias if they are given sympathomimetic drugs. Many general anesthetics also cause dysrhythmias. Beta-adrenergic blocking agents such as propranolol may block the bronchodilatory effects of these beta receptor drugs. Sympathomimetics can block the response of some antihypertensive medications.

 NURSING IMPLICATIONS AND PATIENT TEACHING

▼ Assessment

The nurse should obtain a thorough health history, including whether the patient is pregnant or breast-feeding; has a history of hyperthyroidism, heart disease, hypertension, diabetes, glaucoma, seizures or psychoneurotic disease; is taking other drugs that may interact with the bronchodilators; or has a history of allergy. These conditions may present contraindications or precautions to the use of sympathomimetic bronchodilators.

The patient may have a history of allergies, asthma, bronchitis, emphysema, recurrent acute or chronic attacks of wheezing, and cough. An acute upper or lower respiratory tract infection may precede the onset of acute symptoms.

▼ Planning

To relieve bronchial spasm, beta$_2$ receptors in bronchial smooth muscle cells must be stimulated. One of the drawbacks of adrenergic bronchodilators is that their effects are not limited to beta$_2$ receptors. Some also stimulate beta$_1$ receptors, which increase the rate and force of cardiac contraction, and alpha receptors, which control vasoconstriction. Thus, these drugs should be given with extreme caution to individuals with preexisting cardiovascular, endocrine, or convulsive disorders.

▼ Implementation

The routes of administration of bronchodilators vary according to the acuteness of the disease and the preparation used. They may be given parenterally, orally, or by oral inhalation (nebulizers, IPPB). The patient using the inhalation method of administration should be given demonstrations as well as written instructions for the procedure.

Concurrent administration of more than one sympathomimetic agent is contraindicated.

Refractoriness, or lack of response to a drug, may occur if the drug is administered too frequently.

Patients may get less relief from aerosols if they are used excessively. Irritation of the bronchial tree and oropharynx may occur with use of powdered formulations.

▼ Evaluation

The nurse should monitor the patient's pulse and blood pressure to determine the cardiac effects of the drug. Responses to therapy will vary among patients. The patient should be evaluated frequently to determine whether the respiratory symptoms have improved.

Patients should be monitored for increasing tolerance and resulting diminished response to the drug.

 CRITICAL DECISION:
Monitoring the Dosage

The dosage must be carefully monitored to prevent tachycardia, increased blood pressure, nausea, headache, or other CNS symptoms.

▼ Patient and family teaching

The nurse should provide the patient and family with the following instructions:
1. The patient should take the medication as directed by the physician; the dosage should not be changed.

2. Excessive use of this drug may have severe side effects.
3. The physician should be contacted if the desired effect is not being achieved from the drug.
4. The following symptoms should be reported to the physician: bronchial irritation, dizziness, chest pain, insomnia, or any change in symptoms.
5. Increased fluid intake, especially water, will reduce the thickness of mucus and help the medication work better.
6. The patient must not take any other medications without checking first with the physician.
7. Difficulty in falling asleep may be lessened or avoided by taking the last dose a few hours before bedtime.
8. The drug should be protected from light, and colored solutions should be discarded.

XANTHINE DERIVATIVES

ACTION

The main action of xanthine-derivative bronchodilators is to relax the smooth muscle cells in the bronchi and the blood vessels in the lungs. They act directly on the kidneys to produce diuresis. These drugs produce CNS effects. Other actions include myocardial stimulation, increased respiration, effects on metabolism, and release of epinephrine from the adrenal medulla.

USES

Xanthine derivatives are used to treat the symptoms of bronchospasm occurring in acute and chronic bronchial asthma, bronchitis, and emphysema.

ADVERSE REACTIONS

Adverse reactions to xanthine derivatives include dysrhythmias, flushing, marked hypotension, tachycardia, headache, insomnia, restlessness, diarrhea, epigastric pain, nausea, vomiting, and rash.

Overdosage causes severe adverse reactions, progressing to confusion, respiratory failure, shock, bizarre behavior, extreme thirst, delirium, and hyperthermia. Excessive overdosage may lead to seizures and death without warning symptoms. Children are particularly at risk for this phenomenon.

DRUG INTERACTIONS

Xanthines may enhance the CNS stimulation caused by ephedrine, sympathomimetics, and amphetamines. Erythromycin, lincomycin, and clindamycin may increase blood levels of theophylline. Beta-blocking agents may interfere with (antagonize) the effect of xanthines. These preparations also increase the action of some types of diuretics. Xanthines may increase the risk of toxicity when taken with digitalis glycosides. Large doses of these agents may counteract the effectiveness of oral anticoagulants. Lithium carbonate is excreted more rapidly in the presence of xanthines. The use of furosemide with theophylline increases the serum levels of theophylline and may cause toxicity. Xanthine derivatives shorten prothrombin and clotting times.

 NURSING IMPLICATIONS AND PATIENT TEACHING

▼ Assessment

The nurse should obtain a complete health history, including whether the patient is pregnant or has a history of smoking, hypersensitivity, renal or liver dysfunction, heart disease, cardiac dysrhythmias, peptic ulcer, severe hypertension, or glaucoma. These conditions are contraindications or precautions to the use of xanthines.

▼ Planning

The half-life of xanthine bronchodilators is shorter in smokers than nonsmokers, which may make it necessary to use a higher dosage with smokers.

It is not necessary to use formulations that contain alcohol; they may be harmful.

▼ Implementation

Xanthine products are available in a number of forms: capsules, coated tablets, sustained-release tablets and capsules, aqueous solutions and suspensions, hydro-alcoholic elixirs, suppositories, rectal solutions, and IV and IM injections.

The theophylline-base content varies in xanthine products, and the preparations are not therapeutically equal. This may cause difficulty when the patient is switched from one product to another. The critical factor is to monitor the theophylline blood levels to achieve the desired therapeutic effect.

The rate of absorption of oral theophylline de-

CRITICAL DECISION:
Factors Affecting Blood Levels

The efficacy of the drug is directly related to the theophylline blood levels achieved from its administration. The desired therapeutic range is considered to be 10 to 20 µg per milliliter of serum. The factors affecting blood levels include the following:
1. Differing levels of theophylline in each product
2. Variance in rates of absorption
3. Metabolism and elimination of each drug
4. Age of the patient receiving the medication

pends on the dosage form used. Oral liquids have the fastest absorption time, followed by uncoated tablets. Enteric-coated or sustained-release tablets and capsules produce inconsistent blood levels and should usually be reserved for use at night. Food does not influence the absorption of theophylline. Rectal absorption with suppositories is a slow method of absorption and is sometimes unpredictable. The rate of absorption for rectal solutions and IM injections is usually equivalent to that of an oral solution.

The rates of metabolism and excretion of theophylline are also variable. Xanthines are metabolized in the liver and excreted by the kidneys. The serum half-life of the drugs can range from 3 to 12 hours in adults and 1¼ to 9 hours in children. Heart failure, liver dysfunction, and pulmonary edema can slow excretion, and smoking can increase excretion. Children under 9 years of age require larger doses of theophylline than adults to maintain appropriate therapeutic blood levels of the drug. Thus, the dosage must be prescribed on an individualized basis and be carefully monitored. It is common for an initial loading dose to be indicated. Because of this need for individualized titration of the agents, the use of a fixed combination of bronchodilator products (that is, sympathomimetic, xanthine, and expectorant) is not recommended. Fixed combination products do not allow flexibility in changing dosages for individual drugs, and may increase the toxicity of some of the drugs. Concurrent use of selected sympathomimetic and xanthine dilators administered individually, however, may have a synergistic effect.

See Table 8-3 on page 136 for a summary of bronchodilators.

▼ Evaluation

The patient's respiratory status and symptoms should be monitored for any change or resolution. The nurse should be alert for signs of toxicity, such as development of tachycardia or dysrhythmias, vomiting, dizziness, and irritability.

The drugs should be given according to the therapeutic blood levels of theophylline, the amount of theophylline base in each preparation, and the clinical response of the patient.

Children and elderly patients should be carefully observed for CNS stimulation, since they are particularly sensitive to these drugs.

To minimize GI symptoms, administer the drug with food and water. Rectal irritation may develop from suppository forms.

▼ Patient and family teaching

The nurse should provide the patient and family with the following instructions:
1. The patient should take the medications as ordered; this often means every 6 hours if taking a sustained-release medication.
2. Any unusual symptoms should be reported to the physician, especially seizures, rapid heartbeat, irregular heartbeat, vomiting, dizziness, and irritability.
3. The patient should avoid consuming large amounts of caffeine-containing beverages such as tea, coffee, cocoa, and cola drinks.
4. Some other medications will interfere with the drug action if taken at the same time. The patient should avoid taking any other drugs without first checking with the physician. This includes drugs that patient may buy over the counter, since they may also have an effect on the respiratory system (for example, cough syrups, hayfever and allergy medicine).
5. The patient should take the medicine with a glass of water or with meals to avoid an upset stomach.
6. If a dose is missed and noticed within an hour, take the prescribed dose. If remembered after an hour, skip the dose and stay on the original dosing schedule.
7. Some suppositories must be refrigerated, whereas others may not have this requirement. Check with the pharmacist.
8. Notify the physician if use of suppositories causes burning or irritation of the rectal area.

Table 8-3	Bronchodilators	
Generic name	**Trade name**	**Comments and dosage**

SYMPATHOMIMETIC BRONCHODILATORS

Generic name	Trade name	Comments and dosage
Albuterol	Proventil Ventolin	Selective for beta$_2$ receptors and thus has fewer cardiac side effects than other adrenergic drugs and a long duration of bronchodilation; comes as an inhaler with about 200 doses. *Adults and children:* 1 to 2 inhalations q4 to 6h or 2 to 4 mg PO tid or qid.
Bitolterol	Tornalate	2 inhalations in 1 to 3 minutes, followed by third inhalation if needed.
Ephedrine	Ephedrine sulfate Primatene Mist	Has a long duration; it is used to treat milder forms of chronic obstructive pulmonary disease. *Adults:* 25 to 50 mg PO q3 to 4h or 25 to 50 mg SQ or IM q3 to 4h. *Children 6 to 12 years:* 6.25 to 12.5 mg PO q4 to 6h. *Children 2 to 6 years:* 0.3 to 0.5 mg/kg PO q4 to 6h.
Epinephrine	Adrenalin Medihaler-Epi Sus-Phrine	Reserved for acute attacks of bronchospasm. It has a rapid onset of action (3 to 10 minutes) when given SQ or by inhalation. Light, air, and heat can change color. One to two minutes should be allowed between inhalations if successive dosage is needed. ■ *For Adrenalin and Epinephrine* *Adults:* 0.2 to 1.0 mg SQ or IM. *Children:* 0.01 mg/kg or 0.3 mg/m² to a maximum of 0.5 mg. ■ *For Sus-Phrine* *Adults:* 0.1 to 0.3 ml SQ. *Children:* 0.005 ml/kg SQ.
Ethylnorepinephrine	Bronkephrine Levophed ♣	Nonselective beta-adrenergic bronchodilator; used for patients with severe asthma who do not respond to isoproterenol or epinephrine. *Adults:* 0.5 to 1.0 ml SQ or IM. *Children:* Determined by age and weight; 0.1 to 0.5 ml SQ or IM is average.
Isoetharine	Arm-a-Med	Hand nebulizer: 3 to 7 inhalations undiluted.
Isoproterenol	Isuprel Medihaler-Iso	Selective for beta receptors; helpful for those no longer benefiting from use of epinephrine; may decrease blood pressure; may make saliva pink. *Adults:* 10 to 20 mg SL, not to exceed 60 mg per day. *Children:* 5 to 10 mg SL, not to exceed 30 mg per day. *Inhalation:* 1 to 5 treatments as needed daily.
Metaproterenol	Alupent Metaprel	More selectivity for beta$_2$ receptors of the bronchi and less effect on beta$_1$ receptors of the heart than isoproterenol; well absorbed from the GI tract. *Adults:* 20 mg PO tid or qid. *Children over 9 years or over 60 lb:* 20 mg PO tid or qid. *Children 6 to 9 years or less than 60 lb:* 10 mg PO tid or qid.
Pirbuterol	Maxair	2 inhalations q4 to 6h.
Terbutaline	Brethine Bricanyl	Has a negligible effect on beta$_1$ receptors; has an affinity for beta$_2$ receptors of the bronchial tree, peripheral vascular beds, and the uterus; often effective when other drugs are not. *Adults:* 5 mg PO q6h tid. *Children 12 to 15 years:* 2.5 mg PO tid; or 2.5 mg SQ tid, not to exceed 7.5 mg SQ in 24 hours.

Continued.

Table 8-3   Bronchodilators—cont'd

Generic name	Trade name	Comments and dosage
XANTHINE BRONCHODILATORS		
Aminophylline	Aminophylline	A synthetic preparation that is a prototype for many of the theophylline compounds. It plays a significant role in management of conditions with bronchial constriction and spasm. It is especially useful when differentiation cannot be made between bronchospasm and pulmonary edema. This agent is commonly prescribed by its generic name and contains 78% theophylline and 12% ethylenediamine. IM injection is painful. ■ *Asthma attacks* *Adults:* 500 mg PO stat; 200 to 315 mg PO q6 to 8h maintenance. For rectal suppositories, usual dose is 500 mg qd or bid, not to exceed 1 gm/day, or 500 mg IM as necessary. With rectal solutions use 300 mg qd to tid or 450 mg bid. Timed-release tablets can be given in 300 mg to 600 mg q8 to 12h. *Children:* 7.5 mg/kg PO stat; 5 to 6 mg/kg PO q6 to 8h maintenance; or give 7 mg/kg rectal suppository, or use rectal solutions in 5 mg/kg.
Dyphylline	Dilor Dyflex Protophylline ♣	Few side effects. *Adults:* Give up to 15 mg/kg PO q6h; individualize dosage. For IM dosage, give 250 to 500 mg injected slowly. *Children 40 to 100 lb:* 80 to 240 mg for acute attacks; 27 to 80 mg for maintenance in 3 to 4 hours. *Children under 40 lb:* 40 to 80 mg for acute attacks; 13 to 17 mg in 3 to 4 hours for maintenance. For IM dosage, give 2 to 3 mg/lb qd in divided doses.
Oxtriphylline	Choledyl	Less irritating to gastric mucosa, is readily absorbed from GI tract, and more stable and soluble than aminophylline. Useful for long-term therapy of bronchospasm. *Adults:* 200 mg PO qid. *Children 2 to 12 years:* 100 mg/60 lb qid.
Theophylline	Bronkodyl Elixophyllin Slo-Phyllin Theo-Dur	Popular and effective drug in management of bronchial constriction and spasm. Timed-release capsules slowly provide medication for 8 to 12 or 12 to 24 hours. *Adults:* 200 to 250 mg PO q6h. *Children:* 3 to 6 mg/kg q6h. For timed-release capsules (Theo-Dur): *Adults:* 300 mg PO q12h. *Children 12 to 16:* 200 mg PO q12h. *Children 9 to 12:* 150 mg PO q12h. *Children under 9:* 100 mg PO q12h.

SECTION FIVE: DECONGESTANTS

Objectives

At the conclusion of this section you should be able to:
1. Identify indications for decongestant use.
2. List six common decongestants.

3. Explain why decongestant combination products may not be helpful to the patient.
4. Identify major ideas to present in teaching a patient who is taking a nasal decongestant for a short-term condition.

ACTION

Decongestants directly affect the alpha receptors of blood vessels in the nasal mucosa, causing vasoconstriction. This vasopressor action reduces blood flow, fluid exudation, and mucosal edema. Many agents also act on beta receptors, which may cause **rebound vasodilation,** or an increase in blood flow leading to further congestion. This is commonly seen with prolonged use of the medication.

USES

Decongestants are used to relieve nasal congestion associated with allergies and upper respiratory tract infections. The drugs may also be used as an adjunctive therapy for middle ear infections to decrease congestion around the eustachian tubes. Ear blockage, and pressure and pain caused by air travel may respond to nasal decongestants.

ADVERSE REACTIONS

Stinging and burning as a result of mucosal dryness sometimes follows topical administration. Rebound congestion may occur after prolonged use of topical agents. When the drug is absorbed from the gastrointestinal tract, systemic effects such as nervousness, nausea, dizziness, tachycardia, dysrhythmia, and a transient increase in blood pressure may occur. Rarely, a severe shocklike syndrome with hypotension and coma has been reported in children. Psychologic dependence and toxic psychoses have been reported with long-term high-dose therapy. The severity of overdosage varies widely, resulting in a variety of symptoms.

DRUG INTERACTIONS

The systemic effects of decongestants may be intensified by concurrent use of other sympathomimetics, MAO inhibitors, tricyclic antidepressants, antihistamines, and thyroxine. Decongestants should be used with caution in stable hypertensive patients on guanethidine, bethanidine, and debrisoquine sulfate. Use of decongestants with high doses of digitalis or use of other drugs that may sensitize the heart to dysrhythmias should be avoided, because anginal pain may result when there is coronary insufficiency.

 NURSING IMPLICATIONS AND PATIENT TEACHING

▼ Assessment

The patient may have a history of nasal congestion, postnasal drip, nasal discharge, sneezing, sore throat, headache, itchy eyes, lacrimation, nasal polyps, earache, decreased hearing, upper respiratory tract infection, or allergies.

Take a careful history, including allergy to adrenergic agents, narrow-angle glaucoma, concurrent MAO inhibitor or tricyclic antidepressant therapy, and loss of sensation in the fingers and toes. These are contraindications to the use of decongestants. Use cautiously in patients with hypertension, dysrhythmias, heart disease, angina, hyperthyroidism, diabetes, advanced arteriosclerotic conditions, glaucoma, prostatic hypertrophy, or chronic cough because of the possibility of systemic vasoconstriction and tachycardia. Also use with caution in patients with a long history of asthma and emphysema complicated by degenerative heart disease. Excessive administration of topical decongestants may result in gastrointestinal absorption and cause systemic effects. The safe use of decongestants in pregnancy has not been established.

▼ Planning

Frequent and continual use of the topical decongestants or at dosages greater than recommended may result in a rebound phenomenon. Topical decongestants should be used only in acute states, for no longer than 3 to 5 days, and sparingly in children and the elderly.

▼ Implementation

Oral decongestants are considered to be more effective than nasal preparations because they produce effects in inaccessible parts of the mucous membrane nasal passages. The effects may be more prolonged than those achieved by topical preparations. The disadvantage of the systemic agents is that their effects may be generalized and not limited to the nasal mucosa.

Topical application may take the form of drops, sprays, jellies, and oral inhalation. The advantage of this form of administration is the rapid onset of action and direct stimulation of the nasal mucosa. Drops have a tendency to pass into the hypopharynx and then be swallowed, thus passing into the gastrointestinal tract. Sprays deliver a fine mist that is easily trapped in the upper respiratory tract and are less likely to reach the gastrointestinal tract. Topical preparations should not be used for more than 3 to 5 days because of the risk of rebound phenomenon. Oral preparations are more appropriate for long-term use.

Drops should be given to the patient with the head held back to prevent swallowing of the drug. Use care not to touch the skin while administering topical products. Solutions can become contaminated with use and result in growth of bacteria and fungi.

▼ Evaluation

The nurse should monitor for cessation of symptoms and for development of rebound congestion seen by an increase in symptoms. If headache and nervousness develop, discontinue treatment.

▼ Patient and family teaching

The nurse should provide the patient and family with the following instructions:

1. To administer drops:
   a. Blow the nose gently.
   b. Assume a reclining position with the head tipped back over the edge of the bed.
   c. Put 1 to 2 drops of solution on the lower nasal mucosa.
   d. Breathe through the mouth.
   e. Remain in the position for 5 minutes while turning head from side to side; this will help the drops run back into the nose instead of down the throat.
2. To administer a spray:
   a. Keep the container upright to obtain a fine mist.
   b. Gently blow the nose.
   c. Squeeze the bottle firmly in each nostril.
   d. After 3 to 5 minutes, blow the nose again.
   e. Repeat application if congestion remains.
3. The patient should always rinse the dropper after putting drops into the nose. This will help prevent growth of bacteria and fungi.
4. Each person in the family should use a separate bottle of nasal spray. Topical decongestants should not be shared.
5. To administer jellies:
   a. Put a small amount on the finger.
   b. Apply it to the nasal mucosa.
   c. Snuff deeply through the nose.
6. To administer inhalers:
   a. Insert the open end of the plastic tube in each nostril.
   b. Inhale two times.
7. The patient should avoid excessive use of these medicines or they will cause the symptoms that the patient is trying to reduce.
8. Missed doses may be taken within an hour of the scheduled time and then the regular schedule may be resumed. If more than 1 hour has passed, skip that dose and return to the regular schedule.

• • •

Table 8-4 lists various nasal decongestant products. There are many other decongestants on the market, most available over the counter. Many of these products contain combinations of medications designed to make them attractive to the patient with a variety of symptoms. These drugs may contain a decongestant and one or more antihistamine, analgesic, antitussive, expectorant, or anticholinergic products. Each additional medication increases the precaution with which the drug should be used and the adverse effects that may be found. For example, drugs that contain anticholinergics cause drying of mucus secretions. They should be avoided in patients with asthma or chronic obstructive pulmonary disease. The patient should consider whether there is a need for all the components of the drugs listed. The composition of even well-known drugs changes frequently. Pharmacists are excellent sources of information about over-the-counter medications, and patients should be encouraged to seek their professional advice.

Table 8-4 Nasal decongestants

Generic name	Trade name	Comments and dosage
NASAL DROPS		
Ephedrine	Pretz-D Vatronol	May produce burning, stinging, dryness of nasal mucosa, and sneezing. *Adults and children 6 years and older:* 2 or 3 drops, or application of a small amount of jelly in each nostril q3 to 4h.
Epinephrine	Adrenalin	Stimulates both alpha and beta receptors. Give 1 to 2 drops in each nostril q4 to 6h.
INHALERS		
Propylhexadrine	Benzedrex	May be used as often as needed, but excessive use should be avoided. Rarely causes CNS stimulation. Insert plastic tip in nostril, close other nostril, and inhale two times. Repeat on other side.
Naphazoline	Privine	Has rapid and prolonged effect; produces CNS depression when swallowed. *Adults and children 6 years and older:* 2 drops in each nostril q3h.
Oxymetazoline	Afrin Dristan Duration	Prolonged decongestant effect. Often overused by patients, leading to rebound congestion when used longer than 3 days in succession. *Adults and children 6 years and older:* 2 squeezes each nostril bid, or 2 to 4 drops in each nostril bid.
Phenylephrine	Neo-Synephrine Sinex	Drug ineffective if exposed to air, strong light, or heat. Very effective topical preparation, but it may cause marked local irritation. *Adults:* 0.25% to 1.0% strength, 3 to 4 drops or 1 to 2 sprays q4h. *Children 6 to 12 years:* Use 0.25%, 2 to 3 drops q3 to 4h. *Children 2 to 6 years:* Use 0.167%, 2 to 3 drops q4h. *Infants:* Use 0.125%, 2 to 3 drops q3 to 4h.
Phenylpropanolamine	Propagest Rhindecon	*Adults:* 25 mg PO q4h or 50 mg q6 to 8h; do not exceed 150 mg daily. *Children 2 to 12 years:* 6 to 25 to 12.5 mg PO q4h or 25 mg q8h.
Pseudoephedrine sulfate	Sudafed	*Adults and children 12 years and older:* 60 mg PO tid to qid; or 120 mg timed-release capsule can be given PO q12h. *Children 2 to 12 years:* 15 to 30 mg PO tid or qid.
Tetrahydrozoline	Tyzine	*Adults and children 6 years and older:* 2 to 4 drops of 0.1% solution in each nostril as needed, but no more than q3h. *Children 2 to 6 years:* 2 to 3 drops of 0.05% solution in each nostril no more than q3h.
Xylometazoline	Otrivin Sinutab ♣ sinus spray	Action lasts 8 to 10 hours. Overdose can cause extreme CNS depression in children. *Adults:* Give 2 to 3 sprays or 2 to 3 drops in each nostril. *Children under 12 years:* Use 2 to 3 drops of 0.05% q8 to 10h.

SECTION SIX: EXPECTORANTS

Objectives

At the conclusion of this section you should be able to:

1. Identify products used as expectorants.

2. List two common uses of expectorants.
3. Evaluate the effectiveness of different kinds of expectorants.
4. Describe contraindications to the use of expectorants.

ACTION

Expectorants are agents that decrease the thickness of respiratory secretions and aid in their removal. It is believed they work by increasing the amount of fluid in the respiratory tract. These increased liquid secretions promote ciliary action and decrease the amount of coughing while increasing the amount of sputum produced. There is considerable controversy regarding their therapeutic effectiveness.

USES

Expectorants are used to treat symptoms of productive cough. These products may be useful in chronic respiratory disease when thick mucus is a complication.

ADVERSE REACTIONS

Gastrointestinal upset is a common adverse reaction to expectorants.

DRUG INTERACTIONS

Expectorants with guaifenesin may increase bleeding tendency. Patients on anticoagulants must be closely monitored if they are given expectorants.

 NURSING IMPLICATIONS AND PATIENT TEACHING

▼ Assessment

The nurse should obtain a complete health history, including the history of cough, presence of other respiratory disease, hypersensitivity, and other medications that may cause drug interactions.

▼ Planning

Expectorants are not to be used in persistent cough without the advice of a physician. Chronic or persistent cough may be the result of a serious condition and should not be ignored.

▼ Implementation

The patient should take an increased amount of fluid each day and breathe humidified air. This will help liquefy secretions. Medication should be taken with at least one full glass of water.

See Table 8-5 for a summary of expectorants.

▼ Evaluation

The nurse should monitor for therapeutic effect.

Table 8-5 Expectorants		
Generic name	**Trade name**	**Comments and dosage**
Guaifenesin	Anti-Tuss Robitussin	Although there is a lack of convincing evidence to document clinical efficacy, this is a widely publicized product. *Adults:* 100 to 400 mg PO q4 to 6h; maximum dose 2.4 gm/day. *Children 6 to 12 years:* 50 to 100 mg PO q4 to 6h; maximum dose 600 mg/day. *Children 2 to 6 years:* 50 mg PO q4h; maximum dose 300 mg/day.
Iodinated glycerol	Organidin	Patients may develop dose-related dermatitis, gastrointestinal upset, or rash. Hypersensitivity, thyroid enlargement, and acute parotitis are rare. One drop is approximately equal to 3 mg. *Adults:* 60 mg PO qid with water; one teaspoon (5 ml) elixir qid; or 20 drops of solution qid with water. May also be taken with juice or milk if diet allows. *Children:* Up to half of the adult dose, based on weight.
Iodine products	SSKI Potassium iodide Pima	Do not use continuously, because prolonged use may lead to hypothyroidism. ■ *Potassium Iodide* *Adults:* 300 mg in liquid q4 to 6h. *Children:* 250 to 1000 mg daily in two to four divided doses. ■ *SSKI* *Adults:* 0.3 to 0.6 ml four to twelve times daily, diluted in a glass of water, juice, or milk.

If the patient uses more than the recommended dosage, adverse reactions may occur.

▼ Patient and family teaching

The nurse should provide the patient and family with the following instructions:

1. The patient should be aware that this drug will help make the sputum more liquid. This will make it easier to bring sputum up when the patient coughs.
2. The patient should use a humidifier and drink at least 2 quarts of water daily while taking this product. These will aid the medication in bringing the mucus up.
3. The physician should be notified if the cough is accompanied by high fever, rash, or persistent headaches, or if the cough returns once patient feels it has been under control.
4. The patient should use this medication only in the dosage recommended to decrease chances of side effects.

SECTION SEVEN: INTRANASAL STEROIDS

Objectives

At the conclusion of this section you should be able to:

1. Identify the indications for the use of intranasal steroids.
2. List at least three intranasal steroid products.
3. Describe the proper way to administer intranasal steroids.
4. Identify at least five adverse reactions from intranasal steroids.
5. Present major ideas to cover in teaching a patient about intranasal steroids.

ACTION

The main action of topical intranasal steroids is the antiinflammatory effect of decreasing local congestion.

USES

Topical intranasal steroids are used to treat allergic, mechanical, or chemically induced local nasal inflammation or nasal polyps only when more conventional treatment has been tried and found to be ineffective. They are first-line drugs in treatment of asthma.

ADVERSE REACTIONS

Adverse reactions to topical intranasal steroids include asthma, headache, lightheadedness, loss of sense of smell, nasal irritation and dryness, nausea, nosebleeds, perforation of the nasal septum, rebound congestion, skin rash.

DRUG INTERACTIONS

Intranasal steroids may interact with many products. Consult section on corticosteroids.

 NURSING IMPLICATIONS AND PATIENT TEACHING

▼ Assessment

The nurse should obtain a complete health history, including the presence of hypersensitivity, fungal infections, tuberculosis, ocular herpes simplex, local infections (especially of nose, sinus, or throat), and the possibility of pregnancy. These conditions are contraindications or precautions to the use of topical nasal steroids. The nurse should determine the patient's past experience and response to nasal sprays.

▼ Planning

The patient receiving topical intranasal steroids should not be given smallpox vaccination and immunizations, because the immunologic response may be depressed. In the presence of latent tuberculosis or tuberculosis reactivity, close observation and possible chemoprophylaxis may be indicated. The effects of the drug are enhanced in patients with hypothyroidism and cirrhosis.

▼ Implementation

The recommended dosage must not be exceeded. The dosage should be decreased with subjective improvement of the patient.

See Table 8-6 for a summary of nasal steroids.

▼ Evaluation

The nurse should evaluate the therapeutic action: reduction in nasal stuffiness, obstruction, or discharge, and relief of sinus headaches. The nurse should also monitor the frequency of use and the dosage used. Evidence of cracked or bleeding nasal mucosa should be sought. The nurse should be alert for adverse reactions, such as signs of systemic absorption and fluid retention, elevated blood pressure, weight gain, ankle edema, or evidence of local infection.

Nasal dryness and irritation are side effects and do not usually necessitate discontinuing the drug. The dosage of the drug should be gradually reduced to avoid adrenocortical insufficiency.

The drug may decrease resistance to infection as well as mask some common signs of infection. Elevation of blood pressure, retention of salt and fluid, and increased potassium and calcium loss may occur if the patient takes large doses. This may be treated with dietary salt restriction and potassium supplementation. Loss of the ability to smell, shortness of breath, unrelieved stuffy nose, chest tightness, or wheezing indicates a need for physician intervention.

The patient should be observed for signs of systemic absorption, because fluid retention and temporary inhibition of pituitary-adrenal function may develop.

▼ Patient and family teaching

The nurse should provide the patient and family with the following instructions:

1. The patient should not use this drug if he or she has an infection. Patients should notify the physician if they develop an infection while taking this drug.
2. To avoid the chance of the medication being absorbed into the general circulation, the prescribed dosage and frequency must not be exceeded.
3. Dryness and irritation of the nose may occur temporarily.
4. The drug should be used in the smallest effective dose for the shortest period of time to prevent general absorption.

Table 8-6 Intranasal steroids

Generic name	Trade name	Comments and dosage
Beclomethasone dipropionate	Beclovent Vanceril Beconase Vancenase	Use after other conventional therapy has been found to be ineffective. Symptomatic relief is not immediate, and therapy should be continued even with initial minimal response. Maximal response should be seen within 3 weeks or medication should be discontinued. *Adults and children over 12 years:* One inhalation in each nostril bid to qid. Taper off gradually as relief is obtained.
Dexamethasone	Decadron Turbinaire	The maximum dosage for adults is 12 sprays/day and 8 sprays/day for children. This drug is available by prescription only. *Adults:* 2 sprays bid to tid. *Children 6 years or older:* 1 or 2 sprays bid.
Flunisolide	Aerobid Nasalide Bronalide ✦ aerosol	*Adults:* two sprays in each nostril bid; may increase to tid if warranted. Do not use more than 8 sprays/day/nostril. Maintenance dose may be 1 spray/day/nostril. *Children 6 to 14 years:* 1 spray in each nostril tid; may give 2 sprays in each nostril bid. Maximum dose is 4 sprays/day/nostril. Taper to 1 spray/day/nostril.
Triamcinolone acetonide	Nasacort	*Adults:* two sprays daily in each nostril. Increase doses depending on response.

5. Dosage may need to be tapered slowly and not stopped suddenly, especially if doses have been used for long periods of time.

7. The physician should be notified if symptoms do not improve or if they get worse.

SUMMARY

The following respiratory medications are used to treat allergies or respiratory system disorders: antihistamines, or allergy medications; antitussives, or medications to control cough; asthma medications; bronchodilators; decongestants; expectorants; and nasal steroids. Respiratory medications are available in many forms, as both prescription and over-the-counter medications. Monitoring adverse reactions and teaching the patient about adverse reactions, administration, and dosage considerations are important responsibilities of the nurse in administering respiratory medications.

 ## CRITICAL THINKING QUESTIONS

1. Ms. Allbright comes into your clinic complaining that her antihistamine dosage needs adjustment. You ask her to describe her symptoms, and she gives you the classic symptoms indicating a need for antihistamine. What *are* the signs and symptoms that would indicate antihistamine administration?

2. The doctor listens to your report of Ms. Allbright's complaints and then shakes her head. She tells you that Ms. Allbright has been taking an antihistamine for an extended period of time. The physician suspects that she has built up a possible psychologic dependence, leading to overuse and rebound reactions. What symptoms would lead you to suspect that Ms. Allbright is undergoing the rebound phenomenon? How do you determine if the medication has not been helpful, as Ms. Allbright has claimed from the beginning, or if her symptoms are due to the rebound phenomenon?

3. Mr. Tracy enters the clinic, bringing in with him not only a cold autumn wind, but a nasty cough! He demands loudly in the reception area to be given "cough drops right away!" You understand his discomfort, but tell him you need to ask him some questions

first. What questions will you ask Mr. Tracy about his cough (when it's his turn, of course)? In what situations would you not want to suppress a cough?

4. The physician responds to his examination of Mr. Tracy (and your outstanding assessment notes) by determining that Mr. Tracy should indeed be given something to relieve his coughing. What class of drugs is commonly used to relieve coughing? And what is "symptomatic relief"? Why are these medications used in nonproductive coughs?

5. Mr. Tracy has been prescribed an antitussive. Develop a patient teaching plan that includes a discussion of possible adverse reactions and drug interactions. What will you tell Mr. Tracy?

6. Ms. Henry has just been told she has asthma. She tells you that she has "suspected it for quite some time, but still, well, it is a surprise anyway." She asks you to tell her what causes asthma. Then she asks you to explain why she has to take medication right now, when she hasn't had an "attack" for several weeks. Identify some of the causes to Ms. Henry, explaining that you can't say exactly what caused hers. Then explain the differences between treatment and prophylaxis, and why she needs prophylactic therapy.

7. Ms. Henry has never used a Spinhaler before, but although she is nervous about that, she is willing to learn. Draw up a teaching plan for Ms. Henry, showing her how to properly place the capsules in the Spinhaler and how to inhale. Include strategies in reducing the coughing reaction and care of the Spinhaler itself.

8. Mr. Jeffries enters the clinic coughing and complains of difficulty with breathing. From the way he is holding his chest, you wonder if he is not experiencing bronchospasm. What symptoms and signs will you look for, in physical examination of the chest, to report to the physician?

9. Mr. Jeffries has been prescribed a sympathomimetic. Draw up a nursing care and patient education plan for him; build into the plan ways to monitor regularly for paradoxical bronchospasm, as well as a thorough explanation of the need for hydration.

10. Ms. Rochester has had several nasal polyps removed and has been placed on intranasal steroids. She is worried about taking any kind of steroid and tells you so. "I wouldn't mind as much, I guess, if I just knew what to watch out for," she says. Identify the most common adverse reactions to nasal steroids; compare them to systemic steriods.

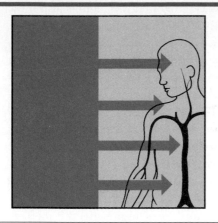

CHAPTER 9

Antiinfective Medications

OBJECTIVES

At the conclusion of this chapter you should be able to:

1. Identify the major categories of drugs used as antiinfective agents and the organisms against which they are effective.

2. Define "spectrum" and give examples of how it is used in antiinfective therapy.

3. List some of the common adverse reactions to medications used to treat infections.

4. Present ideas to teach the patient taking antiinfective medications.

OVERVIEW

This chapter discusses medications used to treat various types of infections. Because of the wide variety of infections and the numerous medications that have been developed to treat them, nurses are commonly involved in giving antiinfective medications and teaching patients about them.

Many organisms are found on the skin and inside the body of healthy individuals. A change in the effectiveness of the skin as a barrier or an increase in the individual's vulnerability may lead to the development of infections. An organism that produces infection is a **pathogen.**

Pathogenic organisms come in a variety of forms. Each infection must be carefully evaluated to determine the specific organism causing the infection and the drug that will be most effective against it. Although some parasites may be observed with the naked eye, most organisms are only visible under the microscope. They must be carefully cultured and tested for medication sensitivity. Organisms can be identified by their shape, and are classed as positive or negative, depending on whether they retain various dyes. Specific identification allows the physician to determine which medication will best control that particular organism.

Antiinfective agents, or **antimicrobials,** are chemicals that kill or incapacitate the pathogenic organisms. Some of these chemicals are produced from other living microorganisms (such as the penicillins), and are classified as **antibiotics.** Other chemicals are synthetically derived (such as sulfonamides) or are combinations of synthetic and naturally occurring microorganisms. Some medications have become more refined, purified, and sensitive as a result of long-term testing. Many new antiinfective medications appear every year because of the research in this area. Thus, there are many **generations** of drugs: drugs, such as cephalosporins, may be classed as first, second, or third generation agents, based on their development from other medications. In general, second and third generation drugs are progressively more effective than first generation agents against a broad group of gram-negative organisms; however, they are progressively less effective against gram-

positive organisms. Third generation agents also show more efficacy against resistant organisms and have increased resistance to beta-lactamase inactivation, but they cost more. Differences among drugs within categories are primarily based on the drug's activity.

Antiinfective medications work in a variety of ways. Usually they interfere with some important life process of a pathogen, thereby making it weaker, or incapable of reproducing; or they actually kill the organism. The term **bacteriostatic** refers to medications that limit the growth of an organism; **bactericidal** refers to drugs that actually destroy the organism.

We describe the number of organisms the medication is effective against in terms of its **spectrum.** Some antiinfective medications are effective against only a few organisms. These are called **narrow-spectrum drugs.** Other medications are effective against a wide variety of organisms. These are known as **broad-spectrum drugs.**

This chapter summarizes the important information about many types of antiinfective medications and is divided into six sections. Section One discusses the broad-spectrum antibiotics. Section Two explores antifungal medications. Section Three describes antitubercular pharmacotherapy, and Section Four discusses medications used to treat parasitic infections, including amebicides, anthelmintics, and antimalarial preparations. Sections Five and Six explore the penicillin and sulfonamide medications.

SECTION ONE: BROAD-SPECTRUM ANTIBIOTICS

Objectives

At the conclusion of this section you should be able to:
1. List the common broad-spectrum antibiotics.
2. Define "spectrum" as it is used in pharmacotherapy.
3. Give examples of common adverse reactions to antibiotics.
4. Identify key elements to include in the patient's teaching plan.

ACTION

Penicillins were the primary antibiotics for many years. They were used for almost every type of infection, including those for which they were not effective. Over the years, overuse and inappropriate use of penicillin has led to the development of penicillin-resistant strains of disease. Penicillin allergy has also become a problem. Although penicillin continues to be an important antibiotic, research concerning penicillin has led to the identification of many other types of antibiotics that may now be used to control infection.

Broad-spectrum antibiotics act in different ways to affect pathogenic bacteria. They may attack a bacterium's internal cell processes, which are vital to its existence, or may destroy the external cell wall. Thus, the antibiotics may be either bactericidal or bacteriostatic.

USES

Broad-spectrum antibiotics are used to treat infections caused by certain susceptible organisms. For the medication to be effective, the organism responsible for the infection should be identified through a culture. The medication effective against that particular organism is determined through sensitivity testing. Organisms are often classified as positive or negative, depending on the dye used to stain them.

Antibiotics are not effective against viral, parasitic, or fungal infections. It is common for a patient with a viral or fungal infection to also develop a bacterial infection, because the body's defenses are weakened. This is a secondary infection, when one infection follows another, or a mixed infection, when both infections are present at the same time. Table 9-1 summarizes the organisms that specific antibiotics are effective against or the primary problems for which the medication might be used.

ADVERSE REACTIONS

There are three primary types of adverse reactions seen with most antibiotics. **Superinfections** (overgrowth of other organisms not sensitive to the medication) may develop, particularly after long-term use. These reactions are usually quite irritating but mild, such as diarrhea, oral thrush, or vaginal itching. At other times, the superinfection may become life threatening. Overgrowth of organisms is commonly seen in AIDS patients, whose immune systems may be totally overwhelmed by a mild superinfection. Oral antibiotics commonly produce mild episodes of nausea, vomiting, and diarrhea, but rarely require discontinuation of therapy. These effects are often dose related, and they result from gastrointestinal irritation, changes in the normal bacterial flora in the bowel, and overgrowth of yeast.

All drugs have the potential to damage the tissue of certain organs. The usual organs that are affected are

 Table 9-1   Sensitivity of specific organisms to antibiotics

Antibiotic	Susceptible organisms and clinical diseases
Tetracyclines	Tetracyclines are used to treat granuloma inguinale, rickettsial diseases, *Mycoplasma* infections, spirochetal relapsing fever, and *Chlamydia trachomatis*. This drug is indicated in patients sensitive to penicillin, especially to treat gonorrhea or syphilis.
Erythromycin	Erythromycin is an alternative treatment for patients hypersensitive to the penicillins.
Chloramphenicol	Chloramphenicol is the drug of choice to treat *Salmonella typhi* (typhoid fever). It is useful in serious infections caused by *Haemophilus influenzae* (ampicillin resistant), in lymphogranuloma, in psittacosis, and in rickettsial and *Salmonella* infections. It is used for meningitis caused by *Neisseria meningitidis* or in cases of streptococcal pneumonia in individuals allergic to penicillin. This drug should be used only in serious infections where other drugs have failed. The patient is usually admitted to the hospital, where adequate monitoring of status can take place.
Clindamycin	Clindamycin is used to treat severe infections caused by streptococci, pneumococci, staphylococci, or anaerobic bacteria when penicillin and erythromycin are contraindicated.
Colistimethate	Colistimethate is used to treat infections caused by *Enterobacter aerogenes*, *Escherichia coli*, *Klebsiella pneumoniae*, and *Pseudomonas aeruginosa*.
Lincomycin	Lincomycin is used to treat severe infections caused by susceptible strains of streptococci, pneumococci, and staphylococci when penicillin and erythromycin are contraindicated.
Spectinomycin	Spectinomycin is the drug of choice to treat gonorrhea in patients who are hypersensitive to the penicillins and to treat penicillinase-producing gonorrhea.
Vancomycin	Vancomycin is used to treat severe infections in patients who are hypersensitive to the penicillins or cephalosporins. It is effective in the treatment of staphylococcal endocarditis, osteomyelitis, pneumonia, soft tissue infections, and methicillin-resistant staphylococcal infections. Oral dosage is effective in the treatment of staphylococcal enterocolitis.
Aminoglycosides	Aminoglycosides are effective in the treatment of gram-negative infections when penicillin is contraindicated.
Polymyxin B	Polymyxin B is effective against all the gram-negative organisms, with the exception of *Proteus*. It is also effective in the treatment of acute infections caused by susceptible strains of *P. aeruginosa*, *H. influenzae*, *E. coli*, *E. aerogenes*, and *K. pneumoniae*.
Bacitracin	Bacitracin is restricted to use in severe illness. It is effective in the treatment of staphylococcal pneumonia or empyema in infants.

CRITICAL DECISION
Antiinfectives

■ *Aminoglycosides* are associated with significant nephrotoxicity or ototoxicity. Patient status must be closely monitored while patient takes this medication.

■ *Bacitracin* may cause renal failure as a result of tubular and glomerular necrosis; therefore patient renal status must be closely monitored.

the auditory nerves of the ear, the kidney, and the liver (producing ototoxicity, nephrotoxicity, and hepatotoxicity). Certain antibiotics are much more likely to produce tissue damage than others. It is important to carefully screen out patients who may have preexisting damage to these organs before medication is started.

Many individuals have demonstrated hypersensitivity or allergy to antibiotics. Allergic reactions may develop within minutes of taking the drug, or may appear days after discontinuing the medication. Hypersensitivity may also develop after repeated use of the

medication. Allergy may range from a mild skin rash or fever to severe and fatal anaphylaxis, characterized by shortness of breath, paralysis of the diaphragm, laryngeal edema, and shock. Patients must be closely questioned each time antibiotic therapy is ordered to determine sensitivity reactions. Cross-sensitivity from one type of antibiotic to another is common.

In addition to these general reactions, some antibiotics have specific adverse reactions associated with their use that should always be monitored. These reactions are summarized in Table 9-2.

DRUG INTERACTIONS

Antibiotics have many common drug interactions. These interactions commonly render the antibiotic ineffective or alter the effectiveness of the other medications. Each antibiotic must be evaluated carefully if the patient is taking other medications. Read about specific drug interactions for each drug in the manufacturer's product information.

Concurrent use of some antacids may impair the absorption of tetracycline. Concurrent use with food, milk, dairy products, or iron preparations may also impair the absorption of antibiotics.

 Table 9-2 Significant adverse reactions produced by specific antibiotics

Antibiotic	Adverse reaction
Tetracycline	Black hairy tongue
Cephalosporins	Painful IM injections, thrombophlebitis with IV therapy; may produce hemolytic anemia and other blood dyscrasias
Erythromycin	GI distress, sensorineural hearing loss, and hepatotoxicity
Chloramphenicol	Severe blood dyscrasias, including aplastic anemia, have been reported with short-term and long-term therapy; irreversible bone marrow depression has also been reported after therapy
Clindamycin	Severe and fatal colitis characterized by abdominal cramps, diarrhea, rectal passage of blood and mucus (these symptoms may not appear until after treatment is completed)
Colistin	Renal toxicity; transient neurologic disturbances have been reported with colistimethate, as well as nephrotoxicity manifested by decreased urinary output and increased serum creatinine
Lincomycin	Severe and fatal colitis characterized by abdominal cramps, diarrhea, or rectal passage of blood and mucus (these symptoms may not develop until treatment is completed); hypotension and cardiac arrest after rapid IV administration
Vancomycin	Nephrotoxicity with toxic effect increased in high serum levels or prolonged therapy; ototoxicity may also occur
Aminoglycosides	Significant renal toxicity, which is usually reversible; risk of toxicity increases in patients with renal impairment; significant auditory and vestibular ototoxicity may occur in patients on prolonged therapy or those taking higher than recommended dosages
Polymyxin B	Nephrotoxicity may develop, evidenced by proteinuria, cellular urinary casts, azotemia, decreased output, or elevated BUN; neurotoxicity may be evidenced by irritability, weakness, drowsiness, ataxia, numbness of extremities, blurring of vision, or respiratory paralysis
Bacitracin	Renal toxicity leading to tubular and glomerular necrosis has been reported; also increased serum drug levels without an increase in drug dosage and severe pain and rash with IM injection are seen

NURSING IMPLICATIONS AND PATIENT TEACHING

▼ Assessment

The patient in need of antibiotic therapy may be asymptomatic to severely ill. The nurse should keep in mind common indicators of infection, such as fever, inflammation, erythema, edema, or pain.

Patients reporting any previous allergy to the penicillins may also be allergic to some cephalosporins. Cephalosporins should be used with extreme caution in these individuals. Nephrotoxicity has been reported with some cephalosporins, and the incidence is greater in the elderly and in individuals with impaired renal function.

 CRITICAL DECISION
Antibiotic Cross-sensitivity

Cross-sensitivity exists within many categories of antibiotics. Any person with a history of multiple drug allergies should be carefully monitored when undergoing any antibiotic therapy.

The nurse should obtain a thorough health history, including prior renal damage, hepatic impairment, systemic lupus erythematosus, or alcoholism; medications that may interact with an antibiotic; pregnancy or breastfeeding; age; and occupation. These problems may be contraindications or precautions to antibiotic drug therapy.

▼ Planning

Many antibiotics cross the placental barrier and are secreted in breast milk. The use of tetracycline in pregnancy and in children under 8 years of age may produce tooth discoloration or inadequate bone or tooth development.

Many antibiotics should be given with extreme caution to patients with impaired renal function. Photosensitivity may occur with tetracycline treatment, so the patient should avoid exposure to the sun or ultraviolet rays.

Many of the parenteral antibiotics should be used with discretion because of their toxic effects. The risk of toxicity is low in patients with normal renal function and if the recommended dosage is not exceeded.

 CRITICAL DECISION
Antibiotic Therapy

Whenever possible, cultures should be drawn before initiation of antibiotic therapy. Usual sites cultured include sputum, urine, blood, wound, or nonhealing topical sites.

▼ Implementation

The nurse should make certain that the medications are taken at the proper time and for the full course of the therapy. The dosage depends on the type and the severity of the infection. All chewable forms of erythromycin must be fully chewed to obtain the complete therapeutic effect.

The strength for erythromycin is expressed as erythromycin base equivalence. Because of differences in absorption, 400 mg ethylsuccinate is required to provide the same free erythromycin serum levels as 250 mg erythromycin base, stearate, or estolate.

Many antibiotics may be administered orally or parenterally. Topical application should be avoided to prevent sensitization. The patient should be kept well hydrated. Forcing fluids to ensure a minimum output of 1500 ml will decrease the chances of renal toxicity.

The nurse should always aspirate before an IM injection to prevent medication from entering a blood vessel.

Lincomycin and tetracycline are best absorbed on an empty stomach, 1 hour before or 2 hours after meals, and should be taken with a full glass of water. In the treatment of syphilis, gonorrhea, or chlamydial infections, the infected partners also must be treated.

Outdated tetracycline should not be used because it may lead to damage of the proximal renal tubules. Tetracycline should be used with caution in patients with hepatic impairment because the drug may cause hepatotoxicity.

See Table 9-3 for a summary of antibiotics.

▼ Evaluation

Hypersensitivity reactions ranging from mild erythema to anaphylaxis have been reported with use of antibiotics. Vertigo may develop with the use of any of the tetracyclines; however, vertigo is more common with the use of minocycline.

Table 9-3 Antibiotics

Generic name	Trade name	Comments and dosage
AMINOGLYCOSIDES		
Amikacin	Amikin	May be used to treat unidentified infections before results of sensitivity tests are known. Do not mix with other drugs. *Adults and children:* 15 mg/kg/day IM or IV in two to three divided doses; do not exceed 1.5 gm/day. *Neonates:* 10 mg/kg loading dose followed by 7.5 mg/kg q12h.
Gentamicin	Garamycin	Used to treat unidentified infections. Do not mix with carbenicillin or other drugs. *Adults:* 1 mg/kg q8h; may use up to 5 mg/kg/day in three to four divided doses parenterally. *Children:* 2 to 2.5 mg/kg q8h.
Kanamycin	Kantrex Kamycine ♣	*Adults:* 3 to 12 gm/day PO in divided doses; 250 mg two to four times a day by inhalation. *Children:* 12.5 mg/kg/day PO in four divided doses. *Suppression of intestinal bacteria:* 1 gm PO qh for 4 hours, followed with 1 gm PO q6h for the next 36 to 72 hours. *Hepatic coma:* 8 to 12 gm/day PO in divided doses.
Neomycin	Mycifradin	Used in urinary tract infections and as preoperative preparation for surgery. *Suppression of intestinal bacteria:* Give 1 gm at 19 hours, 18 hours, and 9 hours before surgery.
Netilmicin	Netromycin	*Adults:* 1.5 to 2 mg/kg q12h.
Paromomycin	Humatin	*Intestinal amebiasis:* 25 to 35 mg/kg/day PO in three divided doses for 5 to 10 days with meals. *Hepatic coma:* 4 gm/day PO in divided doses for 5 to 6 days.
Streptomycin	Streptomycin	Administer deep IM in large muscle mass. *Adults:* 1st week: 1 gm parenterally bid; 2nd week: 0.5 gm parenterally bid with penicillin. ■ *Enterococcal endocarditis* *Adults:* 0.5 to 1 gm parenterally bid with penicillin for 4 weeks.
Tobramycin	Nebcin	May be used in combination with penicillin or cephalosporin in the treatment of unidentified infections before results of sensitivity tests are known. Do not premix with other drugs. *Adults and children:* 3 mg/kg/day IM q8h.
Polymyxin B	Aerosporin	Do not exceed 25,000 units/kg/day. IM administration not recommended because of severe pain at injection site. *Adults and children:* 15,000 units/kg/day IV in two divided doses.
Bacitracin	Bacitracin Bacitin ♣	*Infants under 2.5 kg:* 900 units/kg/day IM in two to three divided doses. *Patients over 2.5 kg:* 1000 units/kg/day IM in two to three divided doses.
Novobiocin	Albamycin	*Adults:* 250 mg q6h or 500 mg q12h PO. *Children:* 15 mg/kg/day to 30 mg/kg/day. Give for 48 hours after temperature returns to normal.

Table 9-3   Antibiotics—cont'd

Generic name	Trade name	Comments and dosage
CEPHALOSPORINS		
First Generation		
Cephalexin	Keflex	*Adults:* 1 to 4 gm/day in divided doses.
		Children: 25 to 50 mg/kg/day in divided doses.
	Keftab	*Adults:* 1 to 4 gm/day in divided doses. Do not use in children.
Cefadroxil	Duricef	*Adults:* 1 to 2 gm/day in single or 2 divided doses.
	Ultracef	*Children:* 30 mg/kg/day in divided doses every 12 hours.
Cephradine	Velosef	Give PO, IM or IV. *Adults:* 250 mg every 6 hours.
		Children: 25 to 50 mg/kg/day in divided doses.
Cephalothin	Keflin	Give IV piggyback or deep IM. *Adults:* 500 mg to 1 gm q4 to 6h.
		Children: 100 mg/kg/day in divided doses.
Cephapirin	Cefadyl	IM or IV use. *Adults:* 500 mg to 1 gm q4 to 6h.
		Children: 40 mg/kg in 4 divided doses.
Cefazolin	Ancef	IM or IV use. *Adults:* 250 mg to 1 gm q8h.
	Kefzol	
	Zolicef	
Second Generation		
Cefaclor	Ceclor	*Adults:* 250 to 500 mg PO q8h.
		Children: Give 20 mg/kg/day in divided doses.
Cefamandole	Mandol	IM or IV. *Adults:* 500 mg to 1 gm q4 to 8h.
		Children: 50 to 100 mg/kg/day in divided doses.
Cefoxitin	Mefoxin	Recommended by CDC in treatment schedules for gonorrhea and acute pelvic inflammatory disease. *Adults:* 1 to 4 gm q6 to 8h.
Cefuroxime	Ceftin	*Adults:* 250 to 500 mg bid.
	Kefurox	See CDC treatment schedules for gonorrhea and acute pelvic
	Zinacef	inflammatory disease.
Cefonicid	Monocid	*Adults:* 1 gm q24h IV or deep IM.
Cefmetazole	Zefazone	*Adults:* 2 gm IV q6 to 12h for 5 to 14 days.
Cefotetan	Cefotan	*Adults:* 1 to 2 gm IV or IM q12h for 5 to 10 days.
Cefprozil	Cefzil	*Adults:* 500 mg PO q24h for 10 days.
		Children: 15 mg/kg PO q12h for 10 days.
Cefpodoxime	Vantin	200 mg PO q12h for 14 days. Reduce dosage in renal insufficiency.
Loracarbef	Lorabid	*Adults:* 200 to 400 mg PO q12h for 7 days.
		Children: 30 mg/kg/day in divided doses for 10 days.
Third Generation		
Cefixime	Suprax	*Adults:* 400 mg/day PO or 200 mg q12h.
		Children: 8 mg/kg/day PO or 4 mg/kg q12h.
Cefoperazone	Cefobid	IM or IV. *Adults:* 2 to 4 gm/day in 2 divided doses.
Cefotaxime	Claforan	Give IV or IM. Maximum daily dose is 12 gm. Dosage depends on severity.
Ceftizoxime	Cefizox	*Adults:* 1 or 2 gm q8 to 12h.
Ceftriaxone	Rocephin	*Adults:* 1 to 2 gm once a day IV or IM.
		Children: 50 to 75 mg/kg/day.
Ceftazidime	Fortaz	*Adults:* 1 gm IV or IM q8 to 12h.
	Tazidime	
	Tazicef	

Continued.

Table 9-3 Antibiotics—cont'd

Generic name	Trade name	Comments and dosage
CHLORAMPHENICOL		
Chloramphenicol	Chloramphenicol Chloromycetin	Give PO on empty stomach. Switch from IV to oral form as soon as possible. Chloramphenicol sodium succinate is effective only if administered IV and must not exceed 100 mg/ml. Administer over 1- to 2-minute interval. Avoid repeated courses of therapy. *Adults:* 50 to 100 mg/kg/day in four divided doses. *Children:* 50 mg/kg/day in four divided doses.
LINCOSAMIDES		
Clindamycin	Cleocin	Give deep IM. Single IM injections that total 600 mg or greater are not recommended. For IV therapy, do not administer as bolus. For oral administration, take on empty stomach with a full glass of water. *Adults:* 150 to 300 mg PO q6h, more severe infections may require 300 to 450 mg PO q6h; 600 to 1200 mg/day parenterally in two to four divided doses, more severe infections may require 1200 to 2700 mg/day in two to four divided doses. *Children:* 8 to 16 mg/kg/day PO in three to four divided doses, more severe infections may require 16 to 20 mg/kg/day PO in three to four divided doses; 15 to 25 mg/kg/day parenterally in three to four divided doses, more severe infections may require 25 to 40 mg/kg/day parenterally in three to four divided doses.
Lincomycin	Lincocin Lincorex	*Adults:* 500 mg PO q8h, with more severe infections requiring 500 mg PO q6h; or 600 mg/day IM as a single dose, more severe infections may require 500 mg IM q12h; 600 mg to 1 gm IV q8 to 12h. Maximum dose is 8 gm/day.
MISCELLANEOUS		
Colistin	Coly-Mycin S	*Adults and children:* 5 to 15 mg/kg/day PO in three divided doses.
Cholistimethate	Coly-Mycin M	*Adults and children:* 2.5 to 5 mg/kg/day parenterally in two to four divided doses. Do not exceed 5 mg/kg/day in patients with normal renal function. Dosage must be altered in patients with impaired renal function.
Spectinomycin	Trobicin	*Adults:* 2 gm IM as a single dose. *For antibiotic resistance:* 4 gm IM divided between two injection sites. *Disseminated gonococcal infections:* 2 gm IM bid for 3 days.
Vancomycin	Vancocin Vancoled	Should be administered IV, not IM. Rapid IV administration may cause hypotension. Dilute solution in 200 ml of glucose or saline solution and infuse over a 30-minute period. IV infusion may cause thrombophlebitis. Drug of choice in treating *Staphylococcus* bacteria. *Adults:* 500 mg q6h or 1 gm PO or IV q12h, lower with renal impairment. *Children:* 20 mg/lb/day PO in divided doses; 44 mg/kg/day IV in divided doses.
FLUOROQUINOLONES		Medications are excreted primarily by renal mechanism. All dosages must be adjusted in patients with impaired renal function. Calculate serum creatinine levels to determine accurate dosage. Keep patients well hydrated.
Ciprofloxacin	Cipro	*Adults:* 250 to 500 mg q12h or 200 to 400 mg IV q12h. Duration depends on severity of infection.

Table 9-3   Antibiotics—cont'd

Generic name	Trade name	Comments and dosage
FLUOROQUINOLONES (cont'd)		
Enoxacin	Penetrex	*Adults:* 200 to 500 mg q12h for 7 to 14 days. Take 1 hour before or 2 hours after a meal.
Lomefloxacin	Maxaquin	*Adults:* 400 mg once daily for 10 to 14 days.
Norfloxacin	Noroxin	*Adults:* 400 mg q12h for 3 to 10 days. Take 1 hour before or 2 hours after meals with glass of water.
Ofloxacin	Floxin	*Adults:* 200 to 400 mg q12h for 7 to 10 days.
MACROLIDES		
Azithromycin	Zithromax	500 mg as a single dose on the first day followed by 250 mg once daily on days 2 through 5 for a total dose of 1.5 gm. Administer 1 hour before or 2 hours after a meal.
Clarithromycin	Biaxin	250 to 500 mg q12h for 7 to 14 days.
Erythromycin	E.E.S. E-Mycin Ilosone	*Adults:* 250 mg (400 mg ethylsuccinate) PO q6h; 15 to 20 mg/kg/day parenterally. Dosage may be increased with the severity of the infection. *Children:* 30 to 50 mg/kg/day PO in three to four divided doses; 15 to 20 mg/kg/day IM.
Troleandomycin	Tao	*Adults:* 250 to 500 mg qid for 10 days. *Children:* 125 to 250 mg (6.6 to 11 mg/kg) q6h for 10 days.
TETRACYCLINES		
Demeclocycline	Declomycin	Frequently associated with photosensitivity and anaphylactoid reactions. *Adults:* 150 mg PO qid or 300 mg PO bid. *Children over 8 years:* 3 to 6 mg/lb/day PO in two or four divided doses.
Doxycycline	Vibramycin	Used to prevent traveler's diarrhea. It may be taken with food. *Adults:* 200 mg PO in two divided doses for the first day; follow with 100 mg/day in two divided doses or as a single dose. *Children over 8 years:* 2 mg/lb/day in two divided doses for the first day; follow with 1 mg/lb/day in two divided doses or as a single dose.
Methacycline	Rondomycin	*Adults:* 150 mg PO qid. *Children over 8 years:* 3 to 6 mg/lb/day in two or four divided doses.
Minocycline	Minocin	Has delayed kidney excretion, as compared with other tetracyclines. Half-life is 11 to 20 hours. *Adults:* 200 mg PO initially, then 100 mg q12h. *Children over 8 years:* 4 mg/kg initially, then 2 mg/kg q12h.
Oxytetracycline	Terramycin	Diarrhea common. Give deep IM in gluteal mass. If pain persists after injection, ice may be applied to the area. Avoid rapid IV administration. *Adults:* 1 to 2 gm/day PO; 100 to 250 mg IM q12h; 100 to 250 mg IV q12h. Do not exceed 500 mg q6h. *Children over 8 years:* 10 to 20 mg/lb/day PO in four divided doses; 15 to 25 mg/kg/day IM in two or three divided doses; 10 to 20 mg/kg/day IV in two doses.
Tetracycline	Achromycin	Administer deep IM. Ice may be applied to the injection site. Avoid rapid IV administration. *Adults:* 1 to 4 gm/day PO; 250 to 500 mg/day or 300 mg IV or IM in divided doses q8 to 12h. *Children over 8 years:* 10 to 20 mg/lb/day PO; or 12 mg/kg/day IM or IV in two divided doses.

Superinfection may occur in the patient undergoing extended antibiotic therapy. The nurse should monitor infections in the mouth and the rectal or vaginal areas.

Because of the possibility of ototoxicity in patients taking vancomycin, the nurse should monitor for tinnitus (ringing in the ears), which may precede deafness.

The nurse should monitor for liver toxicity by checking for abdominal pain, jaundice, dark urine, pale-colored stools, or weakness. Blood or mucus in the stools may indicate colitis. If large doses of antibiotics are given, the patient should be monitored closely for sensorineural hearing loss. The nurse should observe for therapeutic effects, hypersensitivity, and superinfection.

▼ Patient and family teaching

The nurse should provide the patient and family with the following instructions:

1. The patient should take tetracycline and lincomycin on an empty stomach, 1 hour before or 2 hours after eating, and follow with a full glass of water. Most other antibiotics should be taken with meals or food to decrease gastrointestinal upset.
2. If gastrointestinal upset occurs, the patient should eat a few plain crackers with the medicine.
3. The patient should take the medicine exactly as prescribed, even after the symptoms disappear. The medication should not be saved, because taking out-of-date medication may cause rather severe anal irritation.
4. The patient taking tetracyclines should avoid the sun or ultraviolet light.
5. The patient should use care in bathing and when brushing teeth, and watch for signs of infection in the mouth and the anal or vaginal areas.
6. The patient should notify nurse or physician if diarrhea persists for more than 24 hours or if stools have blood or mucus.
8. The patient should not take tetracyclines with any iron preparations, antacids, milk, or dairy products.
9. The patient should watch for dizziness; if it develops, it may be severe enough to limit driving or operating machinery.
10. Liquid medication should be kept in light-resistant containers.
11. The patient with diabetes should be made aware that many antibiotics change the urine glucose test.
12. The patient should be alert to the possibility of bone marrow depression after therapy is completed, and promptly report any bruising, petechiae, sore throat, or weakness.

SECTION TWO: ANTIFUNGALS

Objectives

At the conclusion of this section you should be able to:
1. Identify common antifungal preparations.
2. List adverse reactions associated with antifungal preparations.

ACTION

A fungus is a plant that produces yeastlike or moldlike diseases, called **mycotic infections,** in humans. These can be either superficial infections, such as in the skin or nail, or systemic infections, such as in the lung or liver. **Antifungals** are medications used to treat these infections.

Nystatin is a polyene antibiotic with fungistatic or fungicidal activity. The drug may allow intracellular components to leak through the fungal cell membrane by binding to sterols in the cell membrane.

Griseofulvin is a fungistatic or fungicidal antibiotic derived from *Penicillium griseofulvum*. It deposits in keratin precursor cells where it becomes tightly bound, leaving new keratin cells that are highly resistant to fungal infection as exfoliation occurs.

Ketoconazole is a broad-spectrum antibiotic with fungistatic or fungicidal activity. It impairs the synthesis of the fungus cell membrane, producing increased membrane permeability, which causes the cellular components to leak out.

Flucytosine is a synthetic, fluorinated antifungal

agent with fungistatic activity. The antifungal activity is evident when 5-FC is converted to 5-fluorouracil in the fungus cell, thereby inhibiting nucleic acid synthesis. Flucytosine acts as a fungicidal agent when used in high dosages.

USES

Nystatin is used to treat intestinal, vaginal, and oral fungal infections caused by susceptible strains of *Candida albicans* and other *Candida* species. Griseofulvin is used to treat fungal infections involving the hair, skin, and nails caused by susceptible species of *Epidermophyton, Microsporum,* and *Trichophyton.*

Ketoconazole is used to treat systemic fungal infections caused by candidiasis, chronic mucocutaneous candidiasis, oral thrush, candiduria, blastomycosis, paracoccidioidomycosis, coccidioidomycosis, histoplasmosis, and chromomycosis. It has also been used to treat pityriasis versicolor and vaginal candidiasis. Flucytosine is used to treat serious systemic fungal infections caused by susceptible strains of *Candida* and *Cryptococcus.*

The antifungal drugs have increasingly higher use in the past few years because of their application in treating the opportunistic yeast infections associated with the AIDS virus.

ADVERSE REACTIONS

Adverse reactions of *nystatin* include nausea, vomiting, or diarrhea. The symptoms increase with overdosage.

Griseofulvin may produce headache, vertigo, dizziness, irritability, sore throat, nausea, vomiting, epigastric distress, dryness of mouth, oral thrush, black furry tongue, anorexia, diarrhea, photosensitivity, rash, urticaria, changes in blood cells, angioneurotic edema, arthralgia, blurred vision, proteinuria, fever, malaise, and vaginal discharge. Nausea, vomiting, and diarrhea are symptoms of overdosage.

Metronidazole is carcinogenic in rats. Avoid unnecessary use.

Ketoconazole may produce abdominal pain, diarrhea, dizziness, fever, headache, gynecomastia, impotence, nausea, photophobia, pruritus, and vomiting. Oligospermia has been reported in patients taking excessively high dosages. Severe nausea, vomiting, and diarrhea are symptoms of overdosage.

Flucytosine may produce headache, drowsiness, confusion, vertigo, macular rash, urticaria, nausea, vom-

iting, diarrhea, blood cell changes, and abnormal liver function tests.

CRITICAL DECISION
Antifungals

- *Ketoconazole* has been associated with hepatic toxicity, so patient must be monitored closely.
- *Flucytosine:* Close monitoring of hematologic, renal, and hepatic status is essential.
- *Flagyl and alcohol:* Counsel patients not to drink alcohol or eat alcohol-containing products while taking this medication because a severe GI and cardiovascular response may develop.

DRUG INTERACTIONS

Severe superinfection may result when antifungals are given concurrently with prolonged corticosteroid therapy. Activity of oral anticoagulants is decreased when they are used concomitantly with griseofulvin; it may be necessary to adjust the anticoagulant dosage. Griseofulvin activity is decreased when used concurrently with barbiturates, requiring dosage adjustments of griseofulvin. Use of alcohol while taking antifungals potentiates the effect of the alcohol.

Because antacids, anticholinergics, and H_2 blockers change gastrointestinal pH, at least 2 hours should separate the ingestion of any of these medications and ketoconazole.

Toxicity can result when flucytosine is used concurrently with other drugs that depress bone marrow or when used during radiation therapy. Concomitant use of flucytosine with hepatotoxic or nephrotoxic drugs should be avoided. The use of flucytosine also decreases leukocyte and platelet counts and hemoglobin levels.

Metronidazole and alcohol cause severe disulfiram-like reactions with severe nausea, vomiting, tachycardia, flushing, and confusion.

CRICITAL DECISION:
Drug Interactions with Alcohol

Because of severe drug interactions with alcohol products the nurse should assess the patient's alcohol intake patterns.

NURSING IMPLICATIONS AND PATIENT TEACHING

▼ Assessment

The nurse should obtain a complete health history, including the presence of hypersensitivity, bone marrow depression, concurrent use of other drugs that may produce drug interactions (particularly corticosteroids), or the possibility of pregnancy.

The patient may have a history of fever and chills at the onset of infection. Itching is a common finding, but it may be associated with more systemic symptoms. A history of recent antibiotic therapy is common. The nurse may observe the classic signs of white discharge and erythema associated with thrush. The patient may also have a history of multiple scaly or blistered red patches on the skin, pruritus and soreness of involved areas, and brittle nails with yellow discoloration and separation from the nail bed.

▼ Planning

Individuals allergic to penicillin may exhibit cross-sensitivity to antifungals, although this is rare. The patient may experience a photosensitivity reaction with the drug.

Hepatic toxicity (usually reversible) and a few cases of hepatitis in children have been reported with ketoconazole. Liver function studies must be monitored so that any liver damage may be rapidly detected. The product should be discontinued if even a minor elevation in the liver function studies develops.

▼ Implementation

The absorption rate of griseofulvin is enhanced after the patient eats a fatty meal.

Ketoconazole requires stomach acidity for dissolution and absorption. In patients with achlorhydria (lack of hydrochloric acid), tablets should be dissolved in a small amount of aqueous 0.2 N HCl solution. The patient should drink the solution with a straw to avoid discoloring the teeth and should follow it with a full glass of water. The nurse should explain to the patient how and why this is done.

Because griseofulvin is absorbed over a long period of time, single daily doses are often adequate. The patient must use the medication continuously until the causative organism has been eradicated, as evidenced by both clinical and laboratory examinations. This process may require several weeks to many months of therapy, depending on the causative organism and the site of the infection. Concurrent use of topical antifungal agents may be required to treat some fungal infections, primarily tinea pedis.

See Table 9-4 for a summary of antifungals.

▼ Evaluation

The nurse should observe the patient for therapeutic effects, such as the disappearance of shaking chills and fever, and watch for signs of gastrointestinal distress. The patient should continue to take the medication until the laboratory tests show that normal function has returned. Watch carefully for signs of liver or renal changes. These drugs are very toxic. Report all patient complaints promptly.

▼ Patient and family teaching

The nurse should provide the patient and the family with the following instructions:

1. The patient should take all medication as ordered and not stop treatment when the symptoms disappear. The therapy may need to continue for many weeks before laboratory and clinical tests indicate that the infection is no longer present.
2. The physician should be notified if the patient experiences any nausea, vomiting, or diarrhea, or any bruising, sore throat, or fever. These drugs are very toxic, and no adverse effects should go unreported.
3. The oral suspension of nystatin should be shaken thoroughly before use.
4. Griseofulvin should be taken with meals that are high in fat; this causes more of the medication to be absorbed. Sometimes people taking this drug develop photosensitivity, or an intolerance to the sun. Alcoholic beverages should be avoided while taking griseofulvin or metronidazole.
5. Cleanliness of hair, skin, and nails will aid in controlling and limiting the spread of infection.
6. If skin rash occurs or if nausea, vomiting, or diarrhea becomes pronounced in patients taking flucytosine, they should notify the physician. To avoid or reduce nausea and vomiting, the capsules should be administered several at a time over a period of 15 minutes. If symptoms do not resolve within 2 to 3 days, the physician should be notified.

Table 9-4   Antifungals

Generic name	Trade name	Comments and dosage
Amphotericin B	Fungizone IV	0.25 mg/kg slow IV. Gradually increase if patient tolerates medication. For use only in patients with progressive and potentially fatal fungal infections.
Nystatin	Mycostatin Nilstat	Shake oral suspension well before use. Available for many routes. ■ *Oral thrush* *Adults and children:* 400,000 to 600,000 units (4 to 6 ml), qid, one half the dose is held in each side of mouth a short time before swallowing. *Older infants:* 200,000 units (2 ml) qid, one half the dose is held in each side of the mouth a short time before swallowing. *Neonates:* 100,000 units (1 ml), qid, one half the dose is held in each side of mouth a short time before swallowing. ■ *Intestinal candidiasis* *Adults:* 500,000 to 1,000,000 units, tid, continued for at least 2 days after absence of symptoms. ■ *Vaginitis* 1 to 2 tablets intravaginally for 2 weeks. Can also be treated with oral doses as in intestinal candidiasis.
Griseofulvin microsize	Grifulvin V Grisactin	Divided doses are recommended for those patients unable to tolerate single doses. ■ *Fungal infection* *Adults:* 500 mg PO qd in single or divided doses after meals. *Children:* 10 mg/kg PO qd in single or divided doses after meals.
Griseofulvin ultramicrosize	Fulvicin P/G Grisactin Ultra Gris-PEG	Griseofulvin ultramicrosize has approximately one-and-a-half times the biologic activity as griseofulvin microsize, with no advantage in effectiveness or safety. ■ *Fungal infections* *Adults:* 250 mg qd in single or divided doses after meals. *Children:* 5 mg/kg qd in single or divided doses after meals.
Ketoconazole	Nizoral	*Adults:* Initially give 200 mg qd. May increase up to 400 mg qd, depending on seriousness of the disease and clinical response. *Children older than 2 years:* Give 3.3 to 6.6 mg/kg PO qd. Duration of treatment is not specific and should be based on clinical response. Minimum treatment for candidiasis is 10 days to 2 weeks. May require therapy for up to 6 months.
Flucytosine	Ancobon Ancotil ✦	*Adults and children:* 50 to 150 mg/kg qd in divided doses q6h.
Fluconazole	Diflucan	Give 200 mg PO or IV on first day, then 100 mg qd for 2 to 3 weeks.
Miconazole	Monistat	Give 200 to 3600 mg IV or as bladder instillation, depending on organism.
Metronidazole	Flagyl	Give IV or PO. Dosage varies, depending on site of infection. See package insert.
Itraconazole	Sporanox	Give 200 mg to 400 mg once daily PO. Loading dose of 200 mg tid for first 3 days in life-threatening situations.

SECTION THREE: ANTITUBERCULAR DRUGS

Objectives

At the conclusion of this section you should be able to:
1. Describe the general actions of antitubercular drugs.
2. List the most common adverse reactions of antitubercular drugs.
3. Present key items to teach the patient or family about antitubercular drugs.

OVERVIEW

Tuberculosis is a disease still found among the poor and undernourished. It is most commonly seen in underdeveloped nations where living conditions are crowded and unsanitary. However, it is also increasingly found in the United States among drug users, alcoholics, and in AIDS patients or others with lowered immunity. Currently, most cases of infectious tuberculosis are found in people previously incompletely treated with antitubercular medications and in people who, as a result of reduced immunity from HIV infection, have primary tuberculosis. In these cases, the organisms are often resistant to the antitubercular medications used in the treatment.

CRITICAL DECISION:
Exposure to HIV

Patients who have recurrent vaginal infections that do not easily clear up, and who have been exposed to the HIV virus should be evaluated further.

Tuberculosis is caused by *Mycobacterium tuberculosis*, which infects animals as well as humans. Strains resistant to current medications have been noted.

Multiple drug resistance (MDR) organisms are now common and require vigorous methods of treatment to control infection. New guidelines for treatment of tuberculosis are released from the Centers for Disease Control and Prevention (CDC) in Atlanta, Georgia, on an almost yearly basis. Because there are many new cases of tuberculosis, as well as numerous untreated cases, many new state laws have been passed that take aggressive action against individuals who are infected with tuberculosis and who refuse to take or complete adequate medications. In some states, patients may actually be sent to prison until they have completed the required drug therapy and have been rendered noninfectious.

ACTION

The main action of antitubercular drugs involves an intracellular and/or extracellular bacteriostatic effect against *Mycobacterium tuberculosis*. Most drugs used to treat tuberculosis do not kill the bacterium, but they control the disease and prevent its spread through the patient or to other individuals. The drugs control the bacteria by preventing them from producing new cell walls, so new bacterial cell growth is limited. Some drugs are bactericidal, killing the organism.

USES

Chemoprophylaxis, or taking a drug to prevent disease, is recommended when the patient is highly at risk of developing active tuberculosis. The current duration of prophylactic treatment is 1 year. At present isoniazid is the only drug recommended for prophylactic therapy. Isoniazid prophylaxis is not recommended for healthy individuals over the age of 35, because of their increased risk of developing hepatitis. Prophylaxis is recommended, however, if the patient is at special risk for developing tuberculosis, as indicated in the box on p. 159. Chemotherapy, or taking a drug to treat disease, is recommended for patients with active tuberculosis.

Drugs are classified as primary or retreatment agents, indicating their approximate place and usefulness in treating tuberculosis. Most primary agents are bactericidal and are necessary to sterilize the tuberculosis lesions. Retreatment agents are generally less effective and more toxic than the primary agents. They are used with primary agents for partial or

High-Priority Candidates for Tuberculosis-Preventive Therapy

Patients of all ages with positive tuberculin test, no previous therapy, and
- Known or suspected HIV infection
- Close contacts of individuals with infectious, clinically active TB
- Recent tuberculin skin test converters
- Medical personnel with exposure to large numbers of susceptible individuals
- Medical problems that increase the risk of TB (e.g., diabetes, immunosuppressive therapy, IV drug use, end-stage renal disease, malignancies, hemodialysis)
- Abnormal chest x-rays that show old fibrotic lesions

Patients with positive tuberculin test, < 35 years old, no additional risk factors and
- Foreign-born individuals from high-prevalence countries
- Individuals in long-term care facilities (i.e., prisons, nursing homes)
- Medically underserved low-income populations

complete drug-resistant organisms or to treat extrapulmonary lesions.

ADVERSE REACTIONS

Bacteria build up a resistance to antitubercular drugs. Use of a combination of drugs helps slow the development of bacterial resistance.

Most of the antitubercular medications cause only mild and infrequent symptoms, such as nausea, vomiting, and diarrhea. Most of these symptoms stop when the dosage is reduced. Some of the medications used to treat tuberculosis are toxic to various parts of the body, for example, the ears, kidneys, and liver. The patient must be evaluated closely to detect development of any of these more serious problems.

Capreomycin may cause headache; ototoxicity (hearing loss, tinnitus, vertigo); nephrotoxicity (elevated BUN and nonprotein nitrogen, proteinuria, casts, hematuria, albuminuria, decreased creatinine clearance); changes in blood cells; abnormal liver function tests; maculopapular rash associated with febrile reaction; urticaria; muscle weakness; pain and induration or excessive bleeding at injection site; and sterile abscesses.

Ethambutol is associated with dizziness; headache; confusion; dermatitis; abdominal pain; anorexia; nau-

sea; vomiting; joint pain and swelling; optic neuritis (loss of vision and color discrimination); and loss of visual acuity.

Ethionamide may produce severe postural hypotension; mental depression; rash; anorexia; diarrhea; epigastric distress; jaundice; nausea; and vomiting.

Isoniazide may produce peripheral neuropathies; visual disturbances; optic neuritis; hyperglycemia; hyperkalemia; nausea; constipation; epigastric distress; vomiting; many changes in blood cells; arthritic symptoms; chills; fever; rash; dyspnea; headache; tachycardia; and urinary retention in men. Severe and sometimes fatal hepatitis may develop even after many months of treatment. The drug also interferes with a variety of laboratory tests. Symptoms of overdosage may occur anytime from 30 minutes to 3 hours after the isoniazid is administered. Nausea, vomiting, slurred speech, dizziness, impaired vision, and visual hallucinations may be among the early symptoms. Severe overdosage will result in CNS depression, respiratory distress, coma, and severe intractable seizures.

Pyrazinamide has been associated with photosensitivity; rashes; diarrhea; hepatocellular damage; nausea; vomiting; gout; decreased blood clotting time; and anemia.

Rifampin has produced drowsiness; headache; generalized numbness; transient low-frequency hearing loss; visual disturbances; abdominal pain or cramps; diarrhea; epigastric distress; hepatitis; nausea; sore mouth and tongue; vomiting; and many changes in blood cells. Symptoms of overdosage include nausea; vomiting; increasing lethargy; unconsciousness; liver enlargement and tenderness; and jaundice.

Streptomycin sulfate may produce dizziness; headache; paresthesia; vertigo; anorexia; nausea; stomatitis; vomiting; changes in blood cells; arthralgia; hypertension; hypotension; myocarditis; hepatotoxicity; splenomegaly; ototoxicity; and nephrotoxicity.

DRUG INTERACTIONS

Many drugs should not be given concurrently, sequentially, or topically while the patient is on antituberculosis therapy because of the significant risk for neurotoxicity and nephrotoxicity. All medications taken by the patient should be checked closely for drug interactions. All antitubercular medications have many known interaction potentials.

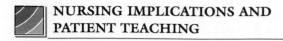
NURSING IMPLICATIONS AND PATIENT TEACHING

▼ Assessment

A tuberculosis infection may develop in a patient's lungs, bones, bladder, or other organs. A patient with active tuberculosis may have symptoms such as productive cough, pain, fever, night sweats, and weight loss, or the patient may be without symptoms. The diagnosis of tuberculosis is made from the patient's history, physical examination, x-ray studies, and laboratory work. Once the diagnosis is confirmed, the patient may be hospitalized while treatment is started. Long-term treatment is required, and much of the treatment will be carried out when the patient is at home.

▼ Planning

Drug resistance is likely to develop if only one drug is administered for active tuberculosis. Two or more drugs should always be given. Drugs that are highly ototoxic should not be given together. Two hepatotoxic drugs should not be given together when clinically active hepatitis is present.

To prevent the development of drug resistance, the nurse should carefully monitor the following:

1. Patient compliance
2. Sputum culture conversions
3. Selection of appropriate drugs

The CDC's Advisory Council for the Elimination of Tuberculosis has issued its recommendations for initial therapy of tuberculosis. Following are the regimen options for children and adults:

■ Daily isoniazid (INH), rifampin (RIF), and pyrazinamide (PZA) for 8 weeks, then 16 weeks of INH and RIF daily or two to three times/week in areas where the INH resistance rate is ≥4%. Add ethambutol (EMB) or streptomycin (SM) to the initial regimen until INH and RIF susceptibility is shown. Continue for ≥6 months and 3 months beyond culture conversion.

■ Daily INH, RIF, PZA, and SM or EMB for 2 weeks, then two times/week of the same drugs for 6 weeks, then two times/week of INH and RIF for 16 weeks.

■ INH, RIF, PZA, and EMB or SM three times/week for 6 months.

For TB patients with HIV infections, use any of the previous 3 treatment options, but continue for 9 months and ≥6 months beyond culture conversion.

Because of the long-term nature of the chemo-therapeutic regimen, drug toxicity is a special problem. Dosages for elderly patients, unusually small adults, and patients with renal impairment should be determined cautiously. All patients should be routinely monitored for symptoms of adverse reactions. If toxic effects, adverse reactions, or hypersensitivity reactions occur, all drugs should be stopped and further evaluation made. Reintroducing drugs after toxic effects or adverse reactions have ceased should be done with caution. In the event of an unsuccessful treatment regimen, two or more drugs should be added to the therapy, never a single drug.

▼ Implementation

Antitubercular drugs should be given in single daily doses unless contraindicated. All drugs, unless stated otherwise, should be taken at the same time each day, preferably in the morning. This is especially important with the combination of isoniazid and rifampin, to decrease the chance of drug resistance occurring. When poor compliance is suspected, the care provider should supervise the administration of the medications.

If parenteral administration is required, the injection sites should be rotated and each site inspected for signs of tenderness, swelling, or redness. Because patients may need to take medications for years, compliance in taking medications should also be assessed.

Many of these medications cause gastric irritation. This may be reduced by taking medication with food. Isoniazid is the only antitubercular medication that is best absorbed on an empty stomach. It should be taken either 1 hour before or 2 hours after a meal as a single daily dose. It should only be taken with food if it cannot be tolerated on an empty stomach.

The chemotherapeutic treatment of choice for uncomplicated pulmonary tuberculosis is the concomitant use of two drugs, isoniazid and rifampin, which are bactericidal both intracellularly and extracellularly. The duration of therapy is usually a minimum of 9 months. Sputum cultured 1 to 3 months after the initiation of isoniazid and rifampin therapy usually will be negative for the bacillus. The therapy usually continues for 6 months after sputum conversion takes place. When necessary, the combination of pyrazinamide and streptomycin may be used to substitute for either one of the bactericidal drugs above. However, there is some controversy over the effectiveness of this shorter, 9-month course of therapy when isoniazid is not used. Currently, intermittent therapy with isoniazid and rifampin is being investigated. The American Thoracic Society recommends that these two drugs be given daily for 2 to 8 weeks. Then the patient is switched to twice per week for a total of 39 weeks. The minimum duration of therapy is 9 months. The daily dosage recommendations for adults are isoniazid 300 mg and rifampin 600 mg. The twice-weekly dosage recommendations for adults are isoniazid 15 mg/kg of body weight and rifampin 600 mg. The American Thoracic Society recommends intermittent therapy only for uncomplicated pulmonary tuberculosis. See new CDC recommendations for multiple drug resistance strains.

Whenever a combination of drugs does not have both an intracellular and an extracellular bactericidal effect, therapy must continue for the traditional 18 to 24 months. This usually occurs when bacteriostatic drugs are used.

See Table 9-5 on p. 162 for a summary of common antitubercular drugs.

▼ Evaluation

Drug resistance should be suspected if the patient has been treated for tuberculosis in the past. Drugs used in the past regimen may be used again while waiting for the results of sensitivity studies, but at least two new drugs should also be prescribed. Drug resistance is low in infections acquired in the United States, but high in tuberculosis infections acquired from Asian, South and Central American, and African sources. Drug resistance is less likely to occur when two bactericidal drugs are given rather than when one bactericidal drug is given in combination with bacteriostatic drugs.

Vital signs should be monitored for recurrence of acute infection. Patients should be weighed on each visit to monitor their general health status. Weight loss should be reported to the physician. Diet changes and nutritional supplements may be indicated.

Some patients taking ethambutol develop psychologic changes. If the patient becomes depressed, anxious, withdrawn, or noncommunicative or shows any changes in personality, these findings should be reported to the physician.

Because of marked toxicity of these drugs, it is essential to carefully and regularly monitor both the bacteriologic studies and the toxic side effects of the drugs. Baseline sputum smears, cultures, and sensitivity studies, chest x-ray studies, weight, and renal, hepatic, and hematopoietic studies should be obtained.

CRITICAL DECISION:
Hepatitis

Hepatitis may develop with the use of isoniazid and pyrazinamide, so symptoms of fatigue, malaise, weakness, fever, nausea, and vomiting may develop. Liver function studies should be monitored periodically. If adverse signs are noted, they should be reported promptly.

▼ Patient and family teaching

Because patients must take their medications for a long time, it is important to establish a good relationship with the patient. Clear instructions should be given about the importance of continuing to take the drugs as ordered and what problems to report to the physician at the scheduled visits. It is important to stress the following instructions:

1. Laboratory and diagnostic tests and frequent office visits are necessary throughout the treatment of tuberculosis. The patient must continue to meet with the physician so progress can be measured.
2. The drug must be taken exactly as directed. The dosage must not be altered without specific instructions from the physician. It is very important to take these drugs as ordered. If a dose is missed, take it as soon as it is remembered, unless it is almost time for the next dose. In that case, the missed dose should not be taken and the regular dosing schedule should be followed. Forgetting to take a dose or failure to continue with one of the medications may cause the organisms to develop a resistance to the medication. This allows the disease process to continue, with continued risk for the patient, close family members, and contacts.
3. Tuberculosis is a disease that must be reported to the local health department. Family members and close contacts will also need to be screened for tuberculosis.

Table 9-5 Common antitubercular drugs

Generic name	Trade name	Dosage and comments
PRIMARY TREATMENT AGENTS		
Ethambutol	Myambutol	Give once every 24 hours. When one other bactericidal drug is used in combination with this medication, therapy will generally last 18 to 24 months. It has been used in twice-weekly regimens. Ethambutol may be taken with food. Watch for optic neuritis, rash. *Initial treatment:* 15 mg/kg PO in a single daily dose. *Retreatment:* 25 mg/kg PO in a single daily dose for 60 to 90 days; dosage is then decreased to 15 mg/kg per day.
Isoniazid	Laniazid Nydrazid Isotamine ♣ PMS Isoniazid ♣	Well absorbed after PO or IM administration. Dosage is determined by weight, with the usual adult dose being 5 mg/kg or 300 mg/day. Children require higher doses than adults. Give with pyridoxine to reduce incidence of peripheral neuropathies. Isoniazid is the drug of choice in the prophylactic treatment of tuberculosis infections. *Adults:* 300 mg/day for 1 year. Watch for hepatic and neurologic toxity.
Pyrazinamide	Pyrazinamide	Should be administered with at least one other antitubercular drug. *Adults:* 20 to 35 mg/kg/day in three or four divided doses. Maximum daily dose is 3 gm. Watch for hepatic toxicity and hyperuricemia, arthralgia and arthritis.
Rifampin	Rifadin Rimactane PMS Pyrazinamide ♣	Used in combination with other antitubercular drugs. Usually given PO, in a single dose, 1 hour before or 2 hours after eating. Peak plasma concentrations occur 2 to 4 hours after ingestion. *Adults:* 600 mg/day PO in a single dose. Dosage range is 450 to 600 mg/day. This is the same whether the therapy is intermittent or daily. *Elderly and debilitated:* 10 mg/kg/day; not to exceed 600 mg/day. *Children 5 years and older:* 10 to 20 mg/kg/day; not to exceed 600 mg/day. Watch for hepatic and hematologic toxicity.
Streptomycin	Streptomycin	Give in combination with other antitubercular agents, except capreomycin. Streptomycin should only be given intramuscularly. Limit quantity in one dose as injections are painful, and sterile inflammatory reactions may occur. Watch for renal and eighth nerve toxicity. *Adults with normal renal function:* 1 gm/day IM (may be given 5 days/week) for 2 to 3 months; then two to three times per week for 4 to 6 weeks. *Elderly patients, unusually small adults, and individuals with renal impairment:* Give reduced dosages, usually 0.5 gm/day IM according to above schedule.
RETREATMENT AGENTS		
P-Aminosalicylate (PAS)	Sodium P.A.S. Nemasol ♣	May produce nausea, vomiting, diarrhea, or abdominal pain. Dosage is usually 14 to 16 gm/day PO in two to three divided doses. Watch for GI distress, hepatitis.
Capreomycin	Capastat	Give deep IM. Watch for renal and eighth nerve toxicity. *Adults:* 1 gm/day IM daily (not to exceed 20 mg/kg/day) for 60 to 120 days, then 1 gm IM two to three times per week. The reduced dosage may continue for 18 to 24 months.
Cycloserine	Seromycin	Usual dose is 500 mg to 1 gm/day PO in divided doses. Watch for psychoses, seizures, rash.
Ethionamide	Trecator-SC	Take with meals or antacids to reduce gastrointestinal distress. High percentage of patients cannot tolerate therapeutic dose. *Adults:* 250 mg PO bid. Every 5 days the dose may be increased by 125 mg/day, until 1 gm/day is given. Dosages should never exceed 1 gm/day. The usual dose is 0.5 to 1 gm/day PO. Watch for hepatitis, GI distress, hypersensitivity.
Kanamycin	Kamtrex	Give 15 mg/kg once daily IM for adults, 7.5 to 15 mg/kg once daily IM for children. Watch for renal and eighth nerve toxicity.
PREVENTION IN HIV PATIENTS		
Rifabutin	Mycobutin	Usual dose: 300 mg once daily. Divided dose, taken with food, may decrease GI distress.

4. During the initial period of illness, patients must remember that they are contagious. Every effort must be made to cover the mouth when coughing, to dispose of sputum and soiled tissues carefully, and to act to protect those nearby.

5. The patient should remember that the whole body is involved in fighting this disease. The body needs adequate rest, nourishing food, and as restful and quiet a recovery environment as possible.

6. Any adverse reactions should be reported promptly. Particular symptoms to report include any episodes of easy bruising, fever, sore throat, unusual bleeding episodes, skin rashes, mental confusion, headache, tremors, severe nausea, vomiting, diarrhea, malaise, yellowish discoloration of the skin, visual changes, severe pain in knees, feet, or wrists, excessive drowsiness, or changes in personality or affect.

7. The patient should not take other medications without the knowledge and permission of the physician.

8. With the exception of isoniazid (which should be taken on an empty stomach) medication should be taken with food or milk. If an aftertaste occurs, a mouthwash, juice, or sugarless gum may be used after taking the medication.

9. The patient should establish a regular time each day to take medication.

10. The medication should be kept in a safe place, away from animals or children.

11. The patient should wear a Medic-Alert tag or other emergency identification indicating the medication being taken.

SECTION FOUR: ANTIPARASITIC MEDICATIONS

Objectives

At the conclusion of this section you should be able to:

1. Identify common parasites.
2. List major categories of medications used to treat parasitic infections.
3. Describe common adverse reactions associated with medications used to treat parasitic infections.
4. Develop specific teaching plans for patients being treated for parasitic infections.

OVERVIEW

Parasites affecting humans are widespread throughout the world. Three major categories of medications used to treat parasites are discussed in this section: amebicides, anthelmintics, and antimalarial products. Each major category will be discussed in detail.

AMEBICIDES

ACTION

Amebiasis is caused by the parasite *Entamoeba histolytica*. In the United States or Canada, this infection is seen primarily in people who have traveled abroad, or those who have eaten unwashed fruit or vegetables imported from other countries. Although the exact mechanism of action is unknown, the main action of an amebicide is to destroy the invading ameba, which may be located within the intestinal lumen or at an extraintestinal site. Extraintestinal amebiasis is much more difficult to treat. The most common extraintestinal infection is hepatic abscess.

USES

Amebicides are the primary therapy for intestinal or extraintestinal amebiasis. The choice of drug depends on the location of the infection.

Diiodohydroxyquin and metronidazole are used to treat *Trichomonas vaginalis*. Chloroquine, primarily an antimalarial agent, is also used for amebiasis and rheumatoid arthritis.

ADVERSE REACTIONS

All drugs may cause nausea, vomiting, headache, anorexia, diarrhea, or GI distress.

Chloroquine may produce dizziness, irritability, pruritus, ototoxicity, tinnitus, vertigo, visual disturbances, abdominal cramps.

Diiodohydroxyquin has been known to cause ataxia, neurotoxicity, peripheral neuropathy, optic neuritis, abdominal cramps, rectal and skin itching, constipation, and hair loss.

Emetine may produce dyspnea, ECG abnormalities, hypotension, cardiac changes, precordial pain, dizziness, mild sensory disturbances, skin lesions, abdominal cramps, and edema.

Metronidazole may cause ECG changes, ataxia, confusion, depression, insomnia, irritability, vertigo, flushing, pruritus, blurred vision, nasal congestion, abdominal cramps, constipation, dysuria, polyuria, pyuria, fever, and metallic taste.

Paromomycin may produce vertigo, rash, ototoxicity, abdominal cramps, constipation, hematuria, and nephrotoxicity.

Symptoms of overdose are also seen with all of these drugs.

DRUG INTERACTIONS

With the exception of metronidazole, there are no significant drug interactions. Combining metronidazole with alcohol can produce headache, flushing, cramps, nausea, and vomiting. If metronidazole is combined with disulfiram, acute psychosis may result.

 NURSING IMPLICATIONS AND PATIENT TEACHING

▼ Assessment

The nurse should obtain a complete health history, including the presence of hypersensitivity to drugs, concurrent use of alcohol or disulfiram, underlying systemic renal, cardiac, thyroid, or liver disease, and the possibility of pregnancy. These conditions are contraindications or precautions to the use of amebicides.

▼ Planning

There are five major drugs used as amebicides. The contraindications for drug use are somewhat different according to the drug chosen. The specific product information should be consulted.

▼ Implementation

The choice of the drug depends on the location of the infection. Some of these drugs are specific for extraintestinal infections. Because of the toxicity of

these drugs, the decision for treatment must be weighed carefully and only the smallest therapeutic dosage possible should be given for the shortest duration of time. If the initial drug is ineffective and the alternative is more hazardous, a repeat treatment with the initial drug may be advisable.

Patients receiving emetine should be as sedentary as possible during the time of treatment. This drug may cause ECG changes that persist for weeks after the therapy is discontinued. The ECG changes are similar to that of a myocardial infarction. Emetine may also decrease potassium levels. The patient should maintain a high-calorie, low-residue diet during therapy and increase the intake of fluids. The nurse should monitor the patient's intake and output during therapy.

The nurse should teach the patient about the method of infection and review specific methods of personal hygiene to prevent reinfection and reduce the risk of spreading infection to others.

See Table 9-6 for a summary of amebicides.

▼ Evaluation

After drug therapy, periodic stool examinations are necessary to make certain that the disease has been eliminated. These examinations may be done on a monthly basis for up to 1 year after therapy.

The nurse should monitor the patient for signs of toxicity. If severe symptoms appear, the drug may have to be discontinued.

▼ Patient and family teaching

The nurse should provide the patient and family with the following instructions:

1. The patient should take all medications as prescribed and not skip any doses or double the medication doses. The patient should not stop taking the medication without being advised to do so by a physician.
2. The patient should take this drug with or after meals to decrease the chances of stomach upset.
3. Some patients experience side effects from this medication. The patient should report any new or troublesome symptoms to the physician.
4. The gastrointestinal system (mouth) is the point of entry for these organisms. Usually infection results from fecal contamination of foods, or by hand-to-mouth contamination. Food should be washed carefully before eating, and hands should be washed after going to the bathroom

Table 9-6   Amebicides

Generic name	Trade name	Comments and dosage
Chloroquine	Aralen	Watch for ototoxicity; obtain baseline audiometry tests; this drug is used primarily in combination with other ambecides to treat hepatic abscess. ■ *Hepatic abscess* *Adults:* Following treatment by emetine (1 mg/kg/day IM for up to 5 days), give 600 mg base (1 gm) qd for 2 days, then 300 mg base (500 mg) qd for 2 to 3 weeks. At the same time, give diiodohydroxyquin 650 mg tid for 20 days. Reduce dosage for children.
Diiodohydroxyquin	Yodoxin Diodoquin ♣	Drug of choice in asymptomatic intestinal amebiasis. *Adults:* 630 to 650 mg PO tid for 20 days. *Children:* 30 to 40 mg/kg/day PO in three doses for 20 days. ■ *Mild, moderate, or severe intestinal amebiasis* *Adults:* In addition to metronidazole (750 mg tid for 5 to 10 days) give 630 to 650 mg PO tid for 20 days. *Children:* In addition to metronidazole (35 to 50 mg/kg/day in three doses for 10 days) give 30 to 40 mg/kg PO in three doses for 20 days.
Emetine HCl	Emetine HCl	Used as alternative drug therapy in severe intestinal or extraintestinal amebiasis therapy. Because of its effects on the heart, ECG monitoring is mandatory while patient is taking this product and patient should be as sedentary as possible during treatment period. ■ *Severe intestinal amebiasis* *Adults:* Give 1 mg/kg/day (maximum 60 mg daily) IM for up to 5 days. Also give 630 to 650 mg diiodohydroxyquin tid for 20 days. *Children:* Give 1 mg/kg/day in two doses (maximum 60 mg daily) IM for up to 5 days. At the same time give 30 to 40 mg/kg/day diiodohydroxyquin in three doses for 20 days.
Metronidazole	Flagyl Protostat	Drug of choice used in mild to severe intestinal amebiasis and in treatment of hepatic abscess. Patient should not take alcohol while on this medication and should not use with disulfiram. ■ *Mild, moderate and severe intestinal amebiasis* *Adults:* Give 750 mg tid for 5 to 10 days, plus diiodohydroxyquin 630 to 650 mg tid for 20 days. *Children:* Give 35 to 50 mg/kg/day in three doses for 10 days, plus diiodohydroxyquin 30 to 40 mg/kg/day in three doses for 20 days.
Paromomycin	Humatin	Used as alternative drug therapy for asymptomatic intestinal amebiasis and mild to moderate infections; may cause ototoxicity, so audiometry tests should be obtained; give medication with meals. ■ *Asymptomatic intestinal amebiasis* *Adults or children:* As alternative to diiodohydroxyquin, give 25 to 30 mg/kg/day in three doses for 7 days. ■ *Mild to moderate intestinal amebiasis* *Adults and children:* Give 25 to 30 mg/kg/day in three doses for 7 to 10 days.

and before preparing foods. This is important to avoid spreading infection.

5. After drug therapy has been completed, it is essential that a stool examination be performed periodically to look for reinfection or for people who may still have amebiasis but are not symptomatic.

ANTHELMINTICS

ACTION

Infestation by worms is called helminthiasis. It is most commonly caused by pinworms, roundworms, hookworms, tapeworms, or whipworms. The worm gains entrance to the body through contaminated food, unwashed hands, or the skin. The diagnosis is made by finding the eggs and/or the parasite in the stool of the infected individual. Once the type of parasite has been identified, the physician may select the appropriate medication for its destruction. The exact mechanism of action of the medication depends on the product used.

The exact action of diethylcarbamazine citrate as an anthelmintic is not known. It is theorized that it sensitizes the parasite's cuticle to allow phagocytosis by the macrophages of the host. Mebendazole blocks the glucose uptake of helminths. Piperazine paralyzes the muscles of parasites by blocking the effects of acetylcholine at the neuromuscular junction, and the parasite is expelled by normal peristalsis.

Quinacrine is used to treat tapeworm infestations. It causes the cestode to temporarily detach from the intestinal wall, thereby dislodging and expelling the intact worm. The exact action of thiabendazole is not known, but it is thought to interfere with the metabolic pathways essential for a variety of helminths.

USES

Thiabendazole is the drug of choice for cutaneous larva migrans (creeping eruption), pinworms, roundworms, *Strongyloides,* and mild cases of hookworm.

Quinacrine is used to treat cestodiasis (tapeworm infestation); however, niclosamide and paromomycin have generally replaced this drug. It is the drug of choice for giardiasis, a protozoan infestation.

Piperazine and pyrantel pamoate are used to treat roundworms and pinworms. Pyrantel is also effective with hookworms.

Diethylcarbamazine citrate is used mostly in tropi-

cal areas, or in patients who have been in areas where these filariae are endemic. It is used to treat *Wuchereria bancrofti* filariasis,* Malayan filariasis, dipetalonemiasis, or loiasis (a filarial worm dwelling in tumors in subcutaneous connective tissue and often affecting the eyes).

Mebendazole is used in single or mixed infections to treat pinworm, roundworm, hookworm, and whipworm infestations.

ADVERSE REACTIONS

Each drug has different side effects. Headache, weakness, anorexia, nausea, vomiting, abdominal pain, arthralgia, lassitude, malaise, myalgia, and skin rash are all common reactions. Allergic reactions may occur as a result of the dead microfilaria, and may be expressed as fever, lymphadenitis, pruritus, and pedal (foot) edema. The incidence of side effects increases with higher dosages and length of treatment.

DRUG INTERACTIONS

Anthelmintics may be antagonistic if they are given together. They also may interfere with a number of specific medications, such as heparin, and a variety of laboratory tests. The specific product information should be consulted.

 NURSING IMPLICATIONS AND PATIENT TEACHING

▼ Assessment

The nurse should obtain a health history, including the presence of hypertension, hypersensitivity, eye disease, intestinal obstruction, inflammatory bowel diseases, severe hepatic, renal, or cardiac disease, malaria, hypersensitivity to helmintics, and the possibility of pregnancy. These conditions are contraindications or precautions to treatment with anthelmintics.

The patient may be asymptomatic or be listless, fatigued, or irritable or have abdominal pain, diarrhea, and weight loss. The patient may also have edema, especially of the lower extremities, and a

---

***Wuchereria bancrofti* is a nematode parasite found in tropical and subtropical countries. It is transmitted by *Culex* mosquitoes, mites, or flies, and produces obstruction of the lymphatic ducts, leading to elephantiasis.

discharge from the eyes. The nurse should learn the signs and symptoms of infestation by the various helminths.

▼ Planning

Severe itching may take place in the treatment of cutaneous larva migrans, and a concomitant administration of an antiinflammatory agent may be necessary.

Patients with a recent history of malaria should be treated with an antimalarial agent before administering anthelmintics in order to prevent a relapse.

Because pinworm infections are easily transferred from person to person, all family members may have to be treated.

Piperazine can be used in the last trimester of pregnancy. However, this drug has potential neurotoxicity; therefore prolonged or repeated treatment in excess of the recommended dosage should be avoided, especially in children.

▼ Implementation

Thiabendazole therapy may cause an asparagus-like odor of the urine. The patient's skin may also have an unusual odor. This medication may cause drowsiness or dizziness; therefore the patient should use caution in driving or performing tasks requiring alertness.

Severe hookworm infestations may produce anemia, so iron supplementation and a diet rich in iron may be required.

The patient should store piperazine syrup and tablets in tightly closed containers to avoid evaporation or decomposition. Liquid preparations are more acceptable for children. Medication is usually administered in the morning before breakfast.

Patients may develop allergic reactions to the dead microfilaria and may need symptomatic treatment. Concomitant administration of antihistamines or corticosteroids may be necessary to reduce allergic effects, particularly in the treatment of ocular onchocerciasis.

Diethylcarbamazine citrate is often used in hospitalized patients, so the patient can be kept recumbent for 48 hours after treatment.

Gastrointestinal reactions from pyrvinium pamoate are more likely to occur in older children and adults who have received large doses. Emesis is more common with the suspension than with the tablets. The drug has staining properties; therefore warn the patient to be careful not to spill it. Have the patient drink the medication through a straw to prevent staining of the teeth.

With quinacrine, treatment may be repeated in 2 weeks if found to be ineffective. Sodium bicarbonate may be given before the drug to reduce nausea and vomiting. The drug imparts a reversible yellow coloration to the skin and urine. Periodic complete ophthalmologic examinations are necessary if the patient is receiving prolonged therapy.

See Table 9-7 for a summary of anthelmintics.

▼ Evaluation

The nurse should observe for compliance with the therapy schedule and suppression of the organism. Follow-up stool specimens should be obtained after treatment. An ophthalmologic examination should be obtained if the patient is being treated for ocular onchocerciasis.

Teach the patient hygienic techniques necessary to prevent reinfestation.

If the patient develops neurologic complications with piperazine therapy, this medication should be abandoned and an alternative should be used.

▼ Patient and family teaching

The nurse should provide the patient and family with the following instructions:

1. The patient must take this medication as ordered. Therapy usually involves an initial treatment that should kill all worms, but in some cases a second course must be taken. It is important to report any symptoms that do not disappear after treatment.
2. Worms passed in bowel movements are still alive and capable of infecting others. Care must be used to avoid transmission. During the next week the patient should:
   a. Wash the toilet seat daily with soap and water.
   b. Boil the sheets and underwear twice in water and disinfectant.
   c. Use special precautions in handling food or drink around others.
3. Good personal hygiene is essential in preventing reinfection. Some worms are transmitted through eating improperly cooked meat or fish, or unwashed fruit or vegetables, or by fecal contamination of food or water. Children who go barefoot may become infected with hookworm from animal droppings. Proper prepara-

Table 9-7   Anthelmintics

Generic name	Trade name	Comments and dosage
Diethylcarbamazine citrate	Hetrazan	Start this oral medication at lowest recommended doses and then gradually increase dosage as needed. ■ *Wuchereriasis:* 2 mg/kg tid after meals for 7 to 14 days. ■ *Loiasis:* 2 mg/kg after meals tid for 10 days. ■ *Onchocerciasis:* 2 mg/kg after meals tid for 14 to 21 days.
Mebendazole	Vermox	No special diets, fasting, or purgation before administration is necessary. Medication is taken orally, by chewing, crushing, and/or mixing with food. ■ *Pinworms:* 100 mg PO as a single dose. ■ *Roundworms, hookworms, and whipworms:* 100 mg PO bid (morning and evening) for 3 days; repeat treatment in 3 to 4 weeks if infestation is still present.
Niclosamide	Niclocide	*Adults:* 2 gm daily for 7 days. *Children:* 1 gm daily for 7 days. Chew tablets and swallow with a little water. Reexamine stool after 7 days and treat again if necessary.
Oxamniquine	Vansil	*Adults:* 12 to 15 mg/kg in single dose. *Children:* 20 mg/kg in 2 divided doses 8 hours apart.
Piperazine	Piperazine Entacyl ♣	■ *Roundworm (ascariasis) infections* *Adult:* 3.5 gm PO as a single daily dose. *Children:* 75 mg/kg PO as a single daily dose; maximum daily dose 3.5 gm; give for 2 consecutive days. ■ *Pinworm (enterobiasis) infections* *Adults and children:* 65 mg/kg PO as a single daily dose.
Praziquantel	Biltricide	Give 3 doses 20 mg/kg as a 1 day treatment. Tablet very bitter if not swallowed promptly.
Pyrantel	Antiminth Reese's Pinworm	Medication can be administered as a single dose for treating roundworms and pinworms; hookworms require longer therapy. No special fasting or diet is necessary before taking medication. Purging is not necessary. Taking drug with fruit juice or milk may make it more palatable. ■ *Roundworm and pinworm therapy* *Adults and children:* 11 mg/kg as a single dose; maximum dose 1 gm; this dose should be repeated after 2 weeks for pinworms. ■ *Hookworms* *Adults and children:* 11 mg/kg for 3 consecutive days; treatment should be repeated after 1 month if necessary.
Quinacrine	Atabrine	■ *Giardiasis:* Take drug after meals with a full glass of water, tea, or fruit juice. *Adults:* 100 mg PO tid for 5 to 7 days. *Children:* 7 mg/kg PO daily in three divided doses (maximum 300 mg/day) for 5 days. ■ *Cestodiasis:* For the treatment of cestodes, the preparation of the patient includes eating a bland, low-residue or liquid diet 1 to 2 days before treatment. The patient should remain fasting after the evening meal. In the morning, omit breakfast and give the medication. The pulverized tablets may be administered with jam or honey to disguise the bitter taste. After 1 to 2 hours give a saline cathartic to flush out the worm. If the worm is expelled, it will be stained yellow.
Thiabendazole	Mintezol	Chew tablets well before swallowing. Take drug after meals. *Adults and children over 150 lb:* 1.5 gm PO. *Adults and children under 150 lb:* 10 mg/lb PO. ■ *Pinworms (enterobiasis):* Give two doses in 1 day; repeat regimen in 7 days. ■ *Cutaneous larva migrans:* Give two doses per day for 2 days. If active lesions are still present after completion of therapy, a second course should be administered. ■ *Roundworms (oscariasis), Strongyloides and hookworms:* Give 2 doses per day for 2 days.

tion and cooking of food and washing of hands after using the toilet and before preparing food are important habits to develop.

4. Worm infestations are easily transmitted, and all family members may need to be tested for their presence.

5. Some people experience diarrhea and abdominal discomfort associated with taking the medication.

6. If the patient develops any signs of headache, tremors, muscle weakness, blurred vision, or an eye that deviates and does not align properly with the other eye, the physician should be alerted.

7. The patient may require iron supplements and a diet rich in iron while being treated for hookworm.

8. If the patient is taking pyrvinium pamoate, the medication is a red dye and therefore urine, stool, emesis, and teeth will be stained from it. If taking the liquid product, the patient should use a straw to decrease staining of the teeth. The staining effects are not permanent. Medication should be stored in a tight container and protected from light. The patient should avoid too much sun or use of a sun lamp when beginning treatment and for a few days after.

9. Quinacrine therapy may produce visual disturbances and a temporary yellow color of the skin and urine. Skin rashes may also occur while taking this drug. Nail pigmentation, along with blue and black skin may also occur. The patient must not drink any alcoholic beverages while taking this medication or he or she will become very nauseated and vomit.

ANTIMALARIALS

ACTION

Although malaria is not commonly seen in the United States or Canada, nurses occasionally see cases among immigrants, refugees, and travelers returning from areas where malaria is endemic. People traveling to or living in areas where malaria is endemic can use antimalarials to prevent and to treat symptoms of malaria.

Malaria is caused by four species of the protozoan *Plasmodium*. These species are *P. falciparum, P. malariae, P. vivax,* and *P. ovale.* The protozoan parasites are transmitted to humans by the *Anopheles* mosquito.

When a mosquito bites a person infected with malaria, the protozoans enter the mosquito's stomach, where they reproduce. The resulting sporozoites make their way to the salivary glands of the mosquito. They are then transmitted to other individuals whenever the mosquito bites. The sporozoites grow and divide in the human host, entering the red blood cells of the person and maturing into the adult form of the protozoan, which then produces infection and the symptoms of malaria.

Antimalarial drugs interfere with the life cycle of *Plasmodium,* usually while it is in the red blood cells, by reducing the ability of the DNA to replicate or serve as a template, thereby decreasing protein synthesis in susceptible organisms. Not all medications are effective against all four species of *Plasmodium.* In addition, many strains of *Plasmodium* have developed resistance to commonly used medications.

Primaquine interferes with the metabolism of parasites by causing mitochondrial swelling, thereby inhibiting protein synthesis. Folic acid antagonists affect the differential growth requirements and the demand for nucleic acid precursors between the host and the parasite. In sulfonamide products, there is a competitive antagonism of para-aminobenzoic acid, which is a component in folic acid synthesis. Quinine is the earliest known medication for malaria, and it reduces the effectiveness of *Plasmodium's* DNA to act as a template in chloroquine-resistant strains of *P. falciparum.* It also decreases the parasite's oxygen use and carbohydrate metabolism, and is a skeletal muscle relaxant, antipyretic, and analgesic.

USES

Antimalarials are used to suppress and treat acute malarial attacks caused by erythrocytic forms of *P. ovale, P. malariae, P. vivax* and most strains of *P. falciparum.* 4-Aminoquinolines are ineffective against the gametocytes of *P. falciparum* but are used with primaquine to attain radical cure of malaria caused by *P. malariae* and *P. vivax.*

ADVERSE REACTIONS

Synthetic *4- and 8-aminoquinolines* may produce hypotension, electrocardiogram changes, mild and transient headaches, pruritus, abdominal cramps, anorexia, diarrhea, nausea, vomiting, blood dyscrasias, visual blurring, reduced hearing, and tinnitus.

Folic acid antagonists may produce anorexia, atrophic glossitis, vomiting, and anemias.

Quinacrine has been associated with dizziness, irritability, mild and transient headaches, nervousness, contact dermatitis, exfoliative dermatitis, abdominal cramps, anorexia, diarrhea, nausea, vomiting, visual blurring, and retinopathy.

Quinine poisoning, or cinchonism, is manifested by diarrhea, dizziness, headache, nausea, tinnitus, visual blurring, apprehension, confusion, excitement, hypothermia, syncope, abdominal cramps, vomiting, anemias, pruritus, rash, urticaria, and night blindness.

All of these medications are associated with occasional development of blood dyscrasias and visual and neurologic changes. Overdosage may produce convulsions and cardiac collapse.

DRUG INTERACTIONS

Concurrent use of any antimalarials with other medications that cause dermatologic, ototoxic, or neurologic symptoms may produce toxicity. There are isolated drugs that interact with these preparations, so the manufacturers' information should be consulted.

 NURSING IMPLICATIONS AND PATIENT TEACHING

▼ Assessment

The nurse should obtain a thorough health history, including whether the patient is pregnant or has a history of allergy, psoriasis, porphyria, or glucose-6-phosphate dehydrogenase deficiency. These conditions are contraindications or precautions to the use of antimalarials.

The patient may have a history of malarial symptoms: periodic fever and chills, profound sweating, headache, nausea, body pains, and exhaustion. The patient may report having been in an area where malaria is endemic. Objective signs of malaria include periodic diaphoresis (sweating) and remittent fever as high as 104° to 105° F.

▼ Planning

The amount of active base varies from product to product. The dosage should be calculated on the basis of the amount of active base in the product. The product package information indicates the tablet's equivalence to base.

Because certain strains of *P. falciparum* are resistant to 4-aminoquinoline compounds, individuals infected with these strains should be treated with other antimalarial drugs, such as quinine.

Individuals taking high dosages or prolonged antimalarial therapy may develop irreversible retinal damage. Children are highly sensitive to 4-aminoquinoline compounds, primarily chloroquine.

Quinine should be used with care in patients with cardiac dysrhythmias. Cardiotoxicity may result with quinine use. In very sensitive individuals, reversible thrombocytopenia may occur with quinine use.

The nurse should make an initial determination of the glucose-6-phosphate dehydrogenase level in black patients and in those of Mediterranean ancestry because antimalarial medications may precipitate hemolysis. The drug should be discontinued if the patient develops any blood dyscrasia that is not associated with the disease.

▼ Implementation

Chloroquine and hydroxychloroquine are administered orally. To treat malaria, an initial loading dose is usually followed by one half that dose on the next 2 days. To suppress malaria, these drugs are usually initiated 2 weeks before the individual enters into a malarious area. The medication is taken once weekly on the same day of the week and is continued for 8 weeks after the individual has left the area.

If the drug's absorption is questionable in cases of acute infection, when the infection is quite severe, or when nausea and vomiting are present, chloroquine may be given parenterally (usually IM).

See Table 9-8 for a summary of antimalarials.

▼ Evaluation

The nurse should watch for the resolution of symptoms. If the patient is to undergo prolonged therapy, periodic complete blood cell counts, urinalysis, and observation for signs and symptoms of hemolysis are necessary. Also, periodic examination of knee and ankle reflexes is necessary to determine the presence of muscular weakness. An electrocardiogram may be desirable before initiating quinine therapy and during treatment if the presence of a cardiac dysrhythmia is possible. Any report of visual disturbances makes ophthalmic examination necessary.

▼ Patient and family teaching

The nurse should provide the patient and family with the following instructions.

Table 9-8 Antimalarials

Generic name	Trade name	Comments and dosage
4-AMINOQUINOLINES		
Chloroquine HCl	Aralen HCl	Parenteral drug of choice for treating acute malarial attacks when oral therapy is ineffective. *Adults:* 200 to 250 mg IM initially, and repeated q6h prn. *Children:* 5 mg/kg (base) initially, repeated in 6 hours prn.
Chloroquine phosphate	Aralen Phosphate	■ *Malaria suppression* *Adults:* 500 mg once weekly on same day of week, beginning 2 weeks before entering malarious area and continued for 8 weeks after departure. *Children:* 5 mg/kg (base) once weekly on same day of week, beginning 2 weeks before entering malarious area and continuing for 8 weeks after departure. ■ *Malaria treatment* *Adults:* 1 gm initially, then 500 mg in 6 hours and 500 mg daily for the next 2 days. *Children:* 10 mg/kg (base) initially, then 5 mg/kg (base) in 6 hours and 5 mg/kg (base) daily for the next 2 days.
Hydroxychloroquine	Plaquenil	■ *Malaria suppression* *Adults:* 400 mg once weekly on same day of week, beginning 2 weeks before entering malarious area and continued for 8 weeks after departure. *Children:* 5 mg/kg (base) once weekly on same day of week, not to exceed adult dosage, beginning 2 weeks before entering malarious area and continued for 8 weeks after departure. ■ *Malaria treatment* *Adults:* 800 mg initially then 400 mg in 6 hours and 400 mg daily for the next 2 days. *Children:* 10 mg/kg (base) initially, then 5 mg/kg (base) in 6 hours and 5 mg/kg (base) daily for the next 2 days.
8-AMINOQUINOLINES		
Primaquine phosphate	Aralen Phosphate with Primaquine Phosphate	Initiate primaquine therapy following a course of chloroquine phosphate suppressive treatment or during the last 2 weeks of therapy with chloroquine phosphate. ■ *Malaria suppression* *Adults:* 26.3 mg once daily for 14 days, beginning immediately after leaving malarious area. *Children:* 0.3 mg/kg (base) once daily for 14 days, beginning immediately after leaving malarious area.
FOLIC ACID ANTAGONISTS		
Pyrimethamine	Daraprim	■ *Malaria suppression* *Adults and children over 10 years:* 25 mg once weekly. *Children 4 to 10 years:* 12.5 mg once weekly. *Children under 4 years:* 6.25 mg once weekly. Therapy should begin 2 weeks before entering malarious area and be continued for 10 weeks after departure.
Sulfadoxine and pyrimethamine	Fansidar	May produce an acute intoxication syndrome. ■ *Malaria prophylaxis* *Adults:* Take 500 mg PO 1 or 2 days before entering an endemic area, and continue 500 mg once a week, or 1000 mg every 2 weeks, for 4 to 6 weeks after departure. Follow with a regimen of primaquine. ■ *Malaria treatment* *Adults:* Take 2 to 3 tablets as a single dose, alone or with quinine or primaquine. *Children:* See product information for schedule.

Continued.

Table 9-8   Antimalarials—cont'd

Generic name	Trade name	Comments and dosage
Mefloquine	Lariam	■ *Treatment* *Adults:* five tablets (1250 mg) as a single dose. ■ *Prophylaxis* *Adults:* 250 mg once weekly for 4 weeks, then every other week up to 4 weeks after leaving travel area.
Quinacrine	Atabrine	■ *Malaria treatment* *Adults and children over 8 years:* 200 mg with 1 gm sodium bicarbonate q6h for 5 days, then 100 mg q8h for 6 days. ■ *Malaria suppression* *Adults:* 100 mg daily for 1 to 3 months. *Children:* 50 mg daily for 1 to 3 months.
Quinine sulfate	Legatrin Quinamm Quinicardine ♣	Concurrent use of pyrimethamine 50 mg daily for the first 3 days of quinine therapy plus sulfadiazine 2 gm daily for the first 6 days is recommended. ■ *Chloroquine-resistant malaria* *Adults:* 650 mg q8h for 10 to 14 days. *Children:* 25 mg/kg q8h for 10 to 14 days.

1. The patient should take all the medication as ordered and not stop when the symptoms disappear.
2. The physician should be notified immediately if the patient has ringing in the ears, hearing difficulties, or visual disturbances.
3. Gastrointestinal upset can be reduced by taking medication with meals. The physician should be notified immediately if nausea, vomiting, anorexia, abdominal cramps, or diarrhea becomes pronounced.
4. This medication should be kept out of the reach of children.
5. Quinine products may cause the skin to appear somewhat yellow.
6. Quinine may cause dizziness and visual blurring. The patient should be cautious when driving.
7. Malaria may recur. The patient should be alert to recurrence of symptoms and see physician immediately if they develop.

SECTION FIVE: PENICILLINS

Objectives

At the conclusion of this section you should be able to:

1. Identify common uses of penicillin products.
2. List common adverse reactions from penicillin products.
3. Describe commonly encountered drug interactions that occur with the use of penicillin products.
4. Use the nursing process when planning to give penicillin products.

ACTION

Penicillin interferes with mucopeptide cell wall synthesis.

USES

Penicillin is the drug of choice for susceptible broad-spectrum gram-positive and gram-negative organisms. The choice of drug depends on the infectious organism (as identified by appropriate cultures or smears) or on the basis of the clinical picture. Penicillin is effective in the treatment of the following susceptible organisms: alpha-hemolytic streptococci, group A beta-hemolytic streptococci, streptococci (groups C, G, H, L, M), *Spirillum minus* (rat-bite fever), *Neisseria gonorrhoeae*, *Treponema pallidum* (syphilis), *Meningococcus meningitidis*, *Clostridium perfringens*, *C. tetani*, *Corynebacterium diphtheriae*, *Staphylococcus*, *Pasteurella meningitidis*, and other less common organisms. Penicillin is also indicated for prophylactic treatment against bacterial endocarditis in patients with rheumatic or congenital heart disease before they undergo dental procedures or surgery of the upper respiratory tract, genitourinary tract, or gastrointestinal tract.

ADVERSE REACTIONS

Adverse reactions to penicillin include neuropathy (with high parenteral dosages), fixed drug eruptions, nausea, vomiting, epigastric distress, anemia, blood dyscrasias, rash, erythema, urticaria, angioedema, laryngeal edema, and anaphylaxis.

DRUG INTERACTIONS

Bacteriostatic antibiotics, such as tetracyclines and erythromycin, may decrease the bactericidal effect of penicillin. Probenecid will prolong blood levels by blocking the renal clearance of penicillin. Concurrent use of ampicillin and oral contraceptives has been associated with menstrual irregularities and unplanned pregnancies. Indomethacin, phenylbutazone, or aspirin may increase serum penicillin levels. Antacids may decrease the absorption of penicillin when they are taken together. Penicillin may interfere with some laboratory tests.

 NURSING IMPLICATIONS AND PATIENT TEACHING

▼ Assessment

The patient in need of antibiotic therapy may be asymptomatic to severely ill. The nurse should look for common indicators of infection, such as fever, inflammation, erythema, edema, or pain.

The nurse should take a thorough health history, including any other medications taken that may interact with penicillin; determine whether there is a prior history of penicillin allergy, multiple allergies, asthma, hypersensitivity to procaine or tartrazine; and determine whether the patient is pregnant or breastfeeding. These conditions are contraindications or precautions to the use of penicillin.

Anaphylaxis has occurred with both oral and parenteral penicillin therapy. Penicillin should be used with caution in patients with multiple allergies.

▼ Planning

Prolonged use may lead to hepatic, renal, or hematologic disorders.

A minimum of 10 days of therapy is indicated to treat group A beta-hemolytic streptococci in order to decrease the risk of rheumatic fever, endocarditis, or glomerulonephritis. The nurse should avoid giving ineffective doses in any therapy, to decrease the risk of developing resistant strains.

▼ Implementation

With IM injections, the nurse should always aspirate to prevent medicine from entering a blood vessel.

The infected partners of patients with syphilis or gonorrhea must be treated also.

Laboratory tests performed while the patient is on penicillin therapy may be inaccurate, because penicillin interferes with the accuracy of many values.

The dosage depends on the type and severity of the infection. Penicillins come in different forms and may be classified as acid-stable, ampicillins, extended-spectrum, penicillin G, or penicillinase-resistant. See Table 9-9 for a summary of penicillins.

▼ Evaluation

A baseline blood pressure and pulse should be obtained before parenteral administration. The patient should be advised to wait 30 minutes after PO or IM administration before leaving outpatient setting. The nurse should observe for signs of hypersensitivity, although some allergic responses may not develop for days after taking the medication.

▼ Patient and family teaching

The nurse should provide the patient and family with the following instructions:

1. The patient should take the medication exactly as prescribed and not stop taking medication just because he or she feels better. Every dose must be taken.
2. The patient should carefully bathe and brush

Text continued on page 176.

Table 9-9 Penicillins

Generic name	Trade name	Comments and dosage

NATURAL PENICILLINS

Penicillin G (potassium or sodium)	Pentids Pfizerpen	Give IM injections deeply, slowly, and steadily to prevent needle blockage; aspirate before injection. Hyperkalemia may develop with large doses. Observe for convulsions, hyperreflexia, or coma. With large doses or extended therapy, monitor renal, cardiovascular, and electrolyte function. IV and PO doses vary with organism. *Adults:* 300,000 units q6 to 8h IM. *Children:* 300,000 to 1,200,000 units/day IM.
Penicillin G (procaine, aqueous)	Crysticillin Wycillin	Contains procaine to decrease injection pain; determine if patient is allergic to procaine. Give deep IM in gluteal muscle; aspirate before injection. Rotate injection sites. This is the drug of choice for gonorrhea. ■ *Pneumonia* (pneumococcal): 600,000 to 1,200,000 units/day IM. ■ *Bacterial endocarditis* (group A beta-hemolytic streptococci): 600,000 to 1,200,000 units/day. ■ *Prophylaxis against bacterial endocarditis:* 1,000,000 units penicillin G with 600,000 units APPG IM 30 to 60 minutes before surgical or dental procedures, then 500 mg penicillin V q6h for 8 doses. ■ *Sexually transmitted diseases* (may vary, depending on disease): 4.8 million units IM (in 2 sites), with 1 gm probenecid, followed by 100 mg oral doxycycline, twice a day, for 10 to 14 days.
Penicillin G benzathine	Bicillin Permapen	Long-acting IM penicillin. In children, administer parenterally in midlateral aspect of thigh. In adults, give IM in gluteal muscle. Oral dosage exhibits poor absorption and is not recommended for routine use. Oral dosages: 400,000 to 600,000 units PO q6h. Parenteral dosages ■ *Prophylaxis for rheumatic fever:* 1.2 million units IM twice a month on a continuous basis. ■ *Streptococcal upper respiratory infection, skin and soft tissue infection, scarlet fever, erysipelas:* *Adults:* 2.4 million units IM. *Children 30 to 60 lbs:* 900,000 to 1.2 million units IM. *Children under 30 lbs:* 600,000 units IM. ■ *Syphilis* *Early:* 2.4 million units IM. *Latent:* 2.4 million units IM once a week for 3 weeks.
Penicillin V	Penicillin V	Stable in gastric juices; however, blood levels are higher when administered on an empty stomach. ■ *Streptococcal, scarlet fever, erysipelas:* 200,000 to 400,000 units PO q6 to 8h for 10 days. ■ *Pneumococcal:* 400,000 to 600,000 units q6h until afebrile for 2 days. ■ *Staphylococcal and fusospirochetosis:* 400,000 to 800,000 units PO q6 to 8h. ■ *Prophylaxis for rheumatic fever/chorea:* 200,000 to 250,000 units PO bid continuously.
Penicillin V (potassium)	Betapen-VK V-Cillin K Pen-Vee K	Used in the treatment of mild to moderately severe infections where patient can take oral medication. *Adults:* 250 to 500 mg PO tid to qid. *Children:* 15 to 50 mg/kg/day in three to six divided doses.

Table 9-9   Penicillins—cont'd

Generic name	Trade name	Comments and dosage

PENICILLINASE - RESISTANT

Cloxacillin	Cloxapen Tegopen	Penicillinase-resistant penicillin. Effective in the treatment of pneumococci. Also effective in the treatment of pneumococci or group A beta-hemolytic streptococci. *Adults and children over 20 kg:* 250 to 500 mg PO q6h. *Children under 20 kg:* 50 to 100 mg/kg/day PO in divided doses q6h.
Dicloxacillin	Dycill Dynapen	Penicillinase-resistant penicillin. It is effective in the treatment of penicillinase-producing staphylococci. *Adults and children over 40 kg:* 125 to 250 mg PO q6h. *Children under 40 kg:* 12.5 to 25 mg/kg/day PO q6h.
Methicillin	Staphcillin	Penicillinase-resistant penicillin. Do not mix with other drugs. *Adults:* 1 gm IM q4 to 6h; 1 gm IV q6h in 50 ml sodium chloride. *Children under 20 kg:* Usual dose is 25 mg/kg q6h.
Nafcillin	Nafcil Unipen	Penicillinase-resistant penicillin. *Adults:* 250 mg to 1 gm PO q4 to 6h; or 500 mg IM q4 to 6h. *Children:* 250 mg PO tid or 25 to 50 mg/kg/day in four divided doses; or 25 mg/kg/day IM in two doses. *IV dosage:* 500 mg q4h in 15 to 30 ml of sodium chloride, injected for 5 to 10 minutes or slow drip to prevent thrombophlebitis.
Oxacillin	Bactocill Prostaphlin	Penicillinase-resistant penicillin. Rare, reversible hepatocellular dysfunction has been reported. *Adults:* 500 to 1000 mg PO q4 to 6h for 5 days, or 250 mg to 1 gm IM q4 to 6h. *Children:* 50 to 100 mg/kg/day PO in divided doses q6h for 5 days; or 50 to 100 mg/kg/day parenterally in four divided doses.

AMINOPENICILLINS

Amoxicillin	Amoxil Polymox Wymox	Extended-spectrum penicillin. *Adults and children over 20 kg:* 250 to 500 mg PO q8h. *Children under 20 kg:* 20 to 40 mg/kg/day PO in divided doses q8h. ■ *Uncomplicated gonorrhea:* 3 gm PO single dose with 1 gm probenecid; follow with tetracycline 500 mg PO qid for 7 days.
Ampicillin	Totacillin Polycillin	Extended-spectrum penicillin. Give with 1 gm of probenecid for treatment of gonorrhea. *Adults:* 250 to 500 mg PO qid. *Children under 20 kg:* 50 to 100 mg/kg/day PO in divided doses q6h. *Children over 20 kg:* 250 to 500 mg PO qid. ■ *Uncomplicated gonorrhea:* 3.5 gm PO with 1 gm of probenecid.
Ampicillin sodium, parenteral	Omnipen-N Polycillin-N Ampicin ♣	Extended-spectrum penicillin. *Adults:* 250 to 500 mg IM or IV q6h. *Children:* 25 to 50 mg/kg/day IM or IV in divided doses q6 to 8h. Used in treatment of serious infections and often used concomitantly with a sodium aminoglycoside or a cephalosporin. ■ *Lower respiratory tract infections, skin infections, bone and joint infections:* 225 to 300 mg/kg/day. Give IV in divided doses of 3 to 4 gm q4 to 6h. ■ *Urinary tract infections:* 100 to 200 mg/kg/day. Give IV in divided doses of 2 to 3 gm q6h.
Bacampicillin	Spectrobid	*Adults:* 400 mg q12h; dose may be doubled in severe infections. *Children weighing less than 25 kg:* 25 mg/kg/day in two equally divided doses q12h; dose may be doubled in severe infections. ■ *Gonorrhea:* Usual adult dosage for males and females is 1.6 gm bacampicillin plus 1 gm probenecid as a single oral dose.

Continued.

Table 9-9 Penicillins—cont'd

Generic name	Trade name	Comments and dosage
AMINOPENICILLINS—cont'd		
Ampicillin sodium and sulbactam sodium	Unasyn	Give either IV or IM. *Adults:* 1.5 to 3 gm q6h.
Amoxicillin and potassium clavulanate	Augmentin	*Adults:* One 250 mg tablet q8h. *Children:* 20 mg/kg/day in divided doses q8h.
EXTENDED SPECTRUM		
Carbenicillin	Geocillin	Extended-spectrum penicillin. Products vary in amount of sodium per gram. ■ *Urinary tract infection* *Adults:* Uncomplicated: 1 to 2 gm IM q6h; serious: 200 mg/kg/day IV drip. *Children:* 50 to 200 mg/kg/day IM in divided doses q4 to 6h. ■ *Septicemia, severe systemic respiratory, or soft tissue infections* *Adults: Pseudomonas* and anaerobes: 400 to 500 mg/kg/day in divided doses or continuous IV. *Proteus* and *E. coli:* 300 to 400 mg/kg/day. *Children:* 400 to 500 mg/kg/day IV divided doses or continuous drip.
Mezlocillin	Mezlin	Extended-spectrum penicillin administered IM or IV. This product is reserved for use in severe or complicated infections. ■ *Urinary tract infections:* 1.5 to 3 gm q6h IV or IM. ■ *Lower respiratory tract infections, intraabdominal infections, skin and gynecologic infections:* 3 to 4 gm q4 to 6h IV or IM.
Piperacillin	Pipracil	Extended-spectrum product effective against a wide number of gram-positive and gram-negative aerobic and anaerobic bacteria. ■ *Urinary tract infections, pneumonia:* 6 to 16 gm/day IV divided into four to six doses. ■ *Uncomplicated gonorrhea infections:* 2 gm IM single dose. ■ *Complicated or serious infections:* 12 to 18 gm/day IV into four to six doses.
Ticarcillin	Ticar	Extended-spectrum penicillin. ■ *Uncomplicated urinary tract infection* *Adults:* 1 gm IM or IV q6h. *Children:* 50 to 100 mg/kg/day IM or IV in divided doses q6 to 8h. ■ *Complicated urinary tract infections:* 150 to 200 mg/kg/day in divided doses q4 to 6h. ■ *Systemic septicemia, respiratory tract infection, soft tissue infection:* 200 to 300 mg/kg/day in three, four, or six divided doses.
Ticarcillin and potassium clavulanate	Timentin	Administer 3.1 gm q4 to 6h by IV infusion. Reduce dosage in renal impairment.

teeth regularly while using this medication and watch for any signs of itching, irritation, or infection.

3. The patient should notify the nurse or physician if rash, hives, decreased urination, diarrhea, or other unusual symptoms develop. Penicillin allergies can develop at any time.

4. If medication is given on an outpatient basis, the patient should go to an emergency room quickly if he or she becomes short of breath or has difficulty breathing.

5. If treatment is for a sexually transmitted disease, the patient should not engage in sexual activity during treatment. All sexual partners should also be tested and treated.

SECTION SIX: SULFONAMIDES

Objectives

At the conclusion of this section you should be able to:

1. Describe the action and uses of sulfonamides.
2. List the adverse reactions associated with various sulfonamides.
3. Construct a plan for teaching the patient and family about the use of sulfonamides.

> **CRITICAL DECISION:**
> *Superinfection*
>
> The nurse should watch for possible superinfection in the oral, vaginal, or rectal areas and monitor for the therapeutic effect of the drug.

ACTION

Sulfonamides exert a bacteriostatic effect against a wide range of gram-positive and gram-negative microorganisms by inhibiting folic acid synthesis.

USES

Sulfonamides are usually used to treat acute and chronic urinary tract infections, particularly cystitis, pyelitis, and pyelonephritis, when caused by *E. coli* or *Nocardia asteroides.* Other indications include trachoma (inclusion conjunctivitis), chancroid, lymphogranuloma venereum, toxoplasmosis, acute otitis media caused by *Haemophilus influenzae,* and prophylactic therapy in cases of recurrent rheumatic fever. Susceptible organisms include *Streptococcus pyogenes, S. pneumoniae,* some strains of *Bacillus anthracis* and *Corynebacterium diphtheriae, Haemophilus ducreyi,* and *Chlamydia trachomatis,* and other less common organisms. Several sulfonamides are useful only in the treatment of ulcerative colitis, preoperative and postoperative therapy for bowel surgery, or dermatitis herpetiformis.

ADVERSE REACTIONS

Adverse reactions to sulfonamides include headache, drowsiness, fatigue, dizziness, vertigo, tinnitus, hearing loss, insomnia, peripheral neuropathy, hypothyroidism, hypoglycemia, anorexia, nausea, vomiting, stomatitis, abdominal pain, drug fever, blood dyscrasias, generalized maculopapular or urticarial rash, fever, malaise, pruritus, dermatitis, local irritation, periorbital edema, anaphylactic shock, crystalluria, hematuria, and proteinuria. Other serious adverse effects, including toxic fever, may develop with overdosage and precede other serious adverse effects.

DRUG INTERACTIONS

Sulfonamides may potentiate the effect of oral anticoagulants, methotrexate, sulfonylureas, thiazide diuretics, phenytoin, and uricosuric agents. Sulfonamides may be displaced from plasma albumin by probenecid, salicylates, phenylbutazone, promethazine, sulfinpyrazone, and indomethacin; this will cause the effects of sulfonamides to be increased. Penicillins may be less effective when used in conjunction with a sulfonamide. The sulfonamide's effect may be antagonized by drugs such as local anesthetics. Antacids may result in decreased absorption of the sulfonamide when they are taken together. Sulfonamides may alter various laboratory tests.

NURSING IMPLICATIONS AND PATIENT TEACHING

▼ Assessment

The nurse should obtain a complete health history, including the presence of allergy to sulfa drugs, aspirin, thiazides, or sulfonylureas; whether the patient is taking any other drugs that may interact with sulfonamides; whether the patient is pregnant or breastfeeding; and whether kidney or liver impairment exists. These conditions are contraindications or precautions to the use of sulfonamides.

The patient in need of antibiotic therapy may be asymptomatic to severely ill. The nurse should keep in mind common indicators of infection, such as fever, inflammation, erythema, edema, or pain.

▼ Planning

The drug should be discontinued if the patient's urinary output is reduced or if a rash develops.

Photosensitivity can occur if the patient is exposed

to excessive amounts of sunlight or ultraviolet light.

The patient should maintain adequate fluid intake to avoid crystalluria or urinary stone formation.

▼ Implementation

Although most sulfonamides are administered orally, several can be given parenterally, primarily intravenously. Other parenteral routes are avoided because they can cause irritation. Some sulfonamides are administered vaginally as creams or suppositories.

Sulfonamide dosage depends on the severity of the infection being treated, the drug used, and the patient's response to and tolerance of the drug. Generally, the short-acting sulfonamides are administered at more frequent intervals than are the intermediate- or long-acting sulfonamides. Also, short-acting sulfonamides usually require an initial loading dose.

If sulfonamides are taken with food, their absorption tends to be delayed but not reduced. See Table 9-10 for a summary of sulfonamides.

▼ Evaluation

A complete blood count, urinalysis, and liver and kidney function tests should be done before initiating sulfonamide therapy and approximately every month thereafter if the patient is on prolonged therapy.

The nurse should observe the patient for signs and symptoms of blood dyscrasias, including sore throat, fever, pallor, purpura, and jaundice, and for renal and/or hepatic failure in high-risk patients.

▼ Patient and family teaching

The nurse should provide the patient and family with the following instructions:

1. Sulfonamides are more fully absorbed when they are taken on an empty stomach. Therefore they should be taken either 1 hour before or 2 hours after meals, along with a full glass of water.
2. To prevent formation of crystals in the urine, the patient must drink large amounts of water while taking this medication.
3. The patient should avoid excessive exposure to sunlight or ultraviolet light to prevent possible photosensitization.
4. The patient should take all the medication prescribed and should not stop taking medication when he or she feels better and the symptoms disappear.
5. The patient should contact the physician if there is no improvement of symptoms within a few days after beginning therapy.
6. The physician should be notified promptly if a skin rash, blood in the urine, bruises, nausea, or other adverse effects of therapy develop.

Table 9-10   Sulfonamides

Generic name	Brand name	Dosage and comments
Sulfacytine	Renoquid	A rapidly absorbed, highly soluble sulfonamide. Used primarily to treat acute, nonobstructive urinary tract infections caused by susceptible organisms. ■ *Urinary tract infection* *Adults and children over 14:* 500 mg PO initially, then 250 mg qid for up to 10 days.
Sulfadiazine	Sulfadiazine	Requires a daily urinary output of at least 1500 ml plus alkalization to prevent crystalluria. SQ and IM routes are contraindicated. ■ *Urinary tract infection, rheumatic fever prophylaxis:* 500 mg qd for patients who weigh less than 30 kg; 1 gm daily for those over 30 kg. ■ *Intraocular infection:* 4 gm initially, then 1 gm q4h. ■ *Intravenous* *Adults:* 100 mg/kg up to total of 5 gm initially, then 30 to 50 mg/kg q6 to 8h. *Children and infants older than 2 months:* 50 mg/kg initially, then 100 mg/kg daily in four divided doses.
Sulfamethoxazole	Gantanol Urobak	An intermediate-acting sulfonamide highly effective in urinary tract infections when used for 7 to 10 days. *Adults:* 2 gm initially, then 1 gm bid to tid. *Children and infants older than 2 months:* 50 to 60 mg/kg initially, then 25 to 30 mg/kg q12h.

Table 9-10	Sulfonamides	
Generic name	**Brand name**	**Dosage and comments**
Sulfamethizole	Thiosulfil	A short-acting, readily soluble sulfonamide effective in the treatment of urinary tract infections. *Adults:* 2 to 4 gm initially, then 2 to 4 gm daily in three to six divided doses. *Children and infants older than 2 months:* 75 mg/kg initially, then 150 mg/kg daily in four to six divided doses, total daily dose not to exceed 6 gm.
Sulfasalazine	Azulfidine SAS Enteric-500 ♣	■ *Ulcerative colitis* *Adults:* 1 to 4 gm daily in four to eight divided doses, then 2 to 3 gm daily in four divided doses as maintenance. *Children and infants older than 2 months:* 40 to 60 mg/kg daily in four to eight divided doses, then 30 mg/kg daily in four divided doses.
Sulfisoxazole	Gantrisin	A highly soluble sulfonamide. ■ *Urinary tract infection* *Adults:* 2 to 4 gm initially, then 4 to 8 gm daily in divided doses. *Children and infants older than 2 months:* 75 mg/kg initially, then 150 mg/kg daily in four to six divided doses, with total daily dose not to exceed 6 gm. ■ *Parenteral use* *Adults and children older than 2 months:* 50 mg/kg initially, then 100 mg/kg daily. ■ *Subcutaneous:* divided into three daily doses. ■ *Intravenous:* divided into four daily doses. ■ *Intramuscular:* divided into two or three daily doses.
Sulfonamide combination products	Triple sulfa	*Vaginal cream:* insert 2.5 to 5.0 ml (one half to one applicator full) cream intravaginally bid for 14 days. Contains equal amounts of sulfadiazine, sulfamerazine, and sulfamethazine, thereby reducing the possibility of crystalluria because the solubility of each sulfonamide exists independently in solution. Used primarily for urinary tract infections. *Adults:* 2 to 4 gm initially, then 2 to 4 gm daily in three to six divided doses. *Children and infants older than 2 months:* 75 mg/kg initially, then 150 mg/kg daily in four to six divided doses, with total daily dose not to exceed 6gm.
Sulfonamide combination vaginal products	Sultrin	Creams contain 3.42% sulfathiazole, 2.86% sulfacetamide, and 3.7% sulfabenzamide. Vaginal tablets contain 172.5 mg sulfathiazole, 143.75 mg sulfacetamide, and 184 mg sulfabenzamide. Full course of therapy is needed to be effective. Sex partners should also be treated. Discontinue medication if burning or local irritation occurs. Effective in about 50% of confirmed *Haemophilus vaginitis* infections. Use one applicatorful of cream intravaginally bid for 4 to 6 days, or one tablet intravaginally bid for 10 days. Treatment may be repeated.
SULFONAMIDE MIXTURES		
Sulfamethoxazole and trimethoprim	Septra Bactrim	Used for acute infections and as prophylaxis. May be used in patients with impaired renal function and for those unable to tolerate sulfonamides alone. ■ *Urinary tract infection* *Adults:* 2 tablets or 20 ml suspension q12h for 10 to 14 days. *Children and infants older than 2 months:* 40 mg/kg sulfamethoxazole and 8 mg/kg trimethoprim daily in two divided doses q12h for 10 days. ■ *Acute otitis media:* Follow pediatric dosage given for urinary tract infection.

SUMMARY

A wide range of medications is available to treat infections. These medications include broad-spectrum antibiotics, antifungals, antitubercular drugs, antiparasitic medications, penicillins, and sulfonamides. Because antiinfectives are so commonly used, the nurse must be familiar with significant adverse reactions and drug interactions, and should know what to teach the patient and family for each type of antibiotic. New antibiotics are continually being developed, partially because of research in this area and also because resistant strains of disease develop (resistant especially to penicillin, which has been in wide use for many years).

 CRITICAL THINKING QUESTIONS

1. After a complete physical, Mrs. Johnson, 87, has just been prescribed a broad-spectrum antibiotic, much to her surprise. Her physician has asked you to administer a first dose for her before she leaves your clinic to head for the pharmacist and then home. After the doctor leaves the room, Mrs. Johnson confides to you, "I'm worried, hon. He shouldn't have given me an antibiotic, should he? I don't have a sore throat. I have a *virus*." Explain to Mrs. Johnson the wide variety of indications for these drugs. Also explain why an antiobiotic is sometimes ordered for a viral infection.

2. Mr. Delavan, a patient in the hospital where you work, has been given metronidazole for a systemic mycotic infection; he also has AIDS and is receiving several other medications as well. Why is it so important to check the ingredients of all other medications Mr. Delavan is taking? What unpleasant interaction can result otherwise?

3. Mr. Delavan had had a number of adverse reactions to a series of treatment trials. He confides in you that he has become wary of ever taking a drug again, saying," All they do is make me sicker, I think. If I take this drug, how do I know it isn't just hurting me in some way?" What adverse reactions should Mr. Delavan be observed for with a fungicide? Write up a treatment and evaluation plan for this patient.

4. A few months later, Mr. Delavan is back. His AIDS has progressed slightly, but a more immediate problem is the discovery that he now has tuberculosis. Mr. Delevan is incredulous, even a little panicky. He tells you that he is anxious to "get rid of it quick before it makes me sicker! How did *this* happen? I thought this disease was eradicated a long time ago!" Explain to Mr. Delavan why TB is easy to catch now and how. Also explain that this a long-term treatment and why compliance is so important. Revise your treatment and teaching plan for this patient.

5. While doing volunteer work overseas, Mr. Johannsen developed malaria and had to come home. His doctor has prescribed chloroquine phosphate. Write out a teaching plan to explain to Mr. Johannsen how to control infection and reinfection, the lifelong possibility of relapses, endemic reactions, how to take his medication, and the need for follow-up exams.

6. Ms. Keaton thinks she is allergic to penicillin, although she has "never been tested," she says. What are the signs and symptoms of hypersensitivity or allergy?

7. What is the difference between bacteriostatic and bactericidal? Using your text, list several drugs that fit into each category. Now add, beneath each drug in your list, indications for the drug's use.

8. Ms. Keaton comes back to the clinic, complaining that she still has the same bladder infection she came to you for the first time. Her doctor switches her to a sulfonamide. "What good will that do?" she asks you. Explain the actions and uses of sulfonamides. Draw up a teaching plan for this patient, stressing the importance of taking the medication properly, symptoms that should be reported immediately to the physician, and symptoms of hypersensitivity.

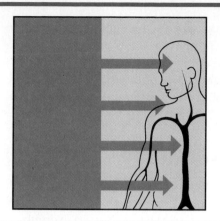

CHAPTER 10
Antineoplastic Agents

OBJECTIVES

At the conclusion of this chapter you should be able to:

1. List the types of drugs used to treat neoplastic disease or cancer.
2. Identify the major adverse effects associated with antineoplastic agents.
3. Develop a teaching plan for a patient taking an antineoplastic drug.

KEY TERMS

alkylating agents, p. 182
antibiotic preparations, p. 182
antimetabolites, p. 182
chemotherapeutic agents, p. 182
male or female hormones, 182
malignancy, p. 181
metastasis, p. 181
mitotic inhibitors, p. 182
neoplasms, p. 181

OVERVIEW

Five types of medications are commonly used to treat neoplastic diseases, including alkylating agents, antibiotics, antimetabolites, hormones, and mitotic inhibitors. These drugs are potentially toxic and should be ordered only by qualified physicians. Adverse effects are common with this group of medications, requiring constant assessment by the nurse.

Most cells in the body grow slowly and at a predictable rate. When cell growth becomes rapid and uncontrolled, **neoplasms** or cancerous tumors may be found. These cells often have the ability to travel throughout the body, spreading this unusually rapid cell growth into other areas (**metastasis**) and robbing other tissues of the nutrients they need to maintain normal health. We call this undisciplined cell growth **malignancy.**

Antineoplastic agents are used to treat malignant diseases. They slow cell growth or delay the spread of the malignant cells throughout the body. Antineoplastic agents, also called **chemotherapeutic agents,** are most often used with other forms of treatment such as surgery and radiation.

Normal cells in the body do not all grow at the same rate. In the gastrointestinal tract, bone marrow, hair follicles, lymph tissue, mouth, and testes or ovaries are rapidly dividing and growing cells. These rapidly growing cells are also affected by antineoplastic drugs, thus producing many of the adverse reactions associated with these drugs.

The types and sites of malignancies vary, and some agents are more effective with some types of malignancies than are other products. The ideal antineoplastic agent will do the most damage to the specific malignant cells of the patient, while preserving the health of the normal cells as much as possible.

There are many new, highly toxic products on the market in this area: interferon, mitotane, asparaginase. These products are used by physicians under strict protocols.

ACTION

There are five major types of antineoplastic agents. They may be used in combination or alone. There are often specific research protocols governing the use of these medications. It is important to accurately report all patient reactions and adverse effects so that the total action of these products can be understood.

Alkylating agents are used to interfere with the normal process of cell division. This effect is found in both malignant and normal cells, although malignant cells seem to be much more susceptible to the medications.

Specific **antibiotic preparations** are used, not for antiinfective properties, but to delay or prevent cell division of the malignant cells. This action is produced through interference with DNA and RNA synthesis.

Antimetabolites disrupt normal cell functions by interfering with various metabolic functions of the cells. This action is most effective in cells that are the most rapidly dividing.

Some tumors may depend on **male or female hormones.** Hormones that counteract these effects may be effective in treating some types of tumors. The mechanism of action is unclear.

Mitotic inhibitors are a special group of medications that interfere with or stop cell division directly.

USES

Antineoplastic drugs are used singly or adjunctively with other types of therapy to treat malignancies. They are usually combined with radiation therapy or are used after surgery. Uses of the drugs are included in the summary of product information presented in Table 10-1.

ADVERSE REACTIONS

Many adverse reactions are produced by the action of the antineoplastic agent on normal cells. Some of these reactions are dose related. Nausea, vomiting, anorexia, and diarrhea are seen with almost all products. Other common reactions include alopecia (hair loss) and bone marrow depression. (Patients with bone marrow depression are more vulnerable to infections and may show evidence of bruising or bleeding.) Some reactions are so severe that the patient feels worse with therapy than with the malignancy. There may be no alternative to the adverse effects except to stop therapy and not treat the malignancy. Knowledge about the most common adverse effects will help the nurse develop a care plan to prevent or reduce as many symptoms as possible. A summary of common adverse effects is presented in Table 10-1.

DRUG INTERACTIONS

Most antineoplastic medications have substantial drug interaction capability. It is very important to consult the manufacturer's guidelines before initiating treatment.

 NURSING IMPLICATIONS AND PATIENT TEACHING

▼ **Assessment**

The nurse must take a careful history regarding the patient's problem and current status, medications taken, surgeries, allergies, and response. Many patients have numerous hospital admissions for a malignancy. Old hospital records should be consulted whenever possible to obtain accurate information and reduce the need for the patient to repeat information. The patient should be asked to review his or her progress since previous hospitalizations. It is

Table 10-1   Antineoplastic agents

Generic name	Trade name	Comments and dosage
ALKYLATING AGENTS		
Busulfan	Myleran	Used in chronic myelogenous leukemia; may produce leukopenia, anemia, thrombocytopenia, hyperpigmentation of skin, and cataracts. Give 1 to 8 mg/day PO.
Carboplatin	Paraplatin	Used in ovarian carcinoma. Give 360 mg/m^2 IV on day 1 every 4 weeks.
Carmustine	BiCNU	Used in brain tumors, Hodgkin's disease, and multiple myeloma; may produce leukopenia, thrombocytopenia, azotemia, nausea, and vomiting; causes burning at injection site. Give 100 to 200 mg/m^2 IV.
Chlorambucil	Leukeran	Used in Hodgkin's disease, chronic lymphocytic leukemia, and malignant lymphomas; may produce hyperuricemia and bone marrow depression. Give 0.03 to 0.2 mg/kg/day PO.
Cisplatin	Platinol	Used in advanced bladder cancer and some metastatic testicular and ovarian tumors; may produce nausea, vomiting, leukopenia, thrombocytopenia, ototoxity, and nephrotoxicity. Give 50 to 70 mg/m^2 IV for bladder cancers and ovarian tumors; 20 mg/m^2 for testicular tumors.
Cyclophosphamide	Cytoxan Neosar	Used in Hodgkin's disease, leukemia, carcinoma of ovary and breast, malignant lymphomas, multiple melanoma, and neuroblastoma; may produce anorexia, nausea, vomiting, diarrhea, cystitis, alopecia, leukopenia, thrombocytopenia, or anemia.
Ifosfamide	Ifex	Used in multiple myeloma. Give 6 mg/day IV in one dose.
Lomustine	CeeNu	Used in Hodgkin's disease, some brain tumors; may produce nausea, vomiting, alopecia, anemia, leukopenia, thrombocytopenia. Give 100 to 130 mg/m^2 PO.
Mechlorethamine	Mustargen	Used in Hodgkin's disease, bronchogenic carcinoma, and lymphosarcoma; may produce nausea, vomiting, jaundice, alopecia, skin rash, diarrhea, lymphocytopenia, granulocytopenia, and thrombocytopenia. Give 0.4 mg/kg IV as a total dose for a course of therapy. Give as a single dose, or divide.
Melphalan	Alkeran	Used in carcinoma of ovary and for multiple myeloma; may produce nausea, vomiting, skin rash, and bone marrow depression. Give 6 to 10 mg/day PO.
Pipobroman	Vercyte	Used in chronic granulocytic leukemia, polycythemia vera; may produce abdominal cramps, nausea, vomiting, diarrhea, and rash. Give 1 to 3 mg/kg/day PO.
Streptozocin	Zanosar	Used in carcinoma of the pancreas; may produce severe nausea, vomiting, and renal toxicity. Give 500 to 1000 mg/m^2 IV.
Thiotepa	Thiotepa	Used in lymphosarcomas or carcinoma of breast, ovary, or urinary bladder; may produce nausea, vomiting, and bone marrow depression; causes pain at injection site. Give 0.3 to 0.4 mg/kg IV. May infiltrate tumor directly.
Uracil mustard	Uracil mustard	Used in non-Hodgkin's lymphomas and chronic lymphocytic or myelogenous leukemias; may produce nausea, vomiting, diarrhea, and bone marrow depression. Give 0.15 mg/kg PO as a single weekly dose.

Table 10-1 Antineoplastic agents—cont'd		
Generic name	**Trade name**	**Comments and dosage**

ANTIBIOTICS

Generic name	Trade name	Comments and dosage
Bleomycin	Blenoxane	Used in testicular carcinoma, lymphomas, and squamous cell carcinomas of head and neck; may cause vomiting, rash, erythema, fever, chills, pulmonary fibrosis, and pneumonitis. Give 0.25 to 0.5 units/kg IV, IM, or SQ.
Dactinomycin	Cosmegen	Used in testicular or uterine carcinoma, Wilms' tumor, and Ewing's sarcoma; may produce anorexia, nausea, vomiting, alopecia, and bone marrow depression. Give 0.5 mg/day IV. Very corrosive to soft tissue.
Daunorubicin hydrochloride	Cerubidine	Used in adult leukemias; may produce nausea, vomiting, fever, chills, alopecia, and bone marrow depression. Give 45 mg/m^2/day IV. Use under strict protocols.
Doxorubicin hydrochloride	Adriamycin Rubex	Used in acute leukemias, Wilms' tumor, carcinomas of breast, ovary, bladder, lymphomas, neuroblastomas, and soft tissue and bone sarcomas; may cause anorexia, nausea, vomiting, alopecia, fever, and bone marrow depression. Give 30 to 75 mg/m^2 IV.
Idarubicin	Idamycin	Used in adult AML. Give 12 mg/m^2 daily for 3 days slow IV.
Mitomycin	Mutamycin	Used in adenocarcinoma of the stomach and pancreas; may cause anorexia, nausea, vomiting, headache, blurred vision, fever, and bone marrow depression. Give 20 mg/m^2 IV as a single dose, or 2 mg/m^2/day IV for 5 days.
Mitoxantrone	Novantrone	Used in combination with other drugs in initial therapy for acute nonlymphatic leukemia; may cause petechiae, nausea, vomiting, diarrhea, stomatitis, sepsis, fungal infections, dyspnea, fever, and alopecia. Give 12 mg/m^2 day on day 1 and day 3; follow with a course of cytosine.
Plicamycin	Mithracin	Used to treat hypercalcemia and hypercalciuria associated with neoplasms and malignant testicular tumors; may produce anorexia, nausea, vomiting, diarrhea, stomatitis, hematemesis, and hemorrhaging of GI tract. Give 25 to 30 µg/kg/day IV for 3 to 4 days.
Pentostatin	Nipent	Used in hairy cell leukemia. Give 4 mg/m^2 IV every other week in well-hydrated patient.

ANTIMETABOLITES

Generic name	Trade name	Comments and dosage
Cytarabine	Cytosar-U	Used in acute myelocytic or lymphocytic leukemia; may cause nausea, vomiting, anorexia, diarrhea, and bone marrow depression. Give 200 mg/m^2/day IV or SQ.
Floxuridine	FUDR	Used in GI adenocarcinoma metastatic to liver; may produce anorexia, nausea, vomiting, diarrhea, alopecia, and bone marrow depression. Give 0.1 to 0.6 mg/kg/day IV.
Fludarabine	Fludara	Used in chronic lymphocytic leukemia. Give 25 mg/m^2 IV over 30 minutes for 5 consecutive days every 28 days.
Fluorouracil	Adrucil	Used in carcinoma of breast, stomach, colon, and pancreas; may cause anorexia, nausea, vomiting, diarrhea, alopecia, and bone marrow depression. Give 3 to 12 mg/kg/day IV.
Mercaptopurine	Purinethol	Used in acute lymphatic leukemia and acute or chronic myelogenous leukemia; may produce hyperuricemia, hepatotoxicity, and bone marrow depression. Give 1.5 to 2.5 mg/kg/day PO.

Continued.

Table 10-1   Antineoplastic agents—cont'd

Generic name	Trade name	Comments and dosage
ANTIMETABOLITES—cont'd		
Methotrexate	Folex	Used in breast cancer, lymphosarcoma, and severe psoriasis; may cause nausea, vomiting, headache, rash, pruritus, stomatitis, bone marrow depression, leukopenia, and renal failure. Give 10 to 50 mg/wk IV, IM, PO or up to 6.5 mg/day PO.
Thioguanine	Thioguanin Lanvis♣	Used in acute nonlymphocytic leukemias and chronic myelogenous leukemia; may produce nausea, vomiting, stomatitis, hyperuricemia, hepatotoxicity, and bone marrow depression. Give 2 to 3 mg/kg/day PO.
HORMONES		
Diethylstilbestrol diphosphate	Stilphostrol Honvol♣	Used in inoperable prostatic carcinoma; may produce pruritus, rash, gynecomastia, thrombophlebitis, and cerebral or pulmonary emboli. Give 50 to 200 mg PO tid; may give IV.
Estramustine	Emcyt	Used in metastatic prostatic carcinoma; may cause nausea, vomiting, diarrhea, anorexia, fluid retention, edema, leukopenia, rash, and thrombocytopenia. Give 15 mg/kg/day PO in three or four divided doses.
Flutamide	Eulexin	Used in metastatic prostatic carcinoma. Give 250 mg tid PO.
Leuprolide	Lupron	Used in advanced prostatic carcinoma; may produce nausea, vomiting, anorexia, dizziness, headache, edema, and bone pain. Give 1 mg/day SQ.
Goserelin acetate	Zoladex	Used in palliative treatment of carcinoma of prostate. Give 3.6 mg SQ every 28 days in upper abdominal wall.
Medroxyprogesterone	Depo-Provera	Used in renal or endometrial carcinoma; may cause pruritus, breast tenderness, and cerebral or pulmonary emboli. Give 400 to 1000 mg/wk IM.
Megestrol acetate	Megace	Used in endometrial or breast carcinoma. Give 40 mg/qid PO for breast carcinoma; 40 to 320 mg/day PO for endometrial cancer.
Polyestradiol phosphate	Estradurin	Used in inoperable, progressing prostate cancer; may cause thrombophlebitis, pulmonary embolism, and cerebral or coronary thrombosis. Give 40 mg deep IM q2 to 4 weeks.
Tamoxifen	Nolvadex	Used in breast cancer in postmenopausal women; may produce hypercalcemia and ophthalmic changes. Give 10 to 20 mg PO bid.
Testolactone	Teslac	Used in breast cancer in postmenopausal women; may cause anorexia, nausea, vomiting, edema, paresthesia, and hypertension. Give 250 mg PO qid.
MITOTIC INHIBITORS		
Etoposide	VePesid	Used in testicular tumors; may produce anorexia, nausea, vomiting, alopecia, and granulocytopenia. Give 50 to 100 mg/m^2/day IV.
Teniposide	Vumon	Used in childhood A.L.L. patients in combination with other products. Extremely corrosive to soft tissue. Give slow IV.
Vinblastine	Velban Velsar	Used in Hodgkin's disease, Kaposi's sarcoma, lymphoma, and testicular carcinoma; may cause nausea, vomiting, malaise, headache, numbness, paresthesias, weakness, depression, and leukopenia. Give 3.7 mg/m^2/week IV as determined by WBC counts.
Vincristine	Oncovin Vincasar PFS	Used in Hodgkin's disease, Wilms' tumor, acute leukemia, lymphosarcoma, neuroblastoma; may produce nausea, vomiting, diarrhea, fever, weight loss, ataxia, headache, and mouth ulcers. Give 1.4 mg/m^2/week IV.

important to evaluate the patient's emotional and physical responses to the illness: cultural beliefs, spiritual and family support, and acceptance of the problem.

▼ Planning

The nurse should consult the latest product information about the preparation, storage, and administration of most antineoplastic medications. All warnings, precautions, and contraindications should be understood and followed. Some preparations should be given only by a physician or a specially trained chemotherapy nurse. New products are released frequently, as well as new suggestions for use based on recently published research.

The initial dosage is often calculated in milligrams per kilogram (mg/kg) or milligrams per square meter of body surface area (mg/m^2 BSA). These calculations are based on surface nomograms, which are usually provided in the manufacturer's product insert. The dosage calculation should be determined by the physician, with future adjustments based on the patient's response as demonstrated by laboratory tests and x-ray studies.

▼ Implementation

The nurse should carefully follow the dosage, frequency, and administration procedures as outlined. Administration of these toxic products may pose a safety hazard to the nurse as well as the patient if the products are not administered properly. The syringes, bottles, and needles must be prepared and disposed of carefully. There usually are special areas designated for mixing these preparations.

See Table 10-1 for a summary of major antineoplastic agents. Additional, more detailed information on hormones may be found in Chapter 19.

▼ Evaluation

The nurse must monitor the patient closely for adverse effects, regularly noting subjective complaints or objective findings on the chart so that the physicians may follow the patient's progress. Patients must be taught which symptoms to report to the physician when medications are given on an outpatient basis.

Nursing or pharmacologic interventions are often needed to reduce adverse effects. Antiemetics may be given for nausea; special skin care may be needed; analgesics or narcotics may be required. Dehydration must be avoided and bowel regularity must be maintained. The nurse must be thorough in the evaluation of the patient's response.

The patient and nurse must cooperate in obtaining needed follow-up laboratory work and x-ray studies to monitor response to medication. The nurse should provide opportunities for patients to discuss their feelings and attitudes about the disease and their therapy.

▼ Patient and family teaching

The nurse should provide the patient and family with the following instructions:

1. Antineoplastic agents are potentially toxic and must be taken as ordered. The reason for their use, the anticipated findings, and the possible adverse reactions must all be explained. The patient may be required to sign a written consent form before many of these drugs can be administered.

2. The possible adverse effects should be explained in detail. Specific plans for preventing or reducing symptoms should be developed.

3. The patient's meals should be made as palatable and attractive as possible because most antineoplastic agents produce anorexia, nausea, and vomiting. The patient may be unable to eat anything at times but may find holding ice chips in the mouth to be helpful.

4. The nurse should be alert to signs of dehydration caused by diarrhea.

5. Hair loss is usually of great concern to the patient. Patients should be given information on wigs and toupees that might be worn until their own hair grows back. Patients with long hair might want to save the hair and have a wig made from their own hair.

6. Patients who have undergone surgery for cancer, such as mastectomy or amputation, should be provided with information about strengthening of muscles following surgery, postoperative recovery period, and prosthesis use and care.

7. There are many support groups available for specific types of cancer, and former patients may visit the hospital and talk to the patient about their colostomy or mastectomy. The nurse can check community resources for further information.

8. The patient should keep any medication that is taken home in a locked cabinet away from children or pets.

SUMMARY

The five types of agents commonly used to treat neoplastic disease are alkylating agents, antibiotics, antimetabolites, hormones, and mitotic inhibitors. Because these drugs are highly toxic, it is especially important for the nurse to monitor adverse reactions in the patient. In addition, dosages must be followed carefully and care must be taken in the preparation and disposal of syringes, bottles, and needles.

 CRITICAL THINKING QUESTIONS

1. What are the five types of medications commonly used in treating neoplastic disease?
2. Describe the development of a malignancy.
3. What common action do all antineoplastic agents share? Are they usually used alone? Describe how treatments (chemotherapy, radiation, or surgery) might be combined and in what order, depending on the circumstances.
4. What healthy, or normal, cells are also affected by antineoplastic agents? Describe the adverse reactions associated with these cells.
5. What is the importance of baseline evaluation in determining therapeutic progress? What factors are taken into consideration? What types of evaluation might be done?
6. What exactly is the nurse's responsibility in each type of evaluation discussed in question 5?
7. Write out a teaching plan for explaining to a patient the correct administration of these powerful agents as well as what to reasonably expect for both therapeutic and adverse effects.
8. What effect might emotional response have on physical response in cancer patients?
9. Describe the typical information that would go on a drug card for a drug in this group.

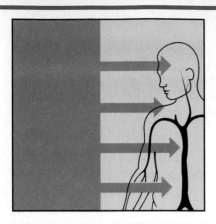

CHAPTER 11

Cardiovascular and Renal-Diuretic Medications

OBJECTIVES

At the conclusion of this chapter you should be able to:

1. Identify the procedures to follow for administration of various forms of antianginal therapy.
2. Discuss the uses and general actions of cardiac drugs used to treat dysrhythmias.
3. Explain the mechanism of action of anticoagulant medications.
4. Describe the common treatment for various types of lipoprotein disorders.
5. Explain the actions of different categories of drugs used to treat hypertension.
6. List the general uses and actions of cardiotonic drugs.

KEY TERMS

action potential duration, p. 196
congestive heart failure, p. 217
depolarization, p. 197
digitalis toxicity, p. 217
digitalizing dose, p. 219
dysrhythmias, p. 196
ectopic beats, p. 197
edema, p. 216
effective refractory period, p. 196
electrocardiogram (ECG), p. 196
end organ damage, p. 210
hyperlipoproteinemia, p. 202
myocardial infarction, p. 196
myocardium, p. 196
normal sinus rhythm, p. 196
pacemaker, p. 196
positive inotropic action, p. 217
primary hypertension, p. 207
secondary hypertension, p. 207

OVERVIEW

This chapter is divided into five major sections, each dealing with an important part of the cardiovascular or circulatory system. Some cardiovascular medications have more than one action and are used for several purposes in the patient with cardiovascular problems. However, they are usually classified into one of several major drug categories.

Section One, antianginal and peripheral vasodilating agents, discusses the medications used to treat angina and occlusive arterial disease. These drugs are widely used, and the nurse has a major responsibility in teaching the patient how to properly store and use the medications.

Section Two discusses the four major classifications of antidysrhythmic medications and the dysrhythmias for which they are most effective. There many adverse reactions associated with some of these medications.

Section Three looks at lipids and the problem of lipoprotein abnormalities. Antihyperlipidemic agents are discussed in the context of overall therapy, including diet, to resolve lipoprotein problems.

Antihypertensive and diuretic drugs are explored in Section Four. This is a major drug category that nurses need to understand thoroughly. The stepped-care approach to antihypertensive therapy is presented, as well as a discussion of common adverse reactions to these medications.

Finally, Section Five examines the cardiotonics—digitalis and related products. These are some of the most frequently prescribed medications, for both the inpatient and the outpatient, and the nurse must clearly understand the mechanisms of action and be able to teach the patient about these medications.

These sections supply basic information about each drug category of cardiovascular medications. A thorough, concurrent study of related anatomy and physiology will help the nurse clearly understand both the cardiovascular problem and the action of the various medications.

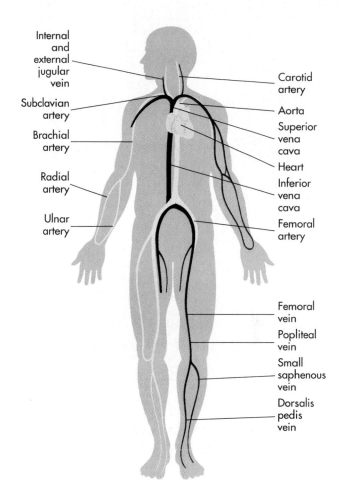

Fig. 11-1   Cardiovascular system.

Cardiovascular System

The cardiovascular system is composed of the heart, blood vessels, and blood (Fig. 11-1). This system transports nutrients, waste products, gases, and hormones throughout the body. It also plays a role in the immune response and the regulation of body temperature.

Using the unique cardiac muscle conduction system, electrical impulses cause the heart to contract, forcing blood from the heart through blood vessels throughout the body. Arteries conduct blood from the heart to tissues using smaller branches called arterioles. Veins conduct blood from tissues toward the heart, with their smaller branches called venules. Capilliaries are extremely small vessels that connect arteries and veins.

The heart is the pump of the circulatory system. It is fed by coronary arteries that nourish it during the resting phase of the cardiac cycle. The heart weakens with disease and advancing age, becoming less efficient. In patients with hypertension the blood vessels become less elastic and the increased pressures that the heart has to pump against cause the heart to work harder. Thus abnormality in the heart, arteries, or veins produces additional stress on the heart itself.

Many of the cardiovascular drugs have either direct or indirect action on the urinary system. The kidneys, urinary bladder, and ducts that carry urine act together to remove waste products from the circulatory system, to regulate blood pH and ion levels, and to maintain water balance. The effective pumping of the heart, the circulatory system efficiency, and the urinary system all work together to produce the body's fluid and electrolyte balance (Fig. 11-2).

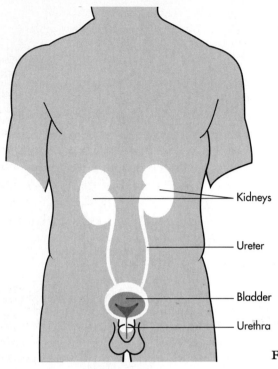

Kidneys

Ureter

Bladder

Urethra

Fig. 11-2   Urinary system.

SECTION ONE: ANTIANGINALS AND PERIPHERAL VASODILATORS

Objectives

At the conclusion of this section you should be able to:
1. Identify the therapeutic goal of antianginal therapy.
2. List systemic effects that may occur when peripheral vasodilating agents are administered.
3. Describe the procedures for administration of various forms of nitroglycerin therapy.
4. Develop a teaching plan that covers the storage and handling of nitroglycerin tablets.

ACTION

Constriction of vascular smooth muscle in the coronary arteries and the peripheral vascular system reduces the amount of blood carried to the heart and the peripheral tissues (Fig. 11-3). Lack of adequate blood supply results in the pain of angina or in peripheral vascular disease. Nitrates are the most effective drugs for treating coronary artery disease, whereas general vasodilating agents are used for pe-

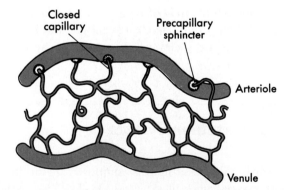

Closed capillary

Precapillary sphincter

Arteriole

Venule

Fig. 11-3   Main components of microcirculation. An arteriole supplies a capillary bed, which drains into a venule.

ripheral vascular disease. Calcium channel blockers are also used to treat angina and hypertension (see the discussion of antihypertensives and diuretics in Section Four).

Nitrates

Nitrate products act directly on vascular smooth muscle and cause it to relax. This effect is felt both in arterial and in venous circulation. Arterial relaxation decreases systemic vascular resistance and cardiac afterload, whereas venous relaxation assists in venous pooling of blood, thereby decreasing venous return to the heart and preload. These effects combine to decrease myocardial oxygen consumption. In addition, nitrates increase the use of coronary collaterals (small blood vessels) so that there is better perfusion of the inner layers of the myocardium. Nitrates are readily absorbed sublingually, through the skin, and orally, but products taken orally are rapidly metabolized in the liver to inactive metabolites, and the half-life is only 1 to 4 minutes. Newer transdermal forms of the medication allow nitrates to pass directly into the bloodstream, thus reaching target organs before being deactivated by the hepatic system.

Calcium channel blockers

Calcium is an electrolyte that helps transmit electrical impulses through cardiac tissue. Calcium channel blockers slow down the movement of calcium ions across the cell membrane, thus lessening the amount of calcium available for impulse conduction. These drugs act directly on vascular smooth muscle to dilate coronary arteries and arterioles, which relieves anginal pain because more oxygen can be delivered to the cardiac tissue. These drugs also reduce the irritability of the cardiac conduction system and are used to treat cardiac dysrhythmias. They are also combined with other medications to treat hypertension (see the sections on antidysrhythmics and antihypertensives, p. 196-199 and 207-216, for a detailed discussion of calcium channel blockers).

Peripheral vasodilators

Some individuals with occlusive arterial disease have been treated with vasodilating drugs, but with only limited success. Patients often have swollen, painful feet with ulcerations around the ankles. Vasodilator medications relax the smooth muscles of peripheral arterial blood vessels, leading to increased circulation to the extremities (Fig. 11-4).

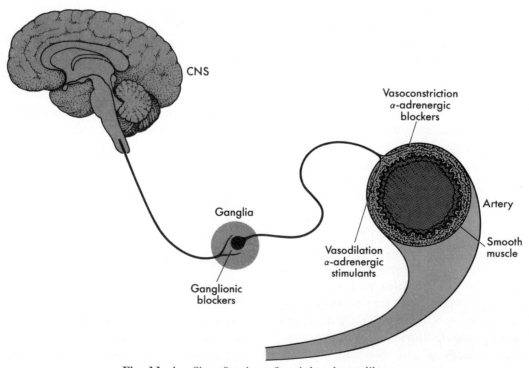

Fig. 11-4   Site of action of peripheral vasodilators.

USES

Rapid-acting nitrates (such as amyl nitrite, sublingual nitroglycerin, and sublingual or chewable isosorbide dinitrate) are used primarily to relieve pain in acute angina. The long-acting nitrates and topical, transdermal, transmucosal, and oral sustained-release nitroglycerin products are used prophylactically to treat predictable anginal attacks and to decrease the severity and frequency of anginal attacks. They are also used to reduce the cardiac workload in cases of myocardial infarction, in congestive heart conditions, and for relief of biliary, gastrointestinal, urethral, and bronchial smooth muscle pain.

It has not been determined whether it is safe to use nitroglycerin in patients with acute myocardial infarctions. When it is used in patients with recent mycardial infarctions, the transdermal systems perform best and patients must be closely evaluated. IV nitroglycerin administration is particularly hazardous and must be performed only when a patient can be monitored carefully.

Peripheral vasodilating agents are used to treat intermittent claudication, arteriosclerosis obliterans, Raynaud's disease, and nocturnal leg cramps, as well as vasospasm associated with thrombophlebitis.

ADVERSE REACTIONS

Some of these products contain tartrazine, which may cause an allergic-type reaction with symptoms similar to bronchial asthma. Patients who are allergic to aspirin have a greater tendency to react to tartrazine.

Tolerance and cross-tolerance may develop to nitrate products that are used for prolonged periods. Excessive doses may produce violent headaches. All nitrates should be given with care to patients with a recent history of cerebrovascular accident (CVA), because of the cerebral vasodilation that occurs.

There are many other common adverse reactions to nitrates, including flushing, postural hypotension, tachycardia, confusion, dizziness, fainting, headache, lightheadedness, vertigo, weakness, drug rash, localized pruritic eczematous eruptions, vesicular and pruritic lesions, conjunctival and oral mucosal edema, local burning in oral cavity, nausea, and vomiting.

Peripheral vasodilating agents may produce dizziness, headache, weakness, tachycardia, flushing, postural hypotension, dysrhythmias, confusion, severe rash, nervousness, tingling, and sweating. The side effects often disappear within a few weeks if they are minimal and if the patient can continue to take the medication.

DRUG INTERACTIONS

Nitrates increase the effects of atropine-like drugs and tricyclic antidepressants, and decrease the effects of all cholinelike drugs. Anticholinergic drugs may be potentiated, especially antihistamines. Nitrates should not be used concurrently with prazosin because of the possibility of interaction. Alcohol, beta blockers, antihypertensives, narcotics, and vasodilators taken with nitrates and nitrites (especially amyl nitrite) may produce severe hypotension and cardiovascular collapse. The vasopressor actions of sympathomimetic drugs may be antagonized. A cold environment or the use of tobacco reduces the effectiveness of nitroglycerin. Cross-tolerance can develop among all nitrates and nitrites. Nitroglycerin also increases urine vanillylmandelic acid (VMA) and catecholamine levels.

Peripheral vasodilating agents are potentiated by antihypertensives and alcohol, leading to hypotension.

 NURSING IMPLICATIONS AND PATIENT TEACHING

▼ Assessment

The nurse should obtain a complete health history to determine the presence of underlying disease, allergy, other drug administration that may produce interactions, and the possibility of pregnancy. A complete description of the anginal attacks should be obtained so that the appropriate therapeutic drug can be selected.

▼ Planning

In choosing the proper preparation for the patient, consider the information found in Table 11-1, comparing the action of various products.

▼ Implementation

Review the procedure for administration of nitroglycerin products in Chapter 4, p. 89.

Excessive dosage may produce violent headaches that can usually be controlled by lowering the dosage and administering analgesics. These headaches will gradually subside.

Table 11-1   Comparison of nitrate-nitrite products

Product	Onset	Duration	Preparation
AGENTS FOR ACUTE ANGINA			
Amyl nitrite	30 sec	3 to 5 min	Inhalant
Isosorbide dinitrate	2 to 5 min	1 to 2 hr	Sublingual/chewable
Nitroglycerin	3 min	30 to 60 min	Sublingual
	3 min	3 to 5 hr	Transmucosal
	Immediately	3 to 5 min	Intravenous
AGENTS FOR ANGINA PROPHYLAXIS			
Erythrityl tetranitrate	5 min	3 hr	Sublingual/chewable
	30 min	6 hr	Oral
Isosorbide dinitrate	15 to 30 min	4 to 6 hr	Oral
	Slow	12 hr	Sustained release, PO
Nitroglycerin	Slow	8 to 12 hr	Sustained release, PO
	30 to 60 min	4 to 6 hr	Topical ointment
	30 to 60 min	24 hr	Transdermal
Pentaerythritol tetranitrate	20 to 60 min	4 to 5 hr	Oral
	30 min	12 hr	Sustained release, PO

See Table 11-2, p. 194, for a summary of antianginal and peripheral vasodilating medications.

▼ Evaluation

The drug should be discontinued if blurring of vision or dry mouth occurs. If the patient reports that portions of the sustained-release medication are being passed in the stool, it is likely that food moves through the GI tract too rapidly to allow the medication to be absorbed. These patients should take oral or sublingual medication.

Elderly patients may have postural hypotension with these drugs and need to be monitored carefully. They may need to have someone with them when they take the medication.

Volatile nitrites are sometimes abused to produce sensations of lightheadedness, dizziness, and euphoria. Abuse may also produce sexual stimulation.

The patient must clearly understand what the uses and limitations are for the nitrate being taken. The patient should understand the dosage schedule and be given instructions about when to seek medical attention during an anginal attack that does not respond to therapy. There are many important considerations in taking this medication by its various routes. Refer to the specific product information sections for details. It is important to note that excessive doses may produce severe headaches. A person using a nitrate for a prolonged period should taper off gradually to avoid precipitating anginal attacks, which may be provoked by stopping the drug suddenly.

 CRITICAL DECISION:

Tolerance with Nitrates

Tolerance and cross-tolerance with other nitrates may develop over time with repeated use. Other coronary vasodilators may have to be used.

▼ Patient and family teaching

The nurse should provide the patient and family with the following instructions:

1. Nitroglycerin breaks down rapidly; sunlight speeds up this process. Even under the best storage conditions these drugs lose their strength in about 3 months after the bottle has been opened. A new prescription should be obtained every 3 months and the old medication should be discarded. A burning sensation

Table 11-2 Antianginal and peripheral-vasodilating medications

Generic name	Trade name	Uses	Adverse reactions	Dose ranges
ANTIANGINALS				
Amyl nitrite	Amyl nitrite	Angina pectoris	Flushing, headache, dizziness, tachycardia, weakness, vertigo	0.18 to 0.3 ml by inhalation
Erythrityl tetranitrate	Cardilate	Prophylaxis of angina	Same as above	5 to 10 mg SL
Isosorbide mononitrate	ISMO	Prophylaxis of angina	Same as above	20 mg bid PO
Isosorbide dinitrate (PO, SL, and chewable)	Isordil Sorbitrate Coradur♣	Prophylaxis of angina Acute angina	Same as above	5 to 30 mg PO qid 2.5 to 30 mg SL; 5 mg chewable and increase as needed
Nitroglycerin (sublingual)	Nitrostat	Prophylaxis, treatment, and management of angina	Same as above	1 tablet SL; repeat in 3 min three times, as needed
Nitroglycerin (sustained release)	Nitro-Bid Nitroglyn Nitrong	Prophylaxis or management of angina	Same as above	1 cap or tab q8 to 12h
Nitroglycerin (topical)	Nitro-Bid Nitrol	Prevention and treatment of angina caused by CAD	Same as above	1 to 5 inches q4 to 8h
Nitroglycerin (transdermal patch)	Nitrodisc Nitro-Dur Transderm-Nitro	Prevention and treatment of angina caused by CAD	Same as above	Apply pad daily
Nitroglycerin (translingual)	Nitrolingual	Prophylaxis and treatment of acute angina	Same as above	1 or 2 metered doses sprayed onto oral mucosa
Nitroglycerin (transmucosal)	Nitrogard	Prophylaxis and treatment of angina	Same as above	Insert buccally 1 mg q3 to 5h during waking hours
Pentaerythritol tetranitrate	Pentylan Peritrate Duotrate	Prophylaxis of angina	Same as above	10 to 40 mg PO tid to qid
PERIPHERAL VASODILATORS				
Cyclandelate	Cyclospasmol Cyclan	Intermittent claudication, arteriosclerosis obliterans	Headache, flushing, GI distress, tachycardia, weakness	200 to 600 mg/day PO ac and hs
Ethaverine	Ethaquin Ethatab	Peripheral and cerebral vascular insufficiency	Nausea, vomiting, GI distress, hypotension, dysrhythmias	100 to 200 mg tid
Isoxsuprine	Vasodilan	Peripheral vascular disease, cerebral vascular insufficiency	Dizziness, hypotension, rash, tachycardia, nausea, vomiting, GI distress, nervousness, weakness, sweating	10 to 20 mg PO tid to qid 5 to 10 mg IM bid to tid
Nylidrin	Adrin Arlidin	Peripheral vascular disease	Nervousness, nausea, weakness, vomiting	3 to 12 mg PO tid to qid
Papaverine	Cerespan Pavabid Papaverine Genabid	Peripheral vascular disease, cerebral ischemia	GI distress, nausea, flushing, vertigo, rash, drowsiness, headache, sedation, sweating	100 to 300 mg PO IM, IV one to five times daily; 3 to 12 mg IM or IV slowly q3h prn

under the tongue is not a reliable indicator that a sublingual medication is still potent, because some drugs are in a much purer form than others. A potent drug always produces the characteristic throbbing headache.

2. Natural and predictable side effects of nitroglycerin include flushing of the face, brief throbbing headache, increased heart rate, dizziness, and lightheadedness when sitting up rapidly. The headache usually lasts no longer than 20 minutes and may be relieved by analgesics. The patient should rest for 10 to 15 minutes after the pain is relieved. The doctor should be notified if blurring of vision, persistent headache, or dry mouth occurs.

3. The medication should be taken on an empty stomach when possible.

4. The patient must not drink alcoholic beverages while taking nitrate products.

5. The active ingredient in nitroglycerin is very easily destroyed. Storage in plastic or in a cardboard box allows the nitrate to escape. Cotton plugs in the top of the container or other drugs stored with nitroglycerin will absorb the nitrate. The medication should be stored in the original dark glass container. All cotton wadding should be removed and the container should be kept tightly capped and out of sunlight; for topical ointment, the tube should be kept tightly closed.

6. Patients using inhalant medication should take it only when lying or sitting down. Because this is a highly flammable product, the patient must not smoke and should avoid using it around fire or sparks.

7. Transmucosal nitroglycerin tablets should not be chewed or swallowed. The patient should put the tablet inside the cheek or under the lip and let it slowly dissolve.

8. The topical ointment should be spread in a thin layer on the skin, using an applicator and a ruler. The ointment should not be rubbed or massaged into the skin. The patient should wash off any medication that might have gotten on the hands.

9. For transdermal application the patient should select a hairless spot (or clip hair) and apply the adhesive pad to the skin. Washing, bathing, or swimming does not affect this system. If the pad should come off, it should be discarded and a new one should be placed on a different site.

10. If the medication does not seem to be as effective after the patient has taken it for a while (requiring the patient to take several pills before getting relief), the patient may be developing a tolerance to the drug. Discontinuing the drug for several days may be long enough to restore sensitivity. The smallest possible dose should be taken to minimize the risk of developing tolerance.

11. The patient should keep a record of the frequency of anginal attacks, the number of pills taken, and any side effects. The patient should bring this record to each appointment.

12. The patient should use nitroglycerin in anticipation of situations in which anginal attacks are likely; taking the medication before the activity may prevent or reduce the degree of pain.

13. This medication is only part of the therapy for angina. The patient should try to avoid situations that precipitate pain (stress, heavy exercise, overeating, smoking), reduce calorie intake if weight loss is desirable, and develop a program of regular and sensible exercise.

14. The patient should avoid excessive intake of foods that stimulate the heart (coffee, tea, caffeinated soft drinks, excessive chocolate).

15. This medication must be kept out of the reach of children and others for whom it is not prescribed.

 CRITICAL DECISION:
Anginal Attacks

For acute anginal attacks, the patient should take one tablet sublingually as soon as the pain begins. The medication should not be chewed or swallowed; it should be dissolved under the tongue. The patient should lie down and rest. If the pain is not relieved within 1 to 3 minutes, a second pill may be taken. If the pain is not relieved within another 3 minutes, a third pill may be taken. If the pain is not relieved, the patient *must* go to an emergency room immediately for evaluation.

SECTION TWO: ANTIDYSRHYTHMICS

Objectives

At the conclusion of this section you should be able to:

1. Discuss the uses and general actions of cardiac depressant drugs used to treat dysrhythmias.
2. Describe the general adverse reactions seen with antidysrhythmic agents.
3. Develop a plan for administering antidysrhythmics.
4. Identify key items to teach the patient and family regarding antidysrhythmics.

ACTION

An individual with heart disease or another disease that secondarily affects the heart muscle has the potential to develop irregular beating of the heart, or cardiac **dysrhythmias.** Dysrhythmias may be fast or slow, with an irregular or regular pattern. The most common causes of dysrhythmias are irritation to the heart tissue after the patient has suffered a heart attack **(myocardial infarction),** or fluid and electrolyte imbalances, diet, hypoxia (reduced blood oxygen), or reactions from drugs.

The heart muscle or **myocardium** is made up of special muscle cells. These muscle cells work together under the direction of a unique group of nerve fibers called the **pacemaker,** located in the sinoatrial (SA) node. The pacemaker cells communicate with the rest of the cardiac cells through a special electrical–nerve transmission system. A person's heart rate is determined by how fast the pacemaker cells direct the heart to pump, and by how quickly this information is spread throughout the heart. The usual path of communication originates in the SA node, passing through the atrium to the atrioventricular (AV) node, through the bundle of His, through the right and left bundle branches, and out through the Purkinje fibers of the myocardium. When the electrical impulse has spread through this pathway, the heart will contract, forcing blood out into the arteries. After a brief rest, the cycle will begin again. This is called **normal sinus rhythm**.

The electrical message directing the heart to contract depends on a special balance of electrolytes in the cardiac tissues and on having the conduction system in good repair. This electrical message is what is recorded by the **electrocardiogram (ECG).** Fig. 11-5 illustrates the conduction system of the heart and the resulting electrocardiogram pattern.

When the cells in the conduction system do not have enough oxygen or are destroyed or damaged through disease, or when the electrolytes become unbalanced, irregular heart action is found. Some patients may describe very slow, regular or irregular heartbeats; some patients may have fast, irregular heartbeats. Some individuals may only feel a little dizzy or report that their heart has "skipped a beat." The nurse may feel an irregular pulse or hear the irregularity with the stethoscope. The exact type of irregular rhythm can only be determined by taking an electrocardiogram. Some patients may wear a heart monitor strapped to their chest, or may be placed in a coronary care unit for close observation and monitoring. The goal of any therapeutic regimen is for the patient's heart to regain a normal rate and rhythm.

Antidysrhythmic medications reduce electrical irregularity of the heart by acting in one of four major ways:

1. Class I drugs (quinidine, procainamide, disopyramide)
   a. Lengthen the **effective refractory period** (time the cells cannot discharge their electrical activity) of atrial and ventricular myocardium by slowing the fast inward current caused by the sodium electrolyte
   b. Make the heart less excitable
2. Class II drugs (beta blockers, such as propranolol, esmolol, and acebutolol) reduce sympathetic excitation to the heart
3. Class III drugs (amiodarone) lengthen the **action potential duration** or the time the electrical impulse is in one cell; class III drugs are currently investigational
4. Class IV drugs (verapamil) selectively block the ability of calcium to come into the myocardium and prolong the effective refractory period (or resting period) in the atrioventricular (AV) node

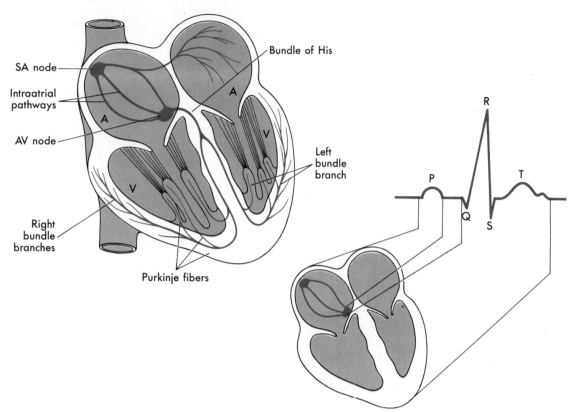

Fig. 11-5   The conduction system and relationship of the electrocardiogram to heart anatomy.

USES

It is important to determine the cause of the dysrhythmia when deciding which drug will be effective. The two basic mechanisms within the heart that cause dysrhythmias are (1) increased sensitivity of electrical cells in the heart resulting in extra or **ectopic beats,** and (2) electrical activity through abnormal conduction pathways.

Two medications commonly used to treat rapid and irregular dysrhythmias are quinidine and procainamide. These medications are chemically unrelated, but both act to quiet the myocardial cells and make them less excitable. This not only decreases the heart rate, but also reduces some of the extra or irregular beats. Conduction cells must rest after passing the electrical message to the next cell and before they can pass another electrical signal. These drugs act to lengthen the resting period (or refractory period) of the cells. This means that it takes longer for each cell to pass the message along to the next cell, slowing the heart rate.

Bretylium is a newer medication used to slow the

conduction rate of ventricular muscle. This medication acts in an unknown manner to slow the release of norepinephrine in the cardiac cells so the heart muscle responds more slowly.

Disopyramide slows the **depolarization** of the cardiac cells. Depolarization is the movement of electrolytes into and out of the cell in preparation for sending another electrical message. The rate of the heart is slowed, because each cell is slower in recovering from the message sent.

A widely used intravenous medication is lidocaine. The electrical impulse sent to the cardiac muscles must be of a certain intensity or it cannot pass along the conduction nerve fibers. Lidocaine increases the level of intensity that the impulse must have to travel the pathway. A diseased heart may have multiple electrical impulses trying to pass, but some impulses are very weak. By increasing the level the impulse must reach before it may be conducted, many weakened impulses will be screened out, and the overall rate will be slower.

Another example of drugs that influence heart

Table 11-3 Acute treatment and chronic prophylaxis of dysrhythmias

	Type of treatment indicated*	
Dysrhythmia	Acute	Chronic prophylaxis
Sinus tachycardia	Propranolol	Propranolol
Premature atrial contractions	Digoxin	Digoxin
		Quinidine, disopyramide, procainamide
		Propranolol
Premature ventricular contractions	Lidocaine	Quinidine, disopyramide, procainamide
	Procainamide	Digoxin
		Propranolol
Atrial flutter/atrial fibrillation	Cardioversion	Digoxin
	Digoxin	Propranolol
		Quinidine, disopyramide, procainamide
		Verapamil
Paroxysmal supraventricular tachycardia	Carotid massage	Propranolol
	Cardioversion	Digoxin
	Propranolol	Quinidine, disopyramide, procainamide
	Digoxin	Verapamil

*Listed in order of suggested use.

activity are the beta-adrenergic blockers, of which propranolol is the most well known. Drugs in this category act very much like quinidine, but they also decrease the response of the heart muscle to epinephrine and norepinephrine by blocking the stimulation of the heart's beta receptors.

There is a wide range of antidysrhythmic medications. Table 11-3 summarizes the suggested treatment of acute and chronic dysrhythmias with these and other cardiotonic medications.

ADVERSE REACTIONS

Most medications given to control dysrhythmias may also cause other dysrhythmias. All patients receiving these medications should have their electrocardiogram closely monitored for change.

Specific symptoms to monitor with each medication include the following:

Bretylium may produce hypotension, postural hypotension, vertigo, lightheadedness, nausea, and vomiting.

Disopyramide may cause dry mouth, constipation, urinary hesitancy, urinary retention, urinary frequency, blurred vision, dryness of mucous membranes, dizziness, headache, hypokalemia, and fatigue.

Lidocaine may produce drowsiness, dizziness, apprehension, euphoria, tinnitus, blurred or double vision, hypotension, cardiac collapse, respiratory depression or arrest, bradycardia, convulsions, and hallucinations.

Procainamide may cause anorexia, rash, itching, nausea, severe hypotension, and ventricular dysrhythmias.

Propranolol may produce bradycardia, dizziness, vertigo, rash, bronchospasm, hyperglycemia or hypoglycemia, hypotension, agranulocytosis, visual disturbances, fatigue, chest pain, joint pain, and itching.

Quinidine may cause cardiac dysrhythmias, hypotension, diarrhea, tinnitus, headache, vertigo, confusion, delirium, disturbances in vision, and abdominal pain. Toxic effects are called cinchonism and produce ringing in the ears, lightheadedness, headache, fever, vertigo, nausea, vomiting, and dizziness.

DRUG INTERACTIONS

Quinidine's effect is enhanced by potassium and is reduced by hypokalemia. Verapamil has an additive effect when used with digitalis and beta blockers. Beta blockers have many interactions. The product information should be consulted for each drug.

NURSING IMPLICATIONS AND
PATIENT TEACHING

▼ Assessment

The nurse should obtain a complete health history, including presence of hypersensitivity, other drugs being taken that may cause drug interactions, and other medical problems, including underlying factors such as hypoxia, acid-base imbalance, increased or decreased potassium, or drug toxicity.

CRITICAL DECISION:
History of Congestive Heart Failure

These drugs often cause or worsen congestive heart failure or urinary retention. Patients with a previous history of heart failure should be monitored carefully.

▼ Planning

A baseline electrocardiogram should be obtained before medications are started.

▼ Implementation

Vital signs should be taken before administering the medication. Hospitalized patients often continue their antidysrhythmia medications when they go home. The nurse should take every opportunity to teach the patient about the medications.

See Table 11-4, p. 200, for a summary of antidysrhythmics.

▼ Evaluation

If the patient is not on a cardiac monitor, the results from routine electrocardiograms must be closely monitored by the physician. Electrolyte levels and other laboratory data should also be obtained as relevant.

▼ Patient and family teaching

The nurse should provide the patient and family with the following instructions:

1. The patient must take this medication exactly as ordered and not skip doses or double the doses.
2. Some people have side effects from these drugs. The patient should report any new or uncomfortable symptoms to the physician, especially any sudden weight gain, trouble breathing, or increased coughing.
3. The patient must return regularly for visits to the physician so that progress on this medication can be followed.
4. The drug may cause dizziness or blurred vision, so the patient should use caution if driving or performing tasks requiring alertness. Alcoholic beverages should be avoided, because they may increase these symptoms.
5. The patient must not take any other medications without the knowledge and approval of the physician, including aspirin, laxatives, cold and sinus products, or other over-the-counter medications.

SECTION THREE: ANTIHYPERLIPIDEMICS

Objectives

At the conclusion of this section you should be able to:

1. Identify the basic types of lipoproteins.
2. Describe the common treatment for various types of lipoprotein disorders.
3. Identify specific drugs helpful in the treatment of type II and type IV hyperlipidemia.

OVERVIEW

Lipids are present in the bloodstream, bound tightly to plasma proteins (albumin and globulins). These lipoprotein complexes contain different proportions of high-density and low-density lipids. The four major types of lipoproteins are:

1. *Chylomicrons.* These are the largest and lightest of the lipoproteins. They are formed during the absorption of dietary fat in the intestine and are normally in plasma only 1 to 8 hours after the last meal. They impart a cloudiness to plasma

Table 11-4	Antidysrhythmics			
Generic name	**Trade name**	**Uses**	**Adverse reactions**	**Dosage ranges**
CLASS I DRUGS				
A				
Disopyramide	Norpace	Treat ectopic ventricular dysrhythmias	Constipation, urinary hesitancy, headache, dry mouth, blurred vision, nausea	100 to 200 mg qid
Procainamide	Pronestyl Procan SR	PVCs, ventricular tachycardias, atrial fibrillation, PAT	Cardiac dysrhythmias, anorexia, urticaria, chills, hypotension	500 to 1000 mg q4 to 6h; or 50 mg/kg/day PO
Quinidine (gluconate, sulfate, or polygalacturonate)	Quinora Quinalan Quinate ♣ Cardioquin	PACs, PVCs, PAT, atrial flutter, atrial fibrillation	Tinnitus, disturbed vision, headache, nausea, dizziness	0.2 to 0.6 mg PO or 330 or 600 mg IM, depending on product; reserve for hospitalized patient
B				
Lidocaine	Xylocaine (without preservatives)	Life-threatening ventricular dysrhythmias	Bradycardia, drowsiness, hypotension, lightheadedness, convulsions	300 mg IM; 50 to 100 mg IV push, 1 to 4 mg/min IV
Mexiletine	Mexitil	Symptomatic ventricular dysrhythmias	GI distress, tremor, lightheadedness, incoordination, hepatic and hematologic effects	600 to 1200 mg/day
Tocainide	Tonocard	Symptomatic ventricular dysrhythmias	Lightheadedness, dizziness, nausea, vomiting, paresthesias, tremor, blood dyscrasias	200 to 400 mg q8h
C				
Encainide	Enkaid	Life-threatening ventricular dysrhythmias	Anorexia, dizziness, nervousness	75 to 200 mg PO qd
Flecainide	Tambocor	Life-threatening ventricular dysrhythmias	Anorexia, dizziness, nervousness, blurred vision, chest pain	100 mg PO q12h
Propafenone	Rythmol	Life-threatening ventricular dysrhythmias	Dizziness, unusual taste, AV block, nausea, vomiting	150 mg q8h

Table 11-4   Antidysrhythmics—cont'd

Generic name	Trade name	Uses	Adverse reactions	Dosage ranges
CLASS I DRUGS **D**				
Moricizine (Does not belong to A, B, or C category but shares some characteristics of each)	Ethmozine	Severe ventricular dysrhythmias	May provoke other dysrhythmias	600 to 900 mg/day in 3 divided doses
CLASS II DRUGS—BETA BLOCKERS (See section on antihypertensives) **A**				
Acebutolol **B**	Sectral	Ventricular tachycardia	Bradycardia, dizziness	200 mg bid
Esmolol **C**	Brevibloc	Supraventricular tachycardia	Bradycardia, dizziness	50 to 200 µg/kg/min
Propranolol	Inderal	Cardiac dysrhythmias, migraine, angina, MI, pheochromocytoma	Bradycardia, dizziness, vertigo, rash, bronchospasm, hyperglycemia, hypotension, agranulocytosis	10 to 30 mg PO tid
CLASS III DRUGS **A**				
Amiodarone **B**	Cordarone	Life-threatening ventricular dysrhythmias	GI distress, CNS symptoms, photosensitivity	800 to 1000 mg/day PO
Bretylium	Bretylol Bretylate ✦	Prophylaxis and treatment of ventricular fibrillation	Hypotension, postural hypotension, nausea, vomiting, lightheadedness, vertigo	5 to 10 mg/kg IV over 10 to 30 min
C				
Sotalol	Betapace	Life-threatening ventricular tachycardia	Proarrhythmic effects	80 mg bid, up to 240 mg/day
CLASS IV DRUGS **A**				
Adenosine **B**	Adenocard	Supraventricular tachycardia	Facial flushing, shortness of breath	6 mg rapid IV bolus
Calcium channel blockers Verapamil	Calan Isoptin	Supraventricular tachydysrhythmias	Cardiac dysrhythmias, CHF, hypotension	80 to 120 mg PO q6 to 8h

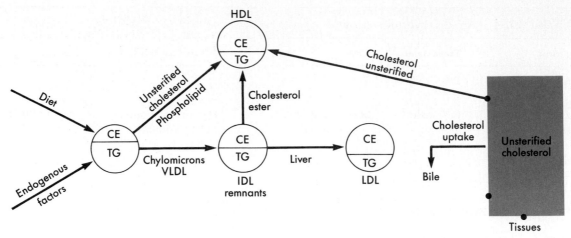

Fig. 11-6 Normal pathway of lipid metabolism. *CE,* Cholesterol esters; *TG,* triglycerides; *IDL,* intermediate-density lipoproteins or remnants; *LDL,* low-density lipoproteins; *HDL,* high-density lipoproteins; *VLDL,* very low–density lipoproteins.

and are primarily triglycerides. If a tube of blood from a fasting patient shows a thick layer of fat or cloudy plasma after several hours, the patient may have an inability to handle dietary fat.

2. *Very low–density lipoproteins (VLDL).* These are made up of large amounts of triglycerides that were synthesized in the liver and are called pre-beta lipoproteins. This is a carrier state for transferring endogenous triglycerides from the liver to the plasma. Practically all the triglycerides in plasma not in chylomicrons are considered to be VLDL.

3. *Low-density lipoproteins (LDL).* When VLDL break down and combine with cholesterol and protein, very little triglyceride is left. This remaining product is then called beta lipoprotein. About 75% of cholesterol concentration in plasma is transported in this form. Elevated serum levels of LDL indicate excess cholesterol levels. Patients with high LDL levels are at high risk for developing atherosclerosis.

4. *High-density lipoproteins (HDL).* These small, dense lipoproteins are called alpha lipoproteins and contain very small parts of triglycerides. They are mostly protein and cholesterol. They serve as the vacuum cleaners of the tissues, clearing out excess cholesterol. They may inhibit atherosclerotic activity by blocking uptake of LDL cholesterol by vascular smooth muscle cells, and may be known among the lay public as "good cholesterol."

Fig. 11-6 illustrates schematically the normal physiology of lipoprotein transport.

Hyperlipoproteinemia is the term used to indicate an increase in levels of one or more of the classes of lipoproteins and may represent an excess of cholesterol, triglycerides, or both. Patients with defects in lipid transport or metabolism can be classified on the basis of the types of lipoproteins that are elevated in the plasma. Accurate diagnosis and treatment prescriptions may be developed through use of these classifications.

The type of hyperlipoproteinemia refers to the abnormal lipoprotein pattern, but does not designate the specific disease. The classification is based on the overload of a particular lipid transport pathway. Types of hyperlipoproteinemia include:

Type I: loss of an enzymatic step in removal of chylomicrons; this is relatively rare. This disorder is seen in infancy, and is marked by abdominal pain. It does not lead to atherosclerosis. It has also been called fat-induced or exogenous hyperlipoproteinemia.

Type II: excess production or inadequate clearance of LDL. Subgroup *a* has characteristics of high levels of LDL, with normal VLDL and slight elevation in triglycerides. Type IIa is fairly common and carries with it an increased risk for development of atherosclerosis. It is also known as familial hypercholesterolemia. Subgroup *b* has high levels of LDL and VLDL, hypercholesterolemia, and hypertriglyceridemia. Xanthomatous lipid deposits are found on knees, feet, elbows, and ears.

Type III: block in metabolism of VLDL to LDL, causing an abnormal "intermediate" form of lipoprotein to circulate in the plasma. Elevated LDL, VLDL, cholesterol, and triglyceride levels are found. This is a recessively inherited disorder and is not as common as some other types. It does carry a risk of developing atherosclerosis.

Type IV: excess production or inadequate clearance of VLDL. Triglycerides are increased, but LDL and cholesterol are normal or slightly elevated. This is also called the carbohydrate-induced or endogenous hyperlipoproteinemia, and it is the most common form. A definite risk for atherosclerosis exists with this type.

Type V: VLDL excess combined with poor chylomicron removal. Elevated levels of VLDL, triglycerides, and chylomicrons are found. It is not associated with a risk of atherosclerosis, and it is a relatively uncommon type.

Although the average cholesterol level for Americans has dropped, there are still a substantial number of people with levels that place them at risk for coronary heart disease (CHD). Recently, a panel of the National Cholesterol Education Program issued a new set of guidelines concerning cholesterol:

1. Establishing therapy based on risk of CHD. Those with existing CHD, men ≥ 45 years old, and women ≥ 55 years old are now considered high-risk patients who would benefit from cholesterol-lowering therapy. Young adult males (< 35 years old) and premenopausal females with elevated total and LDL cholesterol levels are at risk, regardless of their overall health, but should try diet and exercise before resorting to drug therapy.

2. Taking a closer look at HDL levels. HDL levels should be determined at the initial cholesterol test and should be considered when choosing a cholesterol-lowering therapy. Higher HDL levels (e.g., > 60 mg/dl) may in fact be a negative CHD risk factor (i.e., those with lower HDL levels are at higher risk for CHD).

3. Viewing physical activity and diet (reducing intake of saturated fat) as important components of any cholesterol-lowering therapy. In younger patients, it may be the only program necessary.

Lipids are important in the production of atherosclerosis, although the exact mechanism is not clear. It appears that there is a metabolic disturbance in the synthesis, transport, and use of lipids. Patients with

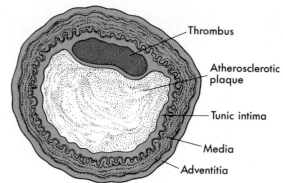

Fig. 11-7   Occlusion of an atherosclerotic coronary artery by a thrombus.

damaged vascular endothelial lining (which occurs in most people in the process of aging and may be made more rapid by other factors) may develop adherence and eventual buildup of fatty deposits within the lining of the vessel walls of the arterial system, resulting in a gradual plugging of the lumen so that blood flow is restricted (Fig. 11-7). The clinical consequences of these lipid deposits include the development of angina resulting from ischemic heart disease, cerebrovascular disease (including stroke), peripheral ischemia, and renovascular hypertension.

It is still a subject of scientific and clinical controversy whether lowering serum lipids or cholesterol has any positive effect on reducing the risk of atherosclerotic disease. Both diet therapy and drug therapy have proponents and opponents. In patients anxious to reduce elevated levels, behavior modification to reduce other risk factors and dietary methods should always be tried first because hypolipemic drugs have risks of their own. The use of medication appears to be primarily prophylactic, slowing or preventing the rate of fatty deposition, without dissolving or removing existing fatty plaques.

ACTION

There are two major types of drugs used to treat hyperlipidemia: bile acid sequestrants and antihyperlipidemic agents.

Bile acid sequestrants, such as cholestyramine and colestipol, work to reduce serum cholesterol levels by forming an insoluble complex with bile salts and thus increase bile loss through the feces. This loss of bile, which is normally recirculated through the enterohe-

Table 11-5 Classification of hyperlipoproteinemias

Type	Diet	Drugs
I	Low fat; no other restrictions	None are effective
IIa	Low cholesterol, low in saturated fats; increased intake of polyunsaturated fats	Cholestyramine, colestipol, probucol, dextrothyroxine, lovastatin, nicotinic acid
IIb	Same as above	Cholestyramine, colestipol, clofibrate, gemfibrozil, lovastatin, nicotinic acid, probucol
III	Low cholesterol, low calorie, low in saturated fats; high protein	Clofibrate, nicotinic acid
IV	Low carbohydrate, low alcohol, low cholesterol, low calorie; maintain protein intake	Clofibrate, gemfibrozil, nicotinic acid
V	Low fat, low carbohydrate, low alcohol; high protein	Clofibrate, gemfibrozil, nicotinic acid

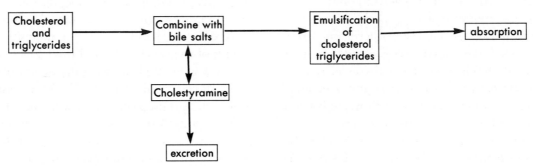

Fig. 11-8 Mechanism of action of bile acid sequestrants.

patic cycle, causes increased oxidation of cholesterol to form bile, a decrease in low-density lipoprotein plasma levels, and a decrease in serum cholesterol levels. Serum triglyceride levels may increase or remain unchanged (Fig. 11-8). These products are generally used to treat type II problems.

Antihyperlipidemic agents such as clofibrate, dextrothyroxine sodium, gemfibrozil, nicotinic acid, and probucol work in similar ways to lower serum triglycerides and very low–density lipoproteins.

1. They inhibit the formation of cholesterol early in the biosynthetic chain.
2. Neutral sterols are excreted in increased amounts.
3. Catabolism of very low–density and low-density lipoproteins is increased through increased breakdown of free fatty acids in liver, decreased release of VLDL from liver to plasma, and interference with binding of free fatty acids to albumin.

4. Hepatic synthesis of very low–density lipoproteins is decreased. Serum cholesterol and low-density lipoproteins are also lowered, but in variable amounts. These drugs also reduce serum fibrinogen levels and platelet adhesiveness.

A summary of the usual diet and pharmacologic regimens in the various types of hyperlipoproteinemias is included in Table 11-5.

ADVERSE REACTIONS

All these medications may affect liver function, and liver function tests should be obtained every 4 to 6 weeks.

Cholestyramine and *colestipol hydrochloride* may cause constipation.

Clofibrate may cause GI upset.

Mevacor should not be given to pregnant women.

Probucol may cause diarrhea, and is reported to produce excessive and foul-smelling perspiration.

DRUG INTERACTIONS

Because these products act by binding, administration with other medications may cause those drugs to be bound to the product. Cholestyramine, colestipol, and gemfibrozil potentiate warfarin anticoagulants. Clofibrate interacts with probenecid, warfarin, and sulfonylureas.

Normal absorption of fat-soluble vitamins may be reduced with bile acid sequestrants, and the patient may show symptoms of vitamin deficiency if the dosage is at high level or for a prolonged time. Bleeding problems resulting from hypoprothrombinemia because of vitamin K deficiency should be anticipated. Normal fat digestion may be impaired. Some patients, especially very young or small patients, may be more susceptible to the development of hyperchloremic acidosis because of the chloride anion exchange.

These products will delay the absorption of cephalexin, clindamycin, chlorothiazide, digitalis preparations, folic acid, iron, penicillin G, phenylbutazone, phenobarbital, thyroid and thyroxine preparations, and trimethoprim. If the patient has been placed on maintenance levels of any of these drugs and then bile acid sequestrant therapy is discontinued, potentially toxic levels may develop once the bile acid resin no longer binds the drug. This would be especially important to consider in digitalis therapy. Mild elevations of levels of alkaline phosphatase and serum glutamic-oxaloacetic transaminase, serum phosphorus, and chloride have been seen, with a decrease in serum sodium and potassium levels.

 ## NURSING IMPLICATIONS AND PATIENT TEACHING

▼ Assessment

The nurse should obtain a complete health history, including the presence of hypersensitivity, other medications taken that may lead to drug interactions, dietary therapy, other attempts to reduce cholesterol levels, and the possibility of pregnancy.

▼ Planning

The nurse should encourage weight reduction, and the patient should be as healthy as possible. The patient must be educated about the long-term nature of this chemical problem and the need for permanent dietary management. The ability of the nurse to establish rapport with the patient, win confidence,

and be sensitive to the patient's reactions will be important in obtaining long-term compliance with diet, medication, and appointment requirements.

▼ Implementation

If the drug is taken for a long period of time, supplemental doses of vitamins A, D, and K should be given. These should be given orally in a water-miscible form, or through parenteral injection.

Bile acid sequestrant preparations should be taken three times a day before meals. (Although there is no evidence that more than twice daily is therapeutic, the patient should get in the habit of taking the medication with each meal as a part of the total dietary modification.) These preparations are powders that will rehydrate when added to a liquid. They may be taken with milk, water, juice, or carbonated beverages, made into gelatin, or put into soups, cereals, or fruits with high moisture content, such as applesauce, nectars, fruit cocktail, or pineapple. The packet or a level scoopful of the powder should be added into the full glass or bowl. Allow the powder to dissolve slowly, without stirring, for at least 1 minute (stirring promotes the formation of lumps). When dissolved, stir to achieve uniform consistency. Rinse the empty glass or bowl with water to ensure taking the full quantity of medicine.

See Table 11-6, p. 206, for a summary of antihyperlipidemics.

▼ Evaluation

The patient may develop constipation and hemorrhoids. Use of a high-bulk diet and a laxative may allow the patient to continue with the dosage regimen. The patient should be evaluated to prevent the development of impaction.

▼ Patient and family teaching

The nurse should provide the patient and family with the following instructions:

1. The patient should take this medication as ordered and not change the dosage or stop taking it without the knowledge of the physician.
2. The most important thing that can be done in learning to live with this problem is to follow the prescribed diet. Restricting dietary intake of cholesterol and saturated fats, reducing calories, and increasing fluids and fiber content are very helpful. The patient should follow the detailed diet that lists the foods that should and should not be eaten.

Table 11-6	Common antihyperlipidemics

Generic name	Trade name	Dosage
BILE ACID SEQUESTRANTS		
Cholestyramine resin	Questran	1 tsp PO tid to qid with meals
Colestipol	Colestid	5 to 30 gm PO qd in two to four doses with meals
HMG-COA REDUCTASE INHIBITORS*		
Lovastatin	Mevacor	20 mg PO qd at PM meal; increase as needed at 4-week intervals; do not exceed 80 mg/day
Pravastatin	Pravachol	Give 10 to 20 mg once daily at bedtime; may increase to 40 mg daily
Simvastatin	Zocor	Start with 5 to 10 mg once daily in the evening; may go up to 40 mg/day; adjust dose at intervals of at least 4 weeks
OTHER PRODUCTS		
Clofibrate	Atromid-S	2 gm PO qd in two to four doses with meals
Dextrothyroxine	Choloxin	1 to 2 mg PO qd, increase in 1 to 2 mg doses q 4 wk to limit of 4 to 8 mg/day
Gemfibrozil	Lopid	600 mg PO 30 minutes before AM and PM meals; do not exceed 1500 mg qd
Nicotinic acid	Niacor	1 to 2 gm PO tid; maximum 6 gm/day
Probucol	Lorelco	500 mg PO at AM and PM meal

*HMG CoA, 3-Hydroxy-3-methylglutaryl coenzyme A.

3. This medicine comes in a powder that *must* be mixed with liquid before being taken. It may be mixed with beverages, soups, fruits, cereals, or gelatin. It should be added to the liquid and not stirred until it is completely dissolved. The container should be rinsed with water so that the patient obtains all of the medication in each dose.

4. Take other medicine 1 hour before or 4 to 6 hours after taking this product. This medicine will delay the absorption of other products if taken at the same time.

5. Some patients experience side effects from these drugs. The patient must notify the physician if any new or troublesome symptoms occur, especially persistent stomach upset, constipation, gas, bloating, heartburn, nausea, vomiting, or bleeding of any type.

6. The patient should keep this medication out of the reach of children and all others for whom it is not prescribed.

7. To decrease constipation, the patient should eat a high-bulk diet (fruit, raw vegetables, bran) and drink at least 2 quarts of fluid per day.

Geriatric Considerations
ANTIHYPERLIPIDEMIC DRUGS

Geriatric patients may be taking other medications in addition to the antihyperlipidemia medications; therefore the nurse should be aware that diuretics such as hydrochlorothiazide and chlorthalidone can increase cholesterol levels by 10%; that beta blockers such as propranolol and estrogen may increase triglyceride serum levels by 25% to 50%.

Dietary modifications and/or recommendations are vital to a successful lipid reduction program. When goals are not obtainable by diet alone, drug therapy may be prescribed.

A common side effect, constipation (sometimes severe), has been reported in geriatric patients taking cholestryramine and colestipol. Encourage the patient to increase daily fluid intake to help reduce the constipating effects of this drug.

Administer the antihyperlipidemic drugs before or with meals (follow manufacturer's instructions) because the drugs are generally not effective if not administered with food. Lovastatin is often given with supper to obtain its maximum beneficial effects, since the highest rate of cholesterol production occurs from midnight to 5 AM.

From McKenry LM, Salerno E: *Mosby's pharmacology in nursing*, ed 18, St Louis, 1992, Mosby.

SECTION FOUR: ANTIHYPERTENSIVES AND DIURETICS

Objectives

At the conclusion of this section you should be able to:
1. Identify the five different types of drugs used to treat hypertension.
2. Explain the stepped-care approach to antihypertensive therapy.
3. Describe actions of different categories of drugs used to treat hypertension.
4. Identify the major adverse reactions of medications used to treat hypertension.

OVERVIEW

Hypertension is a disease in which the patient's blood pressure is elevated above normal values for his or her age. Long-term studies have shown that blood pressures above 140/90 mm Hg are associated with accelerated vascular damage of the heart, the brain, and the kidneys, leading to an increased risk of premature death.

The cause of most hypertension is unknown. This **primary** (or essential) **hypertension** accounts for 80% to 90% of all cases of high blood pressure. In some cases, high blood pressure results from a known disease or other problem. Hypertension in this situation is called **secondary hypertension.**

Approximately 40 million Americans have hypertension, an incurable but controllable disease. Risk factors for hypertension include increasing age, black race, male sex, family history of hypertension, obesity, diabetes mellitus, hypercholesterolemia, and previous history of vascular disease.

ACTION

There are a wide variety of drugs available to treat hypertension. They act at many sites in the body and through many different ways. These drugs fall roughly into the following five main categories:
1. *Diuretics* indirectly reduce blood pressure by producing sodium and water loss and lowering the tone or rigidity of the arteries.
2. *Adrenergic antagonists* are nervous system stimulants and inhibitors that assist in decreasing cardiac output and/or peripheral resistance.
3. *Vasodilators* decrease peripheral resistance.

4. *Inhibitors of the renin-angiotensin system* promote fluid loss.
5. *Slow channel calcium entry blocking agents* reduce peripheral resistance.

Because each of these five drug categories works in a different manner and is also useful in treating problems other than hypertension, each drug category action is discussed separately. Fig. 11-9 illustrates sites of action for antihypertensive medications.

Diuretics

The action of all diuretics is to promote fluid loss from the body. Diuretics have been the cornerstone of modern antihypertensive therapy for the past 25 years. They owe their popularity to the fact that they work quite well, are relatively safe, are well tolerated, and are relatively inexpensive. Many new types of diuretics are currently available. Diuretics may be classified into four related groups: thiazides (for example, chlorothiazide, hydrochlorothiazide, polythiazide), the thiazide-like sulfonamides (for example, chlorthalidone, metolazone, quinethazone, and indapamide), loop diuretics (for example, furosemide, ethacrynic acid, and bumetanide), and the potassium-sparing diuretics (for example, amiloride, triamterene, and spironolactone).

Thiazides and sulfonamide diuretics

Thiazides and sulfonamide diuretics have similar actions. They work by preventing the reabsorption of sodium and chloride through direct action on the thick, ascending portion of the loop of Henle in the distal kidney tubule. In understanding fluid and electrolyte balance, a good rule to remember is that water tends to follow sodium; thus, with sodium loss, water also is pulled out and lost through the urine. The thiazides also act directly to dilate the smooth muscles in the arterioles, the smallest vessels in the arterial system. Because the arterioles are made larger, the heart does not have to pump so hard to get blood into them. This helps keep blood pressure lower.

Loop diuretics

Loop diuretics act by preventing reabsorption of sodium and chloride in the thick, ascending loop of Henle and in both proximal and distal tubules. These

Antihypertensive Agents (Generic and Trade Names)

Diuretics
Thiazides and related sulfonamide diuretics

Bendroflumethiazide (Naturetin)
Benzthiazide (Exna)
Chlorothiazide (Diuril)
Chlorthalidone (Hygroton)
Hydrochlorothiazide (HydroDiuril, Esidrix)
Hydroflumethiazide (Saluron)
Indapamide (Lozol)
Methyclothiazide (Enduron)
Metolazone (Zaroxolyn)
Polythiazide (Renese)
Quinethazone (Hydromox)
Trichlormethiazide (Naqua)

Loop Diuretics

Bumetanide (Bumex)
Ethacrynic acid (Edecrin)
Furosemide (Lasix)

Potassium-sparing agents

Amiloride (Midamor)
Spironolactone (Aldactone)
Triamterene (Dyrenium)

Adrenergic inhibitors
Peripheral adrenergic antagonists

Guanadrel (Hylorel)
Guanethidine (Ismelin)
Rauwolfia alkaloids
   Rauwolfia (whole root) (Raudixin)
   Reserpine (Serpasil)

Central-adrenergic inhibitors

Clonidine (Catapres)
Guanabenz (Wytensin)
Guanfacine (Tenex)
Methyldopa (Aldomet)

Alpha$_1$-adrenergic blockers

Doxazosin (Cardura)
Prazosin (Minipress)
Terazosin (Hytrin)

Beta-adrenergic blockers

Acebutolol (Sectral)
Atenolol (Tenormin)
Betaxolol (Kerlone)
Bisoprolol (Zebeta)
Carteolol (Cartrol)
Esmolol (Brevibloc)
Metoprolol (Lopressor)
Nadolol (Corgard)
Penbutolol (Levatol)
Pindolol (Visken)
Propranolol (Inderal)
Sotalol (Betapace)
Timolol (Blocadren)

Combined alpha- and beta-adrenergic blocker

Labetalol (Normodyne)

Vasodilators

Hydralazine (Apresoline)
Minoxidil (Loniten)

Angiotensin-converting enzyme inhibitors

Benazepril (Lotensin)
Captopril (Capoten)
Enalapril (Vasotec)
Fosinopril (Monopril)
Lisinopril (Zestril)
Quinapril (Accupril)
Ramipril (Altace)

Slow channel calcium entry blocking agents

Amlodipine (Norvasc)
Bepridil (Vascor)
Diltiazem (Cardizem)
Felodipine (Plendil)
Isradipine (DynaCirc)
Nicardipine (Cardene)
Nifedipine (Procardia)
Verapamil (Calan)

drugs are often effective in patients with very low glomerular filtration rates, because they are so efficient in preventing the reabsorption of sodium. The peak diuretic effect is much greater than that observed with any other type of diuretic. They are often used in patients with renal disease, and to treat congestive heart failure, cirrhosis of the liver, and nephrotic syndromes in which a powerful diuretic is indicated.

Potassium-sparing diuretics

Potassium-sparing diuretics increase the excretion of water and sodium, but preserve potassium. They act through competitive binding at receptor sites in the

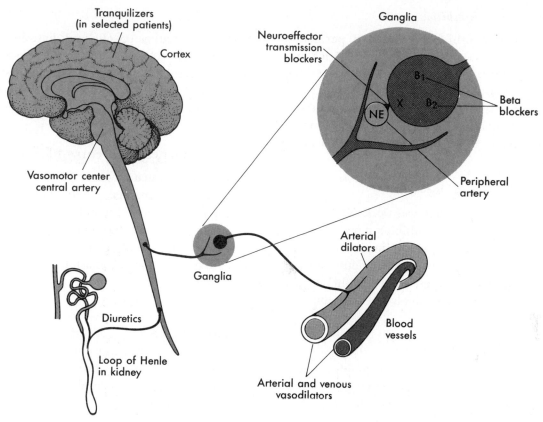

Fig. 11-9   Sites of action for antihypertensive medications.

distal renal tubular cell nucleus, resulting in changes in nuclear protein synthesis that affect the sodium and potassium exchange. These drugs are used in patients with renal disease or in elderly patients with decreased kidney function who have hypokalemia (low potassium levels), or in those with the potential for developing hypokalemia, often because of treatment with other medications, such as digitalis.

Adrenergic inhibitors

Adrenergic inhibitors are also divided into five different categories of drugs:

1. Beta-adrenergic blockers
2. Central adrenergic inhibitors
3. Peripheral adrenergic antagonists
4. Alpha$_1$-adrenergic inhibitors
5. Combined alpha- and beta-adrenergic blockers

The sympathetic nervous system relies on two adrenergic neurohormones or neurotransmitters, epinephrine and norepinephrine, to send its messages. These adrenergic inhibitor drugs plug the adrenergic receptors so that the neurohormones cannot make contact

with the receptor, thus preventing stimulation. Adrenergic nerve fibers have either alpha or beta receptors. Thus, the blockade can be of alpha, beta, or both alpha and beta receptor sites. If the medication blocks all adrenergic receptor sites, we say it is nonselective in its blockade.

Beta blockers

Beta blockers are subdivided into nonselective and selective beta antagonists. The nonselective blocking agents plug up both beta$_1$ and beta$_2$ sites. The selective beta$_1$ blocking agents exhibit action against the beta$_1$ receptors of the heart, but have less influence on the beta$_2$ receptors of the bronchi. There are no selective beta$_2$ inhibitors.

Nonselective beta blockers reduce the heart rate and the force of the contraction, suppress renin release, and decrease the outflow of sympathetic vasoconstrictor and cardioaccelerator messages from the brainstem to the vasomotor center. These drugs block both beta$_1$ and beta$_2$ impulses, and therefore have a wide range of side effects.

Central adrenergic inhibitors

Central adrenergic inhibitors stimulate peripheral alpha-adrenergic receptors, producing a brief and transient vasoconstriction, and then stimulate the presynaptic alpha$_2$-adrenergic receptors in cardiovascular integrating centers in the brainstem. As a result of this, total sympathetic outflow from the brain is decreased, leading to vascular relaxation and lower blood pressure.

Peripheral adrenergic antagonists

Peripheral adrenergic antagonists work as adrenergic neuron blocking agents that inhibit sympathetic vasoconstriction by inhibiting norepinephrine release from neuronal storage sites and by depleting norepinephrine from nerve endings. Total peripheral resistance is thus decreased through the relaxation of vascular smooth muscle.

Alpha$_1$-adrenergic inhibitors

Alpha$_1$-adrenergic inhibitors work through selective blockage of postsynaptic alpha-adrenergic receptor sites, leading to a reduction in peripheral vascular resistance and blood pressure. Both arterioles and venules are dilated by this relaxation of the arteriolar and venous smooth muscles.

Labetalol hydrochloride is a new drug with a combined alpha- and beta-adrenergic blocker action. It works as selective alpha$_1$-adrenergic but nonselective beta-adrenergic in its blocking activity.

Angiotensin-converting enzyme inhibitors

When the juxtaglomerular apparatus of the kidneys is stimulated, renin is released into the circulating blood volume to produce angiotensin I. Angiotensin I is then converted to angiotensin II in the liver and the lungs by an angiotensin-converting enzyme (ACE). Angiotensin II is a powerful vasoconstrictor that acts on the adrenal cortex to increase aldosterone secretion. This renin-angiotensin sequence is important in conserving sodium and water as a compensatory mechanism in maintaining blood pressure in the presence of shock, but it contributes to the increased blood pressure found in hypertension. Although the complete action of the angiotensin-converting enzyme inhibitor is not known, it is thought to prevent the conversion of angiotensin I to angiotensin II by inhibiting ACE in the plasma and vascular endothelium. There may be other complex actions of this medication that also help reduce blood pressure.

Vasodilators

Vasodilators reduce systolic and diastolic blood pressure by direct relaxation of vascular smooth muscle, thus decreasing peripheral vascular resistance. The exact mechanism of action is not known, but it appears to block calcium uptake through the cell membrane.

Slow channel calcium entry blocking agents

Slow channel calcium entry blocking agents selectively inhibit the passage of extracellular calcium ions through specific ion channels of the cell membrane in cardiac, vascular, and smooth muscle cells. This produces a decreased peripheral vascular resistance and a fall in systolic and diastolic blood pressure.

USES

Antihypertensives and diuretics (Table 11-7) are used alone or in combination to decrease elevated systolic and/or diastolic blood pressure. Systolic pressure measures the highest amount of pressure the heart is pumping against, whereas diastolic pressure represents the pressure in the arterial system at its lowest. These pressures are represented with the systolic as the numerator and the diastolic as the denominator when blood pressure is recorded as a fraction. Respected clinical studies suggest that it is beneficial to use a combination of diet, drug therapy, and reduction of risk factors to treat hypertension. The therapeutic goal in the hypertensive patient is to reduce the blood pressure to normal or near normal with a minimum of adverse effects. Reduction of diastolic pressure below 90 mm Hg has been associated with decreased risk of damage to the heart, kidneys, and brain, or **end organ damage.**

The patient with hypertension may have no symptoms or may complain of not feeling well in general. Headaches, frequently associated with hypertension, are often produced by stress, tension, or other reasons, rather than being related to high blood pressure, unless very severe blood pressure elevations are present. In cases of secondary hypertension, there may be reports of getting up at night to go to the bathroom (nocturia), history of renal trauma (producing renal artery stenosis), or a family history of hypertension.

Hypertension is usually classified as mild if the diastolic pressure falls within the range of 90 to 99 mm Hg; moderate if it falls between 100 and 109 mm

Table 11-7　Antihypertensive agents and their dosage ranges

Medication category	Dosage range (mg/day) Initial	Maximum	Medication category	Dosage range (mg/day) Initial	Maximum
DIURETICS			Central adrenergic inhibitors		
Thiazide and related sulfonamide diuretics			Clonidine	0.2	1.2
Bendroflumethiazide	2.5	5	Guanabenz	8.0	32
Benzthiazide	25.0	50	Methyldopa	500.0	2000
Chlorothiazide	250.0	500			
Chlorthalidone	25.0	50	Peripheral adrenergic antagonists		
Cyclothiazide	1.0	2	Guanadrel	10.0	150
Hydrochlorothiazide	25.0	50	Guanethidine	10.0	300
Hydroflumethiazide	25.0	50	Rauwolfia alkaloids		
Indapamide	2.5	5	Rauwolfia (whole root)	50.0	100
Methyclothiazide	2.5	5	Reserpine	0.05	0.25
Metolazone	2.5	5			
Polythiazide	2.0	4	Alpha$_1$-adrenergic blockers		
Quinethazone	50.0	100	Doxazosin	1.0	16
Trichlormethiazide	2.0	4	Prazosin	2.0	15
			Terazosin	1.0	5
Loop diuretics					
Bumetanide	0.5	10	Combined alpha- and beta-adrenergic blocker		
Ethacrynic acid	50.0	200	Labetalol	200.0	1200
Furosemide	80.0	480			
			VASODILATORS		
Potassium-sparing agents			Hydralazine	50.0	300
Amiloride	5.0	10	Minoxidil	5.0	100
Spironolactone	50.0	100			
Triamterene	50.0	100	**ANGIOTENSIN-CONVERTING ENZYME INHIBITORS**		
ADRENERGIC INHIBITORS			Captopril	37.5	150
Beta-adrenergic blockers			Enalapril	10.0	40
Atenolol	25.0	100			
Benazepril	10.0	40	**SLOW CHANNEL CALCIUM ENTRY BLOCKING AGENTS**		
Betaxolol	10.0	40			
Bisoprolol	5.0	20	Amlodipine	5.0	10
Carteolol	2.5	5	Bepridil	200.0	400
Enalapril	2.5	20	Diltiaziem	120.0	360
Fosinopril	10.0	80	Felodipine	5.0	20
Metoprolol	50.0	300	Isradipine	5.0	20
Nadolol	20.0	120	Nifedipine	30.0	60
Pindolol	20.0	60	Verapamil	240.0	480
Propranolol	40.0	480			
Propranolol long-acting	80.0	480			
Quinapril	10.0	80			
Ramipril	2.5	20			
Sotalol	160.0	320			
Timolol	20.0	60			

Hg; and severe if it is 110 to 119 mm Hg. It is considered very severe if the diastolic pressure is greater than 120 mm Hg. Isolated systolic hypertension is systolic pressure more than 140 mm Hg and diastolic pressure less than 90 mm Hg.

The choice of hypertensive drug depends on many factors: the degree of hypertension being treated, the presence of other diseases, the use of other drugs, and the patient's acceptance of the mild but inescapable side effects that may develop.

A stepped-care approach to the use of drugs has become the standard for acceptable therapeutic prescription in hypertension. As recommended by the Joint National Committee on Detection, Evaluation, and Treatment of High Blood Pressure, this approach involves using drugs in a sequence, beginning with a single agent with the least toxicity in a category, gradually increasing the dosage, and adding drugs sequentially from other drug categories to bring the diastolic blood pressure under control. The pharmacologic effects are balanced in this approach to take advantage of differing mechanisms of action. The different antihypertensive medications, classified according to their type of activity, are given in the box above. The stepped-care approach is summarized in Table 11-8.

Step One

Before instituting drug treatment for patients with hypertension, substantial efforts should be made to help patients reduce their risk factors. Life-style modifications to help the patient lose weight, increase physical activity, and reduce fat, salt, and calories in the diet are helpful in reducing hypertension. Behavior modification to assist in smoking cessation and in moderating alcohol intake is also important.

 Table 11-8 Stepped-care treatment regimen for hypertension*

Drug action	Suggested actions/drugs to use
STEP ONE	
Life-style modifications	Weight reduction
	Smoking cessation
	Moderation of alcohol intake
	Regular physical activity
	Reduction of sodium intake
STEP TWO (add to life-style modifications)	*Examples:*
Diuretic	Thiazides, thiazide-like sulfonamides, loop diuretics,
or	potassium-sparing agents
Adrenergic beta blockers	(see below)
Calcium channel blockers, ACE inhibitors	Verapamil
	Nicardipine
	Captopril
	Enalapril
	Lisinopril
STEP THREE (add to regimen)	
	1. Increase drug dose
	2. Substitute a drug
	3. Add a new drug category
Adrenergic-inhibiting agents	Atenolol, clonidine, guanabenz, guanadrel, methyldopa, metoprolol, nadolol, pindolol, prazosin, propranolol, rauwolfia alkaloids, timolol
Vasodilators	Hydralazine, prazosin
Additional adrenergic-inhibiting agents	Guanethidine, captopril, minoxidil
STEP FOUR (add to regimen)	Add additional drugs

*1993 Fifth Report of the Joint National Committee on Detection, Evaluation, and Treatment of High Blood Pressure, *Arch Intern Med* 153:154-183, 1993.

Step two drugs

The drug of choice in beginning antihypertensive therapy is an oral thiazide or thiazide-like sulfonamide preparation or an adrenergic beta blocker. Calcium channel blockers and ACE inhibitors are also primary use drugs. In younger patients a beta blocker, ACE inhibitor, or calcium channel blocker may be favored as initial therapy if they have a rapid resting pulse. Most thiazides or beta blockers are effective as once-a-day therapy. The drug is started in a low dosage and increased to a maximal level as needed. In many cases, one of these preparations used singly will reduce the diastolic blood pressure to an acceptable level. Because these products commonly produce hypokalemia, a potassium supplement may also be used concurrently. Loop diuretics are indicated when hypertension is severe and a prompt response is indicated.

Geriatric Considerations
CALCIUM CHANNEL BLOCKERS

The elderly are more susceptible to these agents and the side effects of increased weakness, dizziness, fainting episodes, and falls.

While nitroglycerin (or other nitrates) may be taken concurrently with these agents, the patient should be advised to report any increase in frequency or intensity of angina attacks to his or her health care provider.

Nicotine may reduce the effectiveness of these agents; thus reduction or avoidance of tobacco smoking is advisable.

Alcohol consumption may result in hypotensive episodes in some patients. Whenever possible, the use of alcohol should be avoided.

These agents should not be discontinued abruptly, since severe rebound angina attacks may result (gradual drug withdrawal is recommended).

From McKenry LM, Salerno E: *Mosby's pharmacology in nursing*, ed 18, St Louis, 1992, Mosby.

Step three drugs

An antiadrenergic agent may be added to the regimen if maximal doses of diuretics or step one drugs fail to lower the blood pressure to the desired level. These two categories of drugs work synergistically to bring down blood pressure and minimize the incidence of side effects, and are superior to the use of an antiadrenergic agent alone. There are a variety of drugs within this category, allowing experimentation to find the most advantageous drug combination for the individual patient. The patient should move on to

the next level only if a variety of these preparations fails to control the blood pressure. One exception is that beta blockers seem to be less effective in blacks and very elderly patients.

Additional drugs to be added to the therapeutic regimen are vasodilators. Vasodilators are most effective when used with a beta-adrenergic blocking agent to control the reflex tachycardia that results from decreased peripheral resistance.

Guanethidine, an additional adrenergic-inhibiting agent, can also be used in refractory hypertension. This drug has marked side effects that make its use as a step two drug inappropriate, leaving it for use in more severe cases of hypertension. The initial dose should be small, with dosage increased under supervision.

Step four drugs

Add a second or third agent or a diuretic if not already prescribed. Although most physicians would follow the stepped-care approach, there is considerably more experimentation and flexibility in recent years as new drugs enter the market and more research findings are published. Some drugs, such as captopril, seem to be less effective in black patients. Some clinicians have suggested that minoxidil and captopril be considered step five drugs and used with other available drugs for antihypertensive therapy, but the Joint National Committee has not followed this suggestion.

ADVERSE REACTIONS

Each category and each individual drug have significant adverse reactions. Hypokalemia (low potassium levels) and drowsiness are commonly seen, and many drugs produce impotence in men. Consult Table 11-9 for a list of the most common adverse reactions to the antihypertensive and diuretic drugs. For example, prazosin may cause a severe syncopal reaction following the first dose.

DRUG INTERACTIONS

The hypertensive patient usually takes many medications for other problems. All of the antihypertensive drugs may be involved in drug interactions. The nurse must check each drug to prevent additive effects that would lower the blood pressure too much or that might make the blood pressure go even higher.

Table 11-9 Adverse drug effects of antihypertensive and diuretic drugs

Drugs	Side effects	Precautions
DIURETICS		
Thiazides and thiazide-related sulfonamides	Hypokalemia, hyperuricemia, glucose intolerance, hypercholesterolemia, sexual dysfunction	May be ineffective in renal failure; hypokalemia increases digitalis toxicity; hyperuricemia may precipitate acute gout
Loop diuretics	Same as for thiazides	Effective in chronic renal failure; cautions regarding hypokalemia and hyperuricemia; may cause hyponatremia, especially in the elderly
Potassium-sparing agents	Hyperkalemia, sexual dysfunction, gynecomastia, mastodynia	Monitor fluid electrolytes
Beta-adrenergic blockers	Bradycardia, insomnia, fatigue, sexual dysfunction, bizarre dreams, decreased HDL cholesterol	Do not use in patients with asthma, chronic obstructive pulmonary disease, CHF, heart block, and sick sinus syndrome Use with caution in patients with diabetes and peripheral vascular disease
Central-acting adrenergic blockers	Drowsiness, fatigue, sexual dysfunction, dry mouth	Clonidine and guanabenz may produce rebound hypertension if abruptly stopped Methyldopa may cause liver damage and a positive direct Coombs' test
Peripheral-acting adrenergic inhibitors	Sexual dysfunction, nasal congestion, orthostatic hypotension, diarrhea, lethargy	Use very cautiously in elderly patients because of the hypotension Rauwolfia and reserpine are not to be given to patients with a history of mental depression
Alpha-adrenergic blockers	"First-dose" syncope with prazosin; orthostatic hypotension, weakness, palpitations, dizziness	Use cautiously in elderly patients because of hypotension
Combined alpha- and beta-adrenergic blockers	Nausea, fatigue, dizziness, asthma, headache	Do not give with sick sinus syndrome or heart block; use with caution in CHF, bronchial asthma, COPD, diabetes mellitus
VASODILATORS		
Vasodilators	Headache, tachycardia, and fluid retention Hydralazine may produce positive ANA Minoxidil may produce abnormal growth of hair, ascites	May produce angina in patients with coronary artery disease Lupuslike syndrome may occur with higher doses of hydralazine May cause or aggravate pleural and pericardial effusions
ANGIOTENSIN-CONVERTING ENZYME INHIBITORS		
ACE inhibitors	Captopril or enalapril may produce rash, problems with taste	Can cause neutropenia with autoimmune-collagen disorders May cause proteinuria or reversible acute renal failure in patients with bilateral renal artery stenosis
SLOW CHANNEL CALCIUM ENTRY BLOCKING AGENTS		
Slow channel blockers	Headache, hypotension, nausea, dizziness, flushing, edema, constipation	Use with caution in patients with CHF or heart block; do not administer immediately after mycardial infarction

NURSING IMPLICATIONS AND PATIENT TEACHING

▼ Assessment

The nurse should obtain a complete health history and physical examination, searching for a secondary cause for hypertension, such as Cushing's disease, Addison's disease, renal artery stenosis, coarctation of the aorta, or pheochromocytoma, and also determine the presence of other underlying diseases, allergies, or medications that may affect antihypertensives and diuretics.

The incidence of drug side effects and complications from inadequately treated hypertension is high, and good record keeping is important in evaluating the patient's status.

▼ Planning

Because there is no cure for high blood pressure, a good deal of patient teaching and education is essential to help the patient understand what is happening and to gain cooperation in the therapy. Although taking the medication is important, it is also important to work on decreasing other risk factors and changing dietary habits.

▼ Implementation

Many patients have difficulty complying with the physician's orders, because this is a silent disease. The patients do not feel ill. In fact, they may have symptoms only when they take their medication. It is

 CRITICAL DECISION:
Collect Data

It is important to collect and record a good initial data base (history, physical, and laboratory findings) to evaluate the progression of end organ damage over the years.

important to establish a realistic teaching plan to help patients understand their disease.

Patients should be encouraged to lose weight, restrict sodium intake, avoid stress and emotional pressures, develop regular and realistic exercise patterns, and engage in hobbies or activities that promote self-esteem. Taking the medications should be emphasized as only a small part of this total regimen.

▼ Evaluation

The most important evidence about the patient's compliance in keeping blood pressure down is in the examination of the fundus of the eye. This is a more reliable indicator than the blood pressure reading in showing long-term effects. The nurse should search for evidence of end-organ damage in the patient with long-term disease, as well as specific problems with medication. Male patients should always be asked about impotence as a result of their antihypertensive medication. They usually will not volunteer this information, and may not even realize that sexual dysfunction may be caused by their medications.

▼ Patient and family teaching

The nurse should provide the patient and family with the following instructions:

1. The patient should take this medication exactly as ordered by the physician. If a dose is missed, it should be taken as soon as it is remembered, if it is within an hour or two of the scheduled time. If it is close to the next scheduled dose, take only the next dose at the regular time; do not double the doses.

2. The patient should take medication with a full glass of orange juice (unless not permitted by diet). Other potassium-rich foods should be eaten daily, including citrus foods (especially oranges and tomatoes), bananas, dried fruits, apricots, cantaloupe, watermelon, nuts, dried beans, beef, and fowl.

3. The patient should know that taking the medication is only one part of the treatment regimen. Reducing other risk factors is also important, such as losing weight (if overweight), reducing sodium intake, stopping smoking, increasing exercise, and avoiding excessive stress and emotional pressures. The patient should avoid foods high in sodium, such as lunch meats, smoked meats, Chinese food, processed cheese, and snack foods. The patient should not salt food when cooking or add salt to food after it is cooked.

4. There are numerous side effects that could develop from use of these preparations. The patient must notify the physician of any new or troublesome symptoms that develop. Medication may need to be changed to find the best drugs. A close working relationship with the physician will be necessary to accomplish this. It

is therefore very important to keep appointments for care.

5. This medication must be kept out of the reach of children and others for whom it is not prescribed, because it is very hazardous for them. The patient should not leave it lying on night tables or low dressers where it might tempt young children.

6. The goal of therapy is to help the patient feel as healthy as possible and to avoid any complications. Generally there is no cure for hypertension and therapy extends for a lifetime. Taking medication and reducing other risk factors will help reduce the chance of serious complications. It is important to keep taking the medicine, even when the patient feels well, and to keep seeing the health care practitioner regularly.

7. The patient should wear a Medic-Alert bracelet and carry a medical identification card specifying that he or she has hypertension and listing the drugs that he or she is taking.

Geriatric Considerations
DIURETICS

Elderly are more susceptible to the development of the adverse reactions of hypotension (orthostatic), impaired mentation, hypokalemia (except with potassium-sparing diuretics), and increased glucose serum levels.

Lower doses are advised in the elderly with dosage increases based on the patient's individual therapeutic response and/or the development of adverse reactions.

When a diuretic is to be discontinued, it is recommended that the drug be reduced gradually to avoid the development of serious fluid retention (edema).

From McKenry LM, Salerno E: *Mosby's pharmacology in nursing*, ed 18, St Louis, 1992, Mosby.

SECTION FIVE: CARDIOTONICS

Objectives

At the conclusion of this section you should be able to:

1. List the general uses and actions of cardiotonic drugs.
2. Describe the most common adverse reactions seen following administration of a cardiotonic drug.
3. Identify symptoms of digitalis toxicity.
4. Explain important signs and symptoms to evaluate in a patient receiving a cardiotonic drug.
5. Identify key ideas to teach the patient or family about cardiotonic drugs.

OVERVIEW

 Cardiotonics make the heart beat stronger and slower. These drugs are also called cardioglycosides (glycosides are sugar-containing substances made from plants). Digitalis and drugs such as digoxin, digitoxin, and deslanoside are common examples of cardiotonics.

ACTION

All cardiotonics have the following two main actions:

1. They increase the strength or force of the contraction of the heart muscle (myocardium).
2. They slow the heart rate.

These actions are especially important in hearts that may be weakened by age or disease.

The normal heart pumps oxygenated blood from the left ventricle out through the body. If the heart is weakened, less oxygenated blood can be pumped out with each contraction of the heart.

When cardiac output (the amount of blood pumped out with each heartbeat) decreases, other organs are affected. For example, the brain reacts to receiving less blood by becoming dizzy, drowsy, or less alert. The kidneys become less effective at removing the waste products, electrolytes, and extra water from the bloodstream. This extra fluid may then pool in the lungs or other tissues (edema). Sometimes the heartbeat itself becomes irregular or too fast. As the body attempts to deal with these changes, the blood

Table 11-10 Symptoms of weakened heart or congestive heart failure

Organ affected	Symptoms
Brain	Dizzy, less alert
Heart	Enlarged heart, murmurs or abnormal heart sounds, irregular heartbeat or dysrhythmias
Lungs	Productive cough, shortness of breath
Kidneys	Edema of tissues of hands and feet
General	Rapid weight gain, weakness, lethargy

Table 11-11 Common signs and symptoms of digitalis toxicity

System	Symptoms
Cardiac	Slow pulse, irregular pulse, fast pulse
Central nervous system	Apathy, confusion, delirium, disorientation, drowsiness, headache, mental depression, visual changes (blurred vision, yellow/green vision, halos around dark objects)
Gastrointestinal	Anorexia, diarrhea, nausea, vomiting
Musculoskeletal	Severe weakness

pressure may increase or a more rapid heart rate may develop. These actions may place further strain on the heart. We call these symptoms of inadequate heart action **congestive heart failure** (CHF) (Table 11-10).

Increasing strength of myocardial contraction

The first action of the cardiotonic drugs is to increase the strength of each heartbeat or the force of the contraction. The stronger heartbeat pumps more blood, or increases the cardiac output. This effect of the drug is called a **positive inotropic action**. As more blood reaches the brain, lungs, kidneys, and other tissues, the signs of inadequate heart action decrease (Figs. 11-10 and 11-11).

Slowing heart rate

The second action of the cardiotonic drugs is to slow the heartbeat. They do this by slowing down the rate at which the pacemaker in the SA node begins the electrical cycle, and also by slowing the rate at which that information is passed through the rest of the heart (see the discussion of conduction pattern on p. 196).

All cardiotonics have the same basic drug action. They differ only in the speed and duration of their action.

USES

Cardiotonics are used to treat congestive heart failure and rapid or irregular heart dysrhythmias (not rhythmic), such as atrial fibrillation, arterial flutter, frequent premature ventricular contractions, and paroxysmal tachycardia.

ADVERSE REACTIONS

Cardiotonics are very powerful and can act as poisons on the heart. The amount of medication that is helpful (therapeutic) and the amount that is harmful (toxic) are not very different. Many things may happen that make even a safe dosage harmful to a patient. When a patient begins to show toxic or harmful reactions to the medication, the term **digitalis toxicity** is used. These symptoms may begin slowly and are often easy to overlook. Some symptoms of digitalis toxicity are included in Table 11-11.

Treatment of digitalis toxicity begins with immediate withholding of the drug and treatment of symptoms as needed. The physician may order blood tests to determine the serum blood digitalis level. Although they have similar names, it is important to keep separate the medications digoxin and digitoxin, because they are quite different in action and dosage. The therapeutic serum level of digoxin is 0.5 to 2 ng/ml (nanogram/milliliter) and the toxic serum level is more than 2.5 ng/ml. Digoxin has a rapid onset and a short duration of action. On the other hand, the therapeutic serum level of digitoxin is 14 to 25 ng/ml and the toxic serum level is more than 35 ng/ml. The action of digitoxin is slower, but it has a longer duration of action. This means that once the medication is withheld, the effects of digoxin will disappear more rapidly than those of digitoxin. Deslanoside is given only parenterally, and so the onset of action is very fast. Medication such as atropine may be ordered to speed up the pulse if the rate is very slow. Potassium may also be given to strengthen the heart's ability to beat regularly.

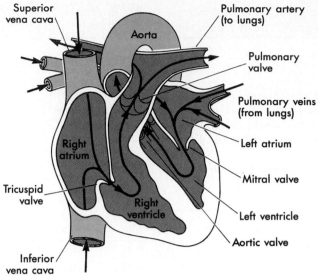

Fig. 11-10   Internal anatomy of the heart.

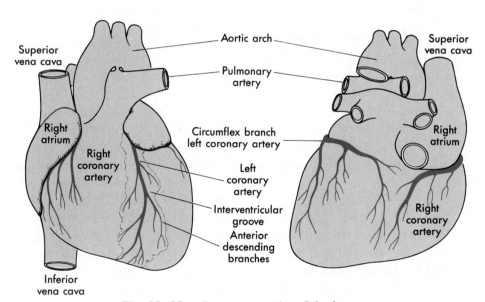

Fig. 11-11   Coronary arteries of the heart.

DRUG INTERACTIONS

Beta-adrenergic blocking agents, calcium gluconate, calcium chloride, succinylcholine, and verapamil increase the therapeutic or toxic effects of cardiotonics.

Cholestyramine reduces the therapeutic effects.

Any medication that influences the electrolyte balance may also precipitate digitalis toxicity.

NURSING IMPLICATIONS AND PATIENT TEACHING

▼ Assessment

Before beginning the medication, the patient should be assessed for the following:
1. History of nausea, vomiting, diarrhea, weakness, shortness of breath, confusion, or depression

2. Presence on physical examination of muscular weakness, confusion, elevated blood pressure, slow heart rate, rapid heart rate, irregular heart rate, abnormal heart sounds or murmurs, unusual lung sounds produced during inspiration or expiration, cyanosis, peripheral edema, distended jugular veins; the patient should also be weighed
3. Abnormalities in laboratory tests, such as ECG, chest x-ray studies, CBC, serum enzymes, serum electrolytes, and renal and hepatic studies.

Planning

There are two different types of dosages for patients taking cardiotonic medications, the initial **digitalizing** (or loading) **dose** and maintenance doses. More frequent and higher doses are given when a patient begins cardiotonic drugs so that a specific level of medication can be achieved in the blood. When the amount of drug in the patient's blood reaches the desired level, smaller regular doses are given once a day to maintain the blood level. How fast the desired drug level is reached is based on the type of medication, the dosage, the diagnosis of the patient, and many other factors.

Because of the risk for overdosage, great care must be taken not to confuse digitoxin and digoxin. Extra care must also be taken in checking the correct dosage. Confusing these medications may cause far-reaching consequences.

Implementation

Before administering each dose, the apical pulse rate should be taken for 60 seconds. If the apical pulse rate is below 60, the medication should be withheld and the physician notified, unless there is a written order giving different instructions. The drug should also be withheld if there are any symptoms of digitalis toxicity or if the patient's condition has worsened since the last time the medication was given. Withholding the medication always means contacting the physician immediately.

Intramuscular administration of cardiotonic drugs is painful. The nurse should take special care in the rotation of injection sites. Warm packs may be necessary to reduce painful swelling.

See Table 11-12 for a summary of cardiotonic medications.

Table 11-12   Cardiotonics

Generic name	Trade name	Uses	Adverse reactions	Dose ranges
Amrinone	Inocor	CHF-short term	Increased ventricular rate	Digitalizing: give 0.75 mg/kg IV bolus over 2 to 3 min Maintenance: 5 to 10 mg/kg min
Deslanoside	Cedilanid-D	Atrial flutter, atrial fibrillation, paroxysmal atrial tachycardia, CHF	Digitalis toxicity	Digitalizing: 1.6 mg IV or IM given at once in 0.8 mg portions
Digitoxin	Crystodigin	Same as for deslanoside	Digitalis toxicity	Digitalizing: 0.6 mg IV, then 0.2 to 0.4 mg q4to 6h; or 0.2 mg PO bid for 4 days Maintenance: 0.05 to 0.3 mg qd
Digoxin	Lanoxin Lanoxicaps	Same as for deslanoside	Digitalis toxicity	Digitalizing: 0.4 to 0.6 mg IV or 500 mg PO Maintenance: based on serum digoxin level
Milrinone	Primacor	CHF-short term	Ventricular arrhythmias	Loading dose followed by continuous IV infusion for severe CHF

▼ Evaluation

Patients must be monitored closely for symptoms of digitalis toxicity. Changes from the initial physical examination should be carefully documented. Vital signs, including daily weights, are very important to record. Patients with other respiratory, gastrointestinal, renal, or CNS problems, patients taking many other medications (especially diuretics and electrolytes), and confused patients who are not eating or drinking well are all at risk for developing digitalis toxicity.

CRITICAL DECISION:
Cardiotonics

Cardiotonics are some of the most commonly ordered medications. Because cardiotonic drugs may reach toxic levels so quickly, it is important for the nurse to closely monitor the patient receiving this medication.

▼ Patient and family teaching

This medication is frequently continued once the patient leaves the hospital.

1. The patient or a responsible family member must be taught to look for the same things for which the nurse observes. This may require teaching the patient or family member how to take the pulse. The procedure the patient is to follow when the pulse is below 60 should be determined by the physician before the patient goes home.
2. The patient should notify the physician if anorexia, nausea, vomiting, diarrhea, unusual weakness, fatigue, vision changes, depression, confusion, or dizziness occurs.
3. The medication must be kept in a safe place, away from animals or small children.
4. The medication must not be discontinued unless the patient is otherwise instructed by the physician. The physician should be called if the patient runs out of medication.
5. It is important to keep scheduled appointments with the physician so that changes in condition can be determined. Diagnostic tests and laboratory work are also important when ordered.

6. The patient should not take other prescription medications or over-the-counter drugs without the approval of the physician. Some drugs interfere with the action of the cardiotonic and may cause potentially serious problems.
7. The patient should take the medication at the same time every day, as directed by the physician; digitalis products are usually taken after meals.
8. The patient should wear a Medic-Alert tag or have other emergency identification indicating the medication being taken.
9. The patient taking cardiotonic drugs may be advised to eat foods rich in potassium. Good sources of potassium include bananas and citrus fruits, dried fruits, dried beans and lentils, all-bran cereal, and decaffeinated coffee (if the patient is not restricted from caffeine products).

Pediatric Considerations
CARDIAC GLYCOSIDES

The digitalis glycosides are reported to be a leading cause of accidental toxicity in children.

Individualized dosing with very close monitoring is necessary, especially in premature and immature infants.

Early signs of toxicity in infants and children may include a slow heart rate (less than 60 beats/minute) and irregular heart rhythms.

From: McKenry LM, Salerno E: *Mosby's pharmacology in nursing*, ed 18, St Louis, 1992, Mosby.

Geriatric Considerations
CARDIAC GLYCOSIDES

The elderly often have a reduced tolerance for these drugs; lower doses of digitalis glycosides may be necessary to reduce the potential for drug toxicity.

Decreased libido and impotence have been reported in approximately 35% of male users because of digoxin's estrogen-type effects. Also, male breast enlargement and breast tenderness have been reported.

From McKenry LM, Salerno E: *Mosby's pharmacology in nursing*, ed 18, St Louis, 1992, Mosby.

SUMMARY

The major classifications of cardiovascular medications are antianginals, peripheral vasodilators, antidysrhythmics, antihyperlipidemics, antihypertensives, diuretics, and cardiotonics. Each major class deals with an important part of the circulatory system. Cardiovascular medications are commonly used by patients, and the nurse has a major teaching responsibility in helping the patient understand the proper storage and use of medications. In addition, a thorough understanding of the anatomy and physiology of the heart is important, since it will assist the nurse in grasping both the cardiovascular problem and the action of the various medications.

 CRITICAL THINKING QUESTIONS

1. Ms. Henson, 70, was admitted to the hospital yesterday with acute angina pectoris. She is a heavy smoker and says that most evenings she drinks either wine or beer with her dinner and coffee with dessert every night. Her physician prescribes sublingual nitroglycerin for anginal pain. Describe major points to teach this patient, especially regarding medication storage, administration, and the results she may expect. Draw up for teaching and reviewing with Ms. Henson a plan of action for receiving medical attention if she has taken three nitroglycerin tablets and continues to have pain.

2. Point out some key distinctions between class I, class II, class III, and class IV antidysrhythmics. Consult Table 11-3 if you get stuck.

3. Define cinchonism and identify the drug associated with this adverse reaction.

4. Explain the need for careful electrocardiographic monitoring of patients taking antidysrhythmic medications. Include what you should be sure to teach about each drug.

5. Divide a large sheet of paper into four columns. You may want to make the fourth column a little wider than the others. Create a chart that identifies (a) the different types of lipoproteins and (b) the various types of hyperlipoproteinemias associated with each. In the third column (c) identify those that are helped by alterations in diet and those that are helped by specific medications from one of two categories. In a fourth column, identify nursing strategies associated with the two different drug categories, particularly how to make these medications more palatable, methods for reducing unpleasant side effects, the need for long-term medication and diet therapy, and regular medical follow-up.

6. Diagram the stepped-care approach for treatment of hypertension. Include for each step (a) appropriate drug categories, (b) their actions, and (c) rationale for moving on to the next step.

7. Develop a generalized, introductory patient teaching plan for the patient with recently diagnosed hypertension. As a first step, be sure to break essential components down into several short lessons, to avoid overwhelming the patient with information. Stress what the patient can do, rather than focusing only on restrictions.

8. Describe the signs and symptoms of congestive heart failure and of the various dysrhythmias.

9. Design a chart that gives easy access to the following information about the major cardiotonic drugs: (a) uses, (b) actions, (c) common adverse reactions and signs of digitalis toxicity.

10. Create a teaching plan for the patient taking a digitalis product. Be sure to include the following elements: (1) why the drug is needed; (2) why it is important to take the drug regularly; (3) what adverse effects to watch out for; (4) how to take a radial pulse; and (5) what to do if the radial pulse falls below 60.

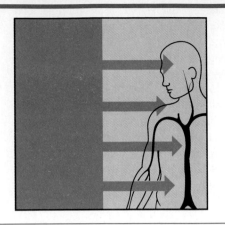

CHAPTER 12
Central Nervous System Medications

OVERVIEW

This chapter contains seven sections dealing with drugs that act on various parts of the central nervous system. Although there are many medications given in central nervous system diseases, the underlying principles of usage, actions of the medications, and adverse reactions are remarkably similar. The nurse will benefit from understanding the commonalities as well as the differences of various categories of drug use.

Sections One and Two discuss how pain is managed with narcotics and nonnarcotic analgesics; antimigraine agents are also discussed. Section Three covers the medications used to treat various types of convulsions. Section Four discusses antiemetics and antivertigo medications, and Section Five presents drugs used to treat Parkinson's disease. Section Six introduces the psychotherapeutic drugs. This section includes subsections dealing specifically with medications used to treat anxiety, depression, and psychosis, and with lithium, a unique medication. The final section discusses sedative-hypnotics and their use in insomnia, anxiety, and sleep disorders.

Nervous System

The major structures of the nervous system include the brain, spinal cord, nerves, and sensory receptors (Fig. 12-1). The central nervous system is a major regulatory and coordinating system. It detects sensation, controls movement, and controls physiologic and intellectual functions.

The nervous system has two divisions, the central and the peripheral. The central nervous system, made up of the brain and the spinal cord, is contained within the cranial cavity of the skull and the vertebral canal of the spinal column. The peripheral nervous system includes all nervous structures (ganglia and nerves) that lie outside the cranial cavity and the vertebral canal. These include the cranial and spinal nerves and the sympathetic division of the autonomic nervous system.

Pathologic conditions located in the brain may produce either local or generalized symptoms; abnormality located peripherally usually causes only localized symptoms. Because of the integration of the nerves and the muscoloskeletal system, it is often difficult to determine if disease lies within the nerves or the structures they innervate.

Although the medications covered in this chapter specifically focus on the actions of the **central nervous system (CNS),** or those actions controlled by the brain and spinal column, many of these agents act through

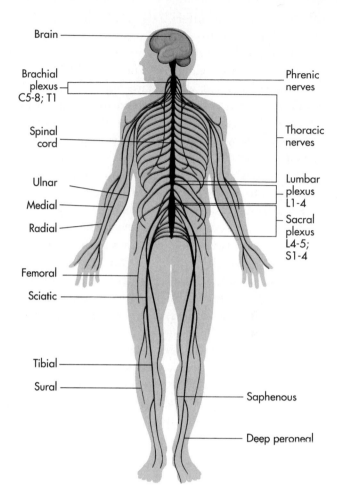

Fig. 12–1   Central nervous system.

the **peripheral nervous system,** or the activity in the body produced by nerves and chemicals of the motor nervous system and the autonomic nervous system as they carry out directions from the CNS.

To learn how medication acts on the CNS, the nurse should understand how nerves transmit information from the brain through chemical **neurotransmitters.** The neurotransmitter chemical is freed at the end of one neuron, passes across a small gap to activate the next neuron in the chain, or at the end of the nerve chain, stimulates an organ, smooth muscle, or gland.

The two major neurotransmitters in the body are **norepinephrine** and **acetylcholine.** There are several other neurotransmitters, especially in the brain. Nerve fibers that free norepinephrine are **adrenergic fibers.** Nerve fibers that free acetylcholine are **cholinergic fibers.** Most organs in the body are influenced by both types of fibers, which have opposite effects. For example, adrenergic agents speed up the heart rate, cholinergic agents slow it down. It is possible to compare this system to a car that is influenced by an accelerator and a brake.

Drugs that produce effects in the body similar to those produced by norepinephrine are called **adrenergic,** or sympathomimetic, **drugs**. These drugs are also referred to as **catecholamines.** There are three naturally occurring catecholamines in the body: norepinephrine, which is secreted from nerve terminals; epinephrine, which is secreted from the adrenal medulla; and dopamine, which is found at selected sites within the brain, kidneys, and gastrointestinal tract.

Those drugs whose action is similar to acetylcholine are called **cholinergic drugs.** Agents that block cholinergic activity are called **anticholinergic agents,** and agents that inhibit the adrenergic system are called **adrenergic blocking agents.** These basic terms are used throughout this chapter. Remembering these terms and definitions will help you understand drug actions.

When neurotransmitters release their chemicals, the chemicals are targeted to act at certain parts of the body. Each neurotransmitter has a certain chemical shape like a key, which produces an action only when it "fits into" a specific **receptor** (lock) for that chemical. These receptors are classified as alpha, beta, or dopaminergic. The alpha and beta receptors are further divided into subparts 1 and 2. When stimulated, alpha and beta receptors often have opposite effects on the heart, blood vessels, GI tract, or eye muscles. The text will often refer to a medication as having alpha or beta properties. For example, some medications are called beta blockers because of their selective action in blocking only the beta effects in the body.

Many of the drugs introduced in the following sections act on more than one type of receptor. Each agent acts differently, making it possible for certain drugs to be given for specific actions without many adverse reactions. It should be clear that if dosages are exceeded, many receptors may be excessively stimulated, causing widespread and serious effects.

SECTION ONE: NARCOTICS

Objectives

At the conclusion of this section you should be able to:

1. Describe common narcotics used to produce analgesia.
2. List common indications for the use of narcotics.
3. Identify major adverse reactions to narcotics.
4. Identify specific signs and symptoms to assess in patients receiving narcotics.
5. Describe differences between narcotic agonists and narcotic agonist-antagonist drugs.

OVERVIEW

This section discusses narcotic agonist analgesics used primarily in preoperative and postoperative care and narcotic agonist-antagonists available for hospital and outpatient use.

NARCOTIC AGONIST ANALGESICS

ACTION

Narcotic analgesics are thought to inhibit painful stimuli in the substantia gelatinosa (gray matter) of the spinal cord, brainstem, reticular formation, thalamus, and limbic system. Opiate receptors in each of these areas interact with neurotransmitters of the autonomic nervous system, producing alterations in reaction to painful stimuli. The narcotic action of the drug is shown through pain relief, sedation, euphoria, mental clouding, respiratory depression, miosis, decreased peristaltic motility, depression of the cough reflex, and orthostatic hypotension.

USES

Narcotic analgesics are used to treat moderate to severe acute pain. They may be used to relieve pain from acute coronary, pulmonary, hepatic, renal, or peripheral vascular origin; for preoperative medications; in severe diarrhea and cramping; for detoxification of narcotic addictions (methadone only); for persistent cough (codeine); for dyspnea related to left ventricular failure or pulmonary edema; in postsurgical trauma; and in labor.

ADVERSE REACTIONS

Adverse reactions to narcotic analgesics include bradycardia, decreased blood pressure, anorexia, constipation, disorientation, dry mouth, euphoria, syncope, vomiting, itching, skin rash, urticaria, slow respirations, and shortness of breath. Overdosage may produce profound respiratory depression, with a rate less than 12 breaths per minute, irregular shallow respirations, deep sleep, stupor or coma, miosis, cyanosis, gradually decreasing blood pressure, oliguria, clammy skin, and hypothermia. Chronic overdosage symptoms seen in drug abusers include constricted pupils, constipation, mood changes, depressed level of consciousness, skin infections, itching, needle scars, and abscesses. Respiratory rate and sedation are the variables most closely monitored for signs of overdosage.

DRUG INTERACTIONS

The CNS depressant effects of narcotic analgesics may be increased by the use of other narcotic analgesics, alcohol, antianxiety agents, barbiturates, anesthetics, nonbarbiturate sedative-hypnotics, phenothiazines, skeletal muscle relaxants, and tricyclic antidepressants. Narcotics act with many other medications to increase or decrease their effects. The nurse should monitor the use of narcotics with any other medications.

 NURSING IMPLICATIONS AND PATIENT TEACHING

▼ Assessment

The nurse should assess the patient's perception of pain, and elicit the history of the pain, including its onset, location, quality and quantity, and aggravating and relieving factors. The nurse's objective evaluation may reveal tensed muscles; alterations in respiration, blood pressure, pulse, perspiration, pupillary reaction; restlessness; affective responses (crying, moaning); and changes in baseline blood pressure and pulse rates.

The nurse should obtain a complete health history, including whether the patient has a history of allergic or adverse reaction to morphine and its congeners, evaluate the patient's pain tolerance, and explore any suspicion of narcotic abuse.

▼ Planning

Whenever possible, pain treatment should begin with nonnarcotic analgesics and supportive pain measures.

Remember that pain relief is maximized if the drug is given before the patient is in intense pain.

The main drawback of using opioids, particularly on a primary care basis, is the associated risk of physical and psychologic dependence for the patient. Extreme caution should be exercised when giving opioids to the elderly, pregnant women, debilitated persons, patients in shock or in acute stages of alcohol intoxication, and to children or newborns.

Pain is often a key symptom necessary for diagnosing acute conditions. Narcotic analgesics can mask this symptom, obscuring the progress of the disease, particularly in abdominal conditions. The use of narcotic analgesics is not recommended in these situations. Narcotic analgesics, as well as any CNS depressants, are contraindicated in persons with increased intraocular pressure, head injury, or loss of consciousness.

▼ Implementation

The nurse should be familiar with regulations concerning the use and dispensation of narcotic analgesics. Narcotic analgesics are classified according to abuse potential as mandated by the Controlled Substances Act of 1970 (see Chapter 2, pp. 11-12).

Once the narcotic analgesic is metabolized, the patient may experience an increased sensitivity to pain. The drugs should be given 2 hours before delivery or surgery to prevent associated respiratory depression in the neonate or the patient.

The cough reflex is suppressed by these products; this may be a problem in patients with pulmonary disease. The ventricular response rate may be increased in patients with supraventricular dysrhythmias. These products may also aggravate preexisting convulsive states. The amount of pain experienced by the patient will determine the dosage of the narcotic and the route of administration. Narcotics may be given orally, rectally, intramuscularly, subcutaneously, and intravenously.

The specific dosage information is summarized in Table 12-1.

Table 12-1 Narcotic agonist analgesics

Generic name	Trade name	Comments and dosage
Codeine	Codeine phospate Codeine sulfate	Schedule II drug. ■ *Pain relief* *Adults:* 15 to 60 mg PO, IM, or SQ q4h prn. *Infants and children:* 0.5 mg/kg PO, IM, or SQ q4h prn. ■ *Antitussive* *Adults:* 5 to 10 mg PO four to six times daily. *Infants and children:* 0.175 to 0.25 mg/kg PO four to six times daily.
Fentanyl	Sublimaze	Schedule II drug; potent, short-acting narcotic. The respiratory depressant effects of fentanyl are particularly dangerous; have resuscitative measures ready. Intravenous medication should be administered slowly. ■ *Preoperative* *Adults:* 0.05 mg to 0.1 mg IM. *Children 2 to 12 years:* 0.02 to 0.03 mg/20 to 25 lb.
	Duragesic	Transdermal system; 25 to 100 mg patch q72h.
Hydromorphone	Dilaudid	Potent synthetic compound that maximizes analgesic effects and minimizes some of the common side effects of morphine; Dilaudid has 7 to 10 times the analgesic action of morphine. *Adults:* 2 to 4 mg IM or SQ q4 to 6h; 2 mg PO q4 to 6h; one suppository bid.
Levomethadyl acetate HCl	Orlaam	Used in managing opioid dependence. Give 20 to 40 mg 3 times weekly, increase by 5 to 10 mg to maintenance of 60 to 90 mg 3 times weekly.
Levorphanol	Levo-Dromoran	Used to relieve moderate to severe pain; often used preoperatively to reduce apprehension and to prolong analgesia. It has a relatively longer onset of action than other narcotic agonist analgesics. *Adults:* 2 to 3 mg PO or SQ. May also be given by slow IV injection.
Meperidine	Demerol	Schedule II drug; synthetic narcotic analgesic with less potency than morphine; each dose of syrup should be taken in one-half glass of water, because if undiluted, it can exert a topical anesthetic effect on mucous membranes. *Adults:* 50 mg to 150 mg IM, SQ, or PO q3 to 4h. *Children:* 0.5 to 0.8 mg/lb IM, SQ, or PO q3 to 4h.
Methadone	Dolophine	Schedule II drug; synthetic narcotic analgesic used primarily in the detoxification, treatment, and maintenance of heroin addicts or for severe pain. When the drug is used for severe pain, it is administered IM. The drug is highly addictive. When used for heroin addicts for more than 3 weeks, methadone moves from a treatment phase to a maintenance phase. ■ *Pain relief* *Adults:* 2.5 to 10 mg IM, SQ, or PO q3 to 4h.
Morphine	Duramorph	Schedule II drug; the primary narcotic analgesic used for relief of severe pain. It is the narcotic analgesic against which all others are compared. It also produces sedation and euphoria when pain is present. Traditionally used for preoperative sedation and postoperative analgesia. Morphine is more effective against dull, continuous pain than sharp, spasmodic pain. IV medication should be given slowly over a 4- to 5-minute period. Protect drug from light and freezing. *Adults:* Administer 5 to 20 mg SQ or IM q4h as indicated; IV administration doses range from 2 to 15 mg/5 ml injected over a 5-minute period. *Children:* 0.1 to 0.2 mg/kg per dose SQ; maximum dose not to exceed 15 mg.

Table 12-1	Narcotic agonist analgesics—cont'd	
Generic name	**Trade name**	**Comments and dosage**
Opium	Pantopon	A highly purified form of opium exhibiting the actions of both morphine and codeine without the side effects; 20 mg equivalent to 15 mg of morphine. *Adults:* 5 to 20 mg IM or SQ q4h prn.
Opium combinations	Brown mixture Paregoric Opium tincture	Schedule II drug. Paregoric is equivalent to 0.04% morphine. Opium tincture is equivalent to 1% morphine. Avoid confusing these two medications. Paregoric is used for cramps, diarrhea, and teething pain in infants (as a topical application to gums). ■ *Diarrhea* *Adults:* Tincture 0.6 to 1.5 ml PO; camphorated tincture 5 to 10 ml PO qid. *Children:* Camphorated tincture 0.25 to 0.5 ml/kg.
Oxycodone	Roxicodone	*Adults:* 5 mg or 5 ml q6h prn.
Oxycodone hydrocodone combinations	Oxycodone Lorcet Percocet Percodan Tylox Vicodin	These agents are similar in action and structure but are not identical; they are opium alkaloids and are morphinelike in action. Used in moderate to severe acute pain. *Adults:* 1 to 2 tablets q4 to 6h prn for pain.
Oxymorphone	Numorphan	*Adults:* 0.5 mg IV; or SQ/IM give 1 to 1.5 mg q4 to 6h.

▼ Evaluation

Generally, oral narcotic analgesics begin to take effect 15 to 30 minutes after they are given. Opioids given subcutaneously may vary considerably in their absorption, because of variations in the drug's solubility. Opioids given orally are considerably less effective than those given parenterally. However, oral narcotic analgesics have a longer duration of action.

The dosage of the narcotic analgesic depends on the severity of pain experienced by the patient, the patient's response to the pain and the medication, and the nature of the illness.

New dosage recommendations released by the Agency for Health Care Policy and Research for treating patients with cancer or chronic pain are much higher than those dosages for preoperative or acute pain. The new guidelines suggest much higher dosages, at more frequent intervals, and for longer periods of time than previous recommendations.

The patient should be checked at regular, frequent intervals. Because narcotic analgesics may depress the cough and sigh reflexes, postoperative patients, particularly long-term smokers, may develop atelectasis and pneumonia.

The nurse should assess the patient's dependency behavior. For example, the patient may be unable to wean from the drug, may make frequent requests for the drug, or may use numerous health providers and health care facilities.

Narcotic analgesics are metabolized by the liver and are excreted through the kidneys; 90% of the drug is excreted during the first 24 hours.

▼ Patient and family teaching

The nurse should provide the patient and family with the following instructions:

1. The patient should take this medication as advised by the physician and not alter the dosage. Although this product is potentially addictive, it is most effective when taken before the patient has severe pain.

2. If the patient is not having substantial pain, other methods for relieving pain should be used whenever possible.

3. The patient should not take any other medications without the knowledge of the physician. Alcohol increases the effect of the medication, and may cause a problem.

4. Some patients experience side effects from this drug, such as suppression of cough reflex, dizziness, lightheadedness, nausea, drowsiness, sweating, and flushing. The patient or family should report any new or troublesome symptoms to the physician.

5. The patient should avoid operating heavy machinery, driving, or performing tasks requiring alertness after taking this medication.
6. The patient should urinate frequently and monitor bowel habits daily.
7. The patient should rise slowly from lying or sitting positions to minimize feelings of lightheadedness and should avoid standing in one position for long periods.
8. When receiving the initial doses of opioids, the patient should lie down for a short period to prevent nausea.
9. The patient should take the medication exactly as prescribed and work to taper the doses down if taken over a long time. The patient should jot down the time when the medication was last taken to prevent overdosing.
10. This medication must be kept out of the reach of children and all others for whom it is not prescribed. All extra medication should be discarded when there is no longer any need for it; it should not be kept for another time.

NARCOTIC AGONIST-ANTAGONIST ANALGESICS

ACTION

Narcotic agonist-antagonist analgesics are potent drugs that act through the CNS, possibly at the limbic system. They also antagonize the action of narcotics. Thus they may produce withdrawal symptoms in patients with narcotic dependency, but they are also less likely to be abused than pure narcotic agonists.

USES

Narcotic agonist-antagonist analgesics are used primarily for the relief of moderate to severe pain. They are also used in the parenteral form for preoperative analgesia and for mothers during active labor. These products may be preferred over narcotics for use in ambulatory patients because their potential for abuse is lower.

Narcotic-analgesic combination drugs work on the pain centers of the CNS. They are combinations of acetaminophen, aspirin, phenacetin, and caffeine, and they contain narcotics such as codeine, oxycodone, or hydrocodone. Some agents also contain a form of barbiturate, which is added for its sedative effects. Narcotics and barbiturates are controlled substances.

Combination drugs are used for the relief of moderate to severe pain of an acute origin, such as postsurgical or postextractional pain. They are often ordered when the patient is discharged from the hospital, or ordered on an outpatient basis. These drugs are addictive and should be used for only a brief time. Table 12-2 lists common combination products used for analgesia.

ADVERSE REACTIONS

Adverse reactions to narcotic agonist-antagonist analgesics include bradycardia, hypertension, hypotension, tachycardia, alteration of mood, blurred vision, confusion, dizziness, headache, lethargy, lightheadedness, nervousness, nystagmus, syncope, tingling, tinnitus, tremor, unusual dreams, pruritus, rash, soft tissue

 Table 12-2 Narcotic-analgesic combination products

Trade name	Chemical components
Acetaminophen with codeine	Codeine, acetaminophen
A.S.A. with codeine compound	Codeine, aspirin (acetylsalicylic acid, ASA)
Duradyne DHC	Hydrocodone, acetaminophen
Empirin with codeine	Codeine, aspirin
Fiorinal with codeine	Codeine, aspirin, caffeine, butalbital
Percocet	Oxycodone, acetaminophen
Percodan	Oxycodone, oxycodone terephthalate, aspirin
Phenaphen with codeine	Codeine, acetaminophen
Tylenol with codeine	Codeine, acetaminophen
Tylox	Oxycodone, acetaminophen
Vicodin	Hydrocodone bitartrate, acetaminophen

induration, stinging on injection, ulceration, anorexia, abdominal cramps, constipation, diarrhea, dry mouth, dyspepsia, nausea, vomiting, depression of white blood cell count, dyspnea, flushing, speech difficulty, and urinary retention or urgency. Overdosage may produce sleepiness and respiratory depression.

DRUG INTERACTIONS

Alcohol and drugs that are depressants should be used cautiously with these products because of the potential for increased CNS depression.

 NURSING IMPLICATIONS AND PATIENT TEACHING

▼ Assessment

The nurse should obtain a complete health history, including the presence of respiratory, hepatic, or kidney disease, pregnancy or breastfeeding, recent myocardial infarction, or evidence of previous emotional instability, drug dependency, or drug misuse. These conditions may be contraindications or precautions to the use of narcotic agonist-antagonist analgesics.

The patient's perception of the pain and the level of tolerance should be assessed, and a history of the pain, including its onset, location, quality and quantity, and aggravating and relieving factors should be obtained. The nurse's objective evaluation may reveal tensed muscles; observable autonomic reactions, such as alterations in respiration, blood pressure, pulse, perspiration, and pupillary reaction; restlessness; affective responses (crying, moaning); and changes in baseline blood pressure and pulse rates.

▼ Planning

Narcotic agonist-antagonist analgesics should be used with extreme caution in patients who are emotionally unstable or in those who have a history of drug abuse. Because both psychologic and physiologic dependence may occur, these drugs should be given under careful supervision and prescribed only in limited amounts.

These drugs should not be given to patients with head injury, because the clinical course must be observed without the confusing effects of the medication. It has not been established whether it is safe to use these drugs in children or in pregnant women (other than during labor).

Because these drugs tend to cause respiratory depression, they should be used cautiously in patients with respiratory impairment (especially asthma), obstructive respiratory conditions, and cyanosis.

These products may produce withdrawal symptoms in patients who have demonstrated dependence to narcotics. These products are also known to provoke seizures, especially in patients with known seizure disorders.

Patients receiving combination drug products may suffer adverse effects from or develop intolerance to any of the drugs used in the medications.

▼ Implementation

All of these narcotic agonist-antagonist analgesics are available in parenteral form, but only pentazocine is available in oral form. These medications should be given by intramuscular injection, because subcutaneous injection may damage tissues.

When frequent injections are needed, each dose should be given in a different site. The injection sites should be rotated to avoid producing tissue injury.

For acute pain, one to two tablets or capsules of drugs with narcotics combined with other medications are given every 4 to 6 hours. These drugs are not recommended for children.

See Table 12-3 for a summary of narcotic agonist-antagonist analgesics.

▼ Evaluation

The nurse should evaluate the patient for relief of pain and the development of adverse effects. If the patient receiving therapeutic doses demonstrates any evidence of hallucinations, confusion, or disorientation, the medication should be discontinued.

The nurse should assess the patient's dependency behavior. For example, the patient may be unable to wean from the drug, may frequently request the drug, or may use numerous health providers and health care facilities.

▼ Patient and family teaching

The nurse should provide the patient and family with the following instructions:

1. The patient should take this medication as advised by the health care provider and not alter the dosage. Although this product has the potential for addiction, it is most effective when

Table 12-3   Narcotic agonist-antagonist analgesics

Generic name	Trade name	Comments and dosage
Buprenophine	Buprenex	Onset of action 15 min, peak 60 min, duration 6 hours. Give 0.3 mg IM or slow IV q6h.
Butorphanol	Stadol	Onset of action is 10 min after IM injection, and almost immediately after IV injection. The respiratory depression effect is similar to that of morphine, is dose related, and is easily reversed with naloxone. *Intramuscular:* 1 to 4 mg, repeated q3 to 4h prn; do not give doses greater than 4 mg. *Intravenous:* 0.5 to 2 mg, repeated q3 to 4h prn.
Dezocine	Dalgan	Onset of action 15 to 30 min; duration 2 to 4 hours. Give 5 to 20 mg IM.
Nalbuphine	Nubain	This product tends to be more expensive than other agonist-antagonist products. *Adults:* 10 mg SQ, IM, or IV, repeated q3 to 6h prn; do not give more than 20 mg in one dose, or more than 160 mg/day. Onset 15 minutes, lasts 3 to 6 hours.
Pentazocine	Talwin	Schedule IV drug; synthetic opioid, used for moderate to severe pain or as a preoperative or preanesthetic medication. Give deep intramuscularly and rotate sites, because subcutaneous injection may produce severe tissue damage at injection site. Do not mix this product with other chemicals during injection. ■ *Pain relief* Onset 15 minutes; duration 3 hours. *Adults:* 50 mg IM, SQ, or IV q3 to 4h; do not exceed doses of 60 mg IM or 30 mg IV. Total daily dose should not exceed 360 mg. For chronic administration, 50 mg oral tablets are recommended q3 to 4h.

taken before the patient has severe pain.

2. As the patient begins to feel better, other methods for relieving pain should be used whenever possible.

3. Some patients experience side effects from these drugs, such as drowsiness, nausea, vomiting, dizziness, blurred vision, sweating, dry mouth, headache, and confusion. The patient should report any new or troublesome symptoms to the physician.

4. The patient should avoid operating heavy machinery, driving, or performing tasks requiring alertness after taking this medication.

5. This medication must be kept out of the reach of children and others for whom it is not prescribed.

SECTION TWO: NONNARCOTIC ANALGESICS

Objectives

At the conclusion of this section you should be able to:

1. Describe at least three groups of nonnarcotics used for analgesia.

2. Discuss use and limitations of antimigraine preparations.

3. Identify common adverse reactions to these products.

4. Develop a teaching plan for patients receiving these agents.

OVERVIEW

This section discusses two types of nonnarcotic analgesics: centrally acting analgesics and preparations used to control or prevent migraine headaches.

Another major category of medications that have analgesic effects, the salicylates, is discussed in Chapter 17, Musculoskeletal and Antiarthritis Medications. Although they could properly be included here, their antiinflammatory and antipyretic actions give them a broader use than analgesia.

CENTRALLY ACTING ANALGESICS

ACTION

These products act centrally, producing analgesia. Although propoxyphene and ethoheptazine are chemically related to narcotic analgesics, they are not comparable in analgesic potency or abuse potential, so they will be included in this section. Methotrimeprazine has potent CNS depressant activity and is a phenothiazine derivative.

Nonnarcotic analgesics are combination drugs used mainly for their analgesic properties. They include combinations of acetaminophen, aspirin, caffeine, phenacetin, antacids, ethoheptazine, or propoxyphene.

USES

These products are used primarily to relieve mild to moderate pain. They are also used in combination with other products for pain alone or when pain and fever are both present.

Combination products are used when additional actions are desired along with mild or moderate analgesia (Table 12-4). Caffeine, a plant extract, has mild cerebral, respiratory, and cardiac stimulant effects, as well as some diuretic activity. It has no analgesic properties, but it is used to treat vascular headaches.

ADVERSE REACTIONS

Adverse reactions to nonnarcotic analgesics include orthostatic hypotension, disorientation, dizziness, euphoria, headache, lightheadedness, minor visual disturbances, sedation, slurring of speech, weakness, skin rashes, abdominal pain, constipation, dry mouth, epigastric distress, nausea, vomiting, difficulty urinating, chills, nasal congestion, and pain at the injection site. Overdosage usually produces sedation, although the patient may have respiratory depression and be comatose. Cyanosis and hypoxia are also present because of the decreased ventilatory rate; hypoten-

Table 12-4   Nonnarcotic analgesic combination products

Trade name	Chemical components
Anacin	Aspirin, caffeine
Anacin Arthritis	Aspirin, antacids
Bromo-Seltzer	Acetaminophen, sodium bicarbonate, citric acid
Excedrin	Aspirin, acetaminophen, caffeine
Fiorinal	Aspirin, caffeine, butalbital
Gemnisyn	Aspirin, acetaminophen
PAC tablets	Aspirin, caffeine
SAC tablets	Acetaminophen, caffeine, salicylamide
Trigesic	Aspirin, acetaminophen, caffeine
Vanquish	Aspirin, acetaminophen, caffeine, antacids

sion and deterioration of cardiac performance may follow. Hepatotoxicity may develop in alcoholics using the drug acetaminophen.

DRUG INTERACTIONS

Nonnarcotic analgesics have CNS depressant effects that add to those of other depressants, including alcohol. Each product has some drug interactions, although they have fewer drug interactions than narcotics. The manufacturer's product information should be consulted.

NURSING IMPLICATIONS AND PATIENT TEACHING

▼ **Assessment**

The nurse should obtain a complete health history, including any respiratory or hepatic disease, pregnancy or breastfeeding, or evidence of previous emotional instability, drug dependency, or drug misuse. These conditions may present contraindications or precautions to the use of nonnarcotic analgesics.

The nurse should assess the patient's perception of pain and elicit the history of the pain, including its onset, location, quality and quantity, and aggravating and relieving factors. The nurse's objective evaluation may reveal tensed muscles, changes in respiration, perspiration, pupillary reaction, restlessness, affective responses (crying, moaning), and changes in baseline blood pressure and pulse rates. The patient's pain tolerance should be assessed.

Table 12-5	Other centrally acting analgesics	
Generic name	Trade name	Comments and dosage
Methotrimeprazine	Levoprome	This product is a phenothiazine derivative with potent CNS depressant activity. Give deep IM injection into large muscles, with rotation of injection sites. ■ *Pain:* 10 to 20 mg deep IM q4 to 6h prn. Although up to 40 mg may be given, start with 10 mg doses until patient response is assessed. Reduce dosage in elderly patients to 5 mg.
Propoxyphene	Darvon Dolene Darvocet-N	Schedule IV drug; a centrally acting opioid, structurally related to methadone. It is used primarily as a weak analgesic, but contains physical and psychologic addictive properties. Often combined with nonnarcotic analgesics. *Adults:* 65 to 100 mg PO q4h prn.

▼ Planning

The nurse should not give nonnarcotic analgesics, including phenothiazines, to patients who are hypersensitive to the products involved. Methotrimeprazine should not be given concurrently with antihypertensive agents, including MAO inhibitors, or to patients with CNS depressant overdosage, comatose states, myocardial infarction, renal or hepatic disease, or severe hypotension.

Methotrimeprazine should not be administered for longer than 30 days, unless narcotics are contraindicated and periodic blood counts and liver function studies can be carried out.

Elderly and debilitated patients may be more sensitive to the effects of many nonnarcotic analgesics. The patient should not perform tasks requiring alertness while on these drugs, because the medication may slow the response time.

▼ Implementation

All of the propoxyphene products are available in oral form; methotrimeprazine also comes as an injection.

Many propoxyphene products are available in combination with other drugs. However, there is no conclusive evidence that propoxyphene combined with other analgesics is more effective than propoxyphene or other analgesics alone.

For combination products, the usual adult dosage is one to two tablets or capsules every 4 to 6 hours for pain. Table 12-5 summarizes important drug information about major nonnarcotic agents.

▼ Evaluation

After methotrimeprazine is given, orthostatic hypotension, fainting, dizziness, or sedation may occur. Patients should be carefully supervised while taking this product, especially for the first 6 hours after the initial dose.

The nurse should check the patient at regular and frequent intervals to assess the action of the medication and to look for symptoms of overdosage. Fatalities from overdosage often occur within the first hour, so it is necessary to monitor the patient carefully. Patients who are emotionally unstable, have abused drugs in the past, or who may be considered unreliable in medication dosage should have their medication restricted.

Dependence may develop when propoxyphene products are taken in high doses over a long time. These drugs should be viewed with the same degree of caution as narcotics.

The nurse should assess the patient's dependency behaviors. For example, the patient may be unable to wean from the drug, may frequently request the drug, or may use numerous health providers and health care facilities.

Because of potential hepatotoxicity in alcoholics using acetaminophen, assess for alcohol abuse.

▼ Patient and family teaching

The nurse should provide the patient and family with the following instructions:

1. The patient should take this medication as advised by the physician and should not alter the

dosage. Although these products are potentially addictive, they are most effective when taken before severe pain occurs.

2. As the patient begins to feel better, other methods for relieving pain should be used whenever possible.

3. Some patients experience side effects from these drugs, such as dizziness, sedation, nausea and vomiting. The patient may also note a feeling of lightheadedness, especially when arising from a lying position; the patient should move slowly to decrease this feeling. The patient should report any new or troublesome symptoms to the physician.

4. The patient should avoid operating heavy machinery, driving, or performing tasks requiring alertness after taking this medication.

5. This medication must be kept out of the reach of children and others for whom it is not prescribed.

ANTIMIGRAINE AGENTS

ACTION

Antimigraine agents block nerve impulses in the receptors of the sympathetic nervous system. The ergot alkaloids used in the prophylaxis and treatment of vascular headaches are adrenergic blocking agents. Adrenergic blocking agents dilate the veins in smooth muscle tissue in the peripheral vascular system and the uterus. This reduces cerebral blood flow and arterial pulsation. Other actions include an increase in contractions of the uterus (oxytocic effect) and a decrease in blood pressure.

USES

Antimigraine agents are used in the prophylaxis and treatment of vascular headaches. They relieve the pain associated with vascular headaches by constricting dilated cerebral arteries. They are also used less commonly for oxytocic and other smooth muscle spasmogenic effects.

ADVERSE REACTIONS

Adverse reactions to antimigraine agents include murmurs, transient tachycardia, confusion, depression, dizziness, drowsiness, fixed miosis, numbness

and tingling in toes, weakness (especially in legs), nausea and vomiting, leg cramps, localized itching and edema, and neutropenia. Symptoms of overdosage include numb, cold, pale extremities, muscle pain at work and at rest, decreased or absent arterial pulses, drowsiness, confusion, depression, convulsions, hemiplegia, and fixed miosis.

DRUG INTERACTIONS

When antimigraine agents are used with other vasoconstrictors, vasoconstriction may be increased.

 NURSING IMPLICATIONS AND PATIENT TEACHING

▼ Assessment

The nurse should obtain a complete health history to identify the type of headache (whether tension, migraine, or cluster), and to rule out contraindications for the use of this drug, such as coronary artery disease or conditions in which a sudden change in blood pressure may be detrimental or dangerous.

The patient may have a history of migraine headaches, vascular headaches, or headache pain of a periodic, throbbing, severe nature. The pain may be unilateral and is commonly felt over one eye. Photophobia (sensitivity to light) and sensitivity to sound may be present, as well as nausea and vomiting. A family history of vascular headaches or history of motion sickness as a child, series of headaches in clusters, history of hypertension, a food allergy, or use of birth control pills may be present. The headache may be relieved or eased by sleep or vomiting.

The nurse may observe signs of sweaty hands and feet, scalp tenderness, autonomic dysfunction (such as miotic pupil), red eye, and unilateral nasal congestion.

▼ Planning

The diagnosis of vascular headaches can be confirmed if the patient's pain is relieved after an IM injection of 1 ml (0.5 mg) ergotamine.

Ergot alkaloids stimulate uterine contraction and are particularly harmful to the pregnant patient.

These migraine medications are slowly and incompletely absorbed from the gastrointestinal tract. Residues of ergotamine remain in various tissues; this accounts for its long-lasting and toxic actions.

▼ Implementation

If migraine agents are used at the onset of an attack, the efficacy of the drugs in relieving migraine pain and symptoms is increased.

These products are available in oral, sublingual, parenteral, and rectal forms, and as a solution for inhalation. Determining which form to use requires the consideration of many factors, including whether the purpose of the agent is to prevent or to treat migraine.

Oral and rectal preparations are absorbed slowly and incompletely from the gastrointestinal tract. To speed up this absorption, caffeine is combined with oral and rectal preparations of ergot alkaloids. Persons who cannot tolerate oral preparations are given rectal forms of the agent. Sublingual tablets are more quickly absorbed than either rectal or oral preparations. Intramuscular and subcutaneous preparations are commonly used, but absorption is often incomplete and slow.

A summary of important dosage information about antimigraine products is presented in Table 12-6.

▼ Evaluation

The nurse should monitor the patient for the therapeutic effect: decrease in number and severity of migraine headaches. To determine whether overdosage, toxicity, or adverse reactions are developing, monitor the patient's blood pressure in standing, sitting, and lying positions and check for peripheral pulses.

Prolonged use of migraine agents can lead to acute overdosage or chronic toxicity because of the wide variability in their absorption, metabolism, and excretion.

Abrupt discontinuation of migraine agents after prolonged use can result in rebound migraine headaches; therefore they should be discontinued slowly.

▼ Patient and family teaching

The nurse should provide the patient and family with the following instructions:

1. The patient should take the medication precisely as ordered and not increase the dosage without consulting the physician, because acute poisoning or overdosage may result.
2. The patient should avoid exposing arms and legs to cold temperatures after taking this medication.
3. The physician should be contacted immediately if numbness, coldness of extremities, or pain in legs during walking occurs.
4. Oral antimigraine agents may produce stomach upset. The medicine should be taken with milk or meals if possible to decrease this effect.
5. Common side effects of antimigraine agents include headache, nausea, vomiting, diarrhea, dizziness, and lightheadedness when changing positions rapidly.
6. After taking this drug, the patient should lie down immediately in a quiet, dark room to help obtain relief of symptoms. Relaxation techniques may also benefit the patient.
7. The physician should be contacted immediately if more than 8 mg of oral ergotamine is needed to relieve migraine pain.
8. This drug should not be used by a patient who suspects she is pregnant.

SECTION THREE: ANTICONVULSANTS

Objectives

At the conclusion of this section you should be able to:

1. Identify at least four groups of drugs used to treat seizure disorders.
2. Describe general nursing assessments that should be made before beginning anticonvulsant therapy.
3. Identify major contraindications to anticonvulsant medications.
4. Describe major adverse reactions associated with anticonvulsant medications.
5. Develop a teaching plan for the family and patient receiving anticonvulsant medications.

ACTION

Seizures are a symptom reflecting abnormal and excessive electrical discharge in the brain. There are a variety of diseases and disorders that produce seizures. The most common diagnosis of chronic and

Table 12-6   Antimigraine preparations

Generic name	Trade name	Comments and dosage
Combination products	Cafergot Cafetrate Ercaf Wigraine Midrin	Cafergot is a combination of ergotamine, caffeine, and other products used to treat migraine and vascular headaches. Caffeine is included to increase absorption of ergot alkaloids. Small amounts of belladonna alkaloids and barbiturates may also be included to control nausea and produce sedation. ■ *Migraine treatment:* 2 tablets PO at the start of an attack, followed by 1 tablet every 30 min to a maximum of 6 tablets per attack, 10 per week; or 1 suppository at the start of an attack. This dosage may be repeated 1 hour later if needed. Do not exceed 2 suppositories per attack, 5 per week.
Dihydroergotamine	DHE 45	An alpha-adrenergic blocking agent with pharmacologic and toxic properties similar to ergotamine used to treat migraine headaches. The drug causes cerebral vasculature to constrict, but it does not have an oxytocic effect and can be used during pregnancy. ■ *Migraine treatment:* 1 mg IM to be repeated at hourly intervals, not to exceed a total of 3 mg; or 1 mg IV to be repeated once. The total weekly dose should not exceed 6 mg.
Ergotamine	Ergostat Medihaler ergotamine	An alpha-adrenergic blocking agent that exerts direct vasoconstriction on cranial blood vessels, relieving pulsations thought to be responsible for vasoconstriction. Dependence on ergotamine may develop, necessitating gradual withdrawal from this product. ■ *Migraine treatment:* 2 mg PO or SL at the start of an attack, followed by 1 mg every 30 min as needed for full relief, up to 6 mg per migraine attack or 10 mg per week; the total amount is then used for subsequent attacks. Or 0.25 mg may be given IM or SQ, repeated in 40 minutes, if needed, for full relief; the total amount needed is then used at the first sign of subsequent attacks. Or 0.36 mg (1 metered spray) may be given by inhalation at the beginning of an attack, then repeated every 5 minutes as needed, up to 2.16 mg (6 metered sprays) per 24 hours, or 12 mg per week; the total amount required may be used at the first sign of subsequent attacks.
Methysergide	Sansert	Used as a migraine prophylactic for patients suffering from one or more severe vascular headaches per week. Thought to block serotonin activity in the CNS, which may be related to vascular headaches. This drug can produce highly toxic effects. Therefore continuous administration should not exceed 6 months. After each 6-month course of therapy, 3 to 4 weeks should be drug free, followed by another 6-month course of medicine. Monitor weight and watch for signs of edema, toxicity, and fibrosis at regular 3-month intervals. Because of significant adverse effects in some individuals, reserve this drug for patients with severe, frequent, uncontrollable headaches. ■ *Migraine prophylaxis:* 4 to 8 mg daily in divided doses with meals or milk.

recurring seizures is epilepsy, which is frequently **idiopathic,** or of an unknown cause. Head injury, brain tumor, stroke, meningitis, temperature elevation, and poisoning, especially from excessive alcohol intake or drugs, are also common causes of seizure activity. The most frequent cause of a seizure is the failure to take medication to control previously diagnosed seizure activity. It is estimated that as many as 10% of all people will have a seizure during their lifetime, although this percentage may rise with the increasing abuse of drugs. The terms epilepsy, convulsions, and seizures are commonly used interchangeably although they each have slightly different medical meanings. The diagnosis of epilepsy often has legal ramifications, which vary among states, including restriction of driver's licenses, operation of heavy machinery, or other activities requiring alertness.

There are a variety of traditional terms used to describe types of seizures, including grand mal (tonic-clonic), petit mal (absence), psychomotor, myoclonic, atonic, and jacksonian types. More recent terminology has been introduced, classifying seizure activity into two broad categories (generalized or focal), based on their clinical presentation and electroencephalographic (EEG) patterns.

Sometimes a surgical or dietary treatment may be used to control symptoms in a patient with a seizure disorder. More commonly, epileptic seizures are treated with medication. The therapeutic goal of this type of therapy is to suppress or reduce the number of seizures experienced by the patient.

There are a number of drugs that control seizures through depression of abnormal electrical discharges in the CNS. These products work in a variety of ways. There is usually one drug that is more effective than another for a patient, depending on the type of seizure activity. Patients with newly diagnosed seizure disorders are usually started on parenteral therapy, and when seizure activity has come under control, oral therapy is initiated.

There are four major anticonvulsant drug groups, as well as a variety of miscellaneous medications used to treat seizure disorders. **Barbiturates,** which have a long duration of action, are the primary category of anticonvulsants and are used for their sedative effect on the brain. They may be used in combination with the other three anticonvulsant medications. Benzodiazepines have selected uses and substantial adverse effects associated with them. Hydantoins have a wide range of use, with phenytoin (Dilantin) by far the most commonly used anticonvulsant. Succinimides

are used to control petit mal seizures. Each of these four groups, along with a variety of other miscellaneous anticonvulsants, will be discussed in this section.

USES

Because of the variety of available medications and the number of possible side effects, the selection of an anticonvulsant medication tends to be a trial or therapeutic experiment for each patient. When seizures are not stopped with one drug, another may be added, or the original drug may be discontinued and another product used instead. See Table 12-7 for a summary of anticonvulsants and their uses.

Because anticonvulsant drugs represent such a range of categories of medications, the major groups of medications will be discussed separately.

BARBITURATES

ACTION

Barbiturates are CNS depressants. They act primarily on the brainstem reticular formation, reducing nerve impulses to the cerebral cortex. Barbiturates depress the respiratory system and slow the activity of nerves and muscles (smooth, skeletal, and cardiac). Barbiturates can also raise the seizure threshold, or the level of electrical activity that must be produced before a seizure will occur.

USES

Long-acting barbiturates are used as anticonvulsants to control and prevent grand mal seizures. They are sometimes used to treat convulsions caused by continuous seizures or status epilepticus, tetanus, fever, or drugs.

ADVERSE REACTIONS

Adverse reactions to barbiturates include worsening of symptoms of certain organic brain disorders in elderly patients, dizziness, drowsiness, hangover, headache, lethargy, paradoxic restlessness or excitement, unsteadiness, photosensitivity, rash, diarrhea, nausea, hepatitis with jaundice, vomiting, anemia, decreased platelet counts, unusual bleeding or bruising, urticaria, joint and muscle pains, tolerance, and withdrawal symptoms when discontinued.

In cases of acute overdose, the patient may show

Table 12-7   Anticonvulsants and their primary uses

Drugs	Primary uses
BARBITURATES	
Amobarbital	All forms of epilepsy, status epilepticus, eclampsia, tetanus, drug reactions
Mephobarbital	Grand mal and petit mal seizures
Phenobarbital	All forms of epilepsy, status epilepticus, severe recurrent seizures, eclampsia
Secobarbital	Status epilepticus, drug reactions, tetanus
Thiopental	Status epilepticus
BENZODIAZEPINES	
Clonazepam	Petit mal, myoclonic seizures
Clorazepate	Focal seizures
Diazepam	All forms of epilepsy, status epilepticus, severe recurrent seizures, tetanus
HYDANTOINS	
Mephenytoin	Grand mal, psychomotor, focal, jacksonian seizures
Phenytoin	Grand mal, psychomotor seizures, status epilepticus
OXAZOLIDINEDIONES	
Paramethadione	Petit mal seizures
Trimethadione	Petit mal seizures
SUCCINIMIDES	
Ethosuximide	Petit mal seizures
Methsuximide	Petit mal seizures
Phensuximide	Petit mal seizures
OTHER DRUGS	
Acetazolamide	Grand mal, petit mal, myoclonic, mixed seizures
Carbamazepine	Grand mal, mixed, psychomotor seizures
Phenacemide	Psychomotor seizures
Primidone	Grand mal, psychomotor, focal seizures
Valproic acid	Petit mal seizures
Felbamate	Partial seizures, Lennox-Gastaut syndrome

exaggerated CNS depression, decreased respiration, constricted pupils, tachycardia, areflexia (absence of reflexes), shock, or coma. Death may occur as a result of cardiorespiratory failure.

DRUG INTERACTIONS

Because barbiturates increase metabolism, they reduce the activity of anticoagulants, corticosteroids, and digitalis preparations. Monoamine oxidase inhibitors may increase the depressant effects of the barbiturates. There may be significant additive effects if barbiturates are used along with alcohol, antihistamines, benzodiazepines, methotrimeprazine, narcotics, and tranquilizers.

BENZODIAZEPINES

ACTION

Benzodiazepines are also CNS depressants. Their exact mechanism of action is not known, but they are thought to act on the hypothalamus and limbic system of the brain, decreasing the vasopressor response and increasing the arousal threshold. Benzodiazepines suppress the spike and wave discharge in seizures and decrease the frequency, amplitude, duration, and spread of the discharge in minor motor seizures.

USES

Benzodiazepines are used to treat minor motor seizures and also to treat Lennox-Gastaut syndrome (petit mal variance) and patients who have failed to respond to succinimides. There are three benzodiazepines approved for use as anticonvulsants. Diazepam is used intraveneously to control scizures and is the drug of choice for treatment of **status epilepticus,** a situation of continuous severe grand mal seizures. Clonazepam is used for oral treatment of petit mal seizures in children, and clorazepate is used with other antiepileptic agents to control partial seizures.

ADVERSE REACTIONS

Adverse reactions to benzodiazepines include hypotension, shortness of breath, difficulty focusing or blurred vision, confusion, drowsiness, flushing, headaches, lightheadedness, paradoxic reactions (excitement, stimulation, hyperactivity), slurred speech, sweating, anorexia, bitter taste, dry mouth, diarrhea, heartburn, nausea, vomiting, pruritus, rash, joint pains, and burning eyes.

Overdosage may produce marked drowsiness, weakness, somnolence, impairment of stance and gait, confusion, and coma.

DRUG INTERACTIONS

Alcohol, other sedatives and hypnotics, antidepressants, anticonvulsants, and narcotics may produce additive sedative effects if used with benzodiazepines. Some combinations of anticonvulsants may result in an antidepressant effect or provoke additional seizures.

HYDANTOINS

ACTION

Hydantoins act primarily on the motor cortex, where they inhibit the spread of seizure activity by either increasing or decreasing the sodium ions across the motor cortex during the generation of nerve impulses.

USES

Hydantoins are used to treat grand mal and psychomotor seizures. Sometimes they are used to treat status epilepticus as well as migraine and trigeminal neuralgia. They are also used in some nonepileptic psychotic patients.

ADVERSE REACTIONS

Adverse reactions to hydantoins include ataxia, dizziness, drowsiness, hallucinations, inattentiveness, nystagmus, ocular disturbances, poor memory, slurred speech, constipation, nausea, vomiting, blood cell disturbances, bruising, acnelike eruptions, gingival hyperplasia, lupus erythematosus, hepatitis with jaundice, and lymph node hyperplasia.

Overdosage may produce ataxia, coma, dysarthria, hypotension, nystagmus, and unresponsive pupils.

DRUG INTERACTIONS

Hydantoin drug interactions are frequent and often substantial. The nurse should carefully monitor the administration of this drug with concomitant use of any other medication or vitamins. It may also alter the results of various laboratory tests.

SUCCINIMIDES

ACTION

Succinimide-type anticonvulsants elevate the seizure threshold in the cortex and basal ganglia and reduce synaptic response to low-frequency repetitive stimulation.

USES

Succinimides are used to control petit mal seizures. Methsuximide is used for refractory petit mal cases.

ADVERSE REACTIONS

Adverse reactions to succinimides include dizziness, headaches, hiccups, hyperactivity, lethargy, mood or mental changes, rashes, blurred vision, photophobia, anorexia, abdominal pain, diarrhea, nausea, vomiting, urinary frequency, vaginal bleeding, blood cell changes, alopecia, muscular weakness, systemic lupus erythematosus, disturbances of sleep, inability to concentrate, mental slowness, and night terrors.

DRUG INTERACTIONS

If succinimides are used with other anticonvulsants, they can result in increased libido or increased frequency of grand mal seizures. Bone marrow–depressing drugs used with succinimides can result in significant and fatal blood dyscrasias.

CARBAMAZEPINE

ACTION AND USES

Carbamazepine has been used as an anticonvulsant, primarily in combination with other anticonvulsants, to control grand mal seizures.

ADVERSE REACTIONS

Adverse reactions to carbamazepine include drowsiness, nausea, vomiting, and dizziness and are often seen when therapy is started. These usually diminish over time. Other major adverse reactions include hypotension, hypertension, edema, nystagmus, visual hallucinations, speech disturbances, pruritus, rashes, alopecia, and skin pigmentation.

DRUG INTERACTIONS

Carbamazepine causes the body to rapidly metabolize many other anticonvulsant medications, estrogen, and birth control pills. It may diminish the anticoagulant effects of warfarin. Propoxyphene increases serum levels of this medication.

PRIMIDONE

ACTIONS AND USES

When primidone is metabolized, it breaks down to two other anticonvulsant agents, phenobarbital and phenylethylmalonamide. This medication is used with other anticonvulsants to treat psychomotor and grand mal seizures.

ADVERSE REACTIONS

Adverse reactions to primidone include nystagmus, blurred vision, sedation, drowsiness, dizziness, paradoxic excitation in children, and blood dyscrasias.

DRUG INTERACTIONS

Primidone may increase the level of phenobarbital, but reduce the level of oral contraceptives.

VALPROIC ACID

ACTION AND USES

Valproic acid is used primarily to treat petit mal seizures, but may be part of combination therapy for other types of seizure disorders. This drug is structurally unrelated to other types of anticonvulsant medications.

ADVERSE REACTIONS

Adverse reactions to valproic acid include nystagmus, blurred vision, nausea, vomiting, indigestion, dizziness, and headache. It occasionally produces blood dyscrasias and hepatic toxicity. In addition, it may produce a false-positive test for urinary ketones.

DRUG INTERACTIONS

Other medications such as alcohol, analgesics, tranquilizers, and CNS depressants taken at the same time produce an exaggerated sedative effect. Interactions with phenobarbital, carbamazepine, and phenytoin may lead to increased seizure activity.

 NURSING IMPLICATIONS AND PATIENT TEACHING

▼ Assessment

The nurse should obtain a thorough health history, including medications that may produce drug interactions, other anticonvulsants, response to anticonvulsants taken in the past, hypersensitivity, and the possibility of pregnancy. Cardiac, respiratory, hepatic, or renal diseases are contraindications or precautions to the use of anticonvulsants.

▼ Planning

Elderly or debilitated patients may be more sensitive to barbiturates and should be started on lower dosages. These patients are more likely to have hangover, confusion, and delirium. Dependence can develop with indiscriminate use, and abrupt withdrawal is dangerous. Several of the anticonvulsant medications may produce blood dyscrasias or systemic lupus erythematosus. Benzodiazepines are changed by the liver into long-acting forms that may remain in the body for 24 hours or more and produce increased sedation; liver function may be impaired with prolonged use. In addition, there is an increased risk of congenital malformations and neonatal depression with most anticonvulsants if used during pregnancy.

▼ Implementation

Barbiturates are controlled substances. Attempts should be made to avoid giving them to patients with a history of abuse or addiction. Barbiturates should not be administered to patients in pain, because they may worsen the pain.

When barbiturates are given parenterally, the nurse should use great caution to avoid accidentally injecting into an artery or tissues, because serious ischemia or gangrene could result.

When benzodiazepines are used in patients who have a mixed type of seizure activity, the drugs may increase or precipitate the onset of generalized tonic-clonic seizures. These drugs should also be used with caution in patients with impaired renal function. Abrupt withdrawal can produce status epilepticus. These drugs may produce increased secretions in patients with some types of respiratory problems.

The dosage of benzodiazepines must be individualized, depending on the patient's response. The onset of action is approximately 30 to 60 minutes. The effects last 7 to 8 hours. The drug should be given 15 to 30 minutes before bedtime. Elderly or debilitated patients should receive reduced dosages of all anticonvulsants. It is important to gradually increase or decrease dosages.

The nurse should counsel the patient and family regarding the possibility of brief and reversible personality changes with succinimide therapy. These should be reported to the physician.

Once the patient is controlled on a particular drug, changing to hydantoin products should be avoided. All dosages must be individualized. The dosage for children is usually larger by weight than for adults. The patient is usually given a single dose within the therapeutic range and then the amount is gradually increased until the seizures are controlled, or until symptoms of overdosage or toxicity make further increases inadvisable.

Oral hydantoin suspension is often difficult to administer accurately. The oral suspension should be shaken well before being given, and the medication should be protected from freezing. Chewable tablets should not be used for once-a-day treatment.

Subcutaneous or perivascular injection of hydantoins should be avoided because of the highly alkaline nature of the solution. It should be administered intravenously very slowly.

Important information about anticonvulsants, including dosages, are summarized in Table 12-8.

▼ Evaluation

It takes several weeks before the success of an anticonvulsant dosage regimen can be assessed. The therapeutic effects should be evaluated, and the nurse should note whether the degree of sedation is compatible with the patient's life-style.

The patient's compliance should be monitored with regard to the amount and times the medication is taken, any pattern of abuse, signs of intoxication, paradoxic reactions, tolerance, dependence, withdrawal, and toxicity (jaundice, rash, sore throat).

The patient should keep a record of uncontrolled seizures: the time, duration, characteristics, and reaction.

Complete blood cell counts and liver function tests should be done as a baseline, and repeated on a set schedule for patients on long-term barbiturate therapy.

Tolerance is usually proportional to the total amount of drug received. Dependence and withdrawal symptoms may occur if these drugs are used for extended periods. Rapid withdrawal following prolonged administration should be avoided.

Hydantoins are metabolized at various rates among patients. Therefore, the nurse must watch carefully for toxic effects. The patient should avoid alcohol while on most anticonvulsants.

Adverse effects are common in long-term therapy. Gum hyperplasia is a typical occurrence with hydantoins and may be distressing to the patient and family. The patient and family must be educated about how to prevent and treat this problem.

Prescriptions are usually written for a particular brand of medication. Once a patient's seizures are controlled with a certain brand, the patient continues to receive that brand. Not all brands are interchangeable.

▼ Patient and family teaching

The nurse should provide the patient and family with the following instructions:

 CRITICAL DECISION:
Oral Hydantoin Therapy

There are two types of oral hydantoin therapy: "prompt" and "extended" capsules. Capsules labeled "extended" are given only once a day. Capsules labeled "prompt" are given two or three times a day.

Table 12-8 Anticonvulsants

Generic drug	Trade name	Comments and dosage
BARBITURATES **Long-acting**		
Phenobarbital	Phenobarbital	Some forms come in sustained-release capsules. Onset 1 hour, effective for 16 hours; give 50 to 100 mg bid or tid.
	Luminal	Give in large muscle mass IM because injection is very painful. Give slowly IV. Give 100 to 300 mg IM.
Mephobarbital	Mebaral	Converts to phenobarbital in body. Onset 1 hour; effective 10 to 16 hours; give 100 to 200 mg PO qd.
Intermediate-acting		
Amobarbital	Amytal	Elixir is 34% alcohol. Store in amber-colored glass bottle. Onset 1 hour, but effective only 4 to 6 hours; give 50 to 200 mg PO.
Amobarbital sodium	Amytal sodium	For IV or IM injection; do not exceed 1 mg/min. Onset 30 to 60 minutes; effective 8 to 10 hours. Give 65 to 200 mg in divided doses qd.
Secobarbital	Seconal	Short acting (3 to 6 hours), so often not used orally. Give 100 mg PO qd.
Secobarbital sodium	Seconal sodium	Give slowly, 50 mg/15 seconds IV; give 100 mg PO; 120 to 200 mg PR; 50 to 250 mg parenterally.
BENZODIAZEPINES		
Clonazepam	Klonopin	*Adults:* Initial dose is 1.5 mg PO divided into three doses per day. After 4 to 9 days, dosage may be increased by 0.5 to 1.5 mg/day every 3 days until the seizures stop or until the side effects preclude any further increase. Maximum recommended daily dose is 20 mg. *Infants and children up to 10 years or 30 kg:* Initial dosage between 0.01 to 0.03 mg/kg/day PO, however *not* to exceed 0.05 mg/kg/day, given in two or three divided doses. Dosage should be increased by not more than 0.25 to 0.5 mg every third day until a daily maintenance rate of 0.1 to 0.2 mg/kg is reached. Whenever possible give in three equally divided doses; if this is not possible, give the largest dose before bedtime.
Clorazepate	Tranxene	*Adults and children over 12 years:* Initial dose is 7.5 mg tid. Increase by no more than 7.5 mg every week. Maximum dose not to exceed 90 mg/day. *Children 9 to 12 years:* Initial dose is 7.5 mg bid. Increase by no more than 7.5 mg every week. Maximum dose not to exceed 60 mg/day.
Diazepam	Valium	*Adults:* 2 to 10 mg PO bid to qid. Give 15 to 30 mg sustained-release capsules qd. *Geriatric or debilitated patients:* 2 to 2.5 mg PO qd or bid; gradually increase dose as needed. *Children older than 6 months:* 1 to 2.5 mg PO tid to qid initially; gradually increase dose as needed. ▪ *Parenteral therapy:* Inject IV medication slowly only into large veins, 1 minute for each 5 mg. *Adults:* Give 5 to 10 mg IV initially, repeated as necessary at 10- to 15-minute intervals; maximum IV dose is 30 mg; therapy may be repeated in 2 to 4 hours as needed. *Children 5 years and older:* Give 1 mg q2 to 5 min; maximum IV dose is 10 mg; repeat in 2 to 4 hours as needed. *Children 30 days to 5 years:* Give 0.2 to 0.5 mg slowly q2 to 5 min; maximum IV dose is 5 mg.

Continued.

| | | Table 12-8   Anticonvulsants—cont'd | | |

Generic drug	Trade name	Comments and dosage
HYDANTOINS		
Phenytoin	Dilantin Diphenylan	*Adults:* 100 mg PO tid initially; gradually increase to achieve level desired; maintenance dosage is 300 to 400 mg. *Children:* 5 mg/kg/day PO in 2 or 3 equally divided doses initially; gradually increase to achieve level desired, up to 300 mg; maintenance dosage is 4 to 8 mg/kg/day. *Children 6 years of age and older:* May require the minimum adult dosage of 300 mg/day.
Mephenytoin	Mesantoin	*Adults and children:* 50 to 100 mg PO qd; can be increased by an additional 50 to 100 mg in three or four divided doses at 1-week intervals. Maximum dosage is 800 mg, 400 mg for children.
SUCCINIMIDES		
Ethosuximide	Zarontin	*Adults and children 6 years and older:* 250 mg bid initially, increase by 250 mg every 4 to 7 days until seizures are controlled or total daily dosage reaches 1.5 gm. The optimal dosage for most children is 20 mg/kg daily. *Children 3 to 6 years:* 250 mg PO qd initially, increase by 250 mg every 4 to 7 days until seizures are controlled or total daily dosage reaches 1 gm.
Methsuximide	Celontin Kapseals	*Adults:* 300 mg qd initially; increase by 300 mg at weekly intervals until seizures are controlled or total daily dosage reaches 1.2 gm. *Children:* Usual adult dosage. Small children may require adjustment using 150 mg capsule.
Phensuximide	Milontin Kapseals	*Adults and children:* 500 mg bid initially, increased by 500 mg at weekly intervals until seizure control or total daily dosage reaches 3 gm. Shake suspension well before pouring. Take drug with meals to decrease gastric discomfort. Efficacy of the drug decreases with prolonged use.
MISCELLANEOUS ANTICONVULSANTS		
Acetazolamide	Diamox	8 to 30 mg/kg/day in divided doses.
Carbamazepine	Tegretol	200 mg bid initially, increasing gradually by 200 mg/day in divided doses at 6- to 8-hour intervals; do not exceed 1200 mg daily.
Primidone	Mysoline	250 mg qd, with weekly increases of 250 mg until therapeutic response or tolerance develops. Usual dosage is 750 to 1500 mg qd; do not exceed 2000 mg qd.
Valproic acid	Depakene Depakote	15 mg/kg/day PO. Increase by 5 to 10 mg/kg/day at weekly intervals; do not exceed 30 mg/kg/day.
Phenacemide	Phenurone	*Adults:* 1.5 gm/day in 3 divided doses.
Oxazolidinedrones		
Paramethadione	Paradione	Give 900 mg to 2.4 gm/day in divided doses.
Trimethadione	Tridione	Give 900 mg to 2.4 gm/day in divided doses.

1. The patient should be aware that there is sometimes a problem with tolerance, dependence, and addiction with anticonvulsant medications.
2. The patient should take the medication exactly as prescribed and not discontinue taking it even if he or she has no seizures and may be feeling well. If a dose is missed, it should be taken as soon as possible. If it is nearly time for the next dose, take only the next dose. Double doses should not be taken. The regular medication schedule should be continued.
3. This medication should be kept in a locked cabinet or out of the reach of children and all others for whom the drug is not prescribed. The medication should not be shared with anyone.
4. Barbiturates may cause drowsiness, and the patient must be cautious when driving, using hazardous machinery, or performing tasks that require alertness.
5. Some medications produce daytime sedation that may interfere with the patient's job or home and child care responsibilities.
6. The physician should be notified immediately if the patient experiences any rash, fever, unusual bleeding, bruising, sore throat, jaundice, or abdominal pain. Some people experience side effects while taking this drug, so the physician should be notified of any new or uncomfortable symptoms.
7. The patient may have excessive dreaming when barbiturates are discontinued; this should lessen each night.
8. Tablets and capsules should be kept in a dry, tightly closed container.
9. Elixirs should be kept in a tightly closed, brown glass bottle.
10. A hangover feeling may sometimes be experienced the day after taking benzodiazepines. It is dangerous to drink alcohol within 24 hours after taking this drug. The patient must take the medication and must not drink any alcohol.
11. Smoking may decrease the length of time benzodiazepines are effective.
12. Succinimides may be taken with food or milk to decrease stomach upset.
13. The liquid form of succinimides should be shaken well before the dose is measured.

14. The patient should maintain good oral hygiene: brush teeth and gums with soft toothbrush twice daily and rinse the mouth well. The patient should see a dentist every 6 months; this is especially true if the patient is taking hydantoin.

CRICITAL DECISION:
Oral Hygiene

The importance of good oral hygiene, especially of gums, should be emphasized when teaching patients taking hydantoins.

15. The patient should wear a Medic-Alert identification or other bracelet or chain that states the medical problem and the medication being taken.
16. Succinimides may make the urine appear pink, red, or red-brown.
17. Chewable tablets must be chewed or crushed before they are swallowed.
18. The patient must not change the brands or dosage forms unless ordered to do so by the physician. Not all brands of the medications are interchangeable.

Pediatric Considerations
ANTICONVULSANTS

The young patient (under age 23) is more susceptible to gingival hyperplasia, especially with phenytoin or mephenytoin therapy. Gingivitis or gum inflammation usually starts during the first 6 months of drug therapy, although severe hyperplasia is unlikely with dosages under 500 mg/day. A dental program of teeth cleaning and plaque control started within 7 to 10 days of initiating drug therapy helps to reduce the rate and severity of this condition.

Coarse facial features and excessive body hair growth are more frequently reported in young patients.

Impaired school performance is reported with long-term, high-dose hydantoin therapy (especially at high or toxic serum levels.)

Children receiving valproic acid, especially those under 2 years old or those receiving multiple anticonvulsant drugs, are at a greater risk for serious hepatotoxicity. This risk decreases with advancing age.

From McKenry LM, Salerno E: *Mosby's pharmacology in nursing*, ed 18, St Louis, 1992, Mosby.

Geriatric Considerations
ANTICONVULSANTS

The elderly tend to metabolize anticonvulsants more slowly; thus drug accumulation and toxicity may occur. Monitor closely as dosage adjustments (lower doses) may be necessary.

Serum albumin levels may be lower in geriatric patients, thus resulting in decreased protein binding of bound drugs, such as phenytoin and valproic acid. Monitor closely as lower drug doses may be necessary.

Administer intravenous doses at a rate slower than the recommended rate for an adult. Elderly rate of administration for phenytoin should be 5 to 10 mg/min up to a maximum of 25 mg/min.

From McKenry LM, Salerno E: *Mosby's pharmacology in nursing*, ed 18, St Louis, 1992, Mosby.

19. When undergoing any kind of surgery, including dental work, the patient should alert the physician or dentist that he or she is taking an anticonvulsant medication.
20. The use of anticonvulsants is not advised in pregnancy. The patient and physician should discuss questions about becoming pregnant.
21. The patient should keep regular follow-up appointments with the physician; this is essential to evaluate reactions to anticonvulsants.

SECTION FOUR: ANTIEMETICS AND ANTIVERTIGO AGENTS

Objectives

At the conclusion of this section you should be able to:

1. Identify the actions of antiemetic and antivertigo drugs.
2. Describe common side effects of anticholinergic drugs.
3. Name at least six medications in this category.

ACTION

Antiemetic or antivertigo products reduce indirect stimulation of the vomiting center (as do anticholinergic agents) and reduce dopamine, which induces vomiting.

USES

Vomiting may be produced by direct action on the vomiting center of the brain, by indirect action through stimulation of the chemoreceptor trigger zone, and through increased activity of chemical neurotransmitters. Nausea and vomiting associated with motion are probably produced by bombardment of impulses to the vestibular network of the labyrinth system of the ear, which is located near the vomiting center. The impulses are conducted to the vomiting center by cholinergic nerve impulses. Thus drugs that inhibit cholinergic nerve impulses should be effective in treating motion sickness.

Some drugs, metabolic disorders, radiation, motion, gastric irritation, vestibular neuritis, or increases in central trigger zone dopamine or vomiting center acetylcholine may provoke vomiting. Antiemetics act by one or more mechanisms to inhibit this response. Antiemetic or antivertigo preparations usually are used to prevent and treat motion sickness or nausea and vomiting with anesthesia and surgery. Antidopaminergic preparations are used almost exclusively to control nausea and vomiting. Anticholinergic medications are used to control motion sickness. Meclizine, dimenhydrinate, and diphenidol are the only products used to control vertigo.

ADVERSE REACTIONS

Drowsiness is the most common side effect of the anticholinergics, but tolerance to this reaction usually develops with prolonged therapy. Patients may also experience dry mouth, stuffy nose, blurred vision, constipation, urinary retention, and other anticholinergic reactions.

DRUG INTERACTIONS

The sedative effect of some antiemetic medications is potentiated by concurrent use of other CNS depressants. They also have an additive effect with anticholinergic drugs. Anticholinergic antiemetics can intensify the anticholinergic side effects of many other drugs. The drug interactions may vary, depending on the type of antiemetic-antivertigo drug, but would be similar to other anticholinergic or antidopaminergic products.

 NURSING IMPLICATIONS AND PATIENT TEACHING

▼ Assessment

The nurse should obtain a health history, including motion sickness, extrapyramidal reactions caused by antipsychotic therapy, labyrinthitis, vertigo, Ménière's disease, radiation therapy, or diabetes. Nausea and vomiting are common adverse reactions to drug therapy, and may occur after taking almost any medication.

The nurse should also find out whether the patient has a history of hypersensitivity, is currently using drugs that would cause drug interactions (especially MAO inhibitors), and is pregnant.

In all cases the underlying cause of vomiting, nausea, or vertigo should be sought. In women of childbearing years, always investigate the possibility of pregnancy. These drugs should not be used for treating morning sickness, because their safe use cannot be ensured.

▼ Planning

Antiemetic and antivertigo agents should be used with extreme caution in patients performing tasks that require mental alertness, because some products produce drowsiness. These preparations are not recommended for use in children because they may contribute to the development, the misdiagnosis, or the severity of symptoms in Reye's syndrome, an encephalopathy often fatal in children.

Vomiting is often an important diagnostic clue and may point to serious underlying problems. The cause of the vomiting or nausea should be determined so that appropriate treatment can be undertaken to eliminate the problem. Antiemetic drugs should not be the only form of therapy in cases of nausea or vomiting. Attempts to maintain hydration, restore electrolyte balance, and reduce accompanying symptoms should be made.

▼ Implementation

Phenothiazine derivatives all turn the urine pink or reddish brown. They also may produce photosensitivity, and the patient should avoid excessive exposure to sunlight. Antiemetic and antivertigo agents generally come in tablets, sustained-release capsules, and concentrates for oral use. For patients who are vomiting or so nauseated that they are unable to take oral medications, injection or suppository forms are usually available.

The dosage should be as low as possible, and therapy should be terminated as quickly as possible. IV preparations should be reserved for severe cases in hospitalized patients. Medications given IM should be switched when the patient can tolerate oral agents.

Table 12-9 summarizes important information about antiemetic-antivertigo agents.

▼ Evaluation

The nurse should monitor for therapeutic effectiveness and side effects.

▼ Patient and family teaching

The nurse should provide the patient and family with the following instructions:

1. The patient should take this medication as instructed by the physician and not double the dosage or alter the medication schedule.
2. If the drug is taken for motion sickness, the patient should take it 30 to 60 minutes before departure and 30 minutes before meals thereafter.
3. The patient should not drive, operate hazardous machinery, or engage in tasks that require alertness while taking these drugs.
4. The patient should not take any other medications without the knowledge of the physician. It is especially important for the patient to avoid other CNS depressants, including alcohol, because of the sedative effect.
5. Although some patients experience drowsiness while taking this medication, this is usually transient and will disappear with continued use of the drug.
6. This medication should be kept out of the reach of children and others for whom it is not prescribed. Overdosage of this medicine may be toxic.

Text continued on p. 250.

Table 12-9 Antiemetic and antivertigo agents

Generic name	Trade name	Comments and dosage

ANTIDOPAMINERGICS
Phenothiazines

Generic name	Trade name	Comments and dosage
Chlorpromazine	Thorazine Ormazine	A phenothiazine derivative used to control nausea and vomiting and to treat intractable hiccups. *Adults:* 10 to 25 mg PO q4 to 6h prn; 50 to 100 mg PR q6 to 8h prn; or 25 mg IM. If no hypotension develops, IM dose may be increased to 50 mg q3 to 4h. *Children over 6 months:* 0.25 mg/lb PO q4 to 6h; 0.5 mg/lb PR q6 to 8h; or 0.25 mg/lb IM q6 to 8h prn. Children up to 5 years should not receive more than 40 mg/day. Children 5 to 12 years should not receive more than 75 mg/day unless severely vomiting.
Triflupromazine	Vesprin	Phenothiazine derivative used to control severe nausea and vomiting. Medication may also change urine color to pink or reddish brown. Activity of drug may last for up to 12 hours after IM administration in children. *Adults:* 20 to 30 mg PO total daily dose for prophylaxis; with 5 to 15 mg IM for vomiting, repeated q4h prn up to 60 mg; or 1 mg IV, up to 3 mg total daily dose. *Children over 2½ years:* 0.2 mg/kg PO, not to exceed 10 mg/day in three divided doses; may give 0.2 to 0.25 mg/kg IM, not to exceed 10 mg/day.
Perphenazine	Trilafon	A phenothiazine derivative used to control severe nausea and vomiting, and for therapy of intractable hiccups in adults. IV use should be reserved for hospitalized patients and given in a slow drip. ■ *Nausea, vomiting, or hiccups:* 8 to 16 mg PO qd in divided doses. Occasionally, as much as 24 mg may be needed. For rapid control of vomiting, 5 mg IM may be given. Higher dosages and IV therapy should be reserved for hospitalized patients.
Prochlorperazine	Compazine	A phenothiazine derivative used to treat vomiting. ■ *Nausea and vomiting* *Adults:* 5 to 10 mg PO tid to qid; or 15 mg sustained-release tablet may be ordered qAM; or a 10 mg sustained-release tablet may be given q12h. Medication may be given PR, 25 mg bid; or 5 to 10 mg IM, repeated in 3 to 4 hours prn. Do not exceed 40 mg/day IM. *Children 40 to 85 lbs:* 2.5 mg tid or 5 mg bid; do not exceed 15 mg/day. *Children 30 to 39 lbs:* 2.5 mg PO or PR bid or tid; do not exceed 10 mg/day. *Children 20 to 29 lbs:* 2.5 mg PO or PR qd or bid; do not exceed 7.5 mg/day. If IM medication is indicated, give 0.06 mg/lb.
Promethazine	Phenergan	A phenothiazine derivative used to treat motion sickness and to prevent and control nausea and vomiting associated with surgery and anesthesia. SQ injection may cause tissue necrosis; intraarterial injection may produce gangrene of the extremity. ■ *Motion sickness* *Adults:* 25 mg 30 to 60 min before travel, repeat 8 to 12 hours later prn. On succeeding days, take 25 mg on arising and again before the evening meal. *Children:* 12.5 to 25 mg bid. ■ *Nausea and vomiting* *Adults:* 12.5 to 25 mg PO, IM, or PR q4 to 6h prn. If parenteral medication is indicated, give 25 mg deep IM. IV medication should be given to hospitalized patients only. *Children:* 0.25 to 0.5 mg/kg IM or PR q4 to 6h prn. For parenteral medication, do not give more than one half the adult dose. Preoperatively, may give equal doses of promethazine and a barbiturate or narcotic, and an atropine-like drug.

Table 12-9   Antiemetic and antivertigo agents—cont'd

Generic name	Trade name	Comments and dosage
Thiethylperazine	Torecan	A phenothiazine derivative that probably acts directly on the trigger zone and the vomiting center to reduce nausea and vomiting. IV use of drug is to be avoided because it will produce severe hypotension. IM use should be limited to deep IM injection, at or shortly before the termination of anesthesia. ■ *Nausea and vomiting:* 10 to 30 mg qd in divided doses.
Other		
Metoclopramide	Reglan Clopra Octamide	10 mg IV or PO before meals and at bedtime.
ANTICHOLINERGICS **Antihistamines**		
Cyclizine	Marezine	Antiemetic, anticholinergic, and antihistaminic agent that also reduces the sensitivity of the labyrinthine apparatus; used primarily for motion sickness. ■ *Antiemetic* *Adults:* 50 mg tablets PO 30 min before travel; repeat q4 to 6h; maximum 200 mg/day. Administer 50 mg IM q4 to 6h.
Meclizine	Antivert Bonine	Antiemetic, anti–motion sickness, and antivertigo agent with anticholinergic properties. ■ *Motion sickness:* 50 mg 1 hour before departure; repeat every 24 hours prn. ■ *Vertigo:* 25 to 100 mg/day in divided doses prn.
Buclizine	Bucladin-S	Antiemetic with central anticholinergic activity; used for nausea and vomiting associated with motion sickness. ■ *Antiemetic* *Adults:* 50 mg tid with a maintenance dose of 50 mg bid.
Diphenhydramine	Benadryl Genahist	Antihistamine that blocks histamine receptors on peripheral effector cells. It has anticholinergic, antitussive, antiemetic, and sedative properties. With IV use, blood pressure should be carefully monitored. *Adults:* 50 mg PO tid to qid or 10 to 50 mg IM or IV; maximum daily dose 400 mg. *Children over 20 lbs:* 12.5 mg to 25 mg PO tid to qid; or 5 mg/kg PO or IM qd.
Dimenhydrinate	Dimetabs Dramamine hydrate	Antiemetic, antivertigo agent used in motion sickness, in radiation sickness, or following anesthesia. It appears to depress motion-induced stimulation of the labyrinthine structures; may alter blood counts. *Adults:* 50 to 400 mg/day PO in divided doses; or 50 mg IM or IV prn. *Children over 3 years:* 1.25 mg/kg tid to qid with a maximum dosage of 300 mg/day PO or IM.
Other		
Trimethobenzamide	Tigan Arrestin	Antiemetic that inhibits the chemoreceptor trigger zone in the medulla; used to control nausea and vomiting. Drug has been linked to the development of Reye's syndrome in children. Give deep IM only, since solution is highly irritating to the tissues. *Adults:* 250 mg PO tid to qid; or 200 mg IM tid to qid; or 200 mg PR tid to qid. *Children between 30 and 90 lbs:* 100 mg PO tid to qid; or 100 to 200 mg PR tid to qid. *Children under 30 lbs:* 100 mg PR tid to qid.

Continued.

Table 12-9 Antiemetic and antivertigo agents—cont'd

Generic name	Trade name	Comments and dosage
Scopolamine	Transderm-Scop	Comes in oral form as well as a transdermal patch, which is placed behind the ear and releases medication at a constant rate over a 3-day interval. The transdermal mechanism allows for lower dosage and produces fewer adverse anticholinergic effects than the oral forms. Scopolamine is used to control motion sickness in adults. Many contraindications. ■ *Motion sickness:* 0.25 to 0.8 mg PO 1 hour before anticipated travel. ■ *Prolonged therapy:* Apply one patch behind ear at least 4 hours before the antiemetic effect is desired; replace every 3 days for continued therapy.
MISCELLANEOUS		
Diphenidol	Vontrol	Used to treat vertigo by acting on the vestibular apparatus, and to inhibit the chemoreceptor trigger zone in controlling nausea and vomiting. It has also been used for nausea and vomiting caused by anesthesia and malignant neoplasms. *Adults:* 25 to 50 mg q4h for nausea or vertigo. *Children over 25 lbs:* 0.4 mg/lb for nausea or vomiting; may repeat in 4 hours as needed; do not exceed 2.5 mg/lb in 24 hours.
Benzquinamide	Emete-Con	Has antiemetic, antihistaminic, sedative, and mild anticholinergic actions. Usually effective within 15 min. Used for prophylaxis and treatment of nausea and vomiting caused by anesthesia and surgery. ■ *Prophylaxis with anesthesia:* 50 mg (0.5 to 1 mg/kg) IM at least 15 min before terminating anesthesia. Repeat in 1 hour, then q3 to 4h prn; may also give 25 mg (0.2 to 0.4 mg/kg) IV as a single dose slowly (1 ml/min), with the following doses given IM.
Hydroxyzine	Atarax Vistaril	Antiemetic and antihistaminic, but is used primarily as an antianxiety agent. ■ *Nausea and vomiting:* 25 to 100 mg IM for adults and 1.1 mg/kg (0.5 mg/lb) IM for children. ■ *Preoperative and postoperative adjunctive medication:* 25 to 100 mg IM for adults and 1.1 mg/kg (0.5 mg/lb) IM for children. ■ *Labor and postpartum adjunctive therapy:* 25 to 100 mg IM.

SECTION FIVE: ANTIPARKINSONIAN AGENTS

Objectives

At the conclusion of this section you should be able to:

1. List signs and symptoms of Parkinson's disease.
2. Identify neurotransmitters that produce the symptoms of Parkinson's disease.
3. Describe the action of anticholinergic and dopaminergic drugs used to treat Parkinson's disease.
4. Identify the therapeutic objective of medications used to treat Parkinson's disease.
5. Identify common adverse reactions to medications used in Parkinson's disease.
6. Identify key items that should be part of a teaching plan for a patient with Parkinson's disease.

ACTION

Antiparkinsonian agents are anticholinergic and dopaminergic medications used to control symptoms by altering the neurotransmitters produced in the brain. The two main actions of the antiparkinsonian agents are (1) to block the uptake of acetylcholine at postsynaptic muscarinic cholinergic receptor sites, and (2) to elevate the functional levels of dopamine in motor regulatory centers. These drugs exert a wide range of effects on all the organs affected by the autonomic nervous system, including the eye, respiratory tract, heart, gastrointestinal tract, urinary bladder, nonvascular smooth muscle, exocrine glands, and the CNS. Antiparkinsonian agents reduce muscle tremors and rigidity, and improve mobility, muscular coordination, and performance.

USES

Paralysis agitans, or **Parkinson's disease,** is a chronic disorder of the CNS. The cause is unknown, but it is thought to involve an imbalance in chemical neurotransmitters within the brain, in which excesses of acetylcholine and an absolute deficit of dopamine in the basal ganglia are found. Common symptoms are fine muscle tremors, slowness of movement, rigidity, muscle weakness, a characteristic shuffling, forward-pitched gait, and resulting changes in posture and equilibrium. There is no known cure for Parkinson's disease. Treatment goals are designed to relieve symptoms and to maintain movement and activity of the patient.

ADVERSE REACTIONS

Dopamine agents may produce dysrhythmias, muscle twitching, psychotic reactions, rigidity, diarrhea, epigastric distress, GI bleeding, nausea, vomiting, blurred vision, alopecia, bitter taste, hot flashes, rash, and urinary retention.

Anticholinergic agents may cause orthostatic hypotension, tachycardia, agitation, confusion, depression, headache, memory loss, muscle cramping, constipation, vomiting, diplopia, increased intraocular pressure, decreased sweating, flushing, and skin rash.

Early signs of toxicity in the patient taking dopaminergic agents include muscle twitching and blepharospasm. Overdosage is a common phenomenon, particularly with long-term drug therapy. It is recognizable because the patient experiences a sudden onset of progressively worsening parkinsonian symptoms. These drugs should be tapered gradually.

DRUG INTERACTIONS

Common drug interactions differ according to whether the preparation is an anticholinergic or a dopaminergic agent. These drugs commonly interact

with many isolated medications; product information must be closely studied.

 NURSING IMPLICATIONS AND PATIENT TEACHING

▼ Assessment

The nurse should obtain a complete health history, including the presence of hypersensitivity, concurrent use of medications that may produce drug interactions, presence of asthma, renal, liver, cardiovascular disease, epilepsy, other contraindications for the drug, and the possibility of pregnancy.

The nurse may elicit a history of either Parkinson's disease or concurrent antipsychotic drug therapy, drooling, or difficulty with coordination and walking. The patient may be middle aged or elderly and have tremors at rest made worse by emotional stress. The arms may fail to move when walking, with rigidity first occurring in the proximal musculature, and the patient may be unable to perform activities of daily living.

▼ Planning

Antiparkinsonian agents are contraindicated for persons with known hypersensitivity, acute narrow-angle glaucoma, asthma, history of epilepsy, peptic ulcer disease, skin lesions, persons on CNS stimulants, those exposed to rubella, those with acute psychoses, history of melanoma, or patients receiving MAO inhibitor therapy. These drugs are known to aggravate many other diseases and must be used with caution.

The anticholinergics and some dopaminergics must be withdrawn slowly, because many of these drugs have a long half-life. When withdrawing a preparation and beginning a new preparation, the new drug should be started in small doses and the old drug should be withdrawn gradually. These agents are usually initiated at the lowest dosage possible and increased gradually until the maximum therapeutic effect has been obtained. The numerous adverse effects of these drugs can be controlled by decreasing the dosage.

▼ Implementation

The anticholinergic drugs include benztropine, biperiden, diphenhydramine, ethopropazine, procyclidine, orphenadrine, and trihexyphenidyl. The dopaminergic agents include amantadine, bromocriptine, carbidopa, and levodopa. These drugs are available in tablets, sustained-release capsules, syrup, elixir, and IV and IM injections. They are generally well absorbed from the gastrointestinal tract. Peak blood levels are achieved in 1 to 6 hours, depending on the route of administration and the type of drug administered, except for the sustained-release capsules, which reach peak plasma blood levels in 8 to 12 hours. Sustained-release capsules are not recommended for initial therapy because they do not allow enough flexibility in dosage regulation.

IV injection of anticholinergics can cause hypotension and incoordination. Carbidopa and levodopa are often administered concurrently. Carbidopa/levodopa retards the peripheral breakdown of L-dopa. If this combination drug is administered after levodopa therapy, the levodopa should be discontinued at least 8 hours before initiating therapy with carbidopa/levodopa. The combination should be substituted at a dosage level that provides 25% of the previous levodopa dose. When these combination doses are excessive, both drugs can be titrated individually.

Table 12-10 summarizes the important medications used to treat Parkinson's disease.

▼ **Evaluation**

Long-term use of dopaminergic and anticholinergic agents often leads to akinesia (loss of movement), tardive dyskinesia (difficulty in performing voluntary movements), and dystonia (impairment of muscle tone). The dosage should be reduced to the minimum effective level to counteract these effects, and dosages should be tapered as necessary to avoid excessive medication.

Numerous laboratory tests may be altered by these medications; this should be taken into account when monitoring patient status.

▼ **Patient and family teaching**

The nurse should provide the patient and family with the following instructions:

1. The patient should take the medication exactly as ordered by the physician. Clinical improvement may take 2 to 3 weeks, so the patient should not stop taking the medication unless advised to do so by the physician.
2. Antiparkinsonian agents should be taken after meals to avoid stomach upset.
3. The patient should avoid taking vitamin preparations with vitamin B_6 (pyridoxine).
4. The physician should be contacted immediately if parkinsonian symptoms become suddenly worse, if intermittent winking or muscle twitching occurs, or if abdominal pain, constipation, distention, or urinary problems occur.
5. Common side effects include dry mouth, dizziness, drowsiness, and gastrointestinal symptoms. Some patients experience dizziness or lightheadedness, especially as they move from lying to standing positions. The patient should avoid driving or tasks requiring alertness or rapid changes of movement.
6. The patient's urine, sweat, and saliva may darken after exposure to air.
7. The patient should avoid overexertion during hot weather.
8. Periodic ophthalmologic examinations are necessary when taking anticholinergic drugs.

SECTION SIX: PSYCHOTHERAPEUTIC AGENTS

Objectives

At the conclusion of this section you should be able to:

1. Identify major categories of drugs used to treat people with anxiety.
2. Recognize common side effects of antianxiety drugs.
3. Give an example of a drug from each of the three major categories of antidepressant drugs.
4. Identify side effects of antidepressant drugs.
5. Identify common psychotic states in which medications are used as part of the therapeutic regimen.
6. List mechanisms of action of major antipsychotic drugs.
7. Describe adverse reactions that may result from antipsychotic drugs.

Table 12-10 Antiparkinsonian drugs

Generic name	Trade name	Dosage and comments
ANTICHOLINERGIC DRUGS		
Belladonna alkaloids	Bellafoline Compound Belladonal	Competes with acetylcholine for muscarinic receptors at the postganglionic fibers of the parasympathetic nervous system; also used to control GI disturbances. Give 0.25 to 0.5 mg PO tid; 0.5 to 1 ml qd to bid parenterally.
Benztropine	Cogentin	Contains anticholinergic and antihistaminic promesylate properties. Pharmacologically, the drug inhibits excessive cholinergic activity in the striatal fibers. Used to treat extrapyramidal symptoms (except tardive dyskinesia) induced by antipsychotic agents. IM injection provides rapid (15 minutes) relief from acute dystonic reactions. Oral doses of the drug are cumulative; therefore therapy should begin with a low dose and increase gradually at 5- to 6-day intervals as necessary. ■ *Parkinsonian symptoms:* 1 to 2 mg/day PO with meals or parenterally; range is 0.5 to 6 mg. ■ *Drug-induced extrapyramidal side effects:* 1 to 4 mg bid with meals.
Biperiden	Akineton	Blocks central cholinergic receptors, restoring the balance between cholinergic and dopaminergic activity in the basal ganglia. IV or IM administration may produce incoordination. ■ *Parkinsonism symptoms:* 1 to 2 mg PO tid to qid, give with meals. ■ *Drug-induced extrapyramidal symptoms:* 2 mg PO qd to tid. Administer 2 mg IM or IV for acute symptoms; repeat q30 min to a maximum of four doses a day.
Diphenhydramine	Benadryl Genahist	Blocks receptor cells on peripheral effector cells. *Adults:* 50 mg PO tid to qid or 10 to 15 mg IM or IV. *Children over 20 lbs:* 12.5 mg to 25 mg PO tid to qid; or 5 mg/kg PO or IM qd.
Ethopropazine	Parsidol	A phenothiazine derivative antiparkinsonian agent with anticholinergic properties; relieves most symptoms, including tremors. Administer initial dose of 10 mg qid; may be increased in 10 mg increments every 2 to 3 days until the desired response is achieved. Moderate symptoms require 100 to 400 mg qd; severe symptoms may require 500 to 600 mg qd.
Procyclidine	Kemadrin	A synthetic antiparkinsonian agent that inhibits hyperactive cholinergic activity in the striatal fibers. It is more effective in the relief of rigidity than tremor and relieves excessive salivation. ■ *Parkinsonism:* 8 to 10 mg PO in 3 to 4 divided doses qd. Dosage may range from 6 to 15 mg qd. ■ *Extrapyramidal symptoms:* 10 to 20 mg in 3 divided doses qd.
Trihexyphenidyl	Artane Trihexy-2	Exerts a direct inhibitory effect on the parasympathetic nervous system. Decreases rigidity, although most symptoms improve to some degree. ■ *Idiopathic parkinsonism:* 6 to 10 mg PO in 3 to 4 divided doses; 1 mg initially and increased in 2 mg increments at intervals of 3 to 5 days until a total dosage of 6 to 10 mg is reached. Once maintenance dose is reached, sustained-release capsule may be used; 5 mg qd to bid.

Continued.

Table 12-10 Antiparkinsonian drugs—cont'd

Generic name	Trade name	Dosage and comments
DOPAMINERGIC DRUGS		
Amantadine	Symmetrel	This drug enhances the release of dopamine from presynaptic nerve endings. The drug has no anticholinergic activity. ■ *Parkinsonism:* 100 mg qd to bid up to a maximum of 400 mg qd. ■ *Drug-induced extrapyramidal reactions:* 100 mg bid up to a maximum of 300 mg qd.
Bromocriptine	Parlodel	Directly stimulates the dopamine receptors in the corpus striatum; this medication is especially helpful in patients who are beginning to deteriorate or develop tolerance to levodopa. Initiate therapy with 1.25 mg tablet, bid with meals. Increase after 2 to 4 weeks prn by 2.5 mg/day; do not exceed 100 mg/day.
Carbidopa/levodopa	Lodosyn Sinemet-10/100 Sinemet-25/100 Sinemet-25/250	This is a fixed combination antiparkinson agent used in all types of parkinsonian treatment, and is composed of both carbidopa and levodopa. *For patients not receiving levodopa:* 1 tablet (10/100 or 25/100) tid initially; increase by 1 tablet daily until a maximum of 8 tablets is given. *Patients receiving levodopa:* Discontinue L-dopa at least 8 hours before initiating therapy with this product. Administer 1 tablet (25/250) tid to qid in patients previously requiring 1500 mg or more of levodopa each day.
Levodopa	Dopar Larodopa	A metabolic precursor of dopamine. It enters the CNS by crossing the blood-brain barrier and is converted to dopamine. Give 0.5 to 1 gm PO qd in two or more doses. Dosage may be increased gradually in increments of 0.75 gm every 3 to 7 days as tolerated. The usual optimum dose should not exceed 8 gm.
Pergolide	Permax	Adjunctive to levodopa/carbidopa therapy. New drug with many adverse effects. Give 0.05 mg for 2 days, gradually increase over 12 days.
Selegiline	Eldepryl	Irreversible MAO inhibitor; new drug. Give 5 mg at breakfast and lunch; allows levodopa/carbidopa dosages to be reduced.

8. Explain the use of lithium to treat patients in manic states.
9. List adverse effects associated with use of lithium.
10. Develop a teaching plan to help family and patients taking psychotherapeutic medications.

ANTIANXIETY AGENTS

OVERVIEW

Anxiety is a common problem associated with many medical and surgical conditions, as well as a primary symptom in many psychiatric disorders. Anxiety is a normal human emotion, but when it is felt too frequently or interferes with a person's ability to perform activities of daily living, it is considered abnormal. Anxiety creates subjective feelings of helplessness, indecision, worry, apprehension, and irritability. Patients may complain of headache, gastric distress, insomnia, and inability to concentrate. It may also produce objective symptoms of restlessness, tremor, constipation, diarrhea, nausea, and muscle tension.

When anxiety is so severe that it must be treated with medication, antianxiety medications or tranquilizers are used to reduce some of the symptoms. They do not prevent the anxiety, because the feelings or problems that produce the anxiety are still there. Therefore, antianxiety medication should be used for only a short time until other remedies may be found.

It is especially important to view the use of these medications as a short-term solution, because of the potential for addiction caused by these medications.

The major products used today for anxiety are the benzodiazepines, accounting for about 75% of the antianxiety prescriptions written today. Although benzodiazepines have a variety of uses, there are particular drugs in this category that are used primarily for treating anxiety. Other antianxiety agents are briefly included.

ACTION

Benzodiazepines apparently act at the limbic, thalamic, and hypothalamic levels of the CNS, producing a calming effect. Benzodiazepines are used to relieve anxiety, tension, and fears that occur alone or as the result of illness. Other indications include management of delirium tremens after alcohol withdrawal; premedication for surgical and endoscopic procedures or electric cardioversion; treatment of convulsive disorders (diazepam only); and relief of muscle spasm.

ADVERSE REACTIONS

Adverse reactions to antianxiety agents include hypotension, tachycardia, clumsiness, confusion, depression, drowsiness, fatigue, headache, insomnia, lightheadedness, paradoxic reactions (excitement, hallucinations, agitation, hostility, or rage), syncope, unsteadiness, visual disturbances, weakness, anorexia, constipation, difficulty swallowing, dry mouth, hiccups, jaundice, nausea, vomiting, urinary retention, blood cell changes, pruritus, skin rash, joint pain, and unexplained sore throat and fever. Overdosage may produce somnolence, confusion, coma, diminished reflexes and hypotension. Tolerance is easily developed.

DRUG INTERACTIONS

Simultaneous administration of benzodiazepines with any of the following substances may increase either agent's effect: alcohol, anesthetics, monoamine oxidase (MAO) inhibitors, or CNS depressants, such as antihistamines, barbiturates, phenothiazines, narcotics, sedatives, tranquilizers, hypnotics, anticonvulsants, or tricyclic antidepressants. Caffeinated products and excessive cigarette smoking can antagonize the anxiolytic effect of these drugs.

 NURSING IMPLICATIONS AND PATIENT TEACHING

▼ Assessment

The nurse should obtain a complete health history, including hypersensitivities, underlying systemic disease (especially pulmonary, cardiac, liver or renal disease, epilepsy or seizures, myasthenia gravis, mental illness, and drug abuse or dependence), possibility of pregnancy, breastfeeding, or concurrent use of medications (both prescribed and over-the-counter) that may present drug interactions. These conditions are contraindications or precautions to the use of antianxiety agents.

The nurse may elicit a history of feelings of apprehension, uncertainty, fear, an unpleasant state of tension, a sense of impending doom, insomnia, irritability, hypersensitivity to stress, difficulty with concentration, or nightmares.

▼ Planning

Elderly patients (over age 60) and those with chronic illnesses may require a decreased initial dosage and may need careful monitoring of individual response before alterations in dosage are made. Benzodiazepines generally have a long half-life and can have cumulative effects. Patients with a history of seizures or epilepsy should have their dosages tapered slowly from benzodiazepines.

 CRICITAL DECISION:
Benzodiazepines

The patient should be given the smallest dosage possible to reduce the opportunity for overdose, particularly in those patients with a history of drug addiction or dependence.

▼ Implementation

Administering the benzodiazepines during or immediately after meals decreases the incidence of gastrointestinal side effects. The manufacturers' instructions for diluting and slowly injecting parenteral medications should be followed to prevent the possibility of respiratory failure.

Depression commonly accompanies anxiety, so patients must be questioned and observed for suicidal tendencies.

Treatment with antianxiety agents should proceed

Table 12-11		Antianxiety medications
Generic name	**Trade name**	**Dosage and comments**

BENZODIAZEPINES

Generic name	Trade name	Dosage and comments
Alprazolam	Xanax	Action peaks in 1 to 2 hours; half-life 12 to 15 hours. Effectiveness and safety in children less than age 18 have not been determined. *Adults:* 0.25 to 0.5 mg PO tid initially; titrate to maximum dose of 4 mg PO qd in divided doses. *Elderly, debilitated patients:* 0.25 mg PO bid to tid initially.
Chlorazepate	Tranxene	Peak effect is in 60 minutes; half-life is 2 days. Some reports indicate a fall in hematocrit with prolonged usage. Can be given once each day. ■ *Anxiety* *Adults:* 30 mg qd; adjust gradually with a range of 15 to 60 mg qd. *Elderly, debilitated patients:* 7.5 to 15 mg qd initially.
Chlordiazepoxide	Librium Mitran	Peak levels in 1 to 4 hours; half-life 5 to 30 hours. Food or antacids slow absorption. Injection IV must be very slow to avoid producing respiratory arrest. ■ *Anxiety Adults:* 5 to 25 mg tid to qid; 5 to 10 mg tid to qid may be given several days preoperatively to allay anxiety. *Elderly, debilitated patients:* 5 mg bid to qid.
Diazepam	Valium Zetran	Peak blood levels are reached within 1 to 2 hours with a half-life of 20 to 50 hours. ■ *Anxiety and management of convulsive disorders:* 2 to 10 mg bid to qid. Sustained-release capsules 15 to 30 mg qd. ■ *Skeletal muscle spasm:* 2 to 10 mg tid to qid. Sustained-release capsules 15 to 30 mg qd. *Elderly, debilitated patients:* 2 to 2.5 mg qd or bid, then gradually increase as tolerated. *Children:* 1 to 2.5 mg tid to qid initially, then gradually increase.
Halazepam	Paxipam	Action peaks in 1 to 3 hours; half-life is 14 hours. Individualize dosages as needed and tolerated. *Adults:* 20 to 40 mg PO tid to qid. Optimal range is 80 to 160 mg PO qd. *Elderly, debilitated patients:* 20 mg PO qd to bid.
Lorazepam	Ativan	Action peaks in 2½ hours; half-life is 10 to 15 hours. Patients may experience withdrawal manifested as insomnia 2 or 3 nights after cessation of therapy. IM injection is used as a preanesthetic agent for adults only. It is also given IV for sedation and relief of anxiety. ■ *Anxiety:* 2 to 3 mg PO bid to tid initially; usual range is 2 to 6 mg qd in divided doses with the largest dose before sleep. ■ *Insomnia:* Single bedtime dose of 2 to 4 mg PO. *Elderly, debilitated patients:* 1 to 2 mg PO qd in divided doses.
Oxazepam	Serax	Peak blood levels at 2 to 4 hours. Half-life is 5 to 20 hours; the incidence of toxicity is low. ■ *Anxiety:* 10 to 30 mg PO tid or qid. *Elderly, debilitated patients:* 10 mg PO tid initially, then increase gradually to 15 mg tid to qid.
Prazepam	Centrax	Peak blood levels at 6 hours after administration. *Adults:* 30 mg PO qd, with dosages gradually adjusted within range of 20 to 60 mg qd. *Elderly, debilitated patients:* 10 to 15 mg PO qd in divided doses. This drug may be given in a single bedtime dose; recommended to start with 20 mg.

Table 12-11   Antianxiety medications—cont'd

Generic name	Trade name	Dosage and comments
OTHER NONBENZODIAZEPINE ANTIANXIETY AGENTS		
Buspirone	BuSpar	Approved for short-term use in anxiety disorders. Mechanism of action unknown; chemically unrelated to other antianxiety medications. *Adults:* 5 mg tid, increased by 5 mg every 2 to 3 days prn; maintenance 20 to 30 mg qd in divided doses.
Doxepin	Sinequan	*Adults:* 75 to 150 mg/day. For oral concentrate, do not mix with grape juice.
Chlormezanone	Trancopal	*Adults:* 200 mg 3 or 4 times daily. *Children:* 50 to 100 mg 3 or 4 times daily.
Hydroxyzine	Atarax Vistaril	Antihistamine for the symptomatic relief of anxiety especially in psychoneurosis. Also has analgesic activity that may be helpful in relieving pruritus caused by allergies. Medication may be used preoperatively for surgery or obstetrical patients to permit decrease in narcotic dosages, reduce anxiety, and control emesis. Product also helps control acutely disturbed or hysterical patients. This product is for IM use only. SQ, intraarterial, or IV use may produce tissue necrosis and hemolysis. *Adults:* 50 to 100 mg PO qid. *Children over 6 years of age:* 50 to 100 mg/day PO in divided doses. *Children under 6 years of age:* 50 mg/day PO in divided doses. ■ *Sedative* *Adults:* 50 to 100 mg PO, or 25 to 100 mg IM. *Children:* 0.6 mg/kg PO, or 1.1 mg/kg IM.
Meprobamate	Equanil Miltown Meprospan	Antianxiety and mild skeletal muscle relaxant, acts on numerous sites in CNS to produce mild sedation; used for short-term relief of anxiety. *Adults:* 400 mg tid or qid; smaller doses in elderly or debilitated patients; do not exceed 2400 mg qd.

slowly in the elderly (over age 60), the debilitated, those with limited pulmonary reserve, and those in whom a hypotensive episode might precipitate cardiac dysfunction.

Table 12-11 summarizes important dosage information about antianxiety medications.

▼ Evaluation

Mental alertness, cognitive functions, and physical abilities may be impaired with the use of antianxiety agents. These drugs should be given in conjunction with counseling or psychotherapy for maximum benefit.

Abrupt termination of these agents may cause delayed withdrawal symptoms (up to 1 week later) of abdominal or muscle cramps, vomiting, diaphoresis, tremor, or convulsions. Tapering the dosage for patients on prolonged therapy helps prevent this occurrence.

The nurse should take lying, sitting, and standing blood pressures when monitoring hypotensive changes.

Alternatives for coping with stress and change should be discussed with the patient, for example, increased regular physical activity, muscle relaxation exercises, and participation in hobbies.

▼ Patient and family teaching

The nurse should provide the patient and family with the following instructions:

1. The patient should take this medication exactly as ordered and not stop taking the medication unless advised to do so by the physician. If a dose is forgotten, it should be taken as soon as it is remembered, if it is within 1 to 2 hours of the regular dosage time. If it is later than 2 hours, the patient should skip the dose

and take the next dose at the regular time. The patient should not double the dosage.

2. The patient must keep regular appointments with the physician so that progress can be checked and side effects of the drug can be monitored.

3. Antianxiety agents can cause dizziness, light-headedness, drowsiness, and unsteadiness. They may decrease the patient's ability to think or react clearly and quickly. The patient should not drive, operate hazardous machinery, or perform activities requiring alertness until response to the drug has been determined. These symptoms will often disappear after the patient has taken the medicine for several weeks. Additionally, the patient should change to sitting or standing positions slowly to minimize these symptoms and prevent falls.

4. The patient should notify the physician if any new or troublesome symptoms occur while he or she is taking this medication, such as ulcers or sores in the mouth, hallucinations, feelings of confusion, difficulty sleeping, skin rash, yellowing of eyes or skin, slow pulse, difficulty with breathing, sore throat and fever, unusual nervousness, excitement, irritability, depression, or eye pain.

5. This medication must be kept out of the reach of children and all others for whom it is not prescribed.

6. The physician should be informed if the patient begins taking any new prescription or nonprescription drugs. Many different medications have interactions with antianxiety agents; therefore the physician may want to increase or decrease the dosage.

7. The patient should not drink any alcohol while taking this medicine.

8. The patient should be aware that cigarette smoking and the use of caffeinated beverages (coffee, tea, cola) can decrease the effect of antianxiety agents.

9. Benzodiazepines are not intended for use by pregnant women. If the patient is pregnant or breastfeeding, or if the patient should become pregnant while taking this medicine, the physician should be informed immediately.

10. This drug may be habit forming; the patient should use it for the least time possible.

ANTIDEPRESSANTS
OVERVIEW

Depression, whether mild or so severe that it interferes with activities of daily living, has been recognized for centuries. Many types of therapy have been explored, but only in the last 30 years have medications been discovered that help to elevate moods.

The antidepressant effects of monoamine oxidase (MAO) inhibitors were initially discovered as side effects of medicine used to treat other diseases. They were then used to treat depressed patients until tricyclic antidepressant therapy became available in the 1960s. MAO inhibitors are now used primarily when tricyclic therapy is unsatisfactory or when other therapy is inappropriate or refused. In the last few years, three other medications, none related chemically to either the tricyclics or the MAO inhibitors, have entered the field for treatment of depressed patients. Each of these groups will be discussed.

Tricyclic Antidepressants
ACTION

The antidepressant effect of tricyclics is not completely understood. It is thought that tricyclic antidepressants inhibit the uptake of norepinephrine and/or serotonin (biogenic amines) by the presynaptic neuronal membrane in the CNS, thereby increasing the concentration of these biogenic amines at the synapse.

USES

Tricyclic antidepressants are used primarily to relieve the symptoms of endogenous depression. They may also be used to treat mild exogenous depression, which is not self-limiting or interfering with usual activities of daily living. They are less commonly used for manic-depressive disorders as **adjunctive** or additional therapy.

ADVERSE REACTIONS

Adverse reactions to tricyclic antidepressants include dysrhythmias, orthostatic hypotension, confusion, headache, prolonged drowsiness, constipation, nausea, vomiting, blood dyscrasias, fever, photosensitivity, pruritus, skin rash, muscle twitching, tremors, urinary hesitancy or retention, altered liver function tests, blurred vision, and nervousness.

Overdosage may initially produce stimulation of the CNS exhibited by irritability, agitation, hallucinations, delirium, twitching, hypertonia, hyperreflexia, nystagmus, hyperpyrexia, hypertension, and seizures (more commonly seen in children). This initial CNS stimulation is followed by CNS depression exhibited by drowsiness, areflexia, hypothermia, hypotension, dysrhythmias, respiratory depression, coma, or cardiorespiratory arrest.

DRUG INTERACTIONS

Tricyclic antidepressants increase the CNS depressant effect of alcohol and other CNS depressants, particularly ethchlorvynol. The effects of anticonvulsants may be decreased when used with tricyclic antidepressants. The antihypertensive effects of guanethidine and clonidine may be blocked when used with most tricyclic antidepressants, with the exception of doxepin. There may be a reduction in the antidepressant effect of tricyclics and an increase in their side effects when used concurrently with estrogen, including oral contraceptives containing estrogen. An increased incidence of cardiac dysrhythmias has been found with concurrent use of thyroid medication and tricyclic antidepressants. Severe hypertension or hyperpyrexia may result when tricyclic antidepressants are used with MAO inhibitors or sympathomimetics.

 NURSING IMPLICATIONS AND PATIENT TEACHING

▼ Assessment

The nurse should obtain a complete health history; allergy, disease, and other medications taken concurrently, including over-the-counter preparations must be considered. Many diseases present contraindications or precautions for the use of tricyclic drugs.

The nurse may elicit a history of insomnia, early morning awakening, anorexia, constipation, loss of motivation, and fatigue. The patient may verbalize feelings of hopelessness and pessimism, degrade self verbally, respond slowly to questions, and have slowed motor movements, decreased facial expression and stooped posture. The nurse should assess the patient thoroughly for any suicidal feelings.

▼ Planning

Tricyclic antidepressants should not be given if the patient has a history of hypersensitivity to a tricyclic antidepressant (cross-sensitivity may occur) or a history of myocardial infarction (during the acute recovery period), narrow-angle glaucoma, or severe hepatic or renal failure. Tricyclic antidepressants should be used very carefully with MAO inhibitors.

Antidepressants may cause manic-depressive patients to convert to the manic phase of their illness; exaggerated symptoms of paranoid ideation and schizophrenia may develop in patients who have these disorders. This may be avoided or treated by reducing the dosage of the tricyclic antidepressant or by using a tranquilizer.

Only the smallest reasonable amount of antidepressants should be given to patients who are possibly suicidal.

▼ Implementation

Because the plasma concentrations of tricyclic antidepressants vary widely and may not correspond well with the dosage or therapeutic effects, the initial and maintenance dosages of these drugs must be carefully determined, based on the patient's age, physical health status, and response to the drug.

The initial dose may cause sedation, especially when the patient is taking a tricyclic known to have moderate to strong sedative effects. Therefore tricyclic antidepressant therapy may be initiated by a single bedtime dose, especially for depressed patients with a sleep disturbance. The drug dosage can then be varied or titrated to achieve the best response with the lowest dosage and minimal side effects. A maintenance dosage, administered in divided doses or as a single bedtime dose, may be continued for 6 months to 1 year.

Table 12-12, page 260, summarizes the important information the nurse should know about tricyclic antidepressant medications.

▼ Evaluation

The desired antidepressant effect of the drug will usually occur within 1 to 4 weeks after therapy is initiated.

If a tricyclic antidepressant is given in large doses or over a prolonged period of time, the drug should be discontinued by gradual reduction for 4 to 8 weeks to avoid withdrawal symptoms of general listlessness, headache, and nausea.

Table 12-12   Tricyclic antidepressants

Generic name	Trade name	Comments and dosage
Amitriptyline	Elavil Endep	Has a strong sedative effect, especially early in therapy. It should be taken at bedtime to decrease daytime drowsiness. Used to treat endogenous depression accompanied by anxiety. *Initial:* 25 mg PO bid to qid. *Maintenance:* 50 to 100 mg/day at bedtime or in divided doses; may also give 20 to 30 mg IM qid.
Amoxapine	Asendin	The antidepressant effect is usually seen within 2 weeks after initiating therapy; used to treat a wide variety of depressions, including reactive, endogenous, and psychotic depressions. *Initial:* 50 mg PO tid; increase to 100 mg PO tid on third day. *Maintenance:* 30 mg/day or less at bedtime.
Clomipramine	Anafranil	Used to treat obsessive-compulsive disorder. Give 25 mg qd and gradually increase to 100 mg over 2 weeks.
Desipramine	Norpramin Pertofrane	Has mild sedative effect; orthostatic hypotension is common during the first few weeks of therapy. Used to treat a variety of depressions, particularly endogenous type. *Initial:* 25 to 50 mg PO tid; give only 25 to 50 mg/day in adolescent and elderly patients. *Maintenance:* Up to 200 mg/day.
Doxepin	Adapin Sinequan	Has marked sedative effect, particularly during initial phase of therapy. Used to treat psychotic and psychoneurotic depression with associated anxiety and somatic symptoms. The oral concentrate should be diluted in milk, fruit juice, or water before administration. *Initial:* 25 mg PO tid. *Maintenance:* 50 to 150 mg/day at bedtime or in divided doses.
Imipramine	Tofranil Janimine	Used to treat endogenous depression; it is the only tricyclic that is also used to treat enuresis in children. *Initial:* 25 mg PO tid and qid; or 25 to 50 mg IM tid to qid; reduce to 30 to 40 mg/day in divided doses for adolescents and elderly patients. *Maintenance:* 50 to 150 mg/day PO at bedtime.
Maprotiline	Ludiomil	Used to treat neurotic depression and manic-depressive disorders, depressed type. Antidepressive effects may occur within 1 week of initiating therapy. *Initial:* 75 mg/day PO in single or divided doses. *Maintenance:* 75 to 150 mg/day.
Nortriptyline	Aventyl Pamelor	Used to treat endogenous depression. *Initial:* 25 mg PO tid to qid; reduce to 30 or 50 mg/day in divided doses for adolescent or elderly patients and increase only as needed and tolerated. *Maintenance:* Up to 100 mg/day PO.
Protriptyline	Vivactil	Used to treat endogenous depression, particularly when the patient is withdrawn or listless. This drug has no sedative effect and stimulates the CNS more than other tricyclics. *Initial:* 5 to 10 mg PO tid to qid; reduce dose in adolescents and elderly to 5 mg tid. *Maintenance:* Not to exceed 60 mg/day.
Trimipramine	Surmontil	This product has a strong sedative effect; used to treat endogenous depression accompanied by anxiety. *Initial:* 25 mg PO tid; reduce dosage to 25 mg bid in adolescent and elderly patients. *Maintenance:* 50 to 150 mg/day at bedtime. In adolescents and the elderly increase dose to maximum of 100 mg/day only as necessary and tolerated.

▼ Patient and family teaching

The nurse should provide the patient and family with the following instructions:

1. The patient should take this medication exactly as ordered. It may be taken with food to avoid gastric distress. It may take up to 8 weeks before the patient begins to feel better. Therefore it is important to take the drug in the exact amount and frequency specified, even though the patient notices no changes initially.
2. Tricyclic antidepressants should never be stopped suddenly, because there could be an increase in symptoms, as well as nausea, headache, and feelings of listlessness. The patient must not stop taking the drug without talking to the physician.
3. Tricyclic antidepressants may cause drowsiness or make the patient feel less alert than usual. If so, the patient should avoid driving or other activities requiring alertness. This feeling should pass after the medication is taken for a short time. The patient should tell the physician if drowsiness or decreased alertness persists longer than 2 weeks and interferes with usual activities.
4. Dryness of the mouth may occur when medication is first started. Chewing sugarless gum, sucking on hard candy, or rinsing the mouth frequently may help relieve the dryness.
5. Tricyclic antidepressants will increase the effects of alcohol, sleeping pills, and some medications for the relief of colds and hay fever. The patient should avoid alcohol and check with the physician before taking any other medications.
6. Tricyclic antidepressants are very powerful drugs and must be kept out of the reach of children and others for whom they are not prescribed. They should not be left on dressers or low bedside tables.
7. Lightheadedness, dizziness, or feelings of faintness occur in some people taking this drug, especially older people. To reduce this feeling, the patient should move slowly, especially when changing from a lying or sitting position to standing upright.
8. Tricyclic antidepressants are usually discontinued several days before the patient undergoes any surgery requiring anesthesia. The physician must develop a plan to gradually discontinue the medicine in the proper manner.
9. The physician should be notified if the patient develops any new or troublesome symptoms, especially the appearance of urinary retention, constipation, blurred vision, or excessive sleepiness.
10. If the patient is taking this medication for a prolonged period of time, it is wise to wear a Medic-Alert bracelet and carry a medical identification card listing this drug.

Monoamine Oxidase (MAO) Inhibitors

ACTION

Monoamine oxidase (MAO) is an enzyme found in the mitochondria of cells located in nerve endings and other body tissues such as the kidney, liver, and intestines. This enzyme normally acts as a catalyst by inactivating dopamine, norepinephrine, epinephrine, and serotonin (biogenic amines) and therefore regulating the intracellular levels of these neurotransmitters. MAO inhibitors block the inactivation of the biogenic amines, resulting in an increased concentration of dopamine, epinephrine, norepinephrine, and serotonin at neuronal synapses. The antidepressant effects of MAO inhibitors are thought to be directly related to this increased concentration of biogenic amines.

USES

MAO inhibitors are used to relieve the symptoms of severe reactive or endogenous depression that have not responded to tricyclic antidepressant therapy, electroconvulsive therapy, or other modes of psychotherapy.

ADVERSE REACTIONS

Adverse reactions to MAO inhibitors include orthostatic hypotension, dysrhythmias, ataxia, drowsiness, hallucinations, headache, hyperactivity, insomnia, seizures, tremors, vertigo, anorexia, constipation, diarrhea, nausea, vomiting, fever, photosensitivity, skin rash, dysuria, incontinence, blurred vision, dry mouth, edema, and impotence.

Overdosage produces mental confusion, restlessness, hypotension, respiratory depression, tachycardia, seizures, and shock, which may persist for 1 to 2 weeks.

DRUG AND FOOD INTERACTIONS

MAO inhibitors have many drug interactions. They may potentiate the CNS depressant effect of alcohol, anesthetics, sedatives, hypnotics, and narcotics and may cause severe hypertension and hyperpyrexia. If they are used with anticonvulsants, they may cause a change in the seizure pattern of the patient and the dosage of the anticonvulsant medication may have to be adjusted accordingly. The hypotensive effects of diuretics and antihypertensives may be enhanced when those agents are used with MAO inhibitors. The hypoglycemic effects of insulin or oral hypoglycemics may be enhanced by MAO inhibitors, and dosages may need to be adjusted accordingly. MAO inhibitors and tricyclic antidepressants are generally not used together because hyperpyrexia, severe convulsions, hypertensive crisis, and death may result.

Sudden and severe hypertension can result when MAO inhibitors are used with the following foods and beverages high in tyramine and other high vasopressor amines: alcoholic beverages such as beer and wines (particularly sherry, hearty red wines, and chianti), yeast extracts, meat tenderizers, soy sauce, beef or chicken liver, other meats; fish, sausage, pickled herring, bean pods, figs, raisins, bananas, avocados, fava beans, sour cream, yogurt, and cheese. Concurrent use of MAO inhibitors and large amounts of caffeine-containing products (coffee, tea, cola, chocolate) can cause hypertension and cardiac dysrhythmias.

 NURSING IMPLICATIONS AND PATIENT TEACHING

▼ Assessment

The nurse should obtain a complete health history, including the presence of any disease conditions that may contraindicate the use of MAO inhibitors. The patient should be asked about concurrent use of medications (especially tricyclic antidepressants) and the possibility of pregnancy. The nurse should also assess the depth of the patient's depression and monitor for suicidal ideas.

▼ Planning

The safe use of MAO inhibitors in pregnant patients or nursing mothers has not been established.

▼ Implementation

MAO inhibitors are only given orally and are well absorbed by this route.

The desired antidepressant effect of MAO inhibitors will usually occur in 1 to 4 weeks of drug therapy; there is no benefit in continuing the drug if results are not obtained after this time. When improvement is noted during the initial period of drug therapy, the dosage should then be reduced gradually over a period of several weeks until an effective maintenance dosage is reached. MAO inhibitors are usually not given in the evening because of their psychomotor stimulating effect, which may produce insomnia.

The maintenance dose of MAO inhibitors can be administered either in single or divided doses.

MAO inhibitors should be discontinued at least 2 weeks before elective surgery. If emergency surgery is indicated, doses of narcotics and anesthetics need to be reduced. All patients treated on an outpatient basis need to be closely monitored. See Table 12-13 for a summary of MAO inhibitors.

▼ Evaluation

All patients taking MAO inhibitors must be monitored for symptoms of postural hypotension. If this occurs, the dosage of the drug should be reduced or the drug should be discontinued.

Patients who are agitated or who have schizophrenia may become more hyperactive. Manic-depressive patients may convert to the manic phase of their illness; this may be treated by discontinuing the drug for a brief period of time and then resuming the drug at a lower dosage.

The effects of MAO inhibitors continue for approximately 2 weeks after the drug is discontinued; therefore all drugs and foods that interact with MAO inhibitors must be avoided during this 2-week period.

▼ Patient and family teaching

The nurse should provide the patient and family with the following instructions:

1. Take this medication exactly as ordered by the physician. It may take up to 4 weeks before the patient begins to feel better. Therefore it is important to take the drug in the exact amount and frequency ordered even though the patient may notice no changes.

2. MAO inhibitors can increase the effects of alcohol and other drugs such as narcotics, sleeping pills, and amphetamines. Alcohol (including beer and wine) should be avoided. The patient should check with the physician before taking any other prescription or over-the-counter medications.

Table 12-13 Monoamine oxidase inhibitors		
Generic name	**Trade name**	**Comments and dosage**
Isocarboxazid	Marplan	Slow onset of action; therapeutic effects may take several weeks to develop; adverse effects can occur within hours. Used to treat neurotic or atypical depression. *Initial:* 30 mg/day PO in single or divided doses. *Maintenance:* 10 to 20 mg PO qd; do not exceed 30 mg/day.
Phenelzine	Nardil	*Initial:* 15 mg PO tid up to 60 to 75 mg maximum. *Maintenance:* Reduce slowly to 15 mg PO qd or qod.
Tranylcypromine	Parnate	Improvement in symptoms is usually seen 1 to 3 weeks after therapy is begun. There is a higher incidence of hypertensive reactions with this drug than other MAO inhibitors. Used to treat endogenous depression. *Initial:* 20 mg to 30 mg PO qd in divided doses (usually 10 to 20 mg in AM and 10 mg in PM). *Maintenance:* 10 to 20 mg PO qd.

3. The effect of MAO inhibitors continues for 2 weeks after the patient stops taking it. Therefore the patient must continue to avoid eating or drinking the above specified foods or beverages during the 2-week time.

4. The patient may experience lightheadedness, dizziness, or feeling of faintness, especially when getting up from a lying or sitting position. To reduce this feeling, the patient should move slowly when changing positions.

5. MAO inhibitors may cause drowsiness or make the patient feel less alert than usual. If so, the patient should avoid driving or other activities requiring alertness.

6. MAO inhibitors should be discontinued 2 weeks before the patient undergoes any surgery requiring anesthesia. The physician must be informed if surgery is planned so that the drug may be discontinued in the proper manner.

7. The physician should be notified immediately or the patient should go to the hospital emergency room if fever, severe headache, nausea, vomiting, chest pain, or rapid heartbeat develops.

8. MAO inhibitors are dangerous drugs that should be kept out of the reach of children and all others for whom they are not prescribed. These drugs must not be left sitting on a dresser or low bedside table.

9. The patient should wear a Medic-Alert bracelet and carry a medical identification card listing this medication.

CRITICAL DECISION:
MAO Inhibitors

MAO inhibitors may cause very dangerous reactions if taken with certain foods or beverages. The patient must not eat foods such as cheese, yogurt, sour cream, raisins, bananas, avocados, bean pods, chicken livers, or pickled herring, and should avoid meat tenderizers and soy sauce. Only very small amounts of coffee, tea, cola drinks, and chocolate are permitted.

Miscellaneous Antidepressants

ACTION

Since the beginning of the 1980s, three new antidepressant medications have been available. They are chemically unrelated to one another, but each is helpful in certain situations. The three medications are bupropion, fluoxetine, and trazodone.

The neurochemical mechanism of bupropion is unknown, but it does not inhibit monoamine oxidase. Its ability to block neuronal uptake of serotonin and norepinephrine is much weaker than that of tricyclics. It does inhibit the neuronal uptake of dopamine to some extent.

Fluoxetine's antidepressant action is thought to be linked to its inhibition of CNS neuronal uptake of serotonin, but not norepinephrine, into human platelets.

Trazodone is a non–tricyclic-tetracyclic and non–MAO inhibitor antidepressant drug that inhibits the uptake of serotonin, a biogenic amine, at the neuronal synaptosomes in the brain and enhances the behavioral changes caused by 5-hydroxytryptophan, a serotonin precursor. The action of this drug is more selective than other types of antidepressants; that is, there is less effect on the cardiac conduction system than with tricyclic-tetracyclic antidepressants and virtually no CNS stimulation, which occurs frequently with MAO inhibitors.

USES

These three drugs are used in short-term treatment (less than 5 weeks) of outpatients with a disease in the DSM-IV category of major depressive disorders; they have not been adequately studied for long-term therapy.

ADVERSE REACTIONS

Adverse reactions to these three drugs include dizziness, tachycardia, dysrhythmias, hypertension, hypotension, rash, pruritus, constipation, weight loss, nausea and vomiting, anorexia, weight gain, diarrhea, appetite increase, dyspepsia, menstrual complaints, impotence, urinary frequency, dry mouth, headache, excessive sweating, tremor, sedation, insomnia, blurred vision, agitation, confusion, hostility, and disturbed concentration.

In nearly 4% of patients taking fluoxetine a rash develops with accompanying fever, leukocytosis, arthralgias, edema, carpal tunnel syndrome, respiratory distress, lymphadenopathy, proteinuria, and mild transaminase elevation.

Trazadone has also produced early menses, hematuria, urinary frequency, and weight changes.

DRUG INTERACTIONS

If bupropion is taken with levodopa, the chance of adverse effects increases. If bupropion is used with carbamazepine, cimetidine, phenobarbital, or phenytoin, the hepatic metabolism of the drugs may be increased. Acute toxicity may develop if bupropion is given with phenelzine.

Fluoxetine increases the half-life of some drugs, may displace drugs bound to protein, such as warfarin

and digitoxin, or may be displaced by them. Concurrent use of trazodone and antihypertensives can cause hypotension. There are many other isolated drug interactions. Trazodone may potentiate the effects of alcohol, barbiturates, and other CNS depressants. The drug should be discontinued as long as possible before general anesthesia, because interactions are unknown.

 NURSING IMPLICATIONS AND PATIENT TEACHING

▼ Assessment

The nurse should obtain a complete health history, including history of hypersensitivity, presence of seizure disorder, current or prior diagnosis of bulimia or anorexia nervosa (these patients tend to have more seizures when receiving bupropion), or recent use of an MAO inhibitor. At least 14 days should elapse between ending MAO-inhibitor therapy and beginning bupropion.

▼ Planning

The incidence of seizures in patients taking bupropion is approximately four times greater than that of those taking other antidepressant medications.

Little is known about the use of fluoxetine with other disease processes. The drug has a relatively long half-life (2 to 3 days), and problems with liver or renal failure may prolong the drug's action in the body.

Dosage levels must be individualized. There is so little information known about these drugs that even suggested dosages may vary widely. The nurse should read the package insert of the medication to make certain that the latest available information is reviewed before administering these drugs.

Constant plasma concentrations are only achieved after 4 to 5 weeks of therapy. Fluoxetine stays in the body for weeks. This is of potential consequence when drug therapy must be discontinued.

Trazodone should not be used concurrently with electroshock therapy.

▼ Implementation

To reduce the risk of seizures while the patient is taking bupropion, the daily dosage should be kept below 450 mg, it should be given in three divided doses, and the dosage should be increased gradually.

Table 12-14   Miscellaneous antidepressants

Generic name	Trade name	Comments and dosage
Bupropion	Wellbutrin	*Initial:* Institute gradually to avoid producing seizures. Begin with 100 mg/day for 3 days. Wait 6 hours between dosages. May require addition of sedative-hypnotic in the first week of therapy. No single dose should be greater than 150 mg.
Fluoxetine	Prozac	*Initial:* 20 mg qd in AM. Consider dose increase after several weeks if no improvement is seen. Do not exceed maximum of 80 mg/day. Full antidepressant effect may not be seen for 4 weeks. Use lower dosage in patients with renal or hepatic impairment, individuals who have multiple diseases or medications, and the elderly. Also effective in reducing symptoms of PMS in women and in treating patients with obsessive-compulsive disorder.
Trazodone	Desyrel	*Initial:* 150 mg PO qd in divided doses, increasing by 50 mg a day q3 to 4 days to a maximum of 400 mg/day. *Maintenance:* Individualize to the lowest dose that is both tolerated and effective.
Sertraline	Zoloft	*Adults:* 50 mg once daily.
Paroxetine	Paxil	*Adults:* Initial dose 20 mg/day. Average dose 30 mg/day.

Trazodone is administered orally and is well absorbed from the gastrointestinal tract. The absorption time is 1 hour on an empty stomach and 2 hours with food.

Important information about these medications is summarized in Table 12-14.

▼ Evaluation

Many patients taking bupropion experience some sort of agitation, increased restlessness, anxiety, and insomnia. If these symptoms cannot be controlled with a sedative-hypnotic, the medication should be discontinued.

The desired antidepressant effect usually occurs within 1 to 2 weeks after initiating therapy.

If drowsiness occurs with trazodone, the larger dose of the drug can be given at bedtime.

These are relatively new drugs; the nurse must be on the alert for adverse reactions that are not known at the present time.

The nurse should watch the patient's level of depression and look for suicide ideation.

▼ Patient and family teaching

The nurse should provide the patient and family with the following instructions:

1. The patient should take these medications exactly as ordered by the physician. It is important that the patient continue to take the drug as ordered, even if the patient feels no improvement, because it may take up to 2 weeks before any changes occur.
2. These are new medications and there is still much to be learned about them. The drugs may produce a variety of side effects, most of them mild. They most frequently cause agitation and restlessness, but may interfere with sleep. In some individuals these drugs can produce seizures. The physician must be contacted immediately if there are any problems that are new or troublesome.
3. These drugs can cause drowsiness or make the patient feel less alert than usual. If so, the patient should avoid driving or other activities that require alertness. If drowsiness persists, the physician should be contacted.
4. These medications must be kept out of the reach of children and all others for whom they are not prescribed.
5. The patient should wear a Medic-Alert bracelet or identification that indicates the name of the medication being taken.
6. The patient should avoid alcohol while taking these medications.

ANTIPSYCHOTIC DRUGS

OVERVIEW

Severe mental illness such as schizophrenia, psychotic depression, mania, or psychotic brain syndrome is commonly treated with major tranquilizers or antipsychotic drugs. These medications are used to sedate or slow the patients down, thereby reducing some of the psychotic symptoms. This allows other therapy to be implemented. Medications are usually given for long periods of time.

Antipsychotic drugs are grouped into two broad categories: (1) the phenothiazines and thioxanthenes, which are chemically and pharmacologically similar and can be used interchangeably, and (2) the nonphenothiazines, including haloperidol, loxapine, and molindone. All antipsychotic agents act by blocking the action of dopamine in the brain. But because they are from different chemical groups, they work at different sites in the brain and also produce side effects on different body systems. The two major categories will be presented separately.

Phenothiazines and Thioxanthenes

ACTION

The major actions of phenothiazine and thioxanthene are:
1. To block dopamine at the postsynaptic receptor sites in the brain, thus enhancing the turnover of the neurotransmitter. Phenothiazines and thioxanthenes also decrease the neuron's uptake of other neurotransmitters, norephinephrine and serotonin. Intraneurally, these drugs decrease the level of cyclic AMP, particularly in areas of the brain that control emotion and behavior. These changes are thought to produce the antipsychotic effects of the phenothiazines.
2. To reduce sensory stimulation of the reticular activating system in the brainstem, thereby producing a sedative effect.
3. To act as an antiemetic by inhibiting action in the chemoreceptor center.

USES

Phenothiazines and thioxanthenes are used primarily for reducing or relieving the symptoms of acute and chronic psychoses, including schizophrenia, schizoaffective disorders, and involutional psychosis. Phe-

nothiazines and thioxanthene derivatives are used interchangeably. However, thioxanthene is preferred for use in psychotic patients who are withdrawn or exhibiting retarded behavior. Clinical evidence has shown that patients with certain types of apathetic psychosis respond well to this drug.

ADVERSE REACTIONS

Adverse reactions to phenothiazines and thioxanthenes include orthostatic hypotension, tachycardia, confusion, drowsiness, hyperactivity, insomnia, amenorrhea, gynecomastia, hyperglycemia, hyperreflexia, tardive dyskinesia, blood cell abnormalities, contact dermatitis, photosensitivity, constipation, dry mouth, dyspnea, enuresis, nasal congestion, opaque deposits on the cornea and lens, and urinary retention.

Overdosage produces exaggerated CNS depression, coma, severe hypotension, and extrapyramidal symptoms, seizures, or cardiac dysrhythmias may appear.

DRUG INTERACTIONS

Phenothiazines taken concurrently with CNS depressants (alcohol, barbiturates, narcotics, and anesthetics) may potentiate and prolong the effects of either the CNS depressant or the phenothiazine. MAO inhibitors and tricyclic antidepressants are potentiated when used concurrently with phenothiazines, and antacids and antidiarrheal drugs reduce the absorption rate. The effects of many other isolated drugs and laboratory tests are altered by phenothiazines and thioxanthenes.

 NURSING IMPLICATIONS AND PATIENT TEACHING

▼ Assessment

The nurse should obtain a complete health history, including the presence of hypersensitivity to any phenothiazines (because cross-sensitivity occurs), the history of cardiac, respiratory, or blood diseases, concurrent use of other medications, and the possibility of pregnancy. These conditions are either contraindications or precautions to the use of phenothiazines and thioxanthenes.

The nurse may elicit a history of emotional unrest, agitation, paranoid ideation, visual, auditory or tactile hallucinations, delusions, inability to think clearly,

Pediatric Considerations
PSYCHOTHERAPEUTIC AGENTS

Children are at a greater risk for neuromuscular or extrapyramidal side effects, especially dystonias. Monitor closely if antipsychotic agents are administered.

Pediatric patients with chickenpox, CNS infections, measles, dehydration, gastroenteritis, or other acute illnesses will be at special risk for adverse reactions and possibly Reye's syndrome. Avoid use of phenothiazine antiemetic therapy in such patients.

The tricyclic antidepressants are usually not recommended for the treatment of depression in children under 12 years old. Some agents, though, such as amitriptyline, desipramine, and imipramine, have been used in children over the age of 6 for major depressions. Several of these agents are also used in the treatment of enuresis and attention deficit disorder. Be aware that children are very sensitive to an acute overdose, which should always be considered very serious and potentially fatal. Adolescents often require a decreased dose because of their sensitivity to this drug category.

Adverse effects reported in children receiving the tricyclic antidepressants include changes in electrocardiogram patterns, increased nervousness, sleep disorders, complaints of tiredness, hypertension, and mild stomach distress.

Lithium may decrease the bone density or bone formation in children. If it is necessary to use this drug, monitor closely serum levels and for signs of toxicity.

From McKenry LM, Salerno E: *Mosby's pharmacology in nursing*, ed 18, St Louis, 1992, Mosby.

Geriatric Considerations
PSYCHOTHERAPEUTIC AGENTS

The elderly tend to have higher serum levels of the antipsychotic and antidepressant drugs because of changes in drug distribution resulting from a decrease in lean body mass, less total body water, less serum albumin, and usually an increase in body fat. Therefore, these patients require a lower drug dose and a more gradual drug dose titration than the adult patient.

Geriatric patients are more prone to have orthostatic hypotension, anticholinergic side effects, extrapyramidal side effects, and sedation. They should be carefully evaluated before starting such potent medications; and if the antipsychotic agents are necessary, close supervision and the prescribing of the lowest dose possible are recommended.

The elderly patient generally should receive half the recommended adult dose. The patient with organic brain syndrome should only receive 33% to 50% of the usual adult dose with increases in dosage at 7- to 10-day periods. When clinical improvement is noted, attempts at tapering and discontinuing the drug should be instituted.

The tricyclic antidepressants may cause increased anxiety in the geriatric patient. If the patient has cardiovascular disease, the use of the tricyclic antidepressants increases the risk of inducing arrhythmias, tachycardia, stroke, congestive heart failure, or myocardial infarction.

From McKenry LM, Salerno E: *Mosby's pharmacology in nursing*, ed 18, St Louis, 1992, Mosby.

severe mood swings, and inability to cope with reality. The patient may or may not verbalize paranoid thoughts and often has difficulty paying attention and responding to the immediate environment. The patient may respond inappropriately to questions and may exhibit inappropriate nonverbal behavior or dress and general appearance.

▼ Planning

Phenothiazines and thioxanthenes are not recommended for use in pregnant women or nursing mothers.

Patients with severe asthma, emphysema, or acute respiratory infections (especially children) may develop reduced respiration as a result of the CNS depressant effects of phenothiazines. Phenothiazines may also depress the cough reflex, putting a patient who is vomiting in danger of aspirating.

▼ Implementation

Phenothiazines can be taken either orally or parenterally. The oral form is fairly well absorbed, but the absorption rate will be delayed if the drug is taken with antacids or antidiarrheal agents.

Stomach upset from the oral form of phenothiazines can be reduced or avoided by taking the drug with bland food or 8 ounces of water.

▼ Evaluation

The desired antipsychotic effects of phenothiazines may take several weeks to appear after therapy is initiated. The initial dose should be the lowest recommended amount, according to the individual's tolerance and the severity of psychosis, until the psychotic symptoms are controlled. The dosage of phenothiazines that controls the patient's symptoms should be maintained for 2 to 3 weeks and then gradually reduced until the lowest effective maintenance dosage is attained. Phenothiazines given in large doses or over a prolonged period of time should be discontinued by gradual reduction over several weeks to avoid symptoms of dyskinesia, nausea, vomiting, dizziness, and trembling.

The patient should have a complete eye examination by a specialist, including inspection of the internal structures and the lens to establish baseline data.

▼ Patient and family teaching

The nurse should provide the patient and family with the following instructions:

1. The patient should take this medication exactly as ordered. It is important that the patient continue to take the drug in the exact amount and frequency specified, even if the patient feels no improvement, because it may take several weeks before any changes occur.
2. Phenothiazines can increase the effects of alcohol, sleeping pills, and many other prescribed medications. The patient should avoid alcohol, and should check with the physician before taking any other prescribed or over-the-counter drugs.
3. Phenothiazines may cause drowsiness or make the patient feel less alert than usual, particularly when first taking the medicine. If so, the patient should avoid driving or other activities that require alertness. The patient should talk with the health practitioner if drowsiness or decreased alertness persists.
4. Lightheadedness, dizziness, or feelings of faintness occur in some people taking phenothiazines. To reduce these feelings, the patient should move slowly when changing from a lying or sitting position.
5. Some people taking phenothiazines become more sensitive to the sun. To avoid sunburn, the patient should use a sunblock and limit exposure to the sun or sunlamps.
6. Patients taking this drug in liquid form should avoid contact of the medicine with the skin or clothes, because it can cause irritation.
7. Gastric distress caused by the medicine may be reduced by taking the drug with food, milk, or 8 ounces of water. The patient should not take any antacids or antidiarrheal medicine within 1 hour of taking the drug.
8. If the drug comes in a bottle with a medicine dropper, the patient should measure the pre-scribed dose as marked on the dropper and then dilute it in a glass of water or juice.
9. Dryness of the mouth may occur when the patient starts taking this drug. Chewing gum, sucking on hard candy, or rinsing the mouth frequently may help relieve this dryness.
10. Phenothiazines may make the patient perspire less than usual. Therefore the patient should avoid becoming overheated in hot and humid weather or when exercising.
11. The physician should be notified promptly if urinary retention, change in vision, sore throat with fever, muscle spasms, trembling or shaking (particularly of hands), skin rash, yellow tinge to skin and eyes, small uncontrollable movements of the tongue, or other new or troublesome symptoms develop.
12. This medication must be kept out of the reach of children and all others for whom it is not prescribed.
13. The patient should wear a Medic-Alert bracelet and carry a medical identification card specifying that he or she is taking phenothiazines.

Nonphenothiazines

Three nonphenothiazine antipsychotic drugs, haloperidol, loxapine, and molindone, will be presented briefly.

Haloperidol

ACTION

Haloperidol's mechanism of action is not well established. It is known that the drug potently and selectively blockades dopamine at receptor sites in the brain, thereby enhancing the turnover of this particular neurotransmitter.

USES

Haloperidol is used primarily to reduce or relieve symptoms of psychoses, including schizophrenia and manic-depressive disorders in the manic phase.

ADVERSE REACTIONS

Adverse reactions to haloperidol include orthostatic hypotension; drowsiness; jerky, ticlike movements of head, face, or neck; shaking hands; shuffling walk;

stiffness of limbs; blurred vision; breast engorgement; constipation; decreased libido; dry mouth; impotence; nausea; and vomiting.

Overdosage may produce severe hypotension, sedation, respiratory depression, and coma.

DRUG INTERACTIONS

Haloperidol may potentiate the CNS depressant effects of alcohol, barbiturates, narcotics, and anesthetics if they are taken concurrently. Severe hypotension may occur when haloperidol is taken concurrently with antihypertensive drugs or epinephrine.

 NURSING IMPLICATIONS AND PATIENT TEACHING

▼ Assessment

The nurse should obtain a complete health history, including the presence of hypersensitivity, history of disease, and other medications taken. These conditions are contraindications or precautions to use of haloperidol.

▼ Planning

Allergic reactions to the tartrazine in the yellow #5 contained in the drug have occurred, especially in patients with a hypersensitivity to aspirin. Haloperidol may elevate prolactin levels. Because approximately one third of breast cancers are prolactin dependent, its use in a patient with breast cancer must be carefully considered. Patients who are in the manic phase of manic-depressive illness may convert to the depressive phase quite rapidly and may be potentially suicidal. Therefore the nurse should monitor these patients closely.

▼ Implementation

Haloperidol is approximately 97% protein bound; therefore its metabolism and excretion may be slow. This drug may be given PO or IM. Very low doses should be given to geriatric patients and children under 12 years of age; the dosage should be titrated slowly.

▼ Evaluation

The desired antipsychotic effect of haloperidol usually takes place within 3 weeks after therapy is begun. Once this desired effect is attained, the dosage should be gradually reduced to a minimum maintenance level.

Haloperidol given over an extended period of time should be discontinued gradually over several weeks to avoid symptoms of nausea, vomiting, trembling, and dyskinesia. The nurse should monitor the patient for suicidal tendencies.

Loxapine

ACTION

Loxapine's mechanism of action is not well established. The drug is thought to inhibit subcortical areas of the brain, thus producing a tranquilizing effect and a decrease in aggressive behavior. This drug is pharmacologically similar to phenothiazine.

USES

Loxapine is used primarily to reduce or relieve symptoms associated with psychosis, particularly with schizophrenia.

ADVERSE REACTIONS

Adverse reactions to loxapine include orthostatic hypotension, tachycardia, drowsiness, hyperactivity, seizures, tardive dyskinesia, skin rash, blurred vision, opaque deposits on the cornea and lens, urinary retention, constipation, dry mouth, headache, and photosensitivity. Overdosage may produce CNS depression, bradycardia, hypotension, increased extrapyramidal symptoms, and coma.

DRUG INTERACTIONS

Loxapine is a relatively new antipsychotic agent, but it is pharmacologically similar to phenothiazine. Therefore, loxapine may have the potential to interact with the same drugs as phenothiazine.

 NURSING IMPLICATIONS AND PATIENT TEACHING

▼ Assessment

The nurse should obtain a complete health history, including the presence of hypersensitivity, other diseases, the possibility of pregnancy, or the concurrent use of other medications. These are contraindications or precautions to the use of loxapine.

The patient should have a complete eye examination, including inspection of external structures and the lens, before beginning therapy.

▼ Planning

Loxapine is not recommended for use in pregnant or breastfeeding women.

▼ Implementation

Loxapine's half-life is 3 to 4 hours, and the effects may last as long as 12 hours.

▼ Evaluation

Elderly, emaciated, or debilitated patients are often unusually sensitive to normal dosages of loxapine and should be started on reduced amounts. They are more prone to extrapyramidal and hypotensive side effects if the medication is not increased slowly.

Dihydroindolone (Molindone)

ACTION

Molindone's mechanism of action is not well established. The primary site of action is the ascending reticular activating system, where stimuli are thought to be blocked. A tranquilizing effect is produced without relaxation of muscles or interference with the coordination of body movements.

USES

Molindone is used primarily to reduce or relieve symptoms associated with psychosis, particularly schizophrenia.

ADVERSE REACTIONS

Adverse reactions to molindone include orthostatic hypotension, depression, drowsiness, tardive dyskinesia, blood cell changes, skin rash, urinary retention, blurred vision, dry mouth, increased libido, heavy menses, and resumption of menses in amenorrheic patients. Overdosage may produce exaggeration of adverse effects, particularly sedation.

DRUG INTERACTIONS

The tablet form of molindone contains calcium sulfate and may interfere with the absorption of tetracycline and phenytoin.

 ### NURSING IMPLICATIONS AND PATIENT TEACHING

▼ Assessment

The nurse should obtain a complete health history, including the presence of hypersensitivity, underlying disease, concurrent use of other medications, and the possibility of pregnancy. These conditions are contraindications or precautions to the use of molindone.

▼ Planning

Molindone is not recommended for use in pregnant or breastfeeding mothers.

▼ Implementation

Molindone is well absorbed from the gastrointestinal tract and the effects of one dose may last for 1 to 1½ days. Elderly and debilitated patients should be started on low dosages and increased slowly. See Table 12-15 for a summary of antipsychotic agents.

▼ Evaluation

Significant drowsiness may occur during initial therapy with molindone. The nurse should monitor the patient for suicidal ideation.

▼ Patient and family teaching

The nurse should provide the patient and family with the following instructions:

1. The patient should take this medication exactly as ordered. It is important that the patient continues to take the drug in the exact amount and frequency ordered, even if the patient feels no improvement, because it may take up to 3 weeks before any changes occur.
2. Molindone can increase the effects of alcohol and other drugs, such as sleeping pills, prescribed pain medication, and some medicines for relief of colds and hay fever. The patient should avoid alcohol and check with the physician before taking any other drugs.
3. Molindone may cause drowsiness or make the patient feel less alert than usual, especially with the initial doses. If the patient experiences these feelings, driving or other activities requiring alertness should be avoided. The patient should talk with the physician if drowsiness or decreased alertness persists.

Table 12-15 Antipsychotic medications

Generic name	Trade name	Comments and dosage
ALIPHATIC PHENOTHIAZINES		
Chlorpromazine	Thorazine	A traditional phenothiazine product, popular and inexpensive. Used in psychotic disorders to control the manic phase of manic-depressive reactions, preoperatively for restlessness, to treat behavioral problems of children who are combative, or for hyperactive children with excessive motor activity.
		Adults: 30 to 300 mg/day PO in divided doses; or 25 to 50 mg IM tid; do not exceed 1000 mg/day.
		Children over 6 months: 0.55 mg/kg PO bid to qid; or 0.55 mg/kg IM q6 to 8h. May also give 1 mg/kg PR tid to qid.
Promazine	Sparine Prozine	Used primarily in the management of psychotic disorders. Oral medication is usually preferred.
		Adults: Give 10 to 200 mg PO q4 to 6h, up to a maximum of 1000 mg/day. May also give 10 to 200 mg IM q4 to 6h.
		Children over 12 years: 10 to 25 mg PO q4 to 6h.
Triflupromazine	Vesprin	*Adults:* 100 to 150 mg/day PO; or 60 to 150 mg/day IM.
		Children over 2 years: 2 mg/kg PO, up to 150 mg/day; or 0.2 to 0.25 mg/kg IM, up to 10 mg/day.
PIPERAZINE PHENOTHIAZINES		
Acetophenazine	Tindal	*Adults:* 20 mg PO tid.
		Children: 0.8 to 1.6 mg/kg/day PO.
Fluphenazine	Permitil Prolixin	*Adults:* Give 0.5 to 10 mg/day PO in divided doses administered at 8-hour intervals initially. Normal maintenance dose is 3 mg PO qd; do not exceed 20 mg/day PO. If given IM, 1.25 mg is usual initial dose, with 2.5 to 10 mg IM divided and given in 6- to 8-hour intervals prn; do not exceed 10 mg/day IM.
		Children: 0.25 to 0.75 mg PO qd to qid; IM dose same as for adult.
		Geriatric: 1 to 2.5 mg/day initially, increase as needed.
Perphenazine	Trilafon	*Adults and children over 12:* 2 to 16 mg PO bid to qid; or 5 to 10 mg IM q6h, up to 15 mg/day.
Prochlorperazine	Compazine	*Adults:* 5 to 10 mg PO tid to qid, up to 150 mg/day; or 10 to 20 mg IM q4 to 6h, up to 200 mg/day. May also give 25 mg PR bid.
		Children over 2 years or 9 kg: 0.1 mg/kg PO qid, not to exceed 10 mg/day on first day or 20 mg/day on subsequent days; or 0.132 mg/kg/day IM; or 2.5 mg PR qd to tid, not to exceed 10 mg/day on first day or 20 mg/day on subsequent days.
Trifluoperazine	Stelazine	Give initial dose, increasing as needed until symptoms are relieved. Then titrate dosage to lowest possible dose, based on individual response. Oral concentrate must be diluted.
		Adults: 1 to 5 mg PO bid, up to 40 mg/day; or may give 1 to 2 mg IM q4 to 6h, up to 10 mg/day.
		Children over 6 years: 1 mg PO qd to bid; or may give 1 mg IM qd to bid.
Mesoridazine	Serentil	Used to treat severe emotional withdrawal, anxiety, tension, hallucinatory behavior, and blunted affect in schizophrenic patients. Reduces hyperactivity and uncooperativeness in some patients with chronic brain syndrome and mental deficiencies. Also used to reduce symptoms present in alcoholism and psychoneurotic manifestations.
		Adults and children over 12 years: 10 to 50 mg PO bid to tid, up to 400 mg/day; or 25 mg IM repeated in 30 to 60 min if necessary, up to 200 mg/day.
		■ *Alcoholism:* 25 mg PO bid initially; maintenance dose is 50 to 200 mg/day.
		■ *Schizophrenia:* 50 mg PO tid; maintenance dose is 100 to 400 mg/day.

Continued.

Table 12-15	Antipsychotic medications—cont'd	
Generic name	**Trade name**	**Comments and dosage**
Thioridazine	Mellaril	Adjunct to short-term therapy in moderate to marked depression and anxiety. May be used in hyperactive children or children with marked behavioral problems. *Adults:* 25 to 100 mg PO tid initially, then 10 to 200 mg PO bid to qid as maintenance; do not exceed 800 mg/day. *Children over 2 years:* 0.25 mg to 3 mg/kg PO; or 10 to 25 mg PO bid to tid.
THIOXANTHENE DERIVATIVES		
Chlorprothixene	Taractan	*Adults:* 25 to 50 mg PO tid to qid, up to 600 mg/day; or 25 to 50 mg IM tid to qid. *Children over 12 years:* 10 mg to 25 mg PO tid to qid. *Children 6 to 12 years:* 25 to 50 mg IM tid to qid.
Thiothixene	Navane	Monitor the patient for early signs of tardive dyskinesia and jerky movements, particularly of the hands. *Adults and children over 12 years:* 2 to 5 mg PO bid or tid initially; maintenance dose is 20 to 60 mg a day in divided doses. 4 mg IM bid to qid may also be given.
BUTYROPHENONE		
Haloperidol	Haldol	*Adults and children over 12 years:* 0.5 mg to 5 mg PO bid to tid, up to 100 mg/day; may also give 2 to 5 mg IM q4 to 8h. *Children 3 to 12 years:* 0.5 mg/day initially with increments of 0.5 mg at 5- to 7-day intervals prn. Total dose may be divided and given bid to tid.
DIBENZODIAZEPINE		
Clozapine	Clozaril	New drug used in severely ill schizophrenic patients who do not respond to standard therapy. Give 25 mg qd to bid to target 300 to 450/mg/day by end of 2 weeks.
DIBENZOXAZEPINE		
Loxapine	Loxitane	The oral concentrate should be diluted with fruit juice just before administration. *Initial:* 10 mg PO bid to tid; or 12.5 mg to 50 mg IM q4 to 6h. *Maintenance:* 20 to 60 mg/day, up to maximum of 250 mg/day.
DIHYDROINDOLONE		
Molindone	Moban	*Initial:* 50 to 75 mg/day PO. *Maintenance:* 5 to 25 mg PO tid to qid, up to a maximum of 225 mg/day.
DIPHENYLBUTYLPIPERIDINE		
Pimozide	Orap	Give 1 to 2 mg/day in divided doses. Increase dose every other day not to exceed 10 mg/day.

4. Lightheadedness, dizziness, or feelings of faintness occur in some people taking this drug. To reduce the possibility of falling, the patient should move slowly when changing from a lying or sitting position.

5. If the drug comes in a bottle with a medicine dropper, the patient should measure the pre-scribed dose as marked on the dropper. The medicine should be taken alone or mixed with food, water, or juice. If the drug causes gastric discomfort, taking it with food may help reduce this problem.

6. Molindone should not be discontinued suddenly, because the patient could experience

nausea, vomiting, trembling, and other symptoms. Therefore, the health care provider should always be contacted before discontinuing this drug.

7. The physician should be notified promptly if the patient develops urinary retention, arm or leg stiffness, shaking of hands, jerking of head or neck, skin rash, yellow tinge to skin and eyes, or small, uncontrollable movements of the tongue.

8. This drug must be kept out of the reach of children and all others for whom it is not prescribed.

9. If the patient misses a dose, it should be taken as soon as possible unless it is close to the next scheduled dose. The doses must not be doubled.

ANTIMANICS

ACTION

Lithium is the primary drug used to treat patients in manic states. The exact mechanism of lithium is not known. The mood-stabilizing effect of the drug may be attributed to its ability to alter sodium transport at the nerve endings, inhibit cyclic AMP formation in nerve cells, and enhance the uptake of serotonin and norepinephrine by nerve cells, thus increasing the inactivation of these neurotransmitters. It has no sedative, depressant, or euphoric actions, making it unique from all other psychiatric drugs.

USES

Lithium is specifically used for patients with manic-depressive psychosis who are in an acute manic phase. It also may be used to prevent recurrent episodes of mania in the manic-depressive patient.

ADVERSE REACTIONS

Adverse reactions to lithium include dysrhythmias, hypotension, ataxia, coma, dizziness, drowsiness, motor retardation, restlessness, slurred speech, tinnitus, pruritus, rash, abdominal pain, anorexia, diarrhea, vomiting, urinary incontinence or retention, polyuria, albuminuria, blurred vision, hyperglycemia, hypothyroidism, leukocytosis, and weight gain.

Overdosage may produce diarrhea, vomiting, muscle weakness, drowsiness, and ataxia.

DRUG INTERACTIONS

Concurrent use of lithium and diuretics can lead to lithium toxicity. There are many significant drug interactions with isolated medications.

 ## NURSING IMPLICATIONS AND PATIENT TEACHING

▼ Assessment

The patient may have a history of excessive talkativeness, restlessness, hyperactivity, aggressiveness, and perhaps delusions of grandeur.

The nurse should obtain a complete health history, including the presence of hypersensitivity, underlying disease, the possibility of pregnancy, and other medications being used. These conditions may be contraindications or precautions to the use of lithium.

▼ Planning

Lithium is not safe to use in pregnant patients and breastfeeding mothers. If a patient receiving lithium becomes pregnant, the drug should be discontinued, especially during the first trimester, because it may cause birth defects.

Elderly patients are often more sensitive to lithium toxicity. It is important to start these patients on lower doses and monitor the therapeutic and adverse effects closely while increasing dosage.

▼ Implementation

The nurse should ensure that the patient maintains adequate hydration and electrolyte balance during lithium therapy.

Table 12-16 summarizes the important information the nurse needs to know about lithium.

▼ Evaluation

The therapeutic level of serum lithium is relatively close to the toxic level, so the serum lithium level must be monitored on a regular basis. Blood should be drawn 12 hours after the dose of lithium is given.

Monitoring should be carried out every few days during the initial therapy and then at least every 2 months after the patient is stabilized. The therapeutic serum lithium level is 1 to 1.5 mEq/L in most laboratories. On each visit the nurse should observe for therapeutic effects and monitor the patient's mental and emotional status.

Table 12-16 Antimanic medications		
Generic name	**Trade name**	**Comments and dosage**
Lithium	Eskalith Lithane Lithotabs Cibalith-S	Lithium administered orally is rapidly absorbed in the GI tract. The desired effect of lithium may take 1 to several weeks to occur. Lithium is excreted by the kidneys, with a half-life of approximately 24 hours in a healthy adult, but in the elderly it may be increased to 36 hours; therefore lower dosages are indicated for this group. Lithium excretion is inhibited in the presence of low serum sodium levels. The therapeutic serum level of lithium is 1 to 1.5 mEq/L. Lithium is not recommended for children under 12 years of age. ■ *Acute mania:* 600 mg PO tid. ■ *Prophylaxis:* 300 mg PO tid to qid.

Lithium is tolerated better when the patient is in an acute manic stage than when in controlled stages where manifestations of mania have subsided. The dosage of lithium may have to be adjusted according to the patient's manifestation of symptoms.

Patients who develop diarrhea or become ill and do not eat are at increased risk of toxicity, and their condition should be followed closely.

▼ Patient and family teaching

The nurse should provide the patient and family with the following instructions:

1. The patient should take this medication exactly as ordered. It is important that the patient continue to take the drug in the exact amount and frequency ordered, even if the patient feels no improvement, because it may take several weeks before any changes occur. Gastric upset caused by the medication may be reduced by taking the drug with milk or food.

2. The serum lithium levels can become toxic if the patient gets too much or if the patient becomes dehydrated from vomiting or diarrhea, or does not eat. The patient should avoid activities that cause excessive sweating (strenuous exercise, sunbathing, hot tub baths) and things that produce excessive urination (consuming large amounts of caffeine in coffee, tea, or cola drinks). The physician should be contacted if the patient becomes ill or does not feel well.

3. Some patients on lithium experience side effects, but they are usually mild and disappear with time. The physician should be notified of any new or troublesome symptoms, such as vomiting, nausea, shakiness, trembling, jerky movements of arms or legs, or generalized weakness.

4. The patient will need to have the level of the drug in the blood measured frequently so that the drug can be kept at the proper level and side effects may be reduced. The patient will need these blood tests every few days when beginning treatment, and then every 1 to 2 months.

5. This medication must be kept out of the reach of children and others for whom it is not prescribed.

6. The patient should wear a Medic-Alert bracelet and carry a medical identification card specifying that he or she is taking lithium.

> *Geriatric Considerations*
> **LITHIUM**
>
> Lithium is more toxic in the geriatric patient, therefore, lower lithium dosages, a lower lithium serum level, and very close monitoring are critical in this age group. The elderly are more prone to CNS toxicity, lithium-induced goiter, and clinical hypothyroidism than the average adult. Generally, excessive thirst and elimination of large volumes of urine may be early side effects of lithium toxicity frequently seen in the elderly.

From McKenry LM, Salerno E: *Mosby's pharmacology in nursing,* ed 18, St Louis, 1992, Mosby.

SECTION SEVEN: SEDATIVE-HYPNOTICS

Objectives

At the conclusion of this section you should be able to:

1. Define sedative and hypnotic.
2. Indicate how the use of sedatives and hypnotics alters normal sleep patterns.
3. List the two common drug groups and other miscellaneous medications used for sedation or hypnosis.
4. Identify common drug interactions caused by sedative-hypnotic medications.
5. Describe the major side effects produced by these medications.
6. Develop a teaching plan regarding use of medications for insomnia.

ACTION

Sedative-hypnotic medications are used in the hospital to relax patients and induce sleep before anesthesia or medical testing procedures, such as electroencephalography; it is also used to treat patients with insomnia caused by mental and physical stress.

Sleep is a normal cyclic process that involves varying levels of unconsciousness from which a patient may be aroused. Normal sleep produces relaxation and relief from stress. Although individual patterns vary, each time a person sleeps, four cyclic stages are encountered for varying times and durations. Stage I and II are very light stages of sleep, during which the person may be easily aroused. Stage III is a transition to stage IV, the period of deepest sleep where basic vital signs slow and the body totally relaxes. It is this period of sleep that makes people feel very refreshed. Approximately every 90 minutes, a period of body arousal is reached, often superimposed on stage I or stage II of sleep. This is called paradoxic sleep, because instead of relaxing, the body is more active. It is also called REM time because dreaming is common, as demonstrated by rapid eye movements (REM). This is an important part of sleeping, when the unconscious mind works out anxieties and tensions. When people do not have adequate REM time each night, they feel anxious and unrested.

USES

At times people may be unable to sleep because of stresses or anxiety. Difficulty falling asleep is termed **initial insomnia.** The inability to stay asleep is termed **intermittent insomnia,** and **terminal insomnia** refers to early awakening with an inability to return to sleep. Terminal insomnia is often associated with depression.

If warm baths, warm drinks, appropriate temperature, and bedding changes do not help the patient to relax, a medication may be prescribed on a short-term basis. A **sedative agent** is a medication that relaxes the patient and allows him or her to rest. A **hypnotic agent** actually produces sleep in the patient. Whether a medication acts as a sedative or hypnotic is often determined not by the drug, but by the dosage used, with smaller dosages producing sedative effects and larger dosages producing hypnotic effects.

The ideal medication would reproduce the normal sleep pattern for the patient: the patient would sleep longer, have no side effects, and arise feeling rested and relaxed with no risk of developing drug dependency. Unfortunately, no ideal medication exists.

Although most sedative-hypnotic medications increase the sleeping time, many of them produce a feeling of lethargy or a "hangover" feeling in the morning. Even a few doses of the medication may reduce the occurrence and duration of REM time, making the patient feel irritable and unrested in the morning. This feeling often leads to the increased desire for more medicine, so that the patient may have a refreshing sleep, with dependency or abuse resulting.

Once a patient has taken sedative-hypnotics, the normal sleep patterns may not return for several weeks. During that time, an increased period of REM will be seen, as if the body is trying to "catch up" for missed time. This may produce long, vivid, or frightening dreams.

Barbiturates are CNS depressants used for a variety of medical problems. All barbiturates act primarily on the brainstem reticular formation, reducing nerve impulses to the cerebral cortex. Barbiturates also depress the respiratory system and the activity of nerves and muscle (smooth, skeletal, and cardiac), thus producing relaxation and sleep.

Barbiturates are used for short-term treatment of anxiety, agitation, and insomnia caused by transient psychosocial stresses, and at times when rest is mandatory, such as before surgery. Large doses of short-acting barbiturates can produce surgical anesthesia (see the section on anticonvulsants, pp. 234-244).

The main action of benzodiazepines is CNS depression; and although the exact mechanism is not known, they are thought to act on the hypothalamus and limbic system of the brain, decreasing the vasopressor response and increasing the arousal threshold. They are used as hypnotic agents to treat insomnia. The therapeutic objective is to prevent insomnia and restore normal sleep patterns. Benzodiazepines are used in patients with acute or chronic medical problems who require restful sleep (see the section on anticonvulsants, pp. 234-244, for more detail).

The nonbarbiturate-nonbenzodiazepine sedative–hypnotics include a variety of chemically unrelated medications. All produce some effects on REM sleep, have a potential for tolerance and habituation, and may produce rebound REM. None are as safe as the benzodiazepines. Therefore they are not as commonly used.

ADVERSE REACTIONS

Nonbarbiturate-nonbenzodiazepine sedative-hypnotics may produce drowsiness, flattened affect, dullness, distortion of mood, impaired coordination, hypersensitivity, lethargy, headache, muscle or joint pain, and mental depression; a feeling of "hangover" commonly occurs.

DRUG INTERACTIONS

Nonbarbiturate-nonbenzodiazepine sedative-hypnotics increase the sedation effects of CNS depressants, including sleeping aids, analgesics, anesthetics, tranquilizers, alcohol, and narcotics. Chloral hydrate may increase the anticoagulant effects of warfarin while glutethimide and ethchlorvynol may diminish the anticoagulant effects of warfarin.

 NURSING IMPLICATIONS AND PATIENT TEACHING

▼ Assessment

The nurse should obtain a thorough health history, including medications that may produce drug inter-

actions, other barbiturates (sometimes present in bronchodilators or antispasmodics), response to barbiturates taken in the past, or hypersensitivity. Sedative-hypnotics are not considered safe in pregnancy. The nurse should determine whether there are any underlying diseases that would represent contraindications to use of sedative-hypnotics.

▼ Planning

If sedative-hypnotics are used for more than 1 week, they may cause further disturbances in the sleep cycle and rebound insomnia. The patient may develop dependence if these drugs are used indiscriminately, and abrupt withdrawal is dangerous. Hypothermia may occur with the use of barbiturates. Alcohol can increase the sedation produced by these drugs and depress vital brain functions.

Flurazepam is increasingly effective on the second or third night of consecutive use. For one to two nights after the drug is discontinued, both the time before the patient falls asleep and the total wake time may still be decreased. These are Schedule IV controlled substances.

▼ Implementation

Benzodiazepines are transformed by the liver into long-acting forms that may remain in the body for 24 hours or more and produce increasing sedation. Liver function may be impaired with prolonged use. The onset of action is approximately 30 to 60 minutes; the effects last 7 to 8 hours. The drug should be given 15 to 30 minutes before bedtime. Table 12-17 summarizes important information regarding benzodiazepine sedative-hypnotics.

Use great caution when parenterally administering barbiturates to avoid intraarterial injection or extravasation, because serious ischemia or gangrene could result. Barbiturates may worsen a patient's pain.

Geriatric or debilitated patients should receive lower than recommended dosages of barbiturates.

All barbiturates exhibit the same sedative-hypnotic effect, but they differ in onset time, duration, and potency. The onset and duration are determined by the lipid solubility of the particular drug. In determining dosage, it is best to begin with the lowest possible effective dose and adjust upward according to the individual patient's response. The amount prescribed should be no greater than that needed for current treatment and less than a potentially lethal dose. See Table 12-18 for a comparison of action of the different medications.

Table 12-17   Benzodiazepine sedative-hypnotic medications

Generic name	Trade name	Dosage and comments
Estazolam	ProSom	*Adults:* 1 mg at bedtime.
Flurazepam	Dalmane	Flurazepam has a longer use period (effective 28 nights) and less REM rebound than some other hypnotics. Markedly suppresses stage IV; increases stage II sleep. ■ *Hypnotic:* 15 or 30 mg PO; 15 mg in elderly or debilitated patients.
Lorazepam	Ativan	This antianxiety agent is usually used for mild or transient situational stress. It is used parenterally as a preanesthetic medication. ■ *Mild anxiety or insomnia:* 2 to 4 mg PO at bedtime; in elderly or debilitated patients use 1 to 2 mg/day in divided doses. ■ *Preanesthesia medications:* 0.05 mg/kg (maximum dose 4 mg) IM at least 2 hours before surgical procedure. ■ *Sedation:* 2 mg total or 0.02 mg/lb IV for adult patients under 50 years.
Temazepam	Restoril	Induces sleep in 20 to 40 minutes. ■ *Hypnotic:* 30 mg PO before bedtime; in elderly or debilitated patients, 15 mg may be sufficient.
Triazolam	Halcion	Used primarily for short-term treatment of insomnia or early morning awakening. *Adults:* 0.25 to 0.5 mg at bedtime, 0.125 to 0.25 mg in elderly.
Quazepam	Doral	*Adults:* 15 mg initially. May reduce to 7.5 mg if response is adequate.

Table 12-18   Comparative action of barbiturates used for sedation-hypnosis

Generic drug	Onset of action (minutes)	Duration (hours)	Sedative dose	Hypnotic dose
LONG ACTING				
Phenobarbital (Barbital, Luminal)	60	10 to 16	30 to 120 mg PO, divided into 2 to 3 doses daily 30 to 120 mg PR or IM, divided into 2 to 3 doses	50 to 320 mg PO 100 to 320 mg PR or IM
Mephobarbital (Mebaral)	60	10 to 16	32 to 200 mg PO, divided into 3 to 4 doses	100 to 200 mg PO
INTERMEDIATE ACTING				
Amobarbital (Amytal)	60	4 to 6	50 to 300 mg PO, divided into 2 to 3 doses	65 to 200 mg PO
Aprobarbital (Alurate)	20	4 to 6	120 to 160 mg PO qd in divided doses	40 to 160 mg PO
Butabarbital (Butisol)	30	6 to 8	40 to 120 mg PO qd in divided doses	50 to 100 mg PO
Talbutal (Lotusate)	20	4 to 6	30 to 180 mg PO qd in divided doses	120 mg PO
SHORT ACTING				
Secobarbital (Seconal)	15 to 30	3 to 6	30 to 90 mg PO divided into 2 to 3 doses qd	100 mg PO
Pentobarbital (Nembutal)	30	3 to 6	90 to 120 mg PO in divided doses 90 to 120 mg PO or PR in divided doses	100 mg PO 100 mg PO, PR; 150 to 200 mg IM

Table 12-19 Miscellaneous sedative-hypnotic medications

Generic name	Brand name	Dosage and comments
CHLORAL DERIVATIVES		
Chloral hydrate	Noctec	Effective in 30 to 60 minutes and lasts 4 to 8 hours. Has a very disagreeable taste and causes gastric irritation; take after meals; take elixir in water, juice, or soda. ■ *Sedative* *Adults:* 250 mg PO tid after meals, or 325 to 650 mg tid PR. *Children:* 25 mg/kg/day PO. ■ *Hypnotic* *Adults:* 500 to 1000 mg PO 15 to 30 minutes before bedtime, or 30 minutes before surgery. *Children:* 50 mg/kg/day; maximum dose 1 gm PO.
CARBAMATES		
Ethinamate	Valmid	Effect lasts 3 to 5 hours. ■ *Hypnosis:* 500 to 1000 mg PO 20 minutes before bedtime.
PIPERIDINE DERIVATIVES		
Glutethimide	Doriden	Effective in 30 minutes and lasts 4 to 8 hours. Should be stored in light-resistant containers. ■ *Sedative:* 125 to 250 mg at bedtime. ■ *Hypnotic:* 250 mg at bedtime.
Methyprylon	Noludar	Induces sleep in 1 hour, lasts 5 to 8 hours. Do not give more than 400 mg daily. Higher doses do not increase hypnotic effects. ■ *Hypnosis* *Adults:* 200 to 400 mg PO at bedtime. *Children:* Begin at 50 mg and increase up to 200 mg if required.
Paraldehyde	Paral Paraldehyde	Sleep induced in 10 to 15 minutes and lasts 6 to 8 hours. ■ *Sedation* *Adults:* 5 to 15 ml PO or PR; 5 ml IM. *Children:* 0.15 ml/kg PO, PR, or IM. ■ *Hypnosis* *Adults:* 10 to 30 ml PO or PR; 10 ml IM. *Children:* 0.3 ml/kg PO.
MISCELLANEOUS		
Acetylcarbromal	Paxarel	*Adults:* 250 to 500 mg bid or tid.
Methaqualone	Quaalude	Effective in 30 minutes and lasts 5 to 8 hours. Drugs may lose their effectiveness after 2 weeks of continued use. ■ *Sedative* *Adults:* 75 mg tid or qid. ■ *Hypnotic* *Adults:* 150 to 400 mg PO at bedtime.
Ethchlorvynol	Placidyl	Sleep produced in 15 to 60 minutes and lasts 5 hours. Do not use longer than 1 week. ■ *Hypnotic:* 500 to 1000 mg PO at bedtime; a single dose of 100 to 200 mg may be given if patient awakens during the night.
Propiomazine	Largon	*Adults:* Give 20 mg with 50 mg meperidine IV or IM preoperatively.
Zolpidem	Ambien	*Adults:* 10 mg before bedtime.

When chloral hydrate or paraldehyde is given orally, it should be diluted in milk or fruit juice to mask the taste and odor. Liquids should be put in a disposable container or in a glass, because plastic will absorb the odor and flavor permanently.

Table 12-19 summarizes miscellaneous sedative-hypnotics.

▼ Evaluation

Sedative-hypnotics should always be discontinued slowly in people who have been on long-term therapy. Tolerance is usually proportional to the total amount of the drug received. Barbiturates are controlled substances, so attempts should be made to avoid giving them to patients with a history of abuse or addiction.

▼ Patient and family teaching

The nurse should provide the patient and family with the following instructions:

1. Sedative-hypnotics are only for short-term use. Sometimes tolerance, dependence, or addiction develops with these drugs.
2. The patient should take the medication exactly as prescribed.
3. The medication should be kept out of reach of children and all others for whom it is not prescribed.
4. A hangover feeling may sometimes be experienced the day after taking the medication. The patient should avoid any driving or activities requiring alertness until all drowsiness has disappeared.
5. It is dangerous for the patient to drink alcohol within 24 hours after taking this drug.
6. Smoking may decrease the length of time the drug helps the patient sleep.
7. The patient should avoid drinking beverages containing caffeine for at least 4 hours before taking the medication, because it reduces the ability of the drug to produce sleep.
8. Some people experience side effects while taking this drug, so the physician should be notified if any new or uncomfortable symptoms appear, such as rash, fever, unusual bleeding, bruising, sore throat, jaundice, or abdominal pain.
9. The patient may develop excessive dreaming when the drug is stopped; this should lessen each night.

10. Tablets and capsules should be kept in a dry, tightly closed container. Elixirs should be kept in a tightly closed brown glass bottle.
11. If using this drug primarily to relax and go to sleep, the patient should investigate alternative methods of relaxation to help reduce the need for medication.

Pediatric Considerations
ANTIANXIETY AGENTS AND SEDATIVES

Young children are more susceptible to the CNS-depressant effects of the benzodiazepines. In neonates, profound CNS depression may result because of the lower rate of drug metabolism by the immature liver.

Chronic use of clonazepam may result in impaired physical or mental functions in the developing child. This may not become apparent until years later.

Buspirone has not been studied in persons under 18 years; therefore it is not recommended for use in that age group.

Although diazepam (Valium) may be used in infants 6 months and over, this drug and other benzodiazepines should not be used to treat a hyperactive or psychotic child.

Methyprylon (Noludar) is not indicated for use in children under 12 years old.

Paradoxic reactions have been reported in children with the use of barbiturates.

From McKenry LM, Salerno E: *Mosby's pharmacology in nursing*, ed 18, St Louis, 1992, Mosby.

SUMMARY

CNS medications include narcotic and nonnarcotic analgesics, antimigraine agents, seizure medications, antiemetics, antivertigo medications, antiparkinsonian agents, antipsychotics, and sedative-hypnotics. It is important to understand how nerves transmit information from the brain through chemical neurotransmitters and how these medications interact with the body. Neurotransmitters fit into receptors in various parts of the body to act on them, and many CNS drugs act on more than one type of receptor. Each agent acts differently. It is extremely important for the nurse to administer dosages carefully, because serious adverse reactions are possible if dosages are exceeded.

CRITICAL THINKING QUESTIONS

1. Mr. Robbins is to be started on a narcotic agonist analgesic immediately after his surgery tomorrow. Plan appropriate nursing strategies to begin as soon as Mr. Robbins comes out of surgery. Explain the importance of good baseline assessment and careful follow-up once Mr. Robbins is taking the medication.

2. Several days after Mr. Robbins' surgery, he seems to be requesting medication more often than you had anticipated. You begin to suspect that he is becoming addicted to the narcotic. How might you be able to tell if this is really what's happening? What is the difference between acute and chronic narcotic overdosage?

3. Mr. Robbins is not addicted to his medication, but both he and his family are concerned about that possibility. Draw up a teaching plan for a narcotic agonist analgesic.

4. Tomorrow Mr. Robbins is going home. He may still be expected to experience some significant pain, so his physician has switched him to a narcotic agonist-antagonist analgesic. Draw up a teaching plan for him and his family before he is discharged. Be sure to highlight the advantage of this drug over the one he was taking initially.

5. Draw up a chart to enable you to easily compare the major types of nonnarcotic analgesics in the following areas: (1) actions, (2) uses, and (3) adverse reactions.

6. Describe the properties of antimigraine products that differentiate them from other nonnarcotic analgesics. Describe the characteristics of a migraine headache in light of the unique actions of these antimigraine agents.

7. Draw up a teaching plan for a patient needing antimigraine medication; be sure to explain the difference between treatment and prophylaxis of pain. Stress the importance of timing, of adverse reactions, as well as other, nonpharmacologic measures for reducing pain, risks of dependency and overdosage, and the effects of certain drugs on pregnancies.

8. Jason is an 8-year-old boy who has recently been hospitalized for evaluation and subsequently diagnosed with a seizure disorder. The physician has prescribed phenobarbital. Jason has never taken this drug before. Develop a nursing care plan, identifying general nursing assessments that should be made before beginning anticonvulsant therapy. Identify possible adverse reactions with this drug. Finally, develop a teaching plan for the family and patient receiving anticonvulsant medications, identifying any properties unique to the drug Jason is taking.

9. Identify at least three different kinds of antiemetics and antivertigo agents, being careful to select agents that differ in their uses or actions. Briefly point out differences and similarities in actions and side effects, and discuss treatment strategies (e.g., when to take a motion sickness medication to obtain maximum effectiveness).

10. Mrs. Davis is being evaluated for possible Parkinson's disease. She asks you what to look for and possible causes. Identify signs and symptoms of Parkinson's disease and suspected contributing factors. Finally, you learn that Mrs. Davis does indeed have Parkinson's disease. Draw up a teaching plan for Mrs. Davis and her husband and son.

11. Lisa, a 17-year-old girl, is brought into the emergency room with suspected overdosage from an antianxiety agent. What are the signs of overdosage in these drugs? How are they distinguished from adverse reactions?

12. Lisa's parents explain that at first they could not tell their daughter was having any adverse reactions, since many of the side effects were the same symptoms Lisa always exhibited when she was anxious. Use this to explain the rationale for obtaining a good baseline interview and assessment before these drugs are prescribed for a patient.

13. Lisa is switched to a tricyclic antidepressant. Draw up a teaching plan for her and her family, identifying common drug interactions, contraindications, precautions, and the overall role this medication plays in the treatment process.

14. What are monoamine oxidase inhibitors used for? What unique interaction is possible with these drugs? What are the contraindications? Draw up an outline of things you would include in a patient and family teaching plan.

15. Create a four-column chart on a large sheet of paper. Down the first column list the following terms, leaving several spaces between them: actions, uses, adverse reactions, interactions, assessment, plannning, and patient teaching. Above the second column write the heading "Haloperidol;" above the third write "Phenothiazine," and above the fourth write "Lithium." Fill out this chart to draw simple comparisons or contrasts among these three types of antipsychotic agents.

16. Develop a teaching plan for the use of medications for treating insomnia, being sure to suggest nonmedicinal strategies as well as drug information.

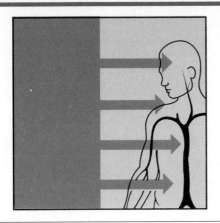

CHAPTER 13

Gastrointestinal Medications

OBJECTIVES

At the conclusion of this chapter you should be able to:

1. Identify uses for antacids and histamine H$_2$-receptor antagonists.
2. Compare and contrast the actions of anticholinergic and antispasmodic medications on the gastrointestinal tract.
3. Compare the action and adverse effects of the five major classifications of laxatives.
4. Identify indications for use of at least two common antidiarrheals, antiflatulents, digestive enzymes, and emetics.
5. Describe indications for disulfiram use, and what is meant by "disulfiram reaction."

KEY TERMS

OVERVIEW

This chapter discusses medications used to treat the many diseases and disorders that affect the gastrointestinal tract. Many of these medications are available over the counter; many others are used, often in combination, to relieve the symptoms of significant problems.

There are three major types of gastrointestinal medications. The first major type includes products designed to help restore or maintain the protective lining of the gastrointestinal tract. These medications include antacids, which act to neutralize or reduce the acidity of the gastric contents, and the histamine H$_2$-receptor antagonists, which reduce gastric acid secretion by inhibiting the action of histamine at the receptor cells in the stomach. These medications are described in Section One.

A second type of medication affects the general motility, or movement, of the gastrointestinal tract. These medications include the anticholinergics and

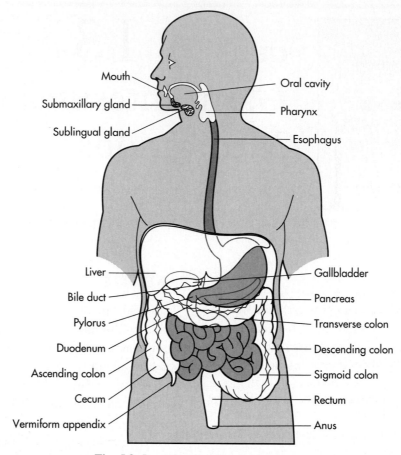

Fig. 13-1 The digestive system.

antispasmodics, which not only reduce gastric motility but decrease the amount of acid secreted by the stomach, and the antidiarrheals, which reduce diarrhea by decreasing the intestinal peristalsis. These preparations are discussed in Section Two.

The third major group of gastrointestinal drugs is the laxatives. These preparations also affect motility, but their action is primarily in the colon. They promote bowel emptying in a variety of ways. They may increase intestinal bulk, lubricate the intestinal walls, soften the fecal mass by increased water retention, or produce increased peristalsis through local tissue irritation or by direct action on the intestine. These drugs are presented in Section Three.

Section Four presents miscellaneous medications. These preparations include antiflatulents, which are used to reduce gas and bloating; digestive enzymes, which are used in deficiency states to break down fats, starches, and proteins in the digestive process; emetics, which are used to produce vomiting, primarily in poisoning or overdosage; and medications used to treat gallstones and alcoholism.

Digestive System

The digestive system is composed of the mouth, esophagus, stomach, intestines, and accessory structures (Fig. 13-1). This system performs the mechanical and chemical processes of digestion, absorption of nutrients, and elimination of wastes.

Digestion begins in the mouth with mastication and the mixing of food with enzyme-containing saliva secreted by salivary glands. The passages and spaces from this point to the anus make up the alimentary canal, in which the complex compounds are reduced to soluble, absorbable substances, the usable food substances being absorbed and the indigestible and waste materials eliminated. The digestive glands secrete enzymes and other chemical components that are essential to the breakdown of food substances and to their absorption into the bloodstream. The salivary glands, liver, and pancreas are included as accessory glands.

Almost all medications use the digestive system as a

means to reach target organs or tissues. Many of the side effects such as diarrhea, nausea, or constipation are results of the direct action of medications on the alimentary tract itself. Medications, as well as all ingested materials, are acted on by the digestive tract, and are metabolized and excreted.

SECTION ONE: ANTACIDS AND HISTAMINE H$_2$-RECEPTOR ANTAGONISTS

Objectives

At the conclusion of this section you should be able to:

1. Describe common actions of antacids and histamine H$_2$-receptor antagonists.
2. Identify indications for the use of antacids and histamine H$_2$-receptor antagonists.
3. List adverse reactions and drug interactions for major antacids and histamine H$_2$-receptor antagonists.
4. Develop a teaching plan for the patient taking antacids or histamine H$_2$-receptor antagonists over a prolonged period of time.

OVERVIEW

The lining of the stomach is usually strong enough to resist the powerful digestive juices and acids that bathe it. When stress or disease provokes oversecretion of gastric acids, or when there is destruction of the protective lining because of alcohol, chemicals, or disease, gastric distress is produced. If the protective lining is not repaired and/or the gastric acid level reduced, ulcerations are produced, which lead to increased pain and bleeding. Duodenal, gastric, or peptic ulcers may be produced. Both antacid therapy and histamine H$_2$-receptor antagonists reduce gastric acidity and promote healing. A variety of products may be used at the same time to help in healing.

ACTION

Antacids are over-the-counter agents that neutralize hydrochloric acid and increase gastric pH, thus inhibiting pepsin (a gastric enzyme). Antacids work in a variety of ways. Some antacids cause hydrogen ion absorption, or buffering of the acid, tightening of the gastric mucosa, and increased tone of the cardiac sphincter. Formation of gas that may be burped up is another way in which antacids work.

Histamine H$_2$-receptor antagonists are unique because they promote healing of ulcers and act with antacids to produce a more alkaline gastrointestinal medium. They block histamine, inhibit the secretion of gastric acid, and are rapidly absorbed; they reach their peak of effectiveness in 45 to 90 minutes.

USES

Antacids are used adjunctively to treat peptic ulcer disease, gastritis, gastric ulcer, peptic esophagitis, hiatal hernia, gastric hyperacidity, and esophageal reflux.

Histamine H$_2$-receptor antagonists promote the healing of duodenal ulcers when used over 6 to 8 weeks. It is common for the patient to have a relapse after the medication is discontinued. It is used in the prophylaxis and treatment of peptic esophagitis, benign gastric ulcers, duodenal ulcers, stress ulcers, and Zollinger-Ellison syndrome.

Most peptic ulcers caused by *Helicobacter pylori* can be cured by antibiotics plus ranitidine.

ADVERSE REACTIONS

Some adverse reactions occur only with a particular category of antacids; others are common to most. Antacids may produce malaise, anorexia, bowel obstruction, constipation, diarrhea, frequent burping, thirst, and muscle weakness. In cases of extreme hypermagnesemia, cardiotoxicity with bradyarrhythmia, asystole, and hypotension may be seen. The most severe reactions include coma, decreased reflexes, and respiratory depression.

With histamine H$_2$-receptor antagonists, side effects are unusual, but the patient may have mild and self-limiting problems, such as dizziness, headaches, somnolence, mild and transient diarrhea, some hematologic changes, rash, impotence, mild gynecomastia, muscle pain, and fever.

DRUG INTERACTIONS

Antacids inhibit the absorption of tetracycline. Enteric coatings of various medications dissolve more quickly in the presence of antacids, leaving the upper gastrointestinal tract more susceptible to irritation. Some antacids have been known to either bind with or alter the absorption rate of digitalis products, anticoagulants, iron, many phenothiazines, antiinflammatory agents, antihypertensives, antiarthritic agents, hydantoin, and possibly propranolol. Aluminum-magnesium hydroxide gel may increase absorption of aspirin. Dicumarol is absorbed 50% faster when taken concomitantly with antacids.

Antacids may increase the absorption of cimetidine, a histamine antagonist agent. Cimetidine may increase the effects of anticoagulants, hydantoins, beta-adrenergic blocking agents, lidocaine, benzodiazepine derivatives, and theophylline. Decreased white blood cell counts have been reported in cimetidine-treated patients who also received other drugs and treatment known to produce neutropenia. Apnea, confusion, and muscle twitching may be produced when cimetidine is administered with morphine. Serum digoxin levels may be reduced when digoxin and cimetidine are administered together. Cigarette smoking may neutralize the action of cimetidine. Ranitidine does not appear to interact with warfarin-type anticoagulants, theophylline, or diazepam, although it does produce false-positive urine protein tests.

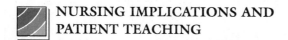

NURSING IMPLICATIONS AND PATIENT TEACHING

▼ Assessment

The nurse should obtain a complete health history, including gastrointestinal symptoms, the presence of underlying disease (especially renal failure), the presence of hypersensitivity to any chemical components of the antacid, and whether any medications that might cause drug interactions are currently being taken by the patient.

▼ Planning

The patient's fluid intake should be increased and the nurse should carefully monitor the patient taking constipative antacids, such as those containing calcium or aluminum. These may be alternated with antacids that have cathartic-like actions, such as those in the magnesium group.

▼ Implementation

Antacids are available in several different forms. Liquids or solutions are the preferred choice whenever possible, because they neutralize acid more rapidly. Suspensions, gels, chewable tablets, effervescent tablets, and powders are also available. If the patient feels unable to accept antacid therapy in another form, tablets should be considered the last alternative. The gastric emptying time of the peptic ulcer patient may vary, so it is wise to individualize the antacid schedule to accommodate this factor. The neutralizing abilities of antacids vary, requiring different quantities of medication, depending on the product. The nurse should discuss flavor preferences with the patient. Many patients discontinue antacid therapy because they dislike the flavor. Products come in many flavors, and various drugs may be tried if compliance becomes a problem.

Antacids with a laxative effect should be taken at bedtime to allow adequate rest before the bowel is stimulated.

The sodium content of various antacids must be carefully assessed before giving them to patients who are on restricted sodium intake (pregnant women, patients with congestive heart failure or other cardiac conditions, hypertension, edema, or renal failure).

Histamine H_2-receptor antagonists may be administered intravenously or orally. Oral preparations should be given with meals and at bedtime. IV injections should be diluted and injected over 1 to 2 minutes or given by infusion, and are usually given to patients with hypersecretion of gastric acid or intractable pain from ulcers. These medications should be given for 2 to 6 weeks, until endoscopy reveals healing. This drug may mask underlying malignancy. See Table 13-1 for a summary of antacids and histamine H_2-receptor antagonists.

▼ Evaluation

The nurse should evaluate the patient for reduction in gastrointestinal distress or the development of any adverse reactions.

▼ Patient and family teaching

The nurse should provide the patient and family with the following instructions:

1. The patient should take the medication exactly as ordered. Antacids are generally taken 1 hour after meals. If the patient is being treated for peptic ulcer, the gastric emptying time (usually

Table 13-1   Antacids and histamine H$_2$-receptor antagonists

Generic name	Trade name	Comments and dosage
ANTACIDS		
Aluminum carbonate gel	Basaljel	Give 1 to 2 tablets or capsules, or 2 teaspoonfuls of suspension in water or fruit juice q2h; may use up to 12 times daily.
Aluminum hydroxide gel	Amphojel ALU-Cap Dialume	Helps delay stomach emptying and binds bile salts. Drug of choice in peptic ulcer disease. *Oral:* 5 to 10 ml q2 to 4h, followed by a sip of water if desired. *Tablets:* 2 tablets (300 mg or 600 mg) five to six times daily; chew thoroughly and follow with water.
Aluminum phosphate gel	Phosphaljel	Preferred for patients with diarrhea or those needing dietary phosphorus. Give 15 to 45 ml PO with water four or more times daily.
Calcium carbonate	Dicarbosil Tums Di-Cal-D ✤	Very effective; promotes prolonged and powerful neutralizing effect greater than aluminum hydroxide. It is primarily suited for short-term therapy and is given in small doses. The constipating effects may be minimized by alternating it with doses of a magnesium-containing antacid, such as magnesium carbonate. Give 2 to 4 gm (30 to 40 gr) qh. Tums should be taken 1 or 2 tablets at a time, chewed or dissolved slowly in the mouth between the cheek and gum.
Dihydroxyaluminum sodium carbonate	Rolaids	Give 1 to 2 tablets, chewed, prn.
Magaldrate	Riopan Lowsium	Combination of magnesium and aluminum hydroxide. Effectiveness depends on GI pH. Give 1 to 2 tablets or 1 to 2 teaspoonfuls between meals and at bedtime; not to be taken for more than 2 weeks or more than 20 tablets in 24 hours.
Magnesium hydroxide	Milk of Magnesia	Helpful because cathartic effect counteracts constipation of aluminum hydroxide. Osmotic diarrhea may occur when given alone. *Adults:* 1 to 3 teaspoonfuls with water up to qid.
Magnesium oxide	Mag-Ox Maox	Acts more slowly than sodium bicarbonate, but has a more prolonged action and increased neutralizing ability. As with other magnesium antacids, osmotic diarrhea may develop, but it may be alleviated if alternated with aluminum or calcium salts. Give 250 mg PO as required.
ANTACID COMBINATIONS		
Aluminum hydroxide and magnesium hydroxide	Maalox ✓	Combined to provide a nonconstipating, noncathartic antacid for relief of hyperactivity of peptic ulcer. Give 2 tablets or 2 teaspoonfuls q4h prn; suspension may be followed by a sip of water.
Aluminum hydroxide, magnesium hydroxide, and simethicone	Gelusil Mylanta ✓	Products use simethicone to reduce gas formation and come in many flavors and a variety of combinations. *Suspension:* 1 to 2 teaspoonfuls qid between meals and at bedtime. *Tablets:* 1 to 2 tablets (chewed well) qid between meals and at bedtime. Do not exceed 24 teaspoonfuls or tablets in a 24-hour period or use the maximum dosage for longer than 2 weeks.
Calcium carbonate and glycine	Titralac	Form an insoluble antacid-protective for the relief of hyperacidity. Give 1 teaspoonful or 2 tablets qh after meals; tablets can be chewed, swallowed, or allowed to dissolve slowly in the mouth; do not exceed 19 tablets or 8 teaspoonfuls in 24 hours.
Calcium carbonate and magnesium hydroxide	Bisodol	Its neutralizing effect is powerful and prolonged. Give 1 to 2 tablets q2h; chew tablets thoroughly and follow with a glass of water.

Continued.

Table 13-1 Antacids and histamine H$_2$-receptor antagonists—cont'd

Generic name	Trade name	Comments and dosage
HISTAMINE H$_2$-RECEPTOR ANTAGONISTS		
Cimetidine	Tagamet	Widely used in prophylaxis and treatment of ulcers. Has more drug interactions than other preparations and a much wider range of actions than other preparations. *Duodenal ulcer:* 300 mg PO qid with meals and at bedtime, or 300 mg q6h IV. Should be taken with antacids.
Famotidine	Pepcid	Relatively new drug. Give 20 to 40 mg qd at bedtime.
Nizatidine	Axid	Relatively new drug. Give 150 to 300 mg qd at bedtime.
Ranitidine	Zantac	Similar in action to cimetidine, but has fewer drug interactions. Headache is a frequent side effect in these patients. *Duodenal ulcer:* 150 mg PO bid. Do not give more than 150 mg/24 hours if creatinine clearance is below 50 ml/min.

between 1 and 3 hours) will dictate when they should take the antacid. The patient should not switch to another antacid or take new drugs without consulting the physician.

2. Antacids may cause diarrhea or constipation. The patient should report any significant difficulty to the physician. A good fluid intake should be maintained, and the amount of fluids in the diet should be increased if constipation becomes a problem.

3. The chewable tablets should be chewed thoroughly before swallowing and followed with a full glass of water.

4. Liquid preparations should be shaken well before taking to ensure accurate dosage.

5. If the patient is taking other medications at the same time, the physician should be consulted as to whether the antacids will affect the medication. Spacing of other medication at different times may eliminate drug interactions.

6. Liquid forms should be stored in a cool place, but not allowed to freeze; refrigeration makes them taste better.

7. Antacids lose their effectiveness over time; the patient should not use old medication.

8. If the physician prescribes an aluminum-containing antacid, the patient's diet must contain adequate amounts of dietary phosphorus (up to 1.5 gm/day). Phosphorus is found in the protein of meat, almonds, beans, barley, bran, cheese, cocoa, chocolate, eggs, lentils, liver, milk, oatmeal, peanuts, peas, walnuts, whole wheat, rye, asparagus, beef, carrots, cabbage,

 Geriatric Considerations
ANTIULCER THERAPIES

Gastrointestinal complaints are very common in elderly patients. Every complaint should be properly evaluated before drug therapy is instituted.

Pain is less frequently the initial complaint, while melena (black stool that contains digested blood) is the more frequent presentation and indication of ulcer disease in the elderly.

Acid secretion reaches its peak during sleep, between the hours of 10 PM and 2 AM. Therefore H$_2$-receptor antagonists prescribed as a daily dose should be administered at bedtime.

Cigarette smoking, which increases the amount of acid produced in the stomach, may decrease the effect of H$_2$-blockers. Clients should be advised to stop smoking if possible, or at least to not smoke after the last daily dose of medication is taken.

Confusion and dizziness are more commonly reported by the elderly than by younger adults with H$_2$ blockers. Mental status changes have been reported with cimetidine (Tagamet), especially in elderly persons who have impaired liver or renal function or who are severely ill. Acute mental changes in the elderly may indicate a need to lower the drug dose or to discontinue the medication.

Antacids effectively neutralize gastric acid; food also serves as a buffer for gastric acid. Thus antacids are most beneficial if administered between meals and at bedtime.

When H$_2$-receptor antagonists are prescribed with antacids, the medications should be scheduled at least 1 hour apart, with the antacid taken first.

celery, cauliflower, chard, chicken, clams, corn, cream, cucumbers, eggplant, fish, figs, prunes, pineapples, pumpkins, raisins, and string beans.

9. The patient with a peptic ulcer will need to make several visits to the physician for examination and laboratory tests; this is done to assess the healing process.

10. Peptic and duodenal ulcers tend to recur, so it is important to determine what causes the problem and to try to correct it. The medication is only part of the therapy. Controlling stress, avoiding sporadic eating and stressful living habits, and eliminating other diseases and infections are also important.

11. Antacids are often taken with histamine H_2-receptor antagonists. The patient should keep all medications at home, at school, or at the office so they can be used at the first appearance of gastric distress.

SECTION TWO: DRUGS AFFECTING MOTILITY

Objectives

At the conclusion of this section you should be able to:

1. Identify appropriate uses of anticholinergics, antispasmodics, and antidiarrheals.
2. Compare actions of anticholinergics, antispasmodics, and antidiarrheals.
3. Describe common side effects of anticholinergics, antispasmodics, and antidiarrheals.
4. Develop a teaching plan for a patient receiving short-term therapy with an anticholinergic, antispasmodic, or antidiarrheal.

OVERVIEW

Motility is the spontaneous but unconscious or involuntary movement of food through the gastrointestinal tract. Much of the discomfort associated with gastrointestinal disease is caused by increased intestinal peristalsis or muscle contraction. Abdominal cramping, bloating, and pain may be related either to acute minor illnesses associated with diarrhea and increased flatulence, or to chronic diseases, such as ulcers or colitis. Also, many drugs have both diarrhea and increased bowel motility as common adverse reactions.

The variety of medications used to treat these problems are classed as anticholinergics, antispasmodics, or antidiarrheals. Their actions are somewhat different, although they are often used interchangeably.

ACTION

The anticholinergic-antispasmodic preparations are parasympatholytic drugs (natural and synthetic) that act with antacids in prolonging the therapeutic benefits of both categories of drugs. **Anticholinergics** reduce spasm and intestinal motility, acid production, gastric motility and consequently, reduce the associated pain. Gastric emptying time is slowed and neutralization is increased. Pancreatic secretions of fluid, electrolytes, and enzymes are also suppressed. However, the adverse reactions resulting from the high dosages necessary to achieve these effects make their use questionable.

Antidiarrheals reduce the fluid content of the stool and decrease peristalsis and motility of the intestinal tract. They increase smooth muscle tone and diminish digestive secretions. The bismuth salts absorb toxins and provide a protective coating for the intestinal mucosa.

USES

Anticholinergic-antispasmodic agents are primarily used to treat peptic ulcer, pylorospasm, biliary colic, hypermotility, hyperacidity, irritable colon, and acute pancreatitis.

Antidiarrheals are used to treat nonspecific diarrhea or diarrhea caused by antibiotics.

ADVERSE REACTIONS

Adverse reactions are common in anticholinergic therapy, because high dosages are usually required. The most common adverse reactions include rapid weak pulse; blurring of vision; difficulty swallowing; difficulty talking; dilation of pupils; drowsiness; excitation; photophobia; confusion; restlessness; staggering; talkativeness; rash primarily over the face, neck, and upper trunk (especially in children); flushing of skin; constipation; dry mouth; great thirst; urinary urgency; and difficulty emptying bladder. Anticholinergics containing phenobarbital may produce convulsions, delirium, excitement, musculoskeletal pain, and various dermatologic and allergic responses.

Antidiarrheals may cause tachycardia, dizziness, drowsiness, fatigue, headache, sedation, pruritus, urticaria, abdominal distention, constipation, dry mouth, nausea, vomiting, urinary retention, and physical dependence.

DRUG INTERACTIONS

Anticholinergics containing phenobarbital may decrease the effects of anticoagulants, requiring higher doses of the anticoagulant. Anticholinergics have many drug interactions; see Chapter 12 for a more specific discussion.

 NURSING IMPLICATIONS AND PATIENT TEACHING

▼ Assessment

The nurse should obtain a complete health history, including the presence of hypersensitivity, underlying diseases, concurrent use of medications, previous gastrointestinal history, and a special history regarding bowel function: regularity, consistency, and frequency. The patient with diarrhea may have frequent loose, watery stools, often with mild, cramping abdominal pain before bowel movements.

Synthetic forms of these drugs are more expensive than the natural forms (belladonna, atropine, scopolamine).

▼ Planning

Preparations containing phenobarbital may be habit forming, so they should not be administered to patients prone to addiction. Initial doses should be small. These drugs should be used with caution in patients who have hepatic dysfunction or prostatic hypertrophy or are at risk for glaucoma.

Opiates, loperamide, and diphenoxylate may cause psychologic or physical dependence if used in high dosages or for long periods. The nonspecific antidiarrheal agents provide symptomatic relief until the cause of the diarrhea can be determined and specific therapy instituted. These agents should not be used in diarrhea caused by poison until the toxin has been removed from the gastrointestinal tract.

▼ Implementation

Anticholinergics may be given orally or parenterally (when oral dosages cannot be retained or when immediate relief is needed). It is generally better to begin the oral dosage as soon as possible. All the antidiarrheal agents are administered orally; individual dosages are determined by need. Dietary modifications are usually a part of the management. The patient's diet is restricted to clear liquids for 24 hours and then foods are gradually added as tolerated. See Table 13-2 for a summary of anticholinergic, antispasmodic, and antidiarrheal medications.

▼ Evaluation

Prolonged diarrhea can result in dehydration and electrolyte imbalance. The nurse should encourage the patient to increase fluid intake to replace the fluid lost in the stool.

Patients being treated with Lomotil or other laxatives with narcotics should be observed for signs of CNS depression. CNS side effects are not to be expected with synthetic anticholinergic therapy, which is one of the advantages of the synthetic products.

Antidiarrheals should not be used on a long-term basis. The nurse should monitor for the therapeutic effect in controlling diarrhea, and for the development of adverse effects.

Long-term anticholinergic therapy may mask or alter the symptoms of gastrointestinal disease, so it may be difficult to determine recurrences.

▼ Patient and family teaching

The nurse should provide the patient and family with the following instructions:

1. Take this medication exactly as ordered by the physician.
2. This medication should be kept out of the reach of children and all others for whom it has not been prescribed.
3. Many people experience mild side effects with these medications. The patient should alert the physician if any new or troublesome problems occur, especially diarrhea, so that they may be evaluated.
4. High environmental temperatures may make the patient feel unusually hot and fatigued. The

Table 13-2   Anticholinergic, antispasmodic, and antidiarrheal medications

Generic name	Trade name	Comments and dosage
ANTICHOLINERGICS Belladonna alkaloids		
Atropine	Atropine Sulfate	Among the most effective of the anticholinergic drugs with minimal side effects. Give 0.4 to 0.6 mg PO or SQ q4 or 6h. *Children:* 0.1 mg to 0.4 mg, depending on size.
Belladonna	Extract or tincture	Same therapeutic action as atropine. ■ *Belladonna extract:* 15 mg PO tid to qid. ■ *Belladonna tincture* *Adults:* 0.6 to 1.0 ml tid to qid. *Children:* 0.03 ml/kg tid.
Levorotatory alkaloids of belladonna	Bellafoline	Used in a variety of smooth muscle spastic conditions and when excessive secretion is present. *Adults:* 0.25 to 0.5 mg PO tid or 0.5 to 1 ml SQ qd to bid. *Children over 6 years of age:* 0.125 to 0.25 mg PO tid.
L-Hyoscyamine	Anaspaz Cystospaz Levsin	Reduces hypermotility and hyperacidity; several contraindications for use. *Adults:* 0.125 to 0.25 mg PO or SQ q4h; use 1 to 2 ml drops q4h prn; use 0.375 mg in sustained-release tablets q12h. In severe cases, use 2 timecaps q12h or 1 timecap q8h. *Children:* calculate dosage based on weight.
Scopolamine	Scopolamine	Similar to atropine in peripheral action, but parenteral dosages cause CNS depression, resulting in drowsiness, euphoria, relief of fear, sleep, relaxation, and amnesia. *Adults:* 0.3 to 0.6 mg SQ or IM, 0.4 to 0.8 mg PO q4 to 6h. *Children:* 0.006 mg/kg PO or SQ.
Quaternary anticholinergics		
Anisotropine	Valpin	Reduces motility and hyperacidity. *Adults:* 50 mg (1 tablet) PO tid.
Clidinium	Quarzan Librax ✦	*Adults:* 2.5 to 5 mg PO tid to qid before meals and at bedtime.
Glycopyrrolate	Robinul	Used orally as adjunctive treatment in peptic ulcer disease. Give 1 to 2 tablets bid to tid.
Hexocyclium	Tral filmtabs Tral gradumets	Used adjunctively as treatment for peptic ulcer disease. Give 25 mg before meals and at bedtime. For timed-release capsule, give 50 mg before lunch and at bedtime; do not chew.
Isopropamide	Darbid	Synthetic anticholinergic that suppresses gastric secretions and reduces hypermotility for 10 to 12 hours. *Adults:* 5 to 10 mg q12h; may use more frequently if symptoms are severe.
Mepenzolate	Cantil	Decreases gastric acid and pepsin secretion while slowing contractions of the colon. *Adults:* 25 to 50 mg PO with meals and at bedtime.
Methantheline	Banthine	This drug is similar in action to atropine. *Adults:* 50 mg initially, then 100 mg q6h. *Children:* 6 mg/kg qd in four divided doses.
Methscopolamine	Pamine	Synthetic substitute for atropine as an antispasmodic. *Adults:* 2.5 mg 30 min before eating and 2.5 to 5 mg at bedtime.
Propantheline	Pro-Banthine	An analog to methantheline, this drug is more effective than methantheline in the reduction of volume and acidity of the stomach's secretions. *PO:* 15 mg with meals and 30 mg at bedtime, adjusted according to therapeutic response. *IM or IV:* 30 mg q6h prn; maintenance is usually 15 mg.

Continued.

Table 13-2 Anticholinergic, antispasmodic, and antidiarrheal medications—cont'd

Generic name	Trade name	Comments and dosage
Tridihexethyl	Pathilon	Synthetic anticholinergic effective in relaxing pain by reducing spasms of the gastrointestinal tract. Also used in irritable bowel syndrome. *PO:* 25 to 50 mg tid to qid, or 75 mg sequels q12h. *IM, IV, or SQ:* 10 to 20 mg q6h; switch to oral preparation as soon as possible.

ANTISPASMODICS

Generic name	Trade name	Comments and dosage
Dicyclomine	Antispas Bentyl Bentyol ♣	Synthetic antispasmodic controls spasms of the gastrointestinal tract; also used in irritable bowel syndrome. *Adults:* 10 to 20 mg PO tid to qid; or 20 mg IM q4 to 6h. *Children:* 10 mg PO tid to qid. *Infants:* 5 mg syrup diluted with an equal volume of water, tid to qid for colic.
Oxyphencyclimine	Daricon	Synthetic antispasmodic used in the adjunctive treatment of peptic ulcers. *Adults and children over 12 years:* 10 mg in AM and at bedtime. Dosage may be increased to tid, or reduced to 5 mg bid prn.

ANTICHOLINERGIC COMBINATION DRUGS

Generic name	Trade name	Comments and dosage
Hyoscyamine, atropine, hyoscine, and phenobarbital	Donnatal	This medication is one of many combination products combining anticholinergic and sedative drugs. Because of the phenobarbital, these products may be habit forming. Give 3 to 8 capsules or tablets in equally divided doses tid to qid. *Elixir:* 15 to 40 ml/day in equally divided doses. *Extentabs:* 2 tablets q12h.

ANTIDIARRHEALS

Generic name	Trade name	Comments and dosage
Bismuth subsalicylate	Pepto-Bismol Bismatrol	Contains salicylates; ask patient about aspirin sensitivity. Has risk of producing Reye's syndrome in children. May cause temporary darkening of the stool and tongue. *Adults:* 30 ml or 2 tablets PO q30 min to 1 hour until symptoms are relieved or until a maximum of eight doses has been given. Give with oral rehydration solution in children with severe diarrhea. *Children:* Calculate dosage by weight.
Difenoxin with atropine	Motofen	*Adults:* 2 tablets, then 1 after each loose stool to a maximum of 8 tablets in 24 hours.
Diphenoxylate and atropine sulfate	Lomotil Logen Lomanate	These are Schedule V controlled substances. Addition of atropine sulfate helps to prevent abuse. *Adults:* 2 tablets or 2 teaspoons qid until diarrhea is controlled. *Children:* Calculate dosage by weight.
Hyoscamine, atropine, and hyoscine	Donnagel	Because of the presence of the belladonna alkaloids, caution must be used in patients with glaucoma or bladder neck obstruction.
Kaolin and pectin	Kaopectate	*Adults:* 2 tablespoons at once and 1 or 2 tablespoons after each bowel movement. *Children:* Calculate dosage by weight. These are nonprescription products widely used in self-treatment of diarrhea; their clinical effectiveness has not been established.

Table 13-2   Anticholinergic, antispasmodic, and antidiarrheal medications—cont'd

Generic name	Trade name	Comments and dosage
Lactobacillus	Bacid Lactinex	Nonprescription product specifically used to treat diarrhea caused by antibiotics. It reestablishes normal intestinal flora and may be used prophylactically in those with a history of antibiotic-induced diarrhea. *Adults:* 2 capsules or 4 tablets of Bacid, or use 1 packet of granules of Lactinex, bid to qid, preferably with milk.
Loperamide	Imodium	This is a Schedule V controlled substance. It is more potent and has a longer duration of action with less CNS depression than diphenoxylate. *Adults:* Initially give 4 mg PO, then 2 mg after each unformed stool; maximum of 16 mg PO qd.
Opium tincture	Brown mixture	This is a Schedule III controlled substance. It is given orally mixed with water. A white, milky fluid forms when they are mixed together.
	Paregoric	■ *Tincture of opium* *Adults:* Give 0.6 ml PO qid. ■ *Camphorated opium tincture* *Adults:* 5 to 10 ml PO qid until diarrhea subsides. *Children:* 0.25 to 0.5 ml/kg PO qid until diarrhea subsides.
Olsalazine	Dipentum	Give 1 gm/day PO in 2 divided doses for ulcerative colitis.
Mesalamine	Asacol Rowasa	Give 800 mg tid for 6 weeks in ulcerative colitis.

patient should avoid becoming overheated while taking this drug.

5. The antidiarrheal agents are used to relieve symptoms and to prevent dehydration until the underlying cause can be found and treated.

6. The patient with diarrhea should be restricted to clear liquids (tea, gelatin, broth, carbonated beverages) for 24 hours; the patient can then begin adding bland foods and continue to add more solid foods if diarrhea does not reappear.

7. Diarrhea that persists more than 48 hours should not be self-treated. The patient should return to the physician for further evaluation and diagnosis.

8. Some antidiarrheal medications contain habit-forming drugs; therefore they should be used only at the dosage recommended, and for the length of time prescribed.

SECTION THREE: LAXATIVES

Objectives

At the conclusion of this section you should be able to:

1. Describe the actions of the five different types of laxatives.
2. List indications and contraindications for laxative use.
3. Identify major adverse effects from laxative usage.
4. Develop a teaching plan to aid the patient and family in appropriate use of laxatives.

OVERVIEW

Laxatives are drugs that change fecal consistency, speed the passage of feces through the colon, and aid in the elimination of stool from the rectum. They are classified in five major categories, based on their mechanism of action. These categories include bulk-forming agents, fecal softeners, hyperosmolar or saline solutions, lubricants, and stimulant or irritant laxatives.

Laxatives are one of the major groups of drugs used as self-treatment for constipation by patients, with use increasing as patients age. Laxatives have a high rate of overuse, destroying the body's natural emptying rhythm when used excessively. Laxatives are used in bowel training of individuals who have lost neurogenic control of the bowel, and are commonly used in preparing patients for x-ray, obstetric, or surgical procedures.

ACTION

Bulk-forming laxatives absorb water and expand, increasing both the bulk and the moisture content of the stool. The increased bulk stimulates peristalsis and the absorbed water softens the stool. These agents are not absorbed systemically.

Fecal softeners soften stool by lowering the surface tension, which allows the fecal mass to be penetrated by intestinal fluids. They also inhibit fluid and electrolyte reabsorption by the intestine.

Hyperosmolar laxatives, such as lactulose and glycerin, produce an osmotic effect in the colon by distending the bowel from fluid accumulation and promoting peristalsis and bowel movement. Saline laxatives also produce an osmotic effect by drawing water into the intestinal lumen of the small intestine and colon.

Lubricant laxatives create a barrier between the feces and the colon wall that prevents the colon from reabsorbing fecal fluid, thus softening the stool. The lubricant effect also eases the passage of feces through the intestine.

Stimulant or irritant laxatives increase peristalsis by several mechanisms, depending on the agent. These mechanisms include primary stimulation of colon nerves (senna preparations), stimulation of sensory nerves in the intestinal mucosa (bisacodyl), or direct stimulation of smooth muscle and inhibition of water and electrolyte reabsorption from the intestinal lumen (castor oil).

USES

Bulk-forming laxatives are used in simple constipation and in atonic constipation from overuse of other cathartics. Bulk-forming laxatives are also particularly useful in postpartum, elderly, and debilitated patients. They have been used to treat diverticulosis and irritable bowel syndrome.

Fecal softeners help relieve constipation produced by a delay in rectal emptying. They are also useful

when it is important to reduce straining at stool, as in patients with hernia or cardiovascular disease, postpartum patients, or after rectal surgery.

Saline laxatives are used to cleanse the bowel in preparation for endoscopic examination, x-ray studies, or surgery. They are used to hasten evacuation of worms after the administration of anthelmintics, and after the ingestion of poisons to hasten elimination of toxic material. Lactulose and glycerin are most commonly used to treat simple constipation.

Lubricant laxatives are used to soften stool in conditions where straining at stool should be avoided, as in myocardial infarction, aneurysm, stroke, hernia, or following abdominal or rectal surgery. They are also used to prevent discomfort and tearing or laceration of hemorrhoids or fissures.

Stimulant or irritant laxatives are used to treat constipation resulting from prolonged bed rest, poor dietary habits, or induced by other drugs. They are also used to cleanse the bowel in preparation for endoscopic examination, x-ray studies, or surgery.

ADVERSE REACTIONS

Bulk-forming laxatives may produce abdominal cramps, diarrhea, strictures, and obstructions when taken without sufficient liquid. Nausea and vomiting are also common. Hypersensitivity may be demonstrated by development of asthma, dermatitis, rhinitis, and urticaria.

Fecal softeners may cause mild cramping or diarrhea.

Hyperosmolar or saline laxatives may produce abdominal cramping, nausea, and fluid and electrolyte disturbance if used daily or in renal impairment. Hypermagnesemia occurs almost exclusively in patients with chronic renal insufficiency and is aggravated by increased intake of magnesium in hyperosmolar laxatives. In patients with cardiac disease or congestive heart failure, the increased sodium intake in the sodium-containing saline cathartics can precipitate or worsen the condition.

Lubricant laxatives may produce abdominal cramps, vomiting, decreased absorption of nutrients and fat-soluble vitamins, diarrhea, and nausea. Lipid pneumonia caused by aspiration and deficiency syndromes reflecting decreased absorption of the fat-soluble vitamins may occur with long-term or excessive use.

Stimulant or irritant laxatives may produce muscle weakness (following excessive use of laxatives), dermatitis, pruritus, abdominal cramps, diarrhea, nausea, vomiting, alkalosis, electrolyte imbalance (with excessive use).

Long-term excessive use of stimulant laxatives may result in irritable bowel syndrome or a severe, prolonged diarrhea. These conditions may lead to hyponatremia, hypokalemia, and dehydration. Cathartic colon, a syndrome resembling ulcerative colitis both radiologically and pathologically, may develop after chronic misuse.

DRUG INTERACTIONS

Antibiotics, anticoagulants, digitalis preparations, and salicylates may have reduced effectiveness if used concurrently with bulk-forming agents, because of binding and hindrance of absorption. A 2-hour interval between dosages of these medications is recommended.

Fecal softeners should never be used concurrently with mineral oil or other laxatives, particularly phenolphthalein. The systemic absorption of the other agents will be enhanced, causing an increased laxative effect and greater risk of toxic effects, especially to the liver. Hyperosmolar saline laxatives should not be taken within 1 to 3 hours of tetracyclines, because they may form nonabsorbable complexes. Lubricant laxatives may reduce the effectiveness of anticoagulants, contraceptives, digitalis, and fat-soluble vitamins if taken concurrently.

Antacids or milk should not be taken with bisacodyl tablets, because they produce a too-rapid dissolving of the enteric coating, resulting in gastric irritation. Some laxatives cause rapid transit through the bowel and so concurrent use of many medications that require time to dissolve may be adversely affected.

 NURSING IMPLICATIONS AND PATIENT TEACHING

▼ Assessment

The nurse should obtain a complete health history, including the presence of underlying disease, allergies, edema, or congestive heart failure, use of a sodium-restricted diet, and other drugs taken concurrently. The patient should be evaluated for potential abuse. Constipation that persists should always be evaluated for serious organic causes. Changes in bowel habits, especially waking up at night to defecate, should always be investigated.

The patient may complain of increased hardness of stool or of difficulty in passing stool. Decreased frequency of stools, mild abdominal discomfort and distention, and occasionally mild anorexia may be present. Confused geriatric patients may only demonstrate increased restlessness.

Laxatives should not be given to patients with abdominal pain, nausea, vomiting, other signs of appendicitis, or acute surgical abdominal conditions. Other contraindications include fecal impaction, intestinal ulcerations, stenosis or obstruction, disabling adhesions, or dysphagia.

▼ Planning

Many bulk-forming products contain significant amounts of dextrose, galactose, and sucrose and should be avoided in patients with diabetes mellitus. Allergic reactions (urticaria, rhinitis, and asthma) may occur as a result of the plant gums present in these agents. This should be considered in patients with a history of allergic reactions, especially to plants.

Bulk-forming agents may become dry, thick, and hardened in the throat or within the intestine if they are swallowed without sufficient water. They can cause esophageal or intestinal obstruction or impaction if this occurs. The drugs should never be chewed or swallowed without one or more full glasses of water. Before giving medication for constipation, make certain that the patient is well hydrated.

Products with sodium salt should be avoided in patients with edema, pregnancy, congestive heart failure, and sodium-restricted diets. Potassium salt should be avoided in patients with renal impairment. Because laxatives are available without prescription, it is especially important to teach the patient about these serious side effects.

The nurse should begin educating the patient by explaining the usefulness of exercise, diet, and liquids in diet to reduce constipation. The patient should be taught the use of bulk-forming foods, fruits, vegetables, and whole grain cereals and encouraged to perform increased physical activities within the patient's capabilities. Proper bowel habits should be discussed and encouraged, and increased fluid intake should be stressed.

Overdosage or overusage of stimulant laxatives may cause excessive fluid loss and electrolyte imbalance, particularly hypokalemia. Overuse of any laxative can lead to atonic constipation and create laxative dependence.

▼ Implementation

All bulk-forming and stimulant laxatives are given orally, with one or more glasses of liquid. Lactulose and the saline laxatives are given orally. Glycerin and bisacodyl may be given by suppository or by enema.

The nurse should plan medication administration to allow the drug's effects to occur at a time that will not interfere with patient's rest or digestion. Time lubricant laxative administration so that it is not given within 2 hours of meals or medicine.

Bisacodyl enteric-coated tablets must be swallowed whole, never chewed or crushed, and never taken with milk or antacids. See Table 13-3 for a summary of laxatives. The need for mixtures of laxatives has not been documented. The actions of various laxatives make it apparent that combinations are unnecessary and may produce harmful or undesirable effects. They also tend to be more expensive than drugs sold individually. A partial listing of available mixtures is provided in Table 13-4, but it is not recommended that combinations be used.

▼ Evaluation

Laxatives should be used only for short periods and should not require any patient monitoring. If for any reason they are used on a long-term basis, question the patient about bowel habits, diet, and exercise and monitor for adverse reactions. Many of the stimulant laxatives discolor alkaline urine red-pink; acid urine yellow-brown. They may give a reddish color to feces.

▼ Patient and family teaching

The nurse should provide the patient and family with the following instructions:

1. Bulk-forming laxatives require large amounts of fluid to work properly; they should never be chewed or swallowed without water. The patient must take at least one full glass of liquid with each dose.
2. Laxatives should be taken exactly as specified by the physician and are indicated for short-term use only. Overuse of laxatives robs the bowel of its ability to perform effectively on its own.
3. Some agents are high in sodium or glucose. The content should be checked if the patient's diet is restricted.
4. Laxatives should be used only as additional

Geriatric Considerations
LAXATIVES, NONPHARMACOLOGIC

Elderly patients often frequently use and abuse laxatives even though studies have indicated that 80% to 90% of persons over 60 years old have at least one bowel movement daily.

To reduce the potential for chronic laxative use and dependency, the patient should be taught nonpharmacologic measures, such as increasing fluid intake to 6 to 8 glasses of water/day if permitted and tolerated. Also recommended is a regular exercise routine, such as a daily walk or active and passive exercise for bedridden patients.

The nurse should obtain a dietary and laxative history from the patient. Consistent intake of a low-fiber diet or a regular intake of foods that tend to harden stools, such as processed cheese, hard-boiled eggs, liver, cottage cheese, high–sugar content foods, and rice, may result in constipation.

High-fiber or high-residue diets along with adequate fluid intake serve to accelerate food transport time in the gastrointentinal tract and exert a mild laxative effect.

High-fiber foods include orange juice with pulp or a fresh orange, bran or whole grain cereals, whole grain or bran breads, leafy vegetables, and fresh fruits. While prunes, bananas, figs, and dates are high in dietary fiber, prunes also contain a laxative substance that stimulates intestinal motility pharmacologically.

McKenry LM, Salerno E: *Mosby's pharmacology in nursing,* ed 18, St Louis, 1992, Mosby.

therapy to good, regular bowel habits, daily exercise, and the use of high-bulk foods and fruits in diet to help maintain regularity.
5. Bulk-forming laxatives should not be taken within 2 hours of any other medications.
6. Allergic reactions may occur. If rash, itching, nasal congestion, or wheezing occurs, the patient should stop taking the medication immediately and contact the physician.
7. The laxative effect of bulk-forming laxatives may occur within 12 hours or may take up to 3 days to appear. Fecal softener preparations act within 24 to 48 hours. Lactulose may require 24 to 48 hours to produce a normal bowel movement. Saline laxatives produce results within 2 to 8 hours and should not be taken at bedtime. The fastest effect of hyperosmolar products is obtained when the drug is taken on an empty stomach with a full glass of water. Mineral oil should not be taken within 2 hours of taking

Table 13-3   Laxatives

Generic name	Trade name	Comments and dosage
BULK-FORMING LAXATIVES		
Methylcellulose	Citrucel Murocel ♣ Unifiber	Produces a laxative effect in 12 to 72 hours. All doses should be taken with one full glass or more of liquid. *Adults:* 5 to 20 ml liquid PO tid with a full glass of water; or 1 to 3 capsules or tablets may be taken PO qid with meals and at bedtime.
Psyllium seed	Fiberall Metamucil	This product is indigestible, nonabsorbed, and does not interfere with absorption of nutrients. These laxatives are least likely to cause laxative abuse. *Adults:* 1 to 2 teaspoonfuls PO in full glass of water qd to tid; follow by second glass of water.
FECAL SOFTENERS OR WETTING AGENTS		
Docusate	Colace Dialose Regutol Modane	Give 50 to 200 mg PO qd.
HYPEROSMOLAR OR SALINE LAXATIVES		
Lactulose	Cholac Cephulac	Available by prescription only. *Adults:* 15 to 30 ml PO qd; may be increased to 60 ml PO qd if necessary.
Magnesium	Milk of Magnesia Magnesium citrate Magnesium sulfate	Magnesium sulfate is the most potent of the products within this group. *Milk of Magnesia:* 30 to 60 ml PO, usually at bedtime. *Magnesium citrate:* 5 to 10 oz PO at bedtime. *Magnesium sulfate:* 15 mg (4 teaspoons) in a glass of water.
Sodium salts	Fleet enema Phospho-soda	Up to 10% of the sodium in these products may be absorbed. *Oral:* 20 ml PO mixed with half a glass of water; follow with another full glass of water; should be taken on arising in the morning. *Enema:* 4 ounces PR for adults; 2½ ounces for children over 2 years.
Glycerin	Sani-Supp	*Suppository:* Use 1 and retain for 15 minutes.
LUBRICANT LAXATIVES		
Mineral oil	Mineral oil	Mineral oil is used orally and also given rectally as an enema for retention and softening. It should be given at least 2 hours after meals. *Adults:* 15 to 30 ml PO at bedtime. *Children over 6 years:* 5 to 15 ml PO; PR: 4 oz given as enema.
STIMULANT OR IRRITANT LAXATIVES		
Bisacodyl	Bisco-Lax Dulcolax	Enteric-coated tablets must be swallowed whole; do not chew or crush. Do not take within 1 hour of antacids or milk. Drink at least one full glass of water with each dose. Suppository should be inserted at time bowel movement is desired; acts within 15 to 60 minutes. Enema is administered rectally at time evacuation is desired. *Adults:* 10 to 15 mg PO in evening or before breakfast. Up to 30 mg PO may be safely used in preparation for special procedures.
Cascara sagrada	Cascara sagrada	The fluid extract contains 18% alcohol. Under various brand names some tablets are sugar coated, others are uncoated. They may discolor alkaline urine red-pink, and acidic urine yellow-brown. *Adults:* Aromatic: 5 ml qd with full glass of water; plain: 1 ml PO qd with glass of water; tablet: one 325 mg tablet at bedtime.
Castor oil	Alphamul Neoloid	Ice held in mouth helps prevent tasting the drug. For best results give on empty stomach. Produces results within 3 hours. For emulsion preparation, shake well. *Adults:* 15 to 60 ml PO.

Continued.

Table 13-3	Laxatives—cont'd	
Generic name	Trade name	Comments and dosage
Phenolphthalein	Ex-Lax Feen-a-mint	The laxative effect may last 3 to 4 days. It may cause a characteristic skin rash, and drug should be discontinued and patient advised to avoid sun exposure until rash has disappeared. *Adults:* 90 to 180 mg tablet, chewed well, night or morning. *Children:* 45 to 90 mg tablet, chewed well, night or morning.
Senna	Senokot	May cause yellow or yellow-green cast to feces, red-pink discoloration of alkaline urine; yellow-brown color in acid urine. Give 1 to 8 tablets/day PO.

Table 13-4	Laxative combination products
Trade name	Chemical combinations
Dialose Plus	Docusate sodium, methylcellulose, casanthranol
Correctol	Docusate sodium, phenolphthalein
Doxidan	Docusate calcium, phenolphthalein
Haley's MO	Milk of magnesia, mineral oil
Peri-Colace	Casanthranol, docusate sodium
Senokot-S	Senna, docusate sodium

food or other medication. The stimulant laxatives act within 6 to 10 hours, except castor oil, which acts within 1 to 3 hours. The laxative effect of phenolphthaleins may last up to 4 days. The stimulant laxatives include many of the chewing gum and chocolate types and are the kind most often abused.

8. Fecal softeners should be used only as additional therapy to good, regular bowel habits, daily exercise, and the use of high bulk in the diet to help maintain regularity. They do not treat preexisting constipation, but prevent constipation from developing.

9. The patient should take milk or fruit juice with fecal softeners to mask the bitter taste. The flavor of the hyperosmolar laxatives may be improved by taking the medication with fruit juice or a citrus-flavored carbonated beverage. Fruit juices or carbonated drinks may help disguise the oily taste of lubricant laxatives.

10. The physician or nurse should give the patient a list of foods high in bulk that can assist in maintaining bowel regularity.

11. Saline laxatives should not be taken daily or used in children under 6 years of age.

12. Large doses of lubricant laxatives may cause a leakage of oil from the rectum. The use of pads to protect clothing may be necessary if tight sphincter control is not present.

SECTION FOUR: MISCELLANEOUS GASTROINTESTINAL MEDICATIONS

Objectives

At the conclusion of this section you should be able to:

1. Identify medications commonly used as antiflatulents.
2. Describe uses of digestive enzymes.
3. Indicate use and adverse effects of emetics.
4. Describe actions of chenodiol on gallstones.
5. Define "disulfiram reaction" and explain when the medication is used.

OVERVIEW

There are many disease processes and symptoms that affect the gastrointestinal tract; there are also many medications used in their treatment. **Antiflatulents,** such as simethicone, disperse and prevent the formation of mucus-surrounded pockets of gas in the intestine. Pancreatic digestive enzymes are used as replacement therapy for individuals with pancreatic enzyme insufficiency. Emetics are used primarily in emergency situations to produce vomiting by direct action on the vomiting center. Chenodiol acts on the liver to increase dissolution of radiolucent cholesterol gallstones. Disulfiram is used in alcoholic patients to produce a severe sensitivity to alcohol. Each of these drugs will be briefly described.

ANTIFLATULENTS

ACTION

Simethicone is an antiflatulent that breaks up gastrointestinal gas bubbles through a defoaming action so that they may be more easily expelled by belching or as flatus. Mucus surrounding the gas bubbles is dispersed, and the gas bubbles coalesce, freeing the gas. Gastric pain is then reduced.

USES

Antiflatulents are used to treat problems that produce bloating, flatulence, or postoperative gas pains. They may also be used for chronic air-swallowing, functional dyspepsia, peptic ulcer, spastic or irritable colon, and diverticulitis. The patient may complain of being bloated or distended, of feeling "full" or gaseous, or of frequent belching. Gas pains may also be noted, especially after surgery. The nurse should determine if the flatulence is of dietary origin and whether changing the diet may decrease the symptoms. Antiflatulents are often used in combination with antacid therapy. This medication is intended for short-term use only. More rigorous evaluation should be undertaken if symptoms do not disappear with therapy.

GALLSTONE SOLUBILIZING AGENTS

ACTION

Gallstone solubilizing agents act on the liver to suppress cholesterol and cholic acid synthesis. Biliary cholesterol desaturation is enhanced, and dissolution of radiolucent cholesterol gallstones eventually occurs. There is no effect on calcified or radiopaque gallstones or radiolucent bile pigment stones.

USES

Gallstone solubilizing agents are useful in selected patients with radiolucent stones in well-opacifying gallbladders. These patients are poor surgical risks because of disease or advanced age. Success is likely to be higher with small and floatable stones.

ADVERSE REACTIONS

Adverse reactions to gallstone solubilizing agents may include dose-related diarrhea, anorexia, constipation, cramps, dyspepsia, epigastric distress, flatulence, heartburn, nausea, nonspecific abdominal pain, and vomiting. Laboratory tests may be altered; nonspecific decreases in white cell count may also develop.

DRUG INTERACTIONS

Biliary cholesterol secretion and incidence of gallstones may be increased by estrogens, clofibrate, and oral contraceptives. Therefore those drugs may counteract the effectiveness of gallstone solubilizing agents. Bile acid sequestering agents such as cholestyramine and colestipol may reduce the absorption of gallstone solubilizing agents. Aluminum-based antacids may absorb bile acids and reduce the absorption of gallstone solubilizing agents also.

These medications should not be used in patients with known liver or other gallbladder disease. If the gallbladder fails to visualize after two consecutive single doses of dye, or if radiopaque or radiolucent bile pigment stones are seen, these medications should not be used. These products may produce hepatic toxicity, ranging from mildly toxic to fatal hepatic failure. They should be used only in patients without previous hepatic problems, and careful monitoring of patient liver function is mandatory. There is also the possibility that chenodiol therapy might contribute to the development of colon cancers in susceptible individuals.

If diarrhea develops, reducing the dosage will usually eliminate the symptoms. The patient is usually able to resume higher dosages without recurrence of diarrhea.

Stone recurrence can be expected within 5 years in 50% of all patients using gallstone solubilizing agents. Low-cholesterol, low-carbohydrate diets with increased dietary bran may help reduce biliary cholesterol. Weight reduction may help to postpone stone recurrence.

Evaluation of patient compliance is important in considering this product as part of the therapeutic regimen. The patient must be reliable in keeping appointments, reporting problems, and undergoing periodic health evaluations.

DIGESTIVE ENZYMES

ACTION

Digestive enzymes promote digestion by acting as replacement therapy when enzymes are lacking, not secreted, or not absorbed properly. They are obtained from pork pancreas. Healthy patients may find a decrease in intestinal gas with medication.

USES

Digestive enzymes are often indicated for individuals with poor digestion, for predigestive purposes, and as replacement therapy. They may be used to relieve the symptoms associated with cystic fibrosis, cancer of the pancreas, or chronic inflammation of the pancreas causing malabsorption syndromes. Patients who have had gastrointestinal bypass surgery may also benefit. Obstruction of the pancreatic or common bile duct by a neoplasm may prompt need for this drug.

ADVERSE REACTIONS

If proper dietary balance of fat, protein, and starch is not maintained, temporary indigestion may develop. Nausea, abdominal cramps, and diarrhea have been reported in patients taking high doses. Inhalation of powder may provoke asthma.

DRUG INTERACTIONS

Antacids containing calcium carbonate or magnesium hydroxide may cancel out the therapeutic effect of digestive enzymes. In addition, serum iron levels caused by iron supplements may be decreased by these preparations.

 NURSING IMPLICATIONS AND PATIENT TEACHING

The patient may complain of sudden intense pain in the gastric region, hiccups, belching of gas, vomiting, constipation, pain radiating to the back, weakness, diarrhea, indigestion, ravenous appetite without weight gain, and chronic cough and infections.

Those individuals hypersensitive to pork protein should avoid this therapy. The patient should avoid inhaling the powdered form or allowing it to come into contact with the skin, because irritation may be produced.

Digestive enzymes are administered with meals or snacks. They are available in tablet or capsule form, which is swallowed, not chewed. It also comes in a powder, or the capsules may be opened and sprinkled on food for those who have difficulty swallowing tablets. Medication granules are not to be taken without food, because this will destroy the enzymes.

The therapeutic dosage may be determined after several weeks of therapy and adjusted accordingly. Different flavors are provided by the product manufacturers.

The nurse should monitor the patient for the therapeutic effect and the absence of adverse reactions. Questioning the patient about the appearance of stools may help evaluate the degree of malabsorption present.

▼ **Patient and family teaching**

The nurse should provide the patient and family with the following instructions:

1. The patient should take this medication exactly as ordered. The capsules or tablets should be swallowed at mealtime, or the capsules of powder can be opened and sprinkled on the food if the patient has difficulty swallowing pills.
2. The granules should always be taken with meals or snacks. The body will destroy the granules and not receive any benefit from them if the patient does not take food with them.
3. The patient must be careful not to inhale the powder or touch it with the hands when opening the powder and pouring it. Direct exposure to the powder produces a strong irritation.
4. The patient should eat a well-balanced diet, with adequate amounts of fat, starch, and protein. The patient should develop and maintain a normal eating routine; this will help prevent indigestion.
5. The patient should experiment with various flavors of medication until he or she finds the ones that are most palatable.
6. The patient should report any discomfort or troublesome symptoms to the practitioner.

DISULFIRAM

ACTION

Disulfiram produces a severe sensitivity to alcohol that results in an extremely unpleasant reaction when even small amounts of alcohol are ingested. This drug promotes excessive accumulation of acetaldehyde by inhibiting the normal liver enzyme activity after the conversion of alcohol to acetaldehyde. Increased levels of acetaldehyde produce the **disulfiram reaction.** The reaction is present until the metabolism of alcohol is completed. The intensity of the reaction is variable, but it is usually proportional to the amounts of disulfiram and alcohol ingested.

A disulfiram reaction may include the following symptoms: flushing and warming of the face, severe throbbing headache, shortness of breath, chest pain, nausea, vomiting, sweating, weakness, hyperventilation, tachycardia, syncope, and confusion. Severe reactions could include dysrhythmias, respiratory distress, cardiovascular collapse, myocardial infarction, acute congestive heart failure, convulsions, and death.

USES

Disulfiram is specific for the management of alcoholism. It is used as a deterrent to alcohol intake, which enables development of a state of enforced sobriety. This drug is an adjunct to psychiatric therapy or alcoholic counseling and is used in patients who are motivated and fully cooperative.

ADVERSE REACTIONS

Disulfiram may produce drowsiness, fatigue, headache, optic neuritis (with impaired vision, decreased color perception, and blindness), psychotic reactions, restlessness, acneiform eruptions, dry mouth, elevation of serum liver enzyme levels, hepatotoxicity, metallic or garliclike aftertaste, and impotence.

DRUG INTERACTIONS

Use of disulfiram with even small amounts of alcohol produces a severe reaction. Concurrent use of disulfiram increases the effects of anticoagulants, phenytoins, and barbiturates and may increase the side effects of isoniazid. Concurrent use with metronidazole and marijuana has an additive effect and may produce

psychotic episodes. Exaggerated clinical effects of diazepam and chlordiazepoxide are produced with concurrent use of this drug. Use with paraldehyde may produce disulfiram-alcohol reactions. Some medications, such as metronidazole, produce a similar reaction when taken with alcohol. Patients must be warned of these disulfiram-like reactions.

 NURSING IMPLICATIONS AND
PATIENT TEACHING

Disulfiram should not be used if the patient has ingested alcohol in any form within the last 12 hours. This includes the use of cough mixtures, tonics, vinegars, sauces, after-shave lotions, backrubbing solutions, creams, or other products containing alcohol. Do not use disulfiram if there has been recent ingestion of paraldehyde or metronidazole. Do not use in the presence of severe myocardial disease or coronary occlusion, psychoses, or hypersensitivity to disulfiram. Do not use disulfiram in pediatric patients.

Disulfiram should be used with extreme caution in patients with any of the following conditions: diabetes mellitus, epilepsy, cerebral damage, hypothyroidism, chronic and acute nephritis, hepatic cirrhosis or insufficiency, conditions requiring multiple drug usage, coronary artery disease, and hypertension. In these patients there is the possibility of an accidental disulfiram reaction.

The patient should give permission for disulfiram therapy. The patient and a responsible family member need to understand the consequences of this therapy. Disulfiram reactions may occur for up to 2 weeks after a single dose of disulfiram. The longer a patient takes this drug, the more sensitive he or she will become to alcohol. The disulfiram reaction may be provoked by even small amounts of alcohol. The patient should be cautioned against hidden forms of alcohol (tonics, cough syrups, after-shave lotions).

Disulfiram users should wear a bracelet or card identifying them as users of this drug and describing the symptoms most likely to occur in the disulfiram reaction. Cards may be obtained from the pharmaceutical company to give to patients on this therapy.

The patient should be actively involved in support and counseling to reduce psychologic dependence and should be monitored for compliance and for development of adverse effects.

EMETICS

ACTION

Emetics are drugs used in emergency situations to remove poisons from the stomach before they can be absorbed. They have largely replaced gastric lavage as the treatment of choice in management of poisoning or drug overdosage. Except in situations for which they are contraindicated, emetics are superior to lavage for rapid elimination of poisons before extensive absorption of gastric contents can occur. There are only two emetics commonly used in current clinical practice: apomorphine and syrup of ipecac. Apomorphine is given by injection and acts directly on the CNS. Syrup of ipecac acts primarily as a gastric irritant to produce vomiting. After ingestion it stimulates the chemoreceptor trigger zone in the brain to induce vomiting.

USES

Ipecac is used when toxic substances are swallowed, to empty the stomach before the toxins can be absorbed.

ADVERSE REACTIONS

Ipecac is not absorbed and has no systemic effect, unless vomiting does not occur within 30 minutes. If the drug is absorbed or an excessive dose is ingested, it may cause cardiac dysrhythmias, atrial fibrillation, or other cardiotoxic effects. For this reason, gastric lavage is necessary if vomiting does not occur within 30 minutes.

DRUG INTERACTIONS

Ipecac should not be given with activated charcoal, because the charcoal will absorb the ipecac, neutralizing the emetic effect.

 NURSING IMPLICATIONS AND PATIENT TEACHING

Vomiting should never be induced after ingestion of corrosive or caustic substances such as lye; regurgitation will only expose the esophagus to additional injury.

Emetics should never be used in unconscious patients, in those who are convulsing, severely inebriated, in shock, or who have loss of the gag reflex.

Always make certain you are giving ipecac *syrup,* not just ipecac, to avoid confusion with the fluid extract, which is 14 times more concentrated.

The nurse should obtain a complete history from the patient or anyone who can give details about what was swallowed, when, and what has happened since that time. A local poison control center should be consulted if the nurse is uncertain how to proceed. If two doses do not produce vomiting within 30 minutes, referral and gastric lavage are necessary.

It is wise for patients to keep 1-oz bottles of syrup of ipecac readily available in their homes in case of a poisoning emergency.

Table 13-5 summarizes the important miscellaneous gastrointestinal medications.

SUMMARY

There are many medications used to treat the variety of diseases or disorders affecting the gastrointestinal tract. The major medications covered in this chapter are antacids, which neutralize or reduce stomach acidity; histamine H_2-receptor antagonists, which inhibit the action of histamine at receptor cells in the stomach; anticholinergics and antispasmodics, which reduce gastric motility and decrease acid secretions; antidiarrheals, which reduce diarrhea; laxatives, which promote emptying of the bowel; antiflatulents, which reduce gas and bloating; digestive enzymes, which break down fats, starches, and proteins; and emetics, which produce vomiting. Many of these medications are used by the patient as self-medications. It is therefore important that the nurse teach the patient or family about significant adverse reactions to watch for and any special administration considerations, such as fluid intake or avoidance of certain foods.

 CRITICAL THINKING QUESTIONS

1. Describe, overall, the differences in actions and uses among the three major types of gastrointestinal medications. Within the second group, compare and contrast the actions of the anticholinergic and antispasmodic medications.

2. Ms. McKelvey has been taking over-the-counter antacids for her stomach ulcer. Now, however, the clinic physician has prescribed the addition of a histamine H_2-receptor

Table 13-5   Miscellaneous gastrointestinal medications

Generic name	Trade name	Comments and dosage
ANTIFLATULENTS		
Charcoal	CharcoCaps	520 to 975 mg after meals or at first sign of discomfort; repeat prn.
Simethicone	Mylanta Gas Mylicon Ovol ♣	Available in both drops and tablet form. Chew tablets thoroughly before swallowing. Shake drops well before using. Give 40 to 80 mg tablets after each meal and at bedtime, or use 40 mg (0.6 ml) drops qid after meals and at bedtime.
GALLSTONE DISSOLUTION		
Chenodiol	Chenix	Recommended dosage range is 13 to 16 mg/kg/day in two divided doses taken morning and evening. Increase dosage by 250 mg/day each week until the recommended or tolerated dose is obtained. Dosages less than 10 mg/kg are usually ineffective and may, in fact, contribute to increased risk of cholecystectomy. Give 3 to 7 tablets/day based on patient's weight.
Monoctanoin	Moctanin	Given by physician as a direct perfusion into biliary tract.
Ursodiol	Actigall	Give 8 to 10 mg/kg/day in two or three divided doses.
DIGESTIVE ENZYMES		
Pancreatin	Dizymes Hi-Vegi-Lip Creon	This product tends to be cheaper than pancrelipase, although it is not as effective. Give 325 mg to 1 gm with meals.
Pancrelipase	Cotazym Cotazym-S Viokase Ku-Zyme HP Pancrease	Pancrelipase is a prescription drug combination of the pancreatic enzymes used in replacement therapy. It works more effectively than pancreatin. It provides a catalyst effect in the hydrolyzation of fats, proteins, and starch. The amount of dietary fat is the key to dosage. For every 17 gm of fat, 300 mg of pancrelipase should be taken. Use 1 to 3 capsules or tablets (or 1 to 2 packets) just before each meal or snack.
ANTIALCOHOLIC PRODUCT		
Disulfiram	Antabuse	The adult dosage is up to 500 mg daily for 1 to 2 weeks, followed by 125 to 500 mg daily for maintenance. It may take up to 3 weeks for the drug to reach full effectiveness, and drug is still effective for up to 2 weeks after therapy is discontinued. The average maintenance dosage is 250 mg daily. Maintenance therapy is needed until the patient is fully recovered socially and a basis for permanent self-control has been established. This may take months or even years.
EMETICS		
Apomorphine	Apomorphine	*Adults:* 5 mg SQ. *Children:* 0.1 mg/kg SQ. Do not repeat.
Ipecac	Syrup of ipecac	Do not confuse with fluid extract ipecac, which is 14 times more concentrated. *Over 1 year:* 1 tablespoon (15 ml) followed by 2 to 3 glasses of water (200 to 300 ml). *Under 1 year:* 2 teaspoons followed by 1 to 2 glasses of water. Dose may be repeated once after 20 minutes if vomiting does not occur.

antagonist. When the physician leaves the room, Ms. McKelvey tells you that she is unhappy about this, because she has prided herself on keeping her "medical costs" down by using only home remedies and over-the-counter drugs. "If they're both for ulcers," she says, "then what's the difference? Why can't I just double my dose of the antacid?" Draw up an informal teaching chart that would make it easy for Ms. McKelvey to see the differences between these two drugs in their actions and uses. Then add appropriate precautions and dietary instructions. (Don't forget to mention constipation and the more serious hypermagnesemia.)

3. Explain why adverse reactions are more frequent with anticholinergics than with antidiarrheals.

4. Mrs. Harris, 82, has been admitted to the hospital for treatment of severe diarrhea. She is placed on antidiarrheal therapy and admitted to your unit for inpatient treatment and observation. Identify signs of dehydration and electrolyte imbalance, as well as any adverse reactions that might be associated with antidiarrheal therapy, particularly in the elderly.

5. On the second day of treatment, Mrs. Harris does show signs of both dehydration and electrolyte imbalance, as you had anticipated. Draw up a treatment plan for this patient.

6. Mr. Weigand has been using fecal softeners on an almost daily basis "for quite a while," he says, but is still having trouble with constipation. The physician has examined Mr. Weigand and tells him that he needs to be switched to a lubricant-type laxative instead of the softeners. Mr. Weigand is uncomfortable with this and asks you why he can't use his "old stand-by." Explain the different actions of the five types of laxatives, the advantages of each, as well as their varying adverse reactions.

7. What is chenodiol, and why is it prescribed? What can contribute to its adverse reactions? In what disorders should this drug be avoided? Why?

8. Mrs. Magid has been prescribed a digestive enzyme. What are the possible indications for this drug? What kind of patient teaching would be necessary to give Mrs. Magid about this drug? How can she minimize adverse reactions?

9. What is a "disulfiram reaction"? Why is disulfiram prescribed? Explain why patient compliance is so important with this drug.

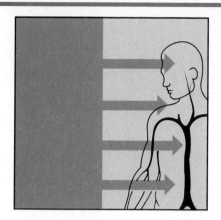

CHAPTER **14**

Hematologic Products

KEY TERMS

anticoagulants, p. 301
fibrin, p. 301
fibrinogen, p. 301
thrombi, p. 301
thromboplastin, p. 301

OVERVIEW

There are three major groups of medications that have hematologic effects. They are the anticoagulants (heparin and coumarin), the heparin antagonist (protamine sulfate), and the vitamins, minerals, or chemicals essential for proper red cell development and function (vitamin K, vitamin B_{12}, iron, and folic acid). This chapter discusses the first two groups and folic acid (the other essential vitamins and minerals are presented in Chapter 19).

ANTICOAGULANTS

One of the body's protective functions is to clot blood in response to tissue injury. Cellular damage results in the formation of **thromboplastin,** which then acts on prothrombin to form thrombin. Calcium must be present for this reaction to occur. Thrombin then acts on **fibrinogen** (a protein found in the blood plasma) to produce **fibrin,** a netlike substance that traps red and white blood cells and platelets and forms the matrix of the clot. Vitamin K must be present to produce prothrombin and other clotting factors produced in the liver. All **anticoagulants** prevent the formation of blood clots, or **thrombi,** by interfering with the complex clotting mechanism of blood. In

301

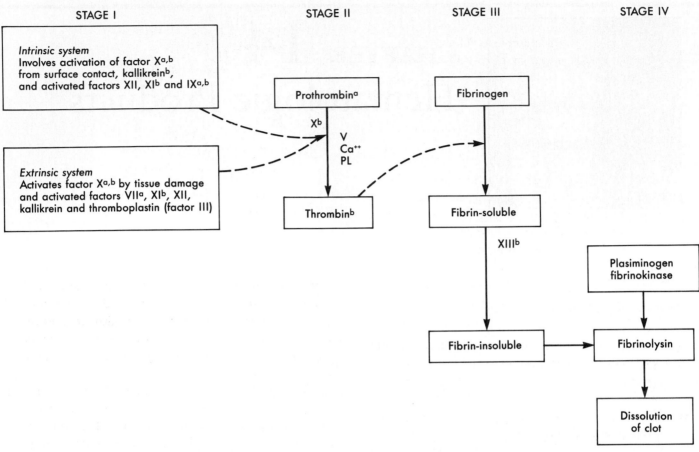

Fig. 14-1 Blood coagulation and clot resolution.

cases of overdosage, protamine sulfate is given to counteract the effect of heparin. In response to some bleeding disorders, vitamin K may be given either orally or parenterally to manufacture prothrombin and serve as an anticoagulant antagonist (see Chapter 19).

ACTION

There are two major categories of anticoagulants. The first category, the coumarin and indandione derivatives, limits formation of blood coagulation factors II, VII, IX, and X in the liver by interfering with vitamin K. These drugs do not destroy existing blood clots; however, they may limit the extension of existing blood clots or thrombi.

The second category, heparin sodium, acts at multiple sites in the normal coagulation system to stop reactions that lead to the clotting of blood and the formation of fibrin clots. It increases the action of antithrombin III (heparin cofactor) on several other

coagulation factors, primarily factor Xa, to slow new clot development. Heparin does not dissolve existing clots either (Fig. 14-1), although new products do.

USES

As part of the circulatory system, the arterial vessels carry oxygenated blood throughout the body. If these small arteries become plugged with clots made of fibrin, platelets, and cholesterol, death may result. Abnormal blood clotting may produce a coronary artery occlusion or blockage, or small emboli may break off from thrombophlebitis in the lower extremities and travel and block areas of the brain or lung (Fig. 14-2). Drugs that can slow or reduce clotting, then, are very helpful.

Anticoagulant therapy is used to prevent new clot formation or the increase in size of existing clots. Anticoagulant therapy is used prophylactically during and after many types of surgery, (especially surgery involving the heart or circulation), in heart valve disease, in some dysrhythmias, and in patients receiving hemodialysis. Any patient on bed rest for a long time is at risk for development of blood clots, especially patients with a history of clotting problems or recent orthopedic, thoracic, or abdominal surgery. Heparin is the anticoagulant of choice when an immediate effect is needed. For long-term therapy, a coumarin or indandione derivative is used. The FDA has classified coumarin preparations as "possibly" effective as part of the therapy for treatment of transient cerebral ischemic attacks. Indandione derivatives (phenindione) are used to treat pulmonary emboli and as prophylaxis to treat deep vein thrombosis, myocardial infarction, rheumatic heart disease with valve damage, and atrial dysrhythmias. Low-intensity coumarin therapy (prothrombin time ratio between 1.2 and 1.5) greatly decreases the risk of stroke from nonrheumatic atrial fibrillation, and has few side effects.

ADVERSE REACTIONS

Warfarin may produce hair loss, rash, urticaria, cramping, diarrhea, intestinal obstruction, nausea, paralytic ileus, vomiting, excessive uterine bleeding, hemorrhage with excessive dosage, leukopenia, and fever.

Heparin sodium may produce elevated blood pressure; headache; hematoma, irritation and pain at the injection site; conjunctivitis; tearing of eyes; rhinitis; frequent or persistent erection; hemorrhage; thrombocytopenia; shortness of breath; wheezing; chills; fever; hair loss; and hypersensitivity reaction.

Early signs of overdosage or internal bleeding include bleeding from gums while brushing teeth, excessive bleeding or oozing from cuts, unexplained bruising or nosebleeds, and unusually heavy or unexpected menses in women. Signs suggesting internal bleeding are abdominal pain or swelling, back pain, bloody or tarry stools, bloody or cloudy urine, constipation (resulting from paralytic ileus or intestinal obstruction), coughing up blood, dizziness, severe or continuous headaches, and vomiting blood or "coffee-ground" substance.

DRUG INTERACTIONS

Other anticoagulants (coumarin or indandione derivatives), methimazole, and propylthiouracil increase the anticoagulant effect of heparin.

Antihistamines, digitalis, nicotine, and tetracy-

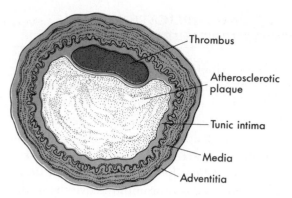

Fig. 14-2   Occlusion of an atherosclerotic coronary artery by a thrombus.

clines decrease the anticoagulant effect of heparin.

Acetylsalicylic acid, coumarin-derivative anticoagulants, dextran, nonsteroidal antiinflammatory-analgesic medications, and other selected drugs increase the risk of bleeding and hemorrhage in a patient receiving heparin.

Acetylsalicylic acid, corticotropin, ethacrynic acid, glucocorticoids, and nonsteroidal antiinflammatory-analgesic medications increase the risk of gastrointestinal bleeding and hemorrhage in a patient receiving heparin.

Allopurinol, aminosalicylic acid, anabolic steroids, antibiotics, androgens, many sedatives, some antacids, dextran, disulfiram, drugs affecting blood elements, glucagon, heparin, narcotics (with prolonged use), phenylbutazone, propylthiouracil, quinidine, quinine, salicylates, thyroid drugs, and vitamin E increase prothombin time response of patients receiving coumarin.

Adrenocorticosteroids, antacids, antihistamines, barbiturates, contraceptives (oral), estrogens, griseofulvin, haloperidol, meprobamate, primidone, rifampin, thiazide diuretics, and vitamin K decrease the prothrombin time response of a patient on coumarin.

Anticoagulant effects may be increased with acute alcohol intoxication and decreased with chronic alcohol abuse. Oral hypoglycemics taken with anticoagulants may increase the effect of either the hypoglycemic or anticoagulant.

Alkylating agents, antimetabolites, corticosteroids, ethacrynic acid, indomethacin, quinidine, and salicylates increase the risk of bleeding in a patient taking coumarin.

NURSING IMPLICATIONS AND
PATIENT TEACHING

Patients requiring rapid anticoagulation are commonly hospitalized. Coagulation and prothrombin tests are ordered when the patient is started on anticoagulants. Heparin is usually started for an immediate effect and then oral anticoagulants are started. Thereafter, the physician orders coagulation and prothrombin tests at regular intervals. When the oral anticoagulant shows proper effect and the prothrombin activity is in the therapeutic range, heparin therapy may be stopped and the oral anticoagulant therapy continued.

The standard tests for determining the general effect of heparin on clotting are the Lee-White whole blood clotting time, the whole blood activated partial thromboplastin time (WBAPTT), and the activated partial thromboplastin time (APTT). The most commonly used test is the APTT. The dosage of heparin is considered adequate when the whole blood clotting time is approximately 2½ to 3 times the control value.

Traditionally, prothrombin tests were used to determine the dosage for coumarin preparations. Initially, prothrombin tests were done daily until the results stabilized in the therapeutic range (1½ to 2½ times the normal control value). After stabilization, the tests were done at 1- to 4-week intervals, depending on patient status.

In the last two years the medical literature has suggested replacing the prothrombin time test with a new monitoring formula that standardizes the clotting time results among different laboratories. The international numerical ratio (INR) uses the patient's prothrombin time, the control prothrombin time, and an international sensitivity index figure to calculate the clotting time. Laboratories throughout the world are switching to this new formula.

▼ Assessment

The nurse should obtain a complete health history, including the presence of hypersensitivity, underlying systemic disease, current nature of the problem, and use of medications, and should inquire about conditions that would contraindicate use of some anticoagulants, such as alcoholism, blood dyscrasias, bleeding tendencies of gastrointestinal, genitourinary, or respiratory tracts, or malignant hypertension. Patients with congestive heart failure may be more sensitive to coumarin anticoagulants and indandione derivatives.

Heparin is derived from animal tissue and should be used with caution in any patient with a history of allergy. This drug should be used cautiously in the presence of hepatic or renal disease or hypertension, during menses, or in patients with indwelling catheters. A higher incidence of bleeding may be seen in women over the age of 60.

Make sure that female patients taking a coumarin or indandione derivative are not pregnant or breastfeeding. These drugs are usually not given to children. There are many medical and surgical contraindications to the use of these drugs, particularly in patients who have recently had surgery, trauma, or obstetric complications.

▼ Planning

The dosages listed for heparin are given in USP heparin units. Heparin is not effective given orally and should be given by intermittent IV injection, IV infusion, or deep SQ (intrafat) injection. Heparin should not be given intramuscularly because of the frequent development of hematomas, irritation, and pain at the injection site. Use a small needle (25 gauge) and a tuberculin syringe.

▼ Implementation

Anticoagulant drugs should not be used if there are inadequate laboratory facilities or if the patient is uncooperative in taking medications or keeping appointments for laboratory and health assessment. Coumarin derivatives should not be used in a patient undergoing diagnostic or therapeutic procedures with potential for uncontrolled bleeding.

The sites of intrafat injections of heparin should be rotated to avoid formation of hematomas. The nurse must not attempt to aspirate blood before injection and must not move the needle while the solution is being injected. Injection sites should not be massaged before or after injection. Patients receiving heparin are not good candidates for IM injections of other medications, because hematomas and bleeding into adjacent areas may occur.

If the solution is discolored or contains a precipitate, it must not be used. Heparin is strongly acidic and is chemically incompatible with many other medications in solution, so it must not be piggybacked with other drugs into an infusion line. Never mix any drug with heparin in a syringe when bolus therapy is given.

If intermittent IV therapy is being given, blood for partial thromboplastin time determination should be drawn ½ hour before the next scheduled heparin dose. Blood for partial thromboplastin time determination can be drawn anytime after 8 hours of continuous intravenous heparin therapy. However, blood should not be drawn from the tubing of the heparin infusion line or from the vein of infusion. Blood should always be drawn from the arm not being used for heparin infusion.

If heparin is being given simultaneously with a coumarin or an indandione derivative, blood should not be drawn for prothrombin time within 5 hours of IV heparin administration, or 24 hours if heparin is given subcutaneously. IV heparin infusions should be checked frequently, even if pumps are in good working order, to ensure that the proper dosage is being administered.

If anticoagulant therapy is initiated with heparin and continued with a coumarin or an indandione derivative, it is recommended that both drugs be given concurrently until the prothrombin time determinations indicate an adequate response to the coumarin or indandione derivative.

See Table 14-1 for a summary of anticoagulants.

▼ Evaluation

If heparin is given by continuous IV infusion, the coagulation time should be determined every 4 hours in the early stages of treatment.

The nurse should watch for signs of overdosage of anticoagulants and internal bleeding as therapy progresses.

▼ Patient and family teaching

The nurse should provide the patient and family with the following instructions:

1. The patient should take the oral medication only as directed. If a dose is missed, it should be taken as soon as possible, but not if it is almost time for the next dose. The doses should not be doubled. The patient should keep a record of all missed doses.
2. The patient will need regular INR time or coagulation tests and regular visits to the physician to ensure that blood clotting stays within special and narrow limits. The dosage may need to be altered from time to time, based on results of laboratory tests.
3. The patient should not take other medication without checking with the physician; this includes aspirin or any over-the-counter medicines.
4. The patient should wear a Medic-Alert bracelet or necklace and carry a medical information card explaining that the patient is taking an anticoagulant.
5. Patients should inform all physicians, dentists, or podiatrists whom they see for care that they are taking an anticoagulant.
6. The patient should use caution in brushing teeth, trimming nails, and shaving (an electric razor should be used when possible).
7. Pressure should be used to stop bleeding from accidental cuts or scrapes; if bleeding persists after 10 minutes, the physician should be called.
8. The patient should not engage in contact sports or other activities that could lead to injuries.
9. The patient should eat a normal, balanced diet, but should avoid eating excessive amounts of foods high in vitamin K (tomatoes, onions, dark leafy greens, bananas, or fish).
10. The patient should avoid alcohol.
11. The patient should know the possible side effects of anticoagulants: active bleeding or signs of bleeding such as tarry stools, blood in the urine, bleeding gums, nosebleeds, dizziness, coughing up blood, abdominal or joint pains, unexplained bruising, or unusually heavy or unexpected menstrual periods in women.
12. After anticoagulation therapy has been stopped, the patient should use caution until the body recovers its blood-clotting abilities.

> **Geriatric Considerations**
> **ANTICOAGULANTS**
>
> The elderly may be more susceptible to the effects of anticoagulants, and a lower maintenance dose is usually recommended for the geriatric patient along with very close supervision and monitoring.
>
> The primary adverse effects of excessive drug usage are prolonged bleeding from gums when brushing teeth or from small shaving cuts, excessive or easy skin bruising, blood in urine or stools, and unexplained nosebleeds. There may be early signs of overdose that indicate the need for medical intervention.
>
> Be aware that administration of concurrent drug therapy that may induce gastric irritation increases the risk for gastrointestinal bleeding. Drugs such as the nonsteroidal antiinflammatory agents (NSAIDs such as ibuprofen, indomethacin) that are commonly prescribed for the elderly patient often cause gastrointestinal effects.

From McKenry LM, Salerno E: *Mosby's pharmacology in nursing*, ed 18, St Louis, 1992, Mosby.

Table 14-1 Anticoagulants and other drugs affecting the blood

Generic name	Trade name	Comments and dosage
COUMARIN AND INDANDIONE DERIVATIVES		
Anisindione	Miradon	Give 300 mg the first day, 200 mg the second day, 100 mg the third day, and 25 to 250 mg daily thereafter, as indicated by prothrombin time or INR levels.
Warfarin (potassium)	Athrombin-K	Preferred anticoagulant if patient is getting antacids or phenytoin. Therapeutic effect in 36 to 72 hours (PO, IM, IV). When the medication is stopped, prothrombin activity returns to normal in 2 to 5 days. Give 10 to 15 mg PO qd for 2 to 4 days, then 2 to 10 mg qd as indicated by prothombin time or INR levels.
Warfarin (sodium)	Coumadin Panwarfin	Dosage same as with warfarin potassium.
HEPARIN		
Heparin	Heparin Liquaemin	Dosage is adjusted according to patient's coagulation time. Deep SQ: 10,000 to 20,000 USP units initially. Then 8000 to 10,000 USP units q8h. IV: 10,000 USP units initially, then 5000 to 10,000 USP units q4 to 6h. Give either undiluted or diluted with 50 to 100 ml of isotonic NaCl. IV infusion: Give 20,000 to 40,000 USP units in 1000 ml of isotonic NaCl solution over 24 hours. Loading dose of 5000 USP units may be given by IV injection. *Children* IV: 50 USP units/kg initially, then 50 to 100 USP units/kg q4h. IV infusion: 50 USP units/kg as a bolus initially, then 100 USP units/kg added and absorbed q4h.
Enoxaparin	Lovenox	Low–molecular weight heparin used to prevent deep vein thrombosis following hip replacement. Give 30 mg SQ bid for 7 to 10 days. Begin immediately following surgery.
FOLIC ACID AND DERIVATIVES		
Folic acid	Folvite	*Dietary supplement:* 100 µg (O.1 mg) per day (up to 1 mg per day in pregnancy); may be increased to 500 µg (0.5 mg) or 1 mg daily if underlying condition causes increased requirements (for example, in tropical sprue 3 to 15 mg daily may be needed). *Treatment of deficiency:* Initially give 250 µg (0.25 mg) to 1 mg daily PO, IM, IV, or deep SQ until hematologic response occurs; for maintenance, give 400 µg (0.4 mg) to 1 mg daily. *Pregnant and lactating women:* 800 µg (0.8 mg) qd.
Leucovorin calcium (folinic acid)	Wellcovorin	*Megaloblastic anemia:* Give up to 1 mg daily IM or PO; greater doses do not lead to increased efficacy.
HEPARIN ANTAGONIST		
Protamine sulfate	Protamine sulfate	The onset of action for protamine sulfate is 0.5 to 1 minute. The duration of action is 2 hours. *Adults and children:* 1 mg of protamine sulfate for every 90 USP units of beef lung heparin or for every 115 USP units of porcine intestinal mucosa heparin to be neutralized. Administer IV at a slow rate over 1 to 3 minutes (limit is 50 mg given in 10 minutes). Additional doses may be given if need is indicated by coagulation studies.

Table 14-1	Anticoagulants and other drugs affecting the blood—cont'd	
Generic name	Trade name	Comments and dosage
OTHER MISCELLANEOUS PRODUCTS		
Alteplase, recombinant	Activase	For lysis of coronary artery thrombi. Best results if given IV within 6 hours of onset of symptoms of MI. Give 6 to 10 mg IV bolus over the first 1 to 2 minutes, 20 mg over the second hour, and 20 mg over the third hour.
Anistreplase	Eminase	For lysis of thrombi obstructing coronary arteries. Give 30 units by IV injection over 2 to 5 minutes.
Antihemophilic factor	Hemofil M Koate-HS Monoclate	Used in treating patients with hemophilia A. Individualize dosage based on needs of patient.
Antiinhibitor coagulant complex	Autoplex T Feiba VH	Individualize dosage based on needs of patient.
Antithrombin III	ATnativ	Used in treating patients with hereditary antithrombin III deficiency. Individualize dosage based on needs of patient.
Pentoxifylline	Trental	Used in intermittent claudication from chronic occlusive arterial disease and in cerebrovascular insufficiency. Give 400 mg tid with meals. Decrease dosage if GI side effects develop.
Streptokinase	Kabikinase Streptase	Used in acute evolving transmural myocardial infarction, deep vein thrombosis, arterial thrombosis and embolism, and occluded AV cannulae. Patients may have severe uncontrolled hypertension or severe allergic reactions. Dosage calculated and administered by physician. Alteplase (above) may be slightly more effective but costs 10 times more than the other products.
Urokinase	Abbokinase	Used to dissolve clots from pulmonary emboli, coronary artery thrombosis, or to clear IV catheters obstructed by clotted blood or fibrin. Physician gives priming dose and follows with a constant infusion pump dosage calculated and administered by physician.

FOLIC ACID

ACTION

Folic acid is required for normal erythropoiesis, or red blood cell formation, and nucleoprotein synthesis. It is metabolized in the liver, where it is converted to its metabolically active form.

USES

Folic acid is used to treat anemias caused by folic acid deficiency; it is also used in alcoholism, hepatic disease, hemolytic anemia, infancy (especially for infants receiving artificial formulas), lactation, oral contraceptive use, and pregnancy. Folic acid supplements may be needed in low-birthweight infants, infants nursed by mothers deficient in folic acid, or infants with infections or prolonged diarrhea.

ADVERSE REACTIONS

Folic acid is reportedly nontoxic. An allergic reaction may consist of bronchospasm, erythema, malaise, pruritus, and rash; large amounts may discolor the urine.

DRUG INTERACTIONS

Chloramphenicol and methotrexate are folate antagonists, and they may cause decreased folic acid activity. Paraaminosalicylic acid and sulfasalazine may cause symptoms of folic acid deficiency. Concurrent use with many anticonvulsants may decrease the anticonvulsant effect, leading to increased seizure activity. Use of oral contraceptives may lead to folic acid deficiency.

NURSING IMPLICATIONS AND PATIENT TEACHING

▼ Assessment

The nurse should obtain a complete health and diet history, including the presence of hypersensitivity, underlying systemic disease, past gastrointestinal surgery, alcoholism, and concurrent use of other medications, especially those that may cause folate deficiency or decrease folic acid activity.

Folic acid is contraindicated as the sole therapeutic agent for the treatment of pernicious anemia. Folic acid will correct the hematologic abnormalities, but the neurologic deficiencies will continue irreversibly.

▼ Planning

The recommended dietary allowances (RDA) of folic acid are as follows:

Adult men and women: 400 µg
Pregnant women: 800 µg
Lactating women: 500 µg
Children 4 to 16 years: 200 µg

These recommended dietary allowances are usually provided by an adequate diet.

▼ Implementation

Folic acid for parenteral use must be protected from light.

Proper nutrition is essential, and dietary measures are preferable to drug therapy. The patient should be counseled to eat foods high in folic acid to prevent a deficiency problem in the future.

▼ Evaluation

Blood for laboratory tests should be drawn before initiating therapy. Drug therapy should provide improvement in the hematologic parameters within 2 to 5 days.

The nurse should stress the importance of remaining under medical supervision while receiving therapy. The patient may need an adjustment in the maintenance dosage. Patients often fail to return for follow-up visits when they begin to feel better.

▼ Patient and family teaching

The nurse should provide the patient and family with the following instructions:

1. The patient should take this medication exactly as ordered by the physician, and should remain under medical supervision while taking this drug. The patient will need to make a return visit to the care provider to confirm that medication is effective.
2. Diet is important in restoring proper folic acid levels and in preventing further deficiencies in the future. The patient should eat foods high in folate, including fresh, leafy green vegetables, other vegetables and fruits, yeast, and organ meats.
3. Vitamins should be stored in a cool, dry place. The folic acid solution should be protected from light.
4. If a dose is missed, the patient should take it as soon as he or she is aware of the missed dose. The patient must take the medication with regularity.

PROTAMINE SULFATE

ACTION

Protamine sulfate is a strongly basic (alkaline) protein that acts as an anticoagulant when it is given alone. It forms a stable salt in the presence of heparin, which is strongly acidic. This cancels out the anticoagulant activity of both drugs. When protamine sulfate is used with heparin, these results occur almost immediately and may persist for 2 hours or more.

USES

Protamine sulfate is used to treat heparin overdosage. It may also be used after surgical procedures to neutralize the effects of heparin given during extracorporeal circulation.

ADVERSE REACTIONS

Adverse reactions to protamine sulfate include bradycardia, dyspnea, lassitude, sudden drop in blood pressure, transitory flushing, and a feeling of warmth. Overdosage may produce anticoagulant effects.

NURSING IMPLICATIONS AND PATIENT TEACHING

▼ Assessment

Because of the anticoagulant activity of protamine sulfate, overdoses of this drug when used as a heparin antagonist may produce additional anticoagulation. The nurse should not give more than 100 mg at a time unless the physician specifies that a larger amount is required.

▼ Planning

Protamine sulfate may be inactivated by blood. Thus there may be a "rebound" effect when a large dose is used to neutralize heparin. This requires an increased dose of protamine. Hyperheparinemia or bleeding may be seen in some patients 30 minutes to 18 hours after open heart surgery, even when adequate amounts of protamine sulfate have been given.

▼ Implementation

Protamine sulfate should only be administered by a physician. It should be given slowly by intravenous injection over 1 to 3 minutes in doses not exceeding 50 mg of protamine sulfate activity (5 ml) during any 10-minute period. Severe hypotension and anaphylactoid-like reactions may be provoked if it is given too rapidly. This drug contains no preservatives, so the unused portion of the medication in the ampule should be discarded.

▼ Evaluation

The nurse should closely monitor the patient for signs of further anticoagulant activity and have equipment readily available to treat shock.

▼ Patient and family teaching

The family and patient should know that this is a routine drug used to neutralize heparin. See Table 14-1 for a summary of hematologic products.

SUMMARY

Hematologic products act in the formation, repair, or function of red blood cells. There are three major groups of hematologic products. They are the anticoagulants, the heparin-antagonist protamine sulfate, and the vitamins, minerals, or chemicals essential for red blood cell development. Patient and family teaching is especially important for the patient undergoing long-term therapy.

 CRITICAL THINKING QUESTIONS

1. Briefly point out the major differences in the three major groups of hematologic agents in actions and uses.

2. For your own understanding, draw a simplified diagram of the blood clotting sequence to illustrate the factors involved. Now, as you review this chapter, graph the points at which oral versus parenteral anticoagulants are needed in this sequence. This will help in understanding the varying actions and indications of these preparations.

3. Mrs. Gardner is being treated for a thrombus. She is concerned about her treatment regimen, pointing out differences in the treatment her sister received for the same thing. As you listen to Mrs. Gardner's worries, you realize she keeps referring to her "embolism." Explain to Mrs. Gardner the difference between a thrombus and an embolism and why this difference may affect methods of treatment.

4. Mr. Pierce is brought to your unit and placed on anticoagulant therapy. Explain the rationale for needing to know *why* this patient is being put on anticoagulation therapy. Why would you need laboratory values to validate accurate dosage?

5. Describe the possible problems that can arise if anticoagulants are used in conjunction with some other specific drugs.

6. In the emergency room, Ms. Zukerman needs an immediate anticoagulant effect. Which is the drug of choice? Why?

7. Ms. Zukerman receives the appropriate medication, as indicated by question 6, but now she exhibits signs of overdosage. What are the signs and symptoms of overdosage with this drug? Describe the needed interventions, both nursing and pharmacologic.

8. Identify the uses of these four tests: prothrombin time, Lee-White clotting time, partial thrombin time, and INR. Which test is most helpful in monitoring the effect of Ms. Zukerman's therapy?

9. Ms. Zukerman's condition is stabilized now, but she is experiencing pain at injection sites. How can you respond?

10. Do some research at your local facility to determine its limitations on who may administer heparin.

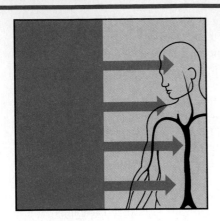

CHAPTER 15
Hormones and Steroids

OBJECTIVES

At the conclusion of this chapter you should be able to:

1. Describe the use of antidiabetic medications.
2. Identify preparations that act on the uterus.
3. Compare and contrast the action of adrenal and pituitary hormones.
4. Describe at least five adverse reactions that may result from the use of glucocortical and mineralocortical steroids.
5. Compare the actions of various male and female hormones.
6. List the indications for the use of thyroid preparations.

KEY TERMS

OVERVIEW

This chapter discusses the various hormones and steroids used in medical therapy. Unlike many other categories of medications, these are natural or synthetic preparations that replace, increase, or decrease naturally occurring substances already present within the patient. At times the body may produce too much of a hormone (for example, hyperthyroidism), and medication is given to correct the situation (such as methimazole to inhibit the synthesis of thyroid hormones). However, in diabetes mellitus the medication is given to replace the hormone insulin, which is not produced in sufficient quantities by the pancreas.

Hormones are chemicals that originate in an organ or gland and are conveyed through the blood to another part of the body, where they stimulate it to increased functional activity or secretion. **Steroids** are a particular chemical group of hormones. They are all part of a complex message system of the body, linking together various organs and systems. Lack of a basic hormone will stimulate the glands to produce more hormone. When the appropriate quantity is reached, the stimulation is turned off, and the gland slows production of the hormone. This feedback mechanism is important in obtaining stability of the body. It also creates a problem if some part of the system does not work properly, because failure in one organ system may then cause changes in other hormonal systems.

This chapter is divided into five basic sections: Section One describes insulin and the oral hypoglycemic agents used to treat diabetes mellitus. The various agents that act on the uterus are presented in Section Two. Section Three describes the pituitary and adrenocortical hormones, the major steroids that act throughout the body. Section Four presents the male and female hormones, and the combination of hormones involved in oral contraceptives. The various preparations used to treat the overproduction and underproduction of the thyroid hormones are described in Section Five.

Endocrine System

The regulation and coordination of body activities are accomplished in two ways: (1) through nervous impulses conducted by the nervous system, and (2) through chemical substances or hormones carried by

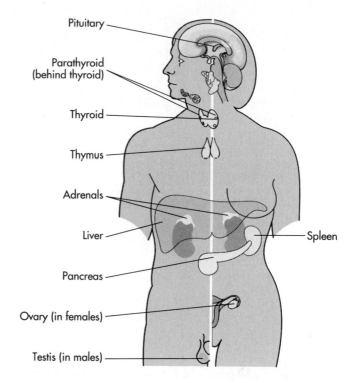

Fig. 15-1   The endocrine system.

the blood and lymph. The organs that secrete hormones are called endocrine glands, or glands of internal secretion. Collectively, these glands constitute the endocrine system (Fig. 15-1). This system includes the pituitary gland, thyroid gland, parathyroid glands, adrenal glands, pancreas, duodenum, testes, ovaries, and placenta. Sometimes the thymus gland and the pineal body are regarded as belonging to the endocrine system.

Endocrine glands are ductless; their secretions are discharged into the blood or lymph and are transported to all parts of the body. In this respect they are differentiated from exocrine glands, such as salivary or sweat glands, whose products are discharged through ducts that open onto a surface.

Of special attention are the hormones that affect the reproductive system. The gonads, accessory structures, and genitals of males and females perform the processes of reproduction and control sexual function and behavior (Figs. 15-2 and 15-3). The development and functioning of these reproductive organs are under hormonal control.

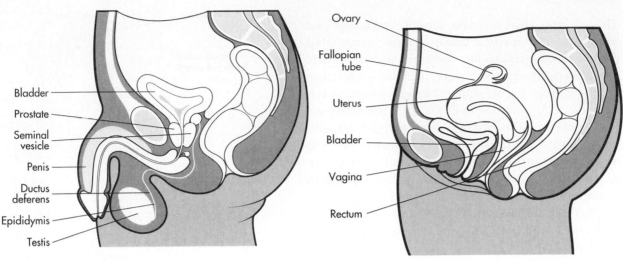

Fig. 15-2 The male reproductive system.

Fig. 15-3 The female reproductive system.

SECTION ONE: ANTIDIABETIC MEDICATIONS

Objectives

At the conclusion of this section you should be able to:

1. Compare and contrast the differences in action of insulin and oral hypoglycemic agents.
2. Compare and contrast the indications for the use of insulin and oral hypoglycemic agents.
3. Identify the adverse effects associated with use of insulin and hypoglycemic agents.
4. Define the terms insulin reaction, insulin dependent, and Somogyi effect.
5. Develop a teaching plan for the patient taking insulin or oral hypoglycemic agents.

OVERVIEW

Insulin is a hormone necessary for the metabolism and use of glucose in the body and is produced by the beta cells of the pancreas. Insulin helps glucose move into fat and striated muscle cells by activating a carrier system.

The patient with **diabetes mellitus** has a pancreas that fails to produce sufficient insulin for the needs of the body. The two major types of diabetes are **type I,** also known as **insulin-dependent diabetes mellitus (IDDM)** or juvenile diabetes, and **type II,** also known

as **non–insulin-dependent diabetes mellitus (NIDDM),** or latent-onset diabetes. Patients with NIDDM usually have a functioning pancreas that can be encouraged by medication to produce more insulin. Patients with IDDM usually have little or no pancreas production of insulin. These patients must have insulin provided to control the symptoms of diabetes mellitus. Since 1922 insulin taken from the pancreas of animals has been used to treat these patients. Insulin may also be necessary for some cases of NIDDM, although diet, weight reduction, and oral hypoglycemic agents are usually effective in controlling symptoms.

INSULIN

ACTION

The main action of insulin is to stimulate carbohydrate metabolism by increasing the movement of glucose and other **monosaccharides** into the cells. Insulin also influences fat and carbohydrate metabolism in the liver and adipose cells. Insulin is commonly obtained from either beef or pork pancreas; however, human insulin is now available, made from a recombinant DNA technology using strains of *Escherichia coli.*

USES

Insulin is used to manage insulin-dependent, ketosis-prone diabetes mellitus (IDDM) and in patients whose symptoms cannot be controlled by diet alone. It is used to treat non–insulin-dependent diabetes mellitus (NIDDM) that fails to respond to oral hypoglycemic therapy.

ADVERSE REACTIONS

Adverse reactions to insulin and oral hypoglycemics include lipodystrophy, local itching, swelling, erythema at the injection site, symptoms of insulin allergy, resistance, hypoglycemia, and hyperglycemia. Overdosage will produce symptoms of hypoglycemia.

DRUG INTERACTIONS

Insulin requirements may be increased by insulin antagonists, such as oral contraceptives, corticosteroids, epinephrine, and preparations used for thyroid hormone replacement therapy. Thiazide diuretics may elevate glucose levels. A variety of other isolated drugs, alcohol, and anabolic steroids may potentiate the hypoglycemic effects of insulin. Insulin promotes the movement of potassium into cells and lowers the serum potassium levels. Propranolol can mask the signs and symptoms of hypoglycemia.

 ## NURSING IMPLICATIONS AND PATIENT TEACHING

▼ Assessment

A patient whose diabetes mellitus was not previously diagnosed or is poorly controlled or out of control may have a history of polyuria, polydipsia, polyphagia, weight loss, blurred vision, and fatigue. In severe cases of hyperglycemia, symptoms of **systemic acidosis,** such as nausea and vomiting, may be present.

In patients taking insulin, look for a history of **hypoglycemia:** sudden onset of nervousness; hunger; weakness; cold, clammy sweat; lethargy; serum glucose levels less than 60 mg/dl; no urine glucose or acetone; pallor; diaphoresis; change in level of consciousness; and shallow respirations. These symptoms are relieved by having the patient eat or drink a source of fast-acting sugar. The nurse may also see signs of **hyperglycemia:** elevated fasting blood sugar blood levels (greater than 150 mg/dl), glycosuria,

ketonuria, Kussmaul's respiration, tachycardia, and acetone breath.

The nurse should monitor the patient for signs of pregnancy, infection, and kidney, liver, or thyroid disease, because these will alter the requirement for insulin. The patient should be asked about previous sensitization to beef or pork and whether the patient is taking other drugs that may interact with insulin.

▼ Planning

The management of diabetes mellitus is dependent on the patient's education. Control and maintenance require that the patient be knowledgeable about his or her diet, the need for weight control, the nature of the disease, urine testing, signs and symptoms of hypoglycemia and hyperglycemia and the appropriate actions to take for each, and the importance of hygiene, exercise, and procedures on sick days.

The patient should be taught about rotation of injection sites to prevent **lipodystrophy,** or shrinkage and atrophy of the fatty tissue when insulin is given in the same spot too frequently.

The patient should be shown the proper injection technique, including the rotation and storage of insulin. Errors in administration are common among patients. Routine follow-up and assessment of technique are important. The patient should periodically give the nurse a demonstration of the technique.

Insulin allergy (transient local itching, swelling, and erythema at the injection site) commonly develops during the initiation of therapy. Insulin resistance (requirements of more than 200 units of insulin per day) is rare and may be attributed to infection, inflammatory diseases, obesity, or stress. The nurse should closely monitor the patient with insulin resistance who is being treated with a concentrated insulin injection to ensure that hypoglycemia is avoided. Long-acting insulins are not adequate in the treatment and management of acidosis and emergencies.

Insulin by aerosol inhaler is currently under investigation. This would allow some diabetic patients to give up injections.

▼ Implementation

Insulin is a protein and therefore is inactivated by gastrointestinal enzymes. Thus insulin is generally administered subcutaneously 15 to 30 minutes before meals. Only regular insulin can be administered intravenously, as is done during ketoacidosis or diabetic coma emergencies.

Table 15-1 Comparison of action of insulin preparations

Action	Preparation	Action in hours			Compatible mixed with
		Onset	Peak	Duration	
Rapid or short	*Insulin injection:* Insulin (regular), Regular Iletin I, Beef Regular Iletin II, Humulin R, Pork Regular Iletin II, Purified Pork insulin, Humulin BR, Novolin R, Velosulin	½ to 1	5 to 10	6 to 8	All
	Prompt insulin, zinc suspension: Semilente Iletin I, Semilente insulin	1 to 1½	5 to 8	12 to 16	Lente
Intermediate	*Isophane insulin suspension:* Humulin N, Insulatard NPH, Isophane insulin (NPH), NPH Iletin I, Beef NPH Iletin II, Pork NPH Iletin II, Novolin N	1 to 1½	4 to 12	24 to 28	Regular
	Insulin zinc suspension: Lente insulin, Lente Iletin I, Lente Iletin II, Purified Pork insulin, Humulin L, Novolin L	1 to 2½	7 to 15	24	Regular, Semilente
Long	*Protamine zinc insulin suspension:* Protamine zinc insulin; Protamine zinc and Iletin I; Beef protamine, zinc and Iletin II; Pork protamine, zinc and Iletin II	4 to 8	14 to 24	36	Regular
	Extended insulin zinc suspension: Ultralente insulin, Ultralente Iletin I, Humulin U Ultralente	4 to 8	10 to 30	36+	Regular, Semilente
High potency	*Concentrated insulin:* Regular Iletin II U-500 (pork)	1 to 1½	5 to 8	24	Given alone

Insulin therapy is individualized according to the patient's response. The dosage should be titrated to gain maximal therapeutic response with the lowest dosage. Controversy exists concerning the degree of control. Generally, the minimal goal of therapy is to avoid extremes of ketoacidosis and hypoglycemia.

The different insulin preparations and their onset, peak, and duration of action are given in Tables 15-1 and 15-2.

The insulin vial in use may be stored outside of the refrigerator for 1 month, provided it is not exposed to extreme temperature. An extra supply of insulin should be stored in the refrigerator. Expiration dates should be checked regularly. Injection of cold insulin may irritate the tissues.

Rapid-acting insulin is used during acidosis and other acute situations (infection, surgery) when the patient's food intake is variable. It is also used in combination with longer-acting insulins to achieve greater control. Regular insulin may be used in divided dose therapy. The dosage is determined by the amount of glucose and acetone in the urine. "Double-voided urines" are used to determine the sliding scale or "rainbow coverage," and a predetermined number of units of insulin is administered for each degree of glycosuria according to a sliding scale.

Table 15-2　Insulin Dosage Regimens

Regimen	Type Insulin Used	Time Administered With Expected Time-Action Curve*	Advantages	Disadvantages
I. Single dose	Intermediate insulin (I)		One injection should cover noon and PM meal; hypoglycemia during sleep is not a problem	No fasting, breakfast, or nighttime coverage of hyperglycemia
II. Split-mixed dose	Intermediate and regular insulin (I) + (R)		Two injections provide coverage over 24-hour period	Two injections required; "locks" patient into set meal pattern
III. Split-mixed dose	Intermediate and regular insulin (I) + (R)		Three injections provide coverage over 24 hours, particularly over early AM hours	Three injections required; evening intermediate insulin dose may potentiate early morning hypoglycemia
IV. Multiple dose	Regular insulin and intermediate insulin (I) + (R)		Allows more flexibility in meal times and amount of food intake	Four injections required; requires before-meal blood glucose checks; establishing and following individualized algorithm; tighter control may predispose to hypoglycemia
V. Multiple dose (insulin delivery via the pump is similar to this regimen)	Regular insulin and longest-acting insulin (R) + (LA)		Provides insulin delivery pattern that more closely simulates normal endogenous insulin pattern; allows for some flexibility in food-intake pattern	Requires three or four injections plus blood glucose checks before meals and on retiring; requires establishing and following individualized algorithm; tight control may predispose to hypoglycemia

From Price MJ *Nurs Clin North Am*, Dec 1983, p. 695.
*Short-acting insulin ———. Long-acting insulin ----------.

For insulin suspensions, the vial is gently rolled and inverted from end to end before withdrawal to return particles to suspension. Vigorous shaking may result in air bubbles that can cause difficult withdrawal.

Most diabetic patients have symptoms controlled with 40 to 60 units of insulin per day. Occasionally a patient will develop resistance to the insulin or become so unresponsive to insulin that several hundred or even thousands of units of insulin may be necessary. Patients who require dosages in excess of 300 or 500 units often have impaired insulin receptors. Concentrated insulin injection allows a higher dosage to be given in a smaller amount of fluid. Each milliliter of the concentrated insulin contains 500 units, rather than the 100 units in the normal products.

▼ Evaluation

The patient's response should be monitored by testing the urine and blood. The physician should inform the patient how frequently the patient needs to be seen, what blood and urine levels are being found, and what the desired levels are. The patient must be encouraged to take responsibility for managing his or her own disease.

The therapeutic objective of insulin therapy is to maintain blood glucose levels within specific limits and to prevent symptoms of hyperglycemia and hypoglycemia. Patients may monitor their blood glucose levels with home **glucometers** or test urine for glucose to measure degree of control. In patients without glucometers, double-voided specimens should be tested before each meal and at bedtime during periods of insulin dosage change, acute illness, or surgery. Patients with glucometers will be told when to check their blood glucose level depending on the type of insulin they are taking. Once control has been achieved, the urine sugar level can be monitored before breakfast and before the evening meal, especially to determine the peak effect of intermediate-acting insulin. Diabetic patients receiving short-acting insulin need to test the sugar level before lunch and at bedtime, depending on when the insulin was taken. Urine ketones should be measured during acute illness or periods of increased glycosuria and in ketosis-prone diabetic patients. The blood and urine records provide information regarding control between office visits.

If hypoglycemia occurs, the patient should be taught to consume a carbohydrate immediately. The family should also be involved in patient teaching

CRITICAL DECISION
Hypoglycemia

Hypoglycemia may develop, especially with insulin overdosage, increased work or exercise, omission or delay of a meal, or an illness associated with vomiting, diarrhea, or delayed digestion. Meals must be correlated with the activity of the insulin (i.e., onset, peak, and duration).

about therapy for hypoglycemia. If the patient is unconscious, honey or Karo syrup may be applied under the tongue or to the buccal mucosa. Additional carbohydrate, such as bread, crackers, or milk should be provided for the next 2 hours, or a sandwich should be eaten if a snack or meal would not be regularly taken within an hour. Glucagon may be administered by a family member or a care provider.

The **Somogyi effect** (rebound elevation of glucose levels triggered by hypoglycemia) can lead to overtreatment of the patient with insulin when less insulin is actually indicated. Patients over 60 are often sensitive to hypoglycemia. They should be observed for confusion and abnormal behavior, because repeated episodes of hypoglycemia may cause brain damage.

▼ Patient and family teaching

The nurse should provide the patient and family with the following instructions:

1. The patient should keep on a diet (regular meals, snacks, and caloric requirements) and maintain an ideal body weight to promote glycemic control and prevent hypoglycemia.
2. The patient must know the signs and symptoms of hypoglycemia (too little sugar) and hyperglycemia (too much sugar), their causes, prevention, and treatment. The patient should notify the physician if any of the symptoms occur.
3. Insulin can cause an increase (hypertrophy) or a decrease (atrophy) in the size of fatty tissue when injected into the same site frequently. A plan for rotation of insulin injection sites should be developed, followed, and recorded.
4. The patient must use the proper syringe and correct type, strength, and dosage of insulin to avoid dosage errors.
5. The patient should avoid alcohol consumption, because a hypoglycemic reaction, severe nau-

sea and vomiting, dizziness, headache, sweating, and flushing may develop.

6. The patient's blood sugar levels can be monitored by daily blood or urine testing. The nurse should teach the patient the proper technique for performing, recording, and interpreting the results. This will help the patient and the physician to manage the disease successfully.

7. Insulin requirements increase when the patient is under stress or becomes ill, especially with an infection. The patient must faithfully test the urine or blood when ill and must not stop taking insulin. The patient may take a liquid diet if he or she has an upset stomach, nausea, or vomiting. The physician should be notified for adjustment of insulin dosage.

8. The patient must be prepared for emergency situations by
   a. Carrying an identification card
   b. Wearing a Medic-Alert bracelet or necklace
   c. Carrying a readily available source of sugar at all times

9. When traveling, the patient should carry an extra supply of insulin, syringes, and needles in case he or she becomes separated from his or her luggage. The patient will need to make adjustments to zone time changes to avoid hypoglycemia.

10. The patient should be alert for hypoglycemia when driving, operating machinery, or engaging in activities that require alertness.

11. The patient taking oral hypoglycemic agents should report jaundice, dark urine, light-colored stools, fever, sore throat, fatigue, or any unusual bleeding or bruising.

12. Allergic skin reactions may develop with initiation of oral hypoglycemic therapy. Red, raised rashes are generally transient and will disappear with continued drug therapy.

ORAL HYPOGLYCEMICS

ACTION

The primary action of the **oral hypoglycemics**, or sulfonylureas, is to stimulate insulin release by the beta cells of the pancreas. Therefore functional islet cell tissue is necessary in patients receiving these drugs. The sulfonylureas also increase the peripheral use of insulin and influence other fat and carbohydrate processes.

USES

Oral hypoglycemics are used to manage NIDDM (non–insulin-dependent) adult-onset diabetic patients who generally are over 40 years of age, whose insulin requirement is less than 20 units per day, whose diabetes mellitus symptoms cannot be adequately controlled by diet and weight loss, and in whom the use of insulin is unacceptable.

ADVERSE REACTIONS

Allergic reactions manifested by urticaria, rash, pruritus, and erythema are generally transient and develop with initiation of therapy. Photosensitivity is a rare adverse reaction. More common reactions include heartburn, nausea, vomiting, abdominal pain, and diarrhea caused by increased gastric acid secretion; occasionally hepatic toxicity and cholestatic jaundice (manifested by jaundice, dark urine, and light-colored stools) are seen.

DRUG INTERACTIONS

The hypoglycemic effects of the sulfonylureas are potentiated by oral anticoagulants and other isolated drugs. Sulfonamide-type antibacterial agents and salicylates displace the sulfonylureas from protein-binding sites, which leads to high blood levels of the active drug. Barbiturates, sedatives, and hypnotics may have a prolonged effect when taken concurrently with the sulfonylureas, because of a decreased rate of elimination from the body. Thiazide diuretics oppose the secretion of insulin from the beta cells and decrease the effectiveness of sulfonylureas.

CRITICAL DECISION
Alcohol Consumption

Alcohol consumption with oral hypoglycemics may result in a disulfiram-like reaction.

 NURSING IMPLICATIONS AND PATIENT TEACHING

▼ **Assessment**

The nurse should obtain a thorough health history and ascertain what other drugs the patient is taking that may interact with the sulfonylureas, and whether

Table 15-3 Comparison of oral hypoglycemics (Sulfonylureas)

Generic name	Trade name	Duration of action (hr)	Serum half-life (hr)	Suggested dosage	Doses/ day
FIRST-GENERATION DRUGS					
Tolbutamide	Orinase	6 to 12	4 to 5	1 gm	1 to 2
Acetohexamide	Dymelor	12 to 24	6 to 8	500 mg	1 to 2
Tolazamide	Tolinase	10 to 15	6 to 8	250 mg	1
Chlorpropamide	Diabinese	60	35	250 mg	1
SECOND-GENERATION DRUGS					
Glipizide	Glucotrol	10 to 16	2 to 4	10 mg	1 to 2
Glyburide	DiaBeta, Micronase	24	4	3 to 5 mg	1 to 2

the patient has any allergy to sulfa drugs, if the patient is pregnant, has renal insufficiency, impaired liver function, or a history of ketoacidosis.

▼ Planning

Some research has created controversy concerning the safety and efficacy of oral hypoglycemic agents. In particular, tolbutamide has been identified as having significant toxicity.

No transition period is necessary when a patient is transferred from one oral hypoglycemic to another.

▼ Implementation

The sulfonylureas are administered orally. The duration of the hypoglycemic effect is the main difference among the various sulfonylureas. The duration of action, serum half-life, dosage range, and approximate doses per day are given in Table 15-3.

▼ Evaluation

The patient's urine and blood levels should be monitored, and the patient should be observed for signs and symptoms of hypoglycemia.

Rashes may develop when therapy begins, but they generally last only a short time. If they persist, the medication should be stopped. Cholestatic jaundice has been reported in a small number of patients on oral hypoglycemic therapy. Discontinuation of the drug reverses any liver damage that may occur.

▼ Patient and family teaching

The patient and family teaching is the same as for insulins (see pp. 316-317).

SECTION TWO: DRUGS ACTING ON THE UTERUS

Objectives

At the conclusion of this section you should be able to:
1. Identify drugs that act on the uterus.
2. List indications for the use of oxytocic drugs.
3. Describe the adverse effects associated with drugs acting on the uterus.

OVERVIEW

There are three types of drugs used for their effect on the uterus. These include oxytocics, uterine relaxants, and abortifacients. These products are used primarily at delivery or to help expel the fetus from the uterus.

ACTION

Oxytocic agents and ergot preparations stimulate the uterus to contract. Oxytocin acts directly on the smooth musculature of the uterus, especially at or near gestation, to produce firm, regular contractions; on the vasculature system to produce vasoconstriction; and on the mammary gland cells in the postpartum phase to stimulate the flow of milk.

USES

Oxytocics are used to stimulate or induce labor at term when there are medical problems threatening the life of the mother or fetus; to assist the delivery of the shoulder of the infant; to assist in the expulsion of the placenta; to control postpartum bleeding or uterine atony; to relieve breast engorgement related to static lactation; to stimulate uterine contraction after a cesarean section birth or other uterine surgery; and adjunctively to treat incomplete abortion. The ergots are used to prevent or control hemorrhage after the delivery of the placenta and in the postpartum period.

Abortifacients are also used to stimulate uterine contractions. Although the mechanism of action is unclear, these products stimulate uterine contractions that will force the pregnant uterus to empty. They are used early in pregnancy.

In contrast to abortifacients, oxytocin, and the ergots, **uterine relaxants** act on the beta-adrenergic receptors to inhibit uterine smooth muscle contractions. This action is used in the management of preterm or premature labor.

ADVERSE REACTIONS

Oxytocin may produce cardiac dysrhythmia, edema, fetal and neonatal bradycardia, anxiety, redness of skin during administration, nausea and vomiting, anaphylaxis, postpartum hemorrhage, cyanosis, and dyspnea.

In the appropriate dosage and in the absence of contraindications, the ergots are fairly safe. The most common adverse reactions are nausea and vomiting. Other, more unusual reactions include allergic reactions, bradycardia, hypotension, elevated blood pressure, or cerebral-spinal symptoms and spasms.

Excessive doses of oxytocics can produce uterine hypertonicity, spasm, tetanic contractions, and ruptures. Lesser overdoses in labor yield a sustained forceful contraction without rest. Overdosage with ergots during labor yields a similar reaction, with cardiovascular and gastrointestinal symptoms progressing to more dangerous problems.

DRUG INTERACTIONS

Vasoconstrictors and local anesthetics increase the effects of oxytocics.

NURSING IMPLICATIONS AND PATIENT TEACHING

▼ Assessment

The patient may be past the anticipated due date for the baby or have a history of engorged breasts. A history of incomplete abortion, cesarean section births, or excessive postpartum bleeding also prompts consideration of oxytocics or ergots. Finally, a patient may also desire to terminate an unwanted pregnancy early in the gestational phase.

▼ Planning

The uterine contractions produced by oxytocics should be comparable to those of spontaneous, normal labor. In women who have been pregnant before, they are used only after the cervix is completely dilated.

There are numerous precautions or contraindications to the use of oxytocics. These medications must be given by qualified nurses under the direct supervision of physicians. Injudicious use of either oxytocic or ergot preparations has caused fetal and maternal death or injury, subarachnoid hemorrhage, and uterine rupture.

▼ Implementation

Oxytocin is the drug of choice for medical induction of labor in many areas of the country. However, prostaglandins are now preferred in some regions. These are usually given by intravenous infusion pump. Buccal tablets are available, but they are not as extensively used as they were at one time, because the effects are more difficult to predict and control.

Ergonovine is now the drug of choice to control postpartum bleeding. It can be given SL, IM, or IV in emergency situations. Methylergonovine is the synthetic homologue of ergonovine and has been found to produce fewer vasoconstrictive or hypertensive side effects than ergonovine. It is noted that intravenous administration of either ergot increases the danger of side effects. See Table 15-4 for a summary of drugs acting on the uterus.

▼ Evaluation

If oxytocin is used during induction, the patient should be monitored for the therapeutic effect and the development of adverse reactions. The blood pressure and pulse should be checked frequently, and continuous monitoring of the fetal heart rate is necessary. The dilation of the cervix and the progres-

Table 15-4 Drugs acting on the uterus

Generic name	Trade name	Comments and dosage
OXYTOCICS		
Ergonovine	Ergonovine	Used to prevent or control postpartum hemorrhage secondary to uterine atony or subinvolution. Note similarity in names between ergotamine (used for migraines) and ergonovine; they are *not* the same although they may be listed the same in some books. Protect the ampule from light, store in a cool place, and discard after 60 days. *SL* (appropriate in nonemergency situations and for prophylaxis after leaving the labor and delivery suite): 200 to 400 µg (0.2 to 0.4 mg) bid to qid for 48 hours post partum. *IM* (postpartally to facilitate uterine contraction and decrease bleeding): 0.2 mg.
Methylergonovine	Methergine	Synthetic ergonovine produces stronger and more prolonged contractions. Protect vials from heat and light and discard colored vials. Onset of action from IV is immediate; after IM it is 2 to 5 minutes, and with PO it is 5 to 10 minutes. *IV:* 0.2 mg over a period of not less than 1 minute with continuous blood pressure monitoring. *IM:* 0.2 mg not more often than every 2 to 4 hours or not more than a total of 5 doses.
Oxytocin	Pitocin Syntocinon	Used to induce or stimulate labor at term and secondarily in the stimulation of milk flow. It is the drug of choice in many areas of the country for medical induction of labor. Syntocinon is a synthetic derivative without the cardiovascular or vasopressor effects. The nasal form is useful for initial milk letdown. Never administer intravenously in undiluted form or in high concentrations. *To induce labor:* 10 units in 1 L D_5W or isotonic saline as an intravenous infusion. Initially give 1 to 2 milliunits/min. If no response within 15 minutes, gradually increase to a maximum of 20 milliunits per minute. The total induction dose ranges from 600 to 12,000 milliunits, with the average being 4000 milliunits. *For postpartum bleeding:* 3 to 10 units IM after delivery of the placenta; or 10 to 40 units in 1000 ml isotonic saline IV at a rate to control the bleeding.
UTERINE RELAXANTS		
Ritodrine HCl	Yutopar	Begin with 0.1 mg/min IV; increase based on patient response and follow with 10 to 20 mg q2 to 6h PO.
ABORTIFACIENTS		
Carboprost	Hemabate	Initially, 250 µg IM; then 250 to 500 µg prn.
Dinoprostone	Prostin E_2	1 suppository high into vagina; repeat prn.

sion of contractions should be monitored, the latter for their frequency, force, duration, and resting uterine tone. Drastic increases in these parameters warrant discontinuation of the drug. The contractions should not be over 50 mm Hg. The nurse should note the urinary output and any edema and should closely watch the rate of IV solution and oxytocin infusion.

The nurse should watch for the symptoms of ergotism: vomiting, diarrhea, unquenchable thirst, tingling, itching and coldness of the skin, a rapid and weak pulse, confusion, and unconsciousness.

Ergonovine might stimulate cramping. If this becomes too uncomfortable, either decrease the dosage or treat symptomatically.

The most common side effects are nausea and vomiting. These can sometimes be alleviated with prior administration of a phenothiazine antiemetic.

If overdosage occurs, producing a continuous contraction, discontinue the drug immediately. It may be necessary to give a general anesthetic to relax the uterus, particularly if the fetus is threatened.

▼ Patient and family teaching

The nurse should provide the patient and family with the following instructions:

1. Oxytocics or ergots are given to augment the body's natural action during and after labor and delivery.
2. The patient will be watched continually throughout this treatment.
3. Contractions should not be more intense than normal contractions.
4. Ergonovine might stimulate cramping; if this becomes intense, the patient should inform the nurse or physician.

SECTION THREE: PITUITARY AND ADRENOCORTICAL HORMONES

Objectives

At the conclusion of this section you should be able to:

1. Identify different hormones produced by the anterior and posterior pituitary gland.
2. Identify hormones produced by the adrenal glands.
3. Describe uses of various pituitary and adrenocortical hormones.
4. Identify common adverse reactions to hormonal replacement or therapy.
5. List at least three important points to cover in teaching the patient who is taking hormones on a long-term basis.

OVERVIEW

The pituitary, or "master" gland, lies in the sella turcica in the sphenoid bone in the skull and is connected to the brain by a slender stalk. The anterior portion of the pituitary, or the adenohypophysis, and the posterior portion of the pituitary, or the neurohypophysis, produce hormones that regulate growth, metabolism, electrolyte balance, water retention or loss, and the reproductive cycle.

The adrenal cortex manufactures the **corticosteroids** and a small amount of the **sex hormones,** which are substances that influence many organs, structures, and life processes of the body. The corticosteroids are composed of the glucocorticoids and the mineralocorticoids.

ANTERIOR PITUITARY HORMONES

ACTION AND USES

The major anterior pituitary hormones include the gonadotropins: the follicle-stimulating hormone (FSH) and the luteinizing hormone (LH). They are called gonadotropins because they influence the gonads, the organs of reproduction. They influence the production of sex hormones, the development of secondary sex characteristics, and the pattern and regularity of the reproductive cycle. An additional hormone, prolactin, stimulates the production of breast milk after childbirth.

There are a number of gonadotropins. Chorionic gonadotropin is taken from human placentas and contains FSH and LH. A purified form of FSH and LH, called menotropin, is taken from the urine of postmenopausal women. These hormones may be given to produce ovulation in women with ovulatory failure, to stimulate production of sperm in men, or to assist in treatment when the testes have failed to descend into the scrotum. Clomiphene is a synthetic nonsteroidal compound that is also used to promote ovulation.

Somatotropic hormone (STH) and adrenocorticotropic hormone (ACTH or corticotropin) are also produced by the anterior pituitary. Somatotropin comes from human pituitary glands removed at autopsy. This hormone regulates the growth of the person during childhood and is given to children who have failed to grow because of a growth hormone deficiency.

Table 15-5 Anterior pituitary hormones

Generic name	Trade name	Comments and dosage
Corticotropin (ACTH)	ACTH Acthar	Very rapid absorption and use necessitates administration q6h to maintain desired production; use 20 to 100 units IM or SQ.
Corticotropin repository	ACTH-40 H.P. Acthar Gel	Slowly absorbed and can be administered in a single daily IM dose. *Adults:* 40 to 80 units IM q24 to 72h.
Corticotropin zinc hydroxide	Cortrophin-Zinc	*Adults:* 40 units IM or SQ q12 to 24h.
Cosyntropin	Cortrosyn	Synthetic subunit of ACTH, but exhibits all the pharmacologic properties of natural ACTH. Cosyntropin 0.25 mg is equivalent in action to 25 units natural ACTH and is less likely to produce allergies. ■ *Adrenocortical insufficiency testing:* 0.25 to 0.75 mg IM or IV; Children less than age 2 may respond to a dose of 0.125 mg.

ACTH stimulates the adrenal cortex to produce and secrete hormones, primarily glucocorticoids. ACTH is used in diagnostic testing and in the treatment of some acute neurologic problems.

ADVERSE REACTIONS

Because all of these medications are hormones, their primary adverse reactions include systemic or local hormonal reactions. Menotropin may produce ovarian enlargement, blood inside the peritoneal cavity, and febrile reactions; when it is used to increase fertility, multiple births may be produced. Clomiphene may produce abdominal discomfort, ovarian enlargement, blurred vision, nervousness, and nausea and vomiting; vasomotor flushes much like those seen in menopause may also occur. Chorionic gonadotropin may cause headache, irritability, restlessness, fatigue, and edema; precocious puberty or onset of sexual development at an early age may result from treatment for undescended testes. Somatotropin may provoke antibody stimulation in some individuals, resulting in failure of the drug to produce any growth. The adrenocorticotropic hormones are involved with numerous adverse reactions, because they stimulate the adrenal gland. For a summary of anterior pituitary hormones, see Table 15-5.

 NURSING IMPLICATIONS AND PATIENT TEACHING

▼ Assessment

The nurse should obtain a thorough history to determine concurrent medication use and the presence of other diseases or conditions that would represent precautions or contraindications to the use of pituitary hormones.

▼ Planning

There are no oral forms of pituitary hormones. They are given IM, SQ, IV, or intranasally.

▼ Implementation

The dosages are individualized to the patient's diurnal rhythm of water metabolism and adequate duration of sleep. Generally, the administration should coincide with the onset of polyuria or excessive thirst and before sleep. The patient should drink one to two glasses of water at the time of administration to reduce the incidence of adverse effects.

▼ Evaluation

The nurse should monitor for a decrease in the frequency and the amount of urination, monitor the specific gravity of the urine, and watch for water intoxication or signs of dehydration.

Table 15-6   Posterior pituitary hormones

Generic name	Trade name	Comments and dosage
Desmopressin	DDAVP Concentraid	Synthetic antidiuretic inhalant. Drug of choice in patients with mild to moderate diabetes insipidus. Offers prolonged antidiuretic activity without vasopressor or oxytocic side effects. Give 2.5 to 10 μg in the evening. Note the effect and increase nightly by 2.5 μg until satisfactory sleep duration is attained.
Lypressin	Diapid	Synthetic derivative of ADH. Use 1 to 2 sprays in one or both nostrils tid to qid or at onset of polyuria or thirst.
Vasopressin	Pitressin	*Adults:* 5 to 10 units (0.25 to 0.5 ml) IM or SQ, bid to qid; maximum 60 units.
	Vasopressin tannate	Water-insoluble derivative of vasopressin that has a longer duration of action and is of use in long-term treatment of diabetes insipidus in children and some adults.
Posterior pituitary injection	Pituitrin	Natural extract of posterior pituitary glands; use is restricted to severe, refractory diabetes insipidus. Give 5 to 20 units IM (preferred) or SQ. For postpartum hemorrhage give 10 units.

POSTERIOR PITUITARY HORMONES

ACTION AND USES

The posterior pituitary gland produces the antidiuretic hormone (ADH) vasopressin, as well as oxytocin, a hormone that stimulates the uterus. Pituitary extract is also given to increase smooth muscle contraction of the digestive tract and vascular bed.

Vasopressin regulates the reabsorption of water by the kidneys. This hormone is specifically released whenever the brain senses that the urine is becoming concentrated because the patient has had severe diarrhea, vomiting, or has become dehydrated through some other condition. Vasopressin may be given when the body inappropriately loses water, as in diabetes insipidus, or when the pituitary fails to secrete vasopressin because of disease or surgical removal. Vasopressin is of secondary use in some gastrointestinal problems.

Oxytocin acts directly on the smooth musculature of the uterus to produce firm, regular contractions as described in Section Two of this chapter.

ADVERSE REACTIONS

Adverse reactions to small doses of vasopressin include abdominal cramps, anaphylaxis, bronchial con-

striction, circumoral pallor, diarrhea, flatus, intestinal hyperactivity, nausea, "pounding" headaches, sweating, tremors, urticaria, uterine cramps, vertigo, and vomiting. Vasopressin given in larger doses may produce death.

DRUG INTERACTIONS

Oral antidiabetic agents, urea, and fludrocortisone increase the effects of vasopressin, and large doses of epinephrine, heparin, and alcohol decrease the effect. The antidiuretic effect of desmopressin is decreased by lithium, large doses of epinephrine, demeclocycline, heparin, and alcohol. The antidiuretic effects of desmopressin may be increased by chlorpropamide, urea, and fludrocortisone.

 NURSING IMPLICATIONS AND PATIENT TEACHING

Nursing implications for posterior pituitary hormones are similar to those for anterior pituitary hormones (see p. 322). For a summary of dosages and drugs, see Table 15-6.

ADRENOCORTICAL HORMONES

ACTION

The adrenal cortex manufactures glucocorticoids, mineralocorticoids and small amounts of sex hormones. Hydrocortisone and cortisone are two of the several glucocorticoids produced by the adrenal glands. These hormones regulate glucose, fat, and protein metabolism, and control the antiinflammatory response and the immune response system. The mineralocorticoids consist of aldosterone and desoxycorticosterone. These hormones work with others to maintain the fluid and electrolyte balance in the body. They conserve sodium and increase the excretion of potassium. They are used in replacement therapy for adrenal insufficiency.

USES

Glucocorticoids may be given in physiologic doses for replacement of missing hormones in adrenal insufficiency (Addison's disease). They are more commonly given in pharmacologic doses for suppression of inflammatory, allergic, or immunologic responses, and with antineoplastics to treat hematologic and malignant diseases.

Examples of situations in which glucocorticoids might be used are acute emergencies, allergic states, collagen diseases, connective tissue disease, diagnostic testing of adrenocortical hyperfunction, edematous states, hematologic and neoplastic diseases, ophthalmologic diseases, respiratory diseases, and miscellaneous conditions such as acute Bell's palsy, chronic kidney disease, chronic ulcerative colitis, and thromboembolic disease.

Local steroids might be used for intraarticular, soft tissue, or intrabursal problems, or for intralesional or subcutaneous dermatologic problems. Steroids might also be used topically for acute and chronic dermatoses, rectal problems, and some eye or ear problems.

ADVERSE REACTIONS

The side effects of systemic corticosteroids in pharmacologic doses are predictable exaggerations of functions of the corticosteroids normally produced by the adrenals, or the results of hypothalamic-pituitary-adrenal axis suppression. Some adverse reactions are quite common, others are more unusual. Adverse reactions that might develop are listed in Table 15-7.

DRUG INTERACTIONS

Corticosteroids increase the effects of barbiturates, sedatives, narcotics, and anticoagulants. They decrease the effects of insulin and oral hypoglycemics,

 Table 15-7   Adverse effects associated with corticosteroids

Biologic System	Potential Adverse Effects
Endocrine	Atrophy of adrenal cortex* (can occur after 10 days); anterior pituitary suppression; diabetes* (catabolism of fat, protein, glycogen, resulting in hyperglycemia); fluid/electrolyte imbalance* (from overlapping mineralocorticoid effect), hypokalemia; muscle cramps, irregular heart rate; redisposition of lipids* (moon face, buffalo hump, truncal obesity, striae, hirsutism, acne), and androgenic effects from sex hormones.
Gastrointestinal	Gastritis,* peptic ulcer* (unrelated to local irritation of oral tablets); esophagitis; and pancreatitis.
Immune	Absence of signs of infection*; uninhibited invasion and proliferation of virus, bacteria, fungus; and inhibition of fibroplasia with delayed wound healing.
Musculoskeletal	Muscle wasting* (catabolism of protein) and osteoporosis.
Neurologic	Mood changes (euphoria, insomnia, nervousness, irritability); emotional lability (psychotic episodes, depression, sense of well-being); and EEG changes.
Ophthalmologic	Induces or aggravates glaucoma by decreasing aqueous outflow; cataracts; optic nerve damage; increased susceptibility to viral or fungal infection; and corneal perforation (when used in conditions that cause cornea to thin).
Vascular	Thrombosis, thromboembolism, thrombophlebitis, hypercholesterolemia, and atherosclerosis; these problems are especially prominent with cortisone.
Miscellaneous	Hypertension; collagen tissue breakdown can activate latent TB by liberating organisms from deposits in pulmonary tissue; hypersensitivity reactions.

*Most common potential adverse effects.

coumarin anticoagulants, isoniazid, aspirin, and broad-spectrum antibiotics. Drugs that increase the effects of steroids are indomethacin, aspirin, and oral contraceptives, especially estrogen. Drugs that decrease the effects of steroids include ephedrine, barbiturates, phenytoin, antihistamines, chloral hydrate, rifampin, and propranolol.

Some drugs produce exaggerated side effects when given with steroids; these include alcohol; aspirin and antiinflammatory drugs; amphotericin B; thiazides and other potassium-wasting diuretics; stimulants such as adrenalin, amphetamines, and ephedrine; anticholinergics; and cardiac glycosides. Steroids also interfere with numerous laboratory tests.

 NURSING IMPLICATIONS AND PATIENT TEACHING

▼ Assessment

These drugs have many contraindications and precautions to use. The nurse should obtain a thorough history to determine the presence of preexisting diseases, concurrent use of other medications, and the presence of infection or pregnancy, and to document the usual pattern of water turnover and sleep duration.

▼ Planning

Although glucocorticoids are exceptionally potent drugs, short-term administration of even extremely large doses is not likely to cause long-term sequelae. However, moderate and long-term administration (longer than 6 days' systemic treatment) places the patient at high risk for a large number of serious adverse effects, and the risk/benefit ratio must be carefully considered. The medication suppresses the steroids normally produced by the body, and any sudden cessation of medication use will leave the body unable to function. The immediate and long-term effects of the drug are exceedingly variable and depend on the individual disease, the route of administration, dosage, duration, and frequency and time of administration.

Generic forms of the drugs are considerably less expensive. Generally, prednisone is considered the drug of choice for an antiinflammatory immunosuppressant effect. It is recommended that antacids be taken with or between doses to minimize peptic ulcer complication. Systemic corticosteroids are administered orally, except in emergency circumstances or when the patient is unable to take oral medication. The onset of action is 2 to 8 hours, and the effects last for 24 hours. Oral corticosteroids are almost completely absorbed in the GI tract.

For conditions requiring a local injection, a single injection yields sufficient antiinflammatory effects to alleviate symptoms in many cases. The slowly absorbed forms (acetate, diacetate, tebutate) of appropriate corticosteroids generally result in relief for 1 to 2 weeks.

▼ Implementation

Corticosteroids may be administered by the following routes: oral, inhalation, intranasal, intravenous, intramuscular, subcutaneous, intrabursal, intradermal, intrasynovial, intralesional, soft tissue injection, topical, and per rectum. Only corticosteroid preparations that are specifically designated should be used for ophthalmologic or otic administration.

Dosages vary radically; they are individualized by the diagnosis, severity, prognosis, and probable duration of the disease, and by patient response and tolerance. Individuals may respond better to one form than another in a somewhat unpredictable manner. The general rule, regardless of route of administration, is to prescribe as high a dose as necessary initially to obtain a favorable response, then decrease the amount gradually to the lowest level that will maintain the therapeutic effect yet minimize complications.

In systemic administration, dosage regimens are of two types: (1) physiologic, for replacement of glucocorticoids in adrenal insufficiency, and (2) pharmacologic, to reduce symptoms.

Corticosteroids cannot be withdrawn without gradual weaning. Sudden withdrawal leads to steroid withdrawal syndrome (anorexia, nausea and vomiting, lethargy, headache, fever, joint pain, desquamation, myalgia, weight loss, and hypotension). Abrupt cessation may also result in rebound of the condition being treated.

When corticosteroids are administered for longer than 1 to 2 weeks at pharmacologic doses, pituitary release of ACTH is suppressed, producing secondary adrenocortical insufficiency. Patients undergoing physiologic, emotional, or psychologic stress may need support via additional amounts of steroids. This suppression may last up to 2 years after discontinuation of the drug.

During tapering to maintenance or withdrawal, the patient must be watched carefully and taught signs of

Table 15-8 Adrenocortical hormones

Generic name	Trade name	Comments and dosage
GLUCOCORTICOIDS		
Short acting		
Cortisone	Cortone	Initially: 25 to 300 mg/day PO, 20 to 300 mg/day IM. ■ *Physiologic replacement:* 0.5 to 0.75 mg/kg/day PO; 0.25 to 0.75 mg/kg/day IM.
Hydrocortisone	Cortef	Initially: 20 to 240 mg/day PO; dosage may be as low as 0.1 mg 3 times/week.
Intermediate acting		
Prednisolone	Delta-Cortef	Initially: 5 to 60 mg/day PO.
Prednisone	Meticorten	Initially: 5 to 60 mg/day PO.
Methylprednisolone	Depo-Medrol	40 to 120 mg IM.
Triamcinolone	Aristocort	Initially: 4 to 60 mg PO.
Triamcinolone diacetate	Aristocort Forte	40 mg/week IM.
Long acting		
Betamethasone	Celestone	0.6 to 8.4 mg/day PO, IM, or IV.
Dexamethasone	Decadron	Initially: 0.75 to 9 mg/day PO.
MINERALOCORTICOIDS		
Fludrocortisone acetate	Florinef Acetate	Used in replacement therapy for adrenal insufficiency; 0.1 mg/day or 0.1 mg 3 times/week.

adrenal insufficiency (weakness, hypotension, anorexia). If this occurs, or if the disease flares up, the steroid dose is increased until symptoms subside. Tapering then begins again on a more gradual regimen. After shorter steroid courses (1 to 2 weeks), reduce the dosage on a daily basis by 50% decrements. Keep the same scheduled intervals.

See Table 15-8 for a summary of adrenocortical hormones.

▼ Evaluation

All patients receiving systemic corticosteroids should be monitored frequently, and the dosage adjusted to reflect remissions, exacerbations, the individual response, or occurrence of stress (injury, infection, surgery, emotional crisis). Patients should be monitored for 1 or 2 years following high-dosage or long-term treatment. While receiving steroids, patients are usually given prescriptions that cannot be refilled to prevent unmonitored steroid consumption.

Corticosteroids mask infection and increase the patient's susceptibility to infection. Corneal fungal infections are particularly likely to develop coincidentally with extensive ophthalmologic corticosteroid use. Corticosteroids are particularly dangerous to use

in patients with a history of tuberculosis, because the disease can be reactivated. Existing active or latent psychologic disorders may be aggravated or activated with prolonged dosage. Prolonged dosage may also produce osteoporosis, leading to vertebral collapse.

▼ Patient and family teaching

The nurse should provide the patient and family with the following instructions:

1. The patient will need to visit the physician frequently to monitor progress during and after steroid therapy.
2. Nicotine raises the blood level of naturally produced cortisone; therefore heavy smoking may add to the expected action.
3. Alcohol may enhance the tendency of steroids to cause ulcers. The patient should avoid alcohol during the course of therapy.
4. Steroids may decrease resistance to infection and the ability to tolerate stress, injury, or surgery (including dental surgery). The patient should inform the physician, dentist, or surgeon that a steroid is being taken.
5. The patient may need an increased dosage of steroids during times of injury, illness, or emotional or psychologic stress for up to 2 years

after prolonged treatment with steroids.

6. The patient and family should know the signs and symptoms of adrenal insufficiency: nausea and vomiting, aching of bones and muscles, headache, increased temperature, and diarrhea. The physician should be notified immediately if any of these problems develop.

7. The patient *must not* stop taking the steroids suddenly. The body will slowly grow to depend on them and cannot survive well without them.

8. The patient should wear a Medic-Alert bracelet or carry other identifying information during and after treatment.

9. The patient should not receive any immunizations without consulting the physician first.

10. The patient should take oral medication with food to minimize stomach upset.

11. The patient may need to eat a diet rich in potassium and low in sodium. The physician should give the patient a list of foods to eat and foods to avoid.

12. The patient should keep the tablets in tightly sealed, brown bottles away from heat.

13. The patient should tell the physician if she becomes pregnant, or if the patient begins to take medications from another health care provider, especially aspirin, diuretics, digitalis preparations, insulin, oral hypoglycemics, phenobarbital, rifampin, phenytoin, and somatotropin.

14. If the patient misses a dose:
    a. If the patient is on an alternate-day schedule, the dose should be taken as soon as possible and the regular schedule should be followed. If the patient remembers in the evening, the dose should be taken the next morning, the next day should be skipped, and a new schedule started.
    b. If the patient is on a daily dose schedule: the dose should be taken as soon as possible. If the patient does not remember until the next day, only the normal dose should be taken and the normal schedule followed.
    c. If the patient is on divided doses (taking medication more than once a day): the dose should be taken as soon as possible, then the normal schedule should be resumed. If the patient forgets until the next dose, that dose should be doubled and then the regular schedule should be resumed.

15. Patients should call the physician if they experience rapid weight gain, black or tarry stools, unusual bleeding or bruising, signs of low potassium or hypokalemia (anorexia, lethargy, confusion, nausea, or muscle weakness).

16. For patients taking ADH, the nurse should teach the patient how to measure fluid intake and the amount and specific gravity of urine, and how to keep accurate records that should be reviewed by the physician. The patient should be aware of the symptoms of water intoxication: drowsiness, listlessness, headache, and convulsions. The drug should be discontinued and the physician notified at once if any of these symptoms develop; also report signs of dehydration: failure to urinate, dry skin and mouth, complaints of thirst, furrowed tongue.

17. Continued appointments to monitor therapy while the patient is taking this drug are important.

SECTION FOUR: SEX HORMONES

Objectives

At the conclusion of this section you should be able to:

1. Explain the use of male and female sex hormones.
2. Identify at least five adverse reactions associated with the male and female sex hormones.
3. Develop a teaching plan for a patient receiving long-term sex hormonal therapy.

OVERVIEW

The sex hormones are produced under the influence of the anterior pituitary gland. The male hormones, testosterone and its derivatives, are called **androgens;** the female hormones are **estrogen** and **progesterone.**

Androgens aid in the development and maintenance of the sex organs at the time of puberty, and secondary sex characteristics in men: facial hair, deep voice, body hair, body fat distribution, and muscle development. They promote the anabolic or tissue-building processes in the body. Anabolic steroids are synthetic drugs with the same use and actions as androgens. These medications may be given as replacement therapy for testosterone deficiency. Androgen therapy may also be given to women as part of the treatment for estrogen-dependent inoperative metastatic breast carcinoma in patients who are past menopause. Androgens are also used to reduce postpartum breast pain and engorgement.

There are two naturally occurring female hormones: estrogen and progesterone. There are also a number of synthetic estrogen and progesterone preparations. Estrogen is secreted by the ovarian follicle and the adrenal cortex. These hormones are responsible for the development and maintenance of the female reproductive system, and the primary and secondary sex characteristics. They also are part of the feedback to the pituitary, providing stimulus for the release of the gonadotropins. Estrogens play a role in the fluid and electrolyte balance in the tissues, especially that involving calcium. They are active in most of the tissue and muscular processes involved in preparation for pregnancy and labor.

Progesterone is produced by the corpus luteum in the ovary, by the placenta, and in small amounts by the adrenal cortex. Progesterones are essential for the development of the placenta and inhibit the pituitary gonadotropins that mature the ovarian follicle to produce ovulation. They play a role in maintaining pregnancy and in preventing pregnancy.

Estrogen, progesterone, and combinations of the two hormones are very effective as oral contraceptives. They prevent ovulation and cause a state that mimics pregnancy in the female.

ANDROGENS

ACTION

The main action of the androgens is the development of secondary male sex characteristics. Androgens are anabolic, increasing the building of tissue. Androgens are also antineoplastic when used to treat certain breast cancers in women. Erythropoiesis, or an increase in red blood cell formation, occurs with the administration of androgens.

USES

Androgens are used in hypogonadism, hypopituitarism, dwarfism, eunuchism, cryptorchidism, oligospermia, and general androgen deficiency in males. They are used to restore a positive nitrogen balance in patients with chronic, debilitating illness or trauma; in treatment of anemia secondary to renal failure and in other blood dyscrasias where increased erythropoiesis is needed; and palliatively for treatment of advanced breast cancer in postmenopausal women and for endometriosis in younger women. Androgens are also used to suppress milk production.

ADVERSE REACTIONS

Adverse reactions to androgens include edema caused by sodium retention (usually only with large doses), acne, hirsutism, male pattern baldness, cholestatic hepatitis with jaundice, buccal irritation, diarrhea, nausea, and vomiting. In women, androgens may produce clitoral enlargement and masculinization. In men, androgens may cause a decrease in sperm count, excessive sexual stimulation, gynecomastia, impotence, and urinary retention. In children, use of androgens may produce precocious puberty, and children may also develop short stature because of premature bone epiphyseal closure.

DRUG INTERACTIONS

Anabolic steroids may increase the effects of anticoagulants, antidiabetic agents, and other drugs. Corticosteroids given concurrently with androgens increase the possibility of edema. Barbiturates decrease the therapeutic effects of androgens because of increased breakdown in the liver. Androgens may affect many laboratory tests.

 NURSING IMPLICATIONS AND PATIENT TEACHING

▼ **Assessment**

The male patient may have a history of impotence, reduced libido, weight loss, male climacteric, or castration, or there may be a history of traumatic castration or failure to develop secondary sex characteristics by 15 to 17 years of age.

The nurse should obtain a complete health history, including the presence of carcinoma, cardiac, renal, or liver dysfunction, other drugs taken concurrently, and the possibility of pregnancy.

▼ Planning

When androgens are given for hypogonadism, careful descriptions of secondary sex characteristics and measurements should be recorded for a baseline to monitor the therapeutic effects.

If cholestatic jaundice develops or liver function decreases, the drug should be discontinued. Stomatitis may result from buccal administration.

▼ Implementation

Androgens can be given by mouth, buccally, and sublingually, depending on the specific drug and the reason for therapy. Dosages vary from 2 to 10 mg daily for replacement therapy. Higher divided doses are given for antineoplastic therapy.

Patients must be instructed not to swallow the pill and not to eat, drink, smoke, or chew until the buccal tablet is absorbed.

See Table 15-9 for a summary of androgens.

▼ Evaluation

The therapeutic response may be slow, requiring 3 or more months to affect symptoms. The nurse should monitor for the development of secondary sex characteristics and improvement in sexual functioning.

▼ Patient and family teaching

The nurse should provide the patient and family with the following instructions:

1. The patient should take this medication as instructed by the physician.
2. Response to the drug may take several weeks or months.
3. The patient should eat a diet high in calories, protein, vitamins, and minerals unless otherwise instructed by the physician.
4. The patient should report any new or troublesome symptoms that may develop. For men: fluid retention, especially in feet and hands;

Table 15-9   Androgens

Generic name	Trade name	Comments and dosage
Danazol	Cyclomen ♣ Danocrine	Synthetic androgen is used to treat endometriosis, fibrocystic breast disease, and hereditary angioedema through suppression of pituitary gonadotropins, and subsequent reduction in menstruation. ■ *Endometriosis:* 400 mg PO bid for 3 to 6 months; may continue for 9 months. Use only for those who cannot tolerate other drugs or who fail to respond; begin therapy during menstruation to rule out pregnancy. ■ *Fibrocystic breast disease:* 50 to 200 mg PO bid for 4 to 6 months; begin during menstruation; use only when pain is severe.
Fluoxymesterone	Halotestin	Gastrointestinal disturbances are more frequent with this product than with other oral androgens. ■ *Hypogonadism:* 2 to 10 mg/day PO. ■ *Breast cancer:* 15 to 30 mg/day PO in divided doses.
Methyltestosterone	Android Metandren ♣ Testred Virilon	Patient should not drink, eat, smoke, or chew until tablet is absorbed buccally. Check mouth each visit for signs of local irritation. ■ *Male eunuchism:* 10 to 40 mg/day PO; 5 to 20 mg buccal. ■ *Androgen deficiency:* 10 to 40 mg/day PO; 5 to 20 mg buccal. ■ *Undescended testicle after puberty:* 30 mg/day PO; 15 mg buccal. ■ *Female breast cancer:* 200 mg/day PO; 100 mg buccal.
Testosterone	Delatest Duratest Histerone Malogen ♣ Testex	■ *Male eunuchism:* 10 to 40 mg/day PO; 5 to 20 mg buccal. ■ *Androgen deficiency:* 10 to 40 mg/day PO; 5 to 20 mg buccal. ■ *Undescended testicle after puberty:* 30 mg/day PO; 15 mg buccal. ■ *Female breast cancer:* 200 mg/day PO; 100 mg buccal.
Androgen hormone inhibitor		
Finasteride	Proscar	Used in benign prostatic hyperplasia and prostatic carcinoma. Give 5 mg once daily. May require 6 months of therapy or more.

enlargement of breasts; shortness of breath; excessive physical or sexual stimulation; prolonged or painful erection of penis; impotence; urinary retention; and yellowing of skin or eyes. For women: yellowing of skin or eyes; fluid retention, especially in feet and hands; shortness of breath; changes in vaginal bleeding; increased sex drive; and masculinization of appearance (signs of masculinization in women usually are reversed when the drug is discontinued).

5. If medicine is taken under the tongue (sublingually) or buccally (putting medicine in cheek), the patient should rinse the mouth and brush the teeth after taking medicine.

ESTROGENS

ACTION

Exogenous estrogens aid in the development of both primary and secondary sex characteristics, including growth and development of the uterine musculature and endothelium, vaginal epithelium, and fallopian tubes; development of breasts; increased cervical mucus and decreased vaginal pH; increased uterine motility; growth of axillary and pubic hair; decreased long-bone growth in prepubertal and pubertal girls; and decreased calcium loss from bones. Estrogens suppress the release of gonadotropins (FSH and LH) from the pituitary or hypothalamus through a feedback mechanism. Estrogens are anabolic and cause retention of salt, water, and nitrogen, an increase in serum lipoproteins and triglycerides, and a decrease in cholesterol. They suppress ovulation when given in adequate doses.

USES

Estrogens are used for therapy in menopause or other conditions in which the natural estrogens are decreased, such as ovarian failure, primary amenorrhea, and oophorectomy. They are used in infertility workups and for palliative therapy in prostatic cancer and breast cancer that is at least 5 years postmenopausal. Estrogens are probably effective for treatment of postmenopausal osteoporosis when used with other measures.

ADVERSE REACTIONS

Adverse reactions to estrogens include edema, hypertension, thrombophlebitis, depression, migraine

headaches, skin rash, decreased glucose tolerance, intolerance to contact lenses, abdominal cramps, diarrhea, nausea, vomiting, breast tenderness and enlargement, changes in vaginal bleeding, exacerbation of estrogen-dependent malignancies, increase in size of uterine fibroids, vaginal candidiasis, and changes in weight and libido. Estrogens have been reported to increase the risk of endometrial carcinoma.

DRUG INTERACTIONS

Rifampin and barbiturates may reduce estrogenic effect. Estrogens may reduce the effects of oral anticoagulants, tricyclic antidepressants, anticonvulsants, and antidiabetic agents. They may potentiate antiinflammatory or glycosuric effects of hydrocortisone and the effect of meperidine. Estrogens alter the results of many diagnostic tests.

PROGESTINS

ACTION

Progestins cause the uterine endometrium to shed during menses after tissue growth stimulated by estrogen. They maintain the endometrium and vaginal epithelium and decrease uterine motility during pregnancy. Acting with estrogen, they cause the breasts to become secretory and more vascular. Some progestins have estrogenic or androgenic effects. Progestins suppress pituitary gonadotropins through a feedback mechanism. They can suppress ovulation, control uterine bleeding caused by hormonal imbalance, increase sodium excretion, and cause a negative nitrogen balance.

USES

Progestins are used for contraception; control of excessive uterine bleeding caused by hormonal imbalance; treatment of secondary amenorrhea, dysmenorrhea, and premenstrual tension; and control of pain in endometriosis. They may be used in the diagnosis and treatment of infertility. Their use is palliative for endometrial cancer. When used for contraception, progestin-only preparations are known as "mini-pills."

ADVERSE REACTIONS

Adverse reactions to progestins include fluid retention; thromboembolic events, including pulmonary embolism; dizziness; headache; mental depression; rashes; decrease in glucose tolerance; weight gain or loss; cholestatic jaundice; diarrhea; nausea; vomiting; amenorrhea; breast tenderness or enlargement; decreased libido; galactorrhea; increased vaginal discharge; spotting; and withdrawal bleeding. Overdosage produces changes in menses, nausea, vomiting, and withdrawal bleeding.

DRUG INTERACTIONS

Progestins alter several laboratory tests.

 ## NURSING IMPLICATIONS AND PATIENT TEACHING

▼ Assessment

For prepubertal ages ask about primary amenorrhea and sexual infantilism. For women of childbearing age, ask about the possibility of pregnancy, history of ovarian failure, need for contraception, and dysmenorrhea. For patients of perimenopausal age, obtain history of hot flashes, menstrual irregularities, dyspareunia, vaginal discharge, vulvar pruritus, urinary frequency, and history of oophorectomy or hysterectomy.

There is an increased dose-related risk of thromboembolic disease, especially in premenopausal women. Progestins should not be used during pregnancy, especially the first 3 months, because of the risk of congenital anomalies and of vaginal adenosis and/or vaginal or cervical cancer when female offspring reach childbearing age. There is an increased risk of gallbladder disease with long-term use. Postmenopausal estrogen therapy is associated with a 5 to 15 times increased risk of endometrial cancer, the risk being related to the length of treatment. Administration of estrogen may result in hypercalcemia in patients with breast or bone cancer.

▼ Planning

Estrogen therapy affects many systems. When estrogens are used before puberty, short stature and decreased growth can result. Use in adult women can increase the risk for migraine headaches, hypertension, diabetes, and certain benign and malignant tumors. Because estrogens are metabolized in the liver and excreted through the kidneys, renal or hepatic dysfunction can alter their actions. Fibroid tumors of the uterus may increase in size. Because

fluid is retained, symptoms of hypertension, asthma, epilepsy, migraine, and heart or kidney dysfunction may be increased. Topical estrogens are readily absorbed and may have systemic effects.

▼ Implementation

Estrogens can be given orally, intramuscularly, or topically. For control of menopausal symptoms, ovarian failure, or postoophorectomy symptoms, they are usually given cyclically with 1 tablet daily for 3 weeks, followed by 1 week off the drug. Usually, the lowest effective dose is given for the shortest period of time. High doses or long-term therapy should be tapered gradually.

Natural progestins are poorly absorbed orally; hence, oral progestins are synthetic products. Tablets are given daily. Progestins are quickly metabolized in the liver, but daily doses are effective.

See Table 15-10 for a summary of estrogens and progestins.

▼ Evaluation

The nurse should monitor for adverse effects. Patients on replacement therapy should be monitored regularly. The nurse should watch for thrombophlebitis and edema in women, and monitor men for feminizing characteristics and impotence.

Timing and characteristics of any vaginal bleeding should be noted to determine if response is therapeutic or adverse.

▼ Patient and family teaching

The nurse should provide the patient and family with the following instructions:

1. Estrogenic drugs, by law, must be dispensed with a patient package insert titled "What You Should Know About Estrogens." When the patient receives a prescription, he or she should look for this package insert and read it thoroughly.
2. Some patients experience side effects when taking this medication. If any of the following symptoms develop, the patient should stop taking the medication and notify the physician immediately: chest pain, abdominal or leg pain or swelling, sudden severe headaches, visual changes, sudden loss of coordination, sudden shortness of breath, or slurred speech.
3. The patient should discontinue the drug immediately if she believes she is pregnant.
4. Less dangerous symptoms that require care or

Table 15-10　Estrogens and progestins

Generic name	Trade name	Comments and dosage
ESTROGENS		
Chlorotrianisene	Tace	A long-acting estrogen retained and released gradually from adipose tissue. Not widely used. Give 12 mg PO qid for 7 days or 50 mg q6h for 6 doses, beginning within 8 hours postpartum. The 72 mg capsule can be given bid for 2 days.
Conjugated estrogens	Premarin	Contains 50% to 65% sodium estrone sulfate and 20% to 35% sodium equilin sulfate; these are naturally occurring and extracted from the urine of pregnant mares. Store in closed containers. Medication should be given for 3 weeks on a daily basis, with 1 week off the medication; 0.3 to 7.5 mg PO qd.
Diethylstilbestrol (DES)	Honuol ♣	Inexpensive product is used primarily in menopausal or postmenopausal women for the control of symptoms. It may also be used in inoperable breast or prostatic cancer that is progressing. Used for postcoital contraception in emergency treatment. ■ *Menopausal-related vasomotor symptoms, atrophic vaginitis:* 0.2 to 0.5 mg qd on cyclic short-term basis only. ■ *Postcoital contraception:* 25 mg bid for 5 consecutive days, beginning within 24 hours after coitus. Do not give later than 72 hours after coitus.
Esterified estrogens	Estratab Menest Menrium ♣	These products contain 75% to 85% sodium estrone sulfate and 6% to 15% sodium equilin sulfate. Store medication in a tightly closed container. ■ *Vasomotor menopausal (natural or surgical) symptoms:* 1.25 to 3.75 mg PO qd. Adjust to lowest dose that controls symptoms.
Ethinyl estradiol	Estinyl	This is the most active synthetic estrogen known. ■ *Vasomotor menopausal symptoms:* 0.02 to 0.05 mg PO qd cycled 3 weeks on, 1 week off. Use decreasing doses as menopause progresses. Use lowest effective dose.
Estradiol	Delestrogen Depogen Estrace Estraderm Gynogen LA	■ *Vasomotor menopausal symptoms, senile vaginitis, kraurosis vulvae, or replacement therapy in hypogonadism or female castration, ovarian failure:* 1 to 2 mg PO qd cycled 3 weeks on and 1 week off. Use lowest therapeutic dosage. Transdermal system: 0.05 mg patch 2 times/week increasing dose until symptoms resolve. May use 3-week cycle on patch, 1 week off.
Estrogen vaginal creams	Dienestrol DV Estrace Ogen Premarin	These preparations are used vaginally and on the vulva to treat atrophic epithelial changes related to low estrogen levels. Can be absorbed systemically and produce side effects. Most effective when used at bedtime. Contain various synthetic estrogens. Give 2 to 4 gm qd. Use applicator that is included, or rub on topically. Use lowest dose for shortest time that will control symptoms.
Estrone	Estronol Gynogen	Give 0.1 to 4 mg IM 2 or 3 times weekly as replacement or to halt abnormal uterine bleeding as a result of hormonal imbalance.
Estropipate or piperazine estrone	Ogen	This drug is composed of crystalline estrone and piperazine for stability. ■ *Prevention of postmenopausal osteoporosis, senile vaginitis or vasomotor menopausal symptoms:* Cycle 3 weeks on, 1 week off with 0.625 to 5 mg qd. Use lowest dose to control symptoms.
Quinestrol	Estrovis	■ *Vasomotor menopausal symptoms, senile vaginitis, female hypogonadism or castration, primary ovarian failure:* 1 tablet qd for 7 days, then 1 tablet weekly. Adjust dose to 2 tablets weekly if needed for therapeutic response.

Table 15-10 Estrogens and progestins—cont'd

Generic name	Trade name	Comments and dosage
PROGESTINS		
Medroxyprogesterone acetate	Amen Curretab Cycrin Provera	Duration of action is long and somewhat variable. ■ *Secondary amenorrhea, abnormal uterine bleeding caused by hormonal imbalance:* 5 to 10 mg PO qd for 5 to 10 days, beginning on 16th or 21st day of menstrual cycle. Maximum therapeutic effect will be seen with 10 mg/day for 10 days beginning on 16th day of cycle. Withdrawal bleeding should occur 3 to 7 days after last dose.
Norethindrone	Norlutin	This medication represents the only ingredient in some "mini-pill" contraceptives (Micronor and Nor-Q.D.). Take with meals to reduce nausea. Store in closed container. ■ *Amenorrhea or uterine bleeding caused by hormonal imbalance:* 5 to 20 mg qd on the 5th to 25th day of the menstrual cycle. ■ *Endometriosis:* 10 mg qd for 2 weeks, increasing 5 mg at 2-week intervals until a total dose of 30 mg is reached. Continue 6 to 9 months or until breakthrough bleeding occurs. Then it can be stopped temporarily.
Norethindrone acetate	Aygestin Norlutate	This medication is twice as strong as norethindrone. It is mildly androgenic. Take with meals to reduce nausea. Store in a closed container. ■ *Uterine bleeding caused by hormonal imbalance:* 2.5 to 10 mg qd on 5th to 25th day of the menstrual cycle. ■ *Endometriosis:* 5 mg for 2 weeks, increasing 2.5 mg at 2-week intervals until a dose of 15 mg per day is reached. Continue 6 to 9 months or until breakthrough bleeding occurs. Then it can be stopped temporarily. The object of therapy is to prevent menstruation.
Hydroxyprogesterone	Duralutin Hylutin Pro Depo	■ *Primary and secondary amenorrhea, dysfunctional uterine bleeding, metrorrhagia:* Give 375 mg IM.

consultation with a physician include changes in vaginal bleeding or discharge, skin rash, breast lumps, jaundice, increased blood pressure, abdominal pain, and mental depression.

5. Nausea and breast tenderness may occur early in therapy, but should lessen after 1 to 3 weeks; taking oral medicines with food may reduce nausea.

6. Less common side effects are changes in libido (sex drive), photosensitivity, chloasma (facial skin changes often seen in pregnancy), and vomiting.

7. Use of estrogens for replacement is associated with an increased risk of developing endometrial cancer. The patient should report any vaginal bleeding after menopause to the physician.

8. If surgery is anticipated, the surgeon should be notified so that doses may be changed or discontinued temporarily.

9. Patients of all ages should be monitored regularly while on any estrogen preparation.

10. The patient should take the pills exactly as directed and keep them out of the reach of children or anyone for whom they are not prescribed.

11. When used for a short period to treat dysfunctional bleeding, progestins should first stop the bleeding and then cause the endometrial lining to shed when the drug is withdrawn. Improvement of heavy bleeding should occur in 24 to 48 hours.

12. Breakthrough or withdrawal bleeding can occur, especially in long-term use for contraception.

13. The patient should report abnormal or unex-

plained vaginal bleeding to the physician.

14. The patient should not take progestins if there is a history of breast or genital cancer, except as palliative treatment in advanced disease.

15. Diabetic patients should tell the physician if they begin developing positive urine tests so that antidiabetic medication can be adjusted.

ORAL CONTRACEPTIVES

ACTION

Most oral contraceptives are combination drugs that contain both an estrogen and a progestin. The principal action is to prevent ovulation by inhibiting the follicle-stimulating hormone (FSH) and the luteinizing hormone (LH). The progestin-only "mini-pill" inhibits ovulation by the same mechanism, but is more variable in suppressing the gonadotropins. The progestins in both types of oral contraceptive pills have several other contraceptive effects: creating a thick cervical mucus hostile to sperm, decelerating ovum transport by decreasing motility of the fallopian tubes, and inhibiting implantation.

USES

Oral contraceptives are used to prevent pregnancy when a highly effective method is needed and heterosexual activity is regular.

ADVERSE REACTIONS

For adverse reactions to oral contraceptives, see estrogen and progestin sections, pp. 330-331. Most adverse reactions are caused by hormonal imbalance. *Estrogen excess* may produce nausea, dizziness, edema, cyclic weight gain, bloating, increase in fibroid size, uterine cramps, irritability, increased fat deposition, poor contact lens fit, vascular-type headache, hypertension, lactation suppression, cystic breast changes, breast tenderness, thrombophlebitis, cerebrovascular infarction, myocardial infarction, and hepatic adenoma.

Progestin excess may cause increased appetite and weight gain (noncyclic), tiredness, weakness, depression and decrease in libido, acne, loss of hair, cholestatic jaundice, decreased length of menstrual flow, hypertension, headaches during "resting" phase of cycle, breast tenderness, decreased carbohydrate tolerance, dilated leg veins, and pelvic congestion syndrome.

Androgen excess may produce increased appetite and weight gain, hirsutism, acne, oily skin, rash, increased libido, cholestatic jaundice, and pruritus.

Estrogen deficiency may cause irritability, nervousness, hot flashes, vasomotor symptoms, uterine prolapse, pelvic relaxation symptoms, early and midcycle spotting, decreased amount of menstrual flow, no withdrawal bleeding, decreased libido, dry vaginal mucosa, atrophic vaginitis and dyspareunia, headaches, and depression.

Progestin deficiency may produce late breakthrough bleeding and spotting, heavy menstrual flow and clots, delayed onset of menses, dysmenorrhea, and weight loss.

DRUG INTERACTIONS

There may be an increase in breakthrough bleeding and a decrease in contraceptive effectiveness in patients taking antitubercular medication, many antibiotics, barbiturates, and anticonvulsants.

Oral contraceptives may decrease the effectiveness of anticoagulants, antihypertensives, anticonvulsants, tricyclic antidepressants, oral hypoglycemics, and vitamins. When oral contraceptives are given with troleandomycin, the effect may be additive in causing jaundice. Oral contraceptives may alter many laboratory test results.

 NURSING IMPLICATIONS AND PATIENT TEACHING

▼ Assessment

To determine the most appropriate type of contraception for a patient, the nurse needs to obtain a thorough menstrual, contraceptive, and reproductive history. This must include any concurrent diseases, the patient's drug history, and whether or not the patient smokes. The nurse must make certain the patient is not breastfeeding or pregnant, assess the patient's sexual activity and knowledge of contraceptive meth-

 CRITICAL DECISION
Obtaining a History

The nurse should obtain a detailed menstrual history and history of any thromboembolic events, migraine headaches, and liver or kidney problems.

Contraindications for oral contraceptives

Absolute contraindications

History or presence of thromboembolic disorders, cerebrovascular accident, coronary artery disease, hepatic adenoma, malignancy of breast or reproductive system, known impairment of liver function, and pregnancy.

Strong relative contraindications

Severe headaches (particularly vascular or migraine),* hypertension (with resting diastolic blood pressure of 90 or greater on three or more separate visits, or an accurate measurement of 110 or more on a single visit),* diabetes,* prediabetes or a strong family history of diabetes, gallbladder disease, including cholecystectomy,* previous cholestasis during pregnancy, congenital hyperbilirubinemia (Gilbert's disease), mononucleosis (acute phase), sickle cell disease (SS) or sickle C disease (SC),* undiagnosed, abnormal vaginal bleeding,† elective surgery (planned in next 4 weeks or major surgery requiring immobilization),* long leg casts or major injury to lower leg, patient over 40 years of age,* patient over 35 years of age with a history of heavy smoking,* and impaired liver function within the past year.

Other relative contraindications

Termination of term pregnancy within past 10 to 14 days,* weight gain of 10 pounds or more while on the "pill,"* failure to have established regular menstrual cycles,* profile suggestive of anovulation and infertility problems (late onset of menses and very irregular, painless menses),* presence of or history of cardiac or renal disease,* conditions likely to make patient unreliable at following dosage instructions (mental retardation, major psychiatric problems, alcoholism, history of repeatedly taking pills incorrectly),* lactation (oral contraceptives may be initiated as weaning begins and may be an aid in decreasing the flow of milk).*

May initiate the pill for women with these problems, but observe carefully for worsening or improvement of the problem: depression,* hypertension (with resting diastolic blood pressure of 90 to 99 mm Hg at a single visit),* presence of or history of chloasma or hair loss related to pregnancy,* asthma,* epilepsy,* uterine fibromyoma,* acne, varicose veins,* history of hepatitis (but liver function tests normal now and for at least 1 year).

*Contraindications to estrogen-containing pills, but may not be contraindications to progestin-only pills or may be less of a contraindication to progestin-only pills than to combined pills.
†Some believe this to be an absolute contraindication.

ods, and determine whether any contraindications for drug use are present (see the box above).

▼ Planning

Although breakthrough bleeding may be a side effect, nonfunctional causes should be investigated. Bleeding irregularities are more common with progestin-only pills.

There is some risk of infertility after discontinuation of oral contraceptives, especially in women who have had irregular or scanty periods before taking pills.

Research suggests many women forget to take pills, resulting in many unintentional pregnancies.

▼ Implementation

To be effective, oral contraceptives must be taken at about the same time each day. This is particularly true with progestin-only pills. Taking medication with meals will reduce the nausea common in the first cycles.

All oral combination contraceptives are to be taken for 21 days. Usually therapy is initiated the 5th day after or the Sunday after menstruation starts. Another method of contraception should be used for the first 7 to 10 days of the first cycle. Pills are packaged in a 1-month packet with the days named or numbered. Some preparations contain 28 pills to be taken daily, 7 of which contain an inert substance or iron. Others require the patient to go 7 days without pills before starting another 28-day cycle. During the "rest," vaginal bleeding should occur.

Combination pills vary in the type and relative amounts of estrogen and progestin (see box on p. 336). All contain a combination of one estrogen and one progestin. Two estrogens, ethinyl estradiol and mestranol, are used. Mestranol is half as strong as ethinyl estradiol. Several progestins are used in combination with them. Some progestins are estrogenic, antiestrogenic, and/or androgenic in effect. A dose of 50 µg or less of estrogen is used to initiate therapy. Less than this dose may cause breakthrough bleeding,

Content of Oral Combination Contraceptive Pills

Estrogen and Progestin

Mestranol and norethindrone

Genora 1/50
Nelova 1/50M
Norethin 1/50M
Norinyl 1 + 50
Ortho-Novum 1/50

Estradiol and norethindrone

Brevicon
Genora 1/35; 0.5/35
Modicon
N.E.E. 1/35
Nelova 1/35E; 0.5/35E
Norcept-E 1/35
Norethin 1/35E
Norinyl 1+35
Ortho-Novum 1/35
Ovcon-50; -35

Estradiol and norethindrone biphasic or triphasic pills

Nelova 10/11 (Norethindrone dose increases phase 2)
Ortho-Novum 10/11 (Norethindrone dose increases phase 2)
Ortho-Novum 7/7/7 (Norethindrone dose increases phase 2 and 3)
Tri-Levlen (Norethindrone dose increases phase 2 and 3)
Tri-Norinyl (Norethindrone dose increases phase 2 and 3)
Triphasil (Norethindrone dose increases phase 2 and 3)

Estradiol and norethindrone acetate

Loestrin 21 1.5/30; Fe 1.5/30; 21 1/20; Fe 1/20
Norlestrin 1/50; Fe 1/50; 21 2.5/50; Fe 2.5/50

Estradiol and ethynodiol diacetate

Demulen 1/35; 1/50

Estradiol and levonorgestrel

Levlen
Nordette

Estradiol and norgestrel

Lo/Ovral
Ovral

Estradiol and desogestrel

Ortho-Cept

but increasingly, doses of less than 50 µg are being prescribed. New combinations are introduced frequently. For the progestin-only pills, the medication is taken daily on a continuous basis.

See Table 15-11 for a summary of oral contraceptives.

▼ Evaluation

The nurse should monitor for adverse effects, which may vary in severity. They may be a result of the relative strengths of estrogen and progestin. Side effects may be eliminated by changing to a different combination of estrogen and progestin. Some spotting can be tolerated in younger women.

The nurse should evaluate the patient's compliance in taking medications. Patients who have trouble remembering to take other medications are not good candidates for oral contraceptives.

Patient and family teaching

The nurse should provide the patient and family with the following instructions:

1. The patient must take the pills exactly as prescribed. If a pill is missed, the patient should follow the directions given by the physician. Usually the patient takes 2 pills the next day or discards 1 tablet and takes 1 tablet the next day. Risk for bleeding and/or conception increases with 2 or more pills missed. The patient may need to use a backup method of contraception for a period of time. Another method should also be used in the first 3 weeks of the first cycle and if vomiting for several days occurs because of illness.

2. Certain side effects should be reported to the physician immediately: pain in chest, groin, or legs; sudden, severe headaches; sudden slurring

Table 15-11 Oral contraceptives

Generic name	Trade name	Comments and dosage
Oral forms		
Estrogen and progestin combinations	■ *Monophasic* Brevicon Demulen Genora Loestrin Lo/Ovral Modicon N.E.E. Nelova Norcept-E Nordette Norethin Norinyl Norlestrin Ortho-Cept Ortho-Novum Ovcon Ovral ■ *Biphasic* Nelova 10/11 Ortho-Novum 10/ll ■ *Triphasic* Ortho-Novum 7/7/7 Tri-Levlen Tri-Norinyl Triphasil	The patient should take one pill each day for 21 days, beginning with the regimen the physician suggests, either starting the Sunday after a period begins or starting 5 days after the onset of the period. If there are 7 inert pills, they should be taken after the 21-day cycle. If not, the patient should start a new pack after 7 days. If one pill is missed, the forgotten one should be taken and a backup contraceptive method used. If 2 pills are missed, 2 should be taken for 2 consecutive days and another method used until the end of the cycle. If 3 are missed, a new pack should be started on the 8th day or the first Sunday after the last pill was taken. Another birth control method must be used for 7 to 14 days, depending on the dosage.
Progestin-only (mini-pills)	Micronor Nor-Q.D. Ovrette	Pills must be taken at the same time each day to be most effective. Only the most reliable patients should use these. Slightly less effective than combination products in preventing pregnancy. Incidence of pregnancy is highest in the first 6 months of use. Breakthrough bleeding is more common than with combination pills; therefore undiagnosed genital bleeding is an important contraindication, especially in older women. The patient should take one pill at the same time every day continually. Do not stop during menses.
Other conctraceptive forms		
Levonorgestril implants	Norplant	Medication implanted in a set of six flexible closed capsules made of Silastic, each containing the progestin levonorgestril. This is an implantable system effective in contraception for up to 5 years and completely reversible. Contraindicated in abnormal bleeding, thrombophlebitis, pregnancy, liver disease, and carcinoma of the breast. Implant subdermally in the midportion of the upper arm about 8 to 10 cm above the elbow crease during the first 7 days after the onset of menses. Breakthrough bleeding is a common occurrence.
Progesterone intrauterine insert	Progestasert	A T-shaped unit containing a reservoir of 38 mg progesterone with barium sulfate dispersed in a silicone fluid is inserted into the uterine cavity. Contraceptive effectiveness is maintained for 1 year and then the unit must be replaced. Bleeding and cramps may occur during the first few weeks after insertion, sometimes requiring removal.
Medroxyprogesterone acetate	Depo-Provera	Long-term injectable contraceptive. Give 150 mg every 3 months after the onset of normal menses. Give in gluteal or deltoid muscle. Make certain that the patient is not pregnant.

of speech; sudden loss of coordination; sudden visual changes; sudden shortness of breath. Other symptoms may require attention, but are not emergencies: changes in vaginal bleeding; hypertension; breast lumps; jaundice; vaginal discharge; stomach or side pains; mental depression. Other side effects may be present, but not serious: nausea, loss of appetite, acne, stomach cramps, edema of ankles and feet, breast swelling and tenderness, tiredness, brown spots on skin, changes in libido, changes in weight, increased body hair, some hair loss on scalp, sensitivity to the sun.

3. The patient must return for scheduled check-ups.
4. The patient should immediately stop taking the pill if she thinks she is pregnant or if she misses two periods. The patient must not take oral contraceptives while breastfeeding.
5. The patient should keep one extra month's supply of pills on hand so there is no chance of running out and breaking the cycles.
6. The patient should not smoke while taking the pill.
7. All other medications the patient is taking should be reported to the physician because of possible drug interactions.
8. For women under 40, the risk of death from complications from the pill is less than the risk of death from complications of pregnancy. (Patients should not be so frightened of taking the pill that they fail to recognize that it is safer

CRITICAL DECISION:
Adverse Effects of Smoking

Patients should be questioned about smoking while taking the pill. Patients who smoke while taking oral contraceptives are at increased risk of adverse effects.

CRITICAL DECISION:
Other Medications

Patients should be cautioned about taking other medications while taking contraceptives. For example, antiobiotics may reduce the effectiveness of contraceptives, thus placing the patient at risk for pregnancy.

statistically to take the pill than to be pregnant.)
9. For patients using the Norplant or the Progestasert systems, special instructions are needed. Patient should watch for signs of infection or excessive bleeding following insertion. Difficulties should be reported to the health care provider immediately.

Each visit to the care provider should include an interim history of possible side effects or adverse reactions, a review of proper administration, and a reminder of signs and symptoms to report.

SECTION FIVE: THYROID PREPARATIONS

Objectives

At the conclusion of this section you should be able to:

1. List at least three medications that act on the thyroid gland.
2. Describe the use of thyroid medications.
3. Compare adverse effects of various thyroid preparations.
4. Develop a teaching plan for patients who are taking thyroid preparations on a long-term basis.

OVERVIEW

The thyroid gland, located in the neck in front of the trachea, produces the hormones thyroxine (T_4) and triiodothyronine (T_3), which influence almost every organ and tissue of the body. Although their exact mechanism of action is unknown, their primary action is to determine the metabolic rate of the tissues.

The anterior pituitary gland secretes thyroid-stimulating hormone (TSH), which tells the thyroid gland to release the hormones that it has stored. When the level of circulating thyroid hormones is high, TSH from the anterior pituitary gland is withheld; when the circulating level falls, this information is also communicated and TSH is once again released. This type of arrangement is called a feedback mechanism, because physiologic action returns to influence the organ sending the signals.

Two general types of diseases can influence the hormone-producing activity of the thyroid gland. A decrease in the amount of thyroid hormones manufactured or secreted is called hypothyroidism. An increase in the amount of thyroid hormones manufactured and secreted is called hyperthyroidism.

Synthetic hormones, natural hormones, or a combination product may be given to increase the level of thyroid hormone in hypothyroid conditions, or given as replacement therapy when the thyroid gland has been surgically removed. In hyperthyroid conditions, other preparations are given that slow the rate of thyroid production. Both thyroid supplements and antithyroid medications will be described.

THYROID SUPPLEMENTS OR REPLACEMENTS

ACTION

The main action of the thyroid hormones is to increase metabolic rate. This results in an increase in tissue oxygen consumption, body temperature, heart and respiratory rate, cardiac output, and carbohydrate, lipid, and protein metabolism. In addition, thyroid hormones influence growth and development of the skeletal system, especially ossification in the epiphyses of long bones.

USES

Thyroid hormones are used in replacement therapy to manage hypothyroidism, myxedema, cretinism, and/or nontoxic goiter caused by deficiency of thyroid hormones, atrophy, congenital defects, the effects of surgery, antithyroid products, or radiation. They are also used to treat chronic thyroid infections and tumors that are dependent on thyrotropic hormone.

ADVERSE REACTIONS

Adverse reactions to thyroid replacements include dysrhythmias, hypertension, tachycardia, hand tremors, headache, insomnia, nervousness, diarrhea, vomiting, weight loss, menstrual irregularities, rash, glycosuria, hyperglycemia, increased prothrombin time, increased serum cholesterol levels. Overdosage produces signs of **hyperthyroidism** (weight loss, decreased or absent menstruation, rapid or pounding heart, heat intolerance, nervousness, irritability, diarrhea, sweaty skin, inability to fall asleep, fever, or chest pain).

DRUG INTERACTIONS

Thyroid preparations may increase the patient's requirement for antidiabetic agents. Anticoagulant effects may be potentiated by thyroid replacement because of increased hypoprothrombinemia. Corticosteroid requirements are increased for patients taking thyroid preparations because of increased tissue demands. Effects of tricyclic antidepressants are enhanced by thyroid hormones. Many other isolated medications may be affected.

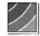 **NURSING IMPLICATIONS AND PATIENT TEACHING**

▼ Assessment

The patient may have a history of **hypothyroidism,** including fatigue, weakness, lethargy, moderate weight gain (around 10 pounds) with minimal appetite, cold intolerance, menorrhagia, dry skin, coarse hair, hoarseness, impaired memory, and constipation.

On examination, the nurse may find skin changes associated with **myxedema,** including nonpitting edema, doughy skin, puffy face, large tongue, decreased body hair, and cool, dry skin. The thyroid gland may be normal in size, enlarged, or not palpable, depending on the cause of hypothyroidism. Neurologic signs include slow mentation, muscle weakness, slowed relaxation phase of the deep tendon reflexes, dull facial expression, or carpal tunnel syndrome. Cardiac signs include bradycardia and decreased blood pressure.

Laboratory findings in thyroid disease may include reduced free T_4 index and elevated serum TSH; other tests may be abnormal.

The nurse should obtain a complete health history including other drugs being taken that may produce drug interactions, and the possible presence of diabetes mellitus, cardiovascular disease, adrenocortical insufficiency, or pregnancy; these conditions are precautions to the use of thyroid supplements.

Table 15-12 Thyroid supplements or replacements

Generic name	Trade name	Comments and dosage
Liothyronine (T_3)	Cytomel Triostat	A synthetic hormone; has rapid effect and short duration of action, which allow fast dosage adjustment and quick reversibility of overdosage. The therapeutic effects are achieved in 24 to 72 hours and persist up to 72 hours after withdrawal of drug. ■ *Mild hypothyroidism:* Initiate therapy at 25 µg daily and increase by 12.5 to 25 µg q 1 to 2 weeks until effects are achieved. Maintenance dosage is usually 25 to 100 µg/day.
Levothyroxine	Levoxine Synthroid Levothroid	Synthetic preparation; drug of choice because effect is predictable. *Initial therapy:* Give 0.05 to 0.1 mg PO qd with increases in dosage of 0.05 to 0.1 mg at 2-week intervals until therapeutic effect is achieved. Maintenance is 0.1 to 0.2 mg/day PO.
Liotrix	Euthroid Thyrolar	Liotrix is a combination of synthetic levothyroxine sodium (T_4) and liothyronine sodium (T_3) in a 4:1 ratio. Predictable therapeutic effect is an advantage. Initiate therapy with one ½ tablet and increase by one ½ tablet at 1- to 2-week intervals.
Thyroglobulin	Proloid	Contains levothyroxine (T_4) and liothyronine (T_3). Because it is a natural product, its hormonal content is variable. Start with 16 to 32 mg/day PO and increase q2 weeks until therapeutic effect is achieved. Maintenance dosage is usually 32 to 200 mg/day.
Thyroid, desiccated	Thyrar Armour USP Strong S-P-T	Desiccated thyroid contains T_4 and T_3 thyroid hormones in their natural state. Because these drugs are composed of desiccated animal thyroid glands, the hormonal content is variable and T_3 and T_4 levels fluctuate; therefore, avoid varying brands. ■ *Myxedema without hypothyroidism:* Initiate therapy at 30 mg/day with increases of 60 mg/month until therapeutic effects are achieved. Maintenance is usually 60 to 180 mg/day.

▼ Planning

Patients over 50 are often sensitive to thyroid hormones. It is important to begin the patient on a small dose and observe for signs and symptoms of cardiovascular disease before increasing dosage.

▼ Implementation

Patients with hypothyroidism are sensitive to thyroid preparations; therefore treatment should begin in small doses and be increased gradually. A reduction in dosage and gradual upward adjustment may be necessary when side effects occur; therapy should be withdrawn for 2 to 6 days, then resumed at a lower dosage.

The patient's age, the presence of cardiac disease, and the severity of symptoms should be considered when initiating therapy. Titration of dosage to gain maximal therapeutic response with the lowest dosage is the objective. The usual maintenance dosage in the treatment of hypothyroidism is 0.5 to 2 gm as a single daily dose before breakfast.

T_4 (thyroxine) is the treatment of choice for hypothyroidism, because of its purity and long duration of action. Because T_4 has a slow onset of action, therapeutic effects may not occur for 3 to 4 weeks. T_3 (triiodothyronine), which has a rapid onset, may be administered if rapid correction of hypothyroidism is necessary. The equivalent strengths of the various thyroid products vary, and care must be used in changing from one product to another. Patients should take the medication at the same time every day, preferably before breakfast. If medication is taken late in the day, insomnia may result.

See Table 15-12 for a summary of thyroid supplements or replacements.

▼ Evaluation

Response to therapy is not immediate. Most patients begin to feel better within 2 weeks, and the therapeutic results are often achieved in 3 months.

The nurse should teach patients the signs and symptoms of hypothyroidism and hyperthyroidism so that they can monitor underdosage or overdosage themselves.

If symptoms of overdosage occur, the medication should be stopped for several days and therapy should be resumed at a lower dosage.

Periodic blood tests should be done before initiating thyroid hormone therapy and once the patient is on a maintenance dose.

▼ Patient and family teaching

The nurse should provide the patient and family with the following instructions:

1. The patient should take the medication exactly as directed by the physician. The medication should be taken at the same time every day, preferably before breakfast. If it is taken too late in the day, the patient may have difficulty going to sleep.
2. Response to this medicine is not immediate; symptoms should improve within 2 weeks. The patient should not increase the dosage unless instructed to do so by the physician. Taking the medication and compliance with therapy are extremely important.
3. If the patient is being treated concurrently for diabetes mellitus, any changes in urine sugar and acetone test results should be reported to the physician.
4. If the patient is receiving anticoagulant therapy, bleeding or excessive bruising should be reported to the physician.
5. Check with the physician before taking any other medications; this will decrease the chance of drugs interacting.

Geriatric Considerations
THYROID HORMONES

Since the elderly are usually more sensitive to and experience more adverse reactions to thyroid hormones than other age groups, it is recommended that thyroid replacement doses be individualized. In some patients the dose should be 25% lower than the usual adult dose.

Hypothyroidism, the second most common endocrine disease in the elderly, is often misdiagnosed. Only one third of geriatric patients exhibit the typical signs and symptoms of cold intolerance and weight gain. Most often the symptoms are nonspecific, such as failing to thrive, stumbling and falling episodes, weight loss, incontinence, and if neurologic involvement has occurred, the patient may be misdiagnosed as having dementia, depression, or a psychotic episode.

From McKenry LM, Salerno E: *Mosby's pharmacology in nursing*, ed 18, St Louis, 1992, Mosby.

6. Report signs and symptoms of overdosage (hyperthyroidism) or underdosage (hypothyroidism) to the physician promptly (these signs and symptoms are summarized earlier).

ANTITHYROID PRODUCTS

ACTION

The main action of antithyroid products is to inhibit the synthesis of thyroid hormones. They are the main drugs used to treat hyperthyroidism. These agents do not inactivate or inhibit the thyroid hormones, thyroxine or triiodothyronine, that are already stored or circulating in the blood.

USES

These products are used to treat hyperthyroidism or to improve hyperthyroidism in preparation for surgery or radioactive iodine therapy.

ADVERSE REACTIONS

Adverse reactions to antithyroid products include drowsiness, headaches, neuritis, paresthesia, vertigo, epigastric distress, jaundice, nausea, vomiting, skin rash, urticaria, myalgia, edema, loss of hair, and lymphadenopathy. Hypothyroidism may occur as a result of prolonged therapy. Agranulocytosis is a rare but serious occurrence. In addition, other, more serious problems may develop.

DRUG INTERACTIONS

The effects of anticoagulants are potentiated by propylthiouracil. Caution should be taken in administering antithyroid drugs to patients who are receiving additional drugs known to cause agranulocytosis (e.g., hydantoins).

NURSING IMPLICATIONS AND PATIENT TEACHING

▼ Assessment

The patient may have a history of hyperthyroidism, including nervousness and/or tremor, weight loss with increased appetite, heat intolerance and excessive sweating, emotional lability, and muscle weakness. On physical examination the nurse may find exophthalmos; thyroid enlargement; tachycardia; in-

Table 15-13 Antithyroid products

Generic name	Trade name	Comments and dosage
Methimazole	Tapazole	Does not inhibit peripheral conversion of thyroxine to T_3. It is more potent than propylthiouracil (PTU), and doses are one tenth those of PTU. It acts more rapidly but less consistently than PTU. Initial dosage is 15 to 60 mg PO qd; maintenance is usually 5 to 15 mg qd.
Propylthiouracil	Propylthiouracil	PTU interferes with synthesis of thyroxine and blocks peripheral conversion of thyroxine to T_3. It may cause hypoprothrombinemia and bleeding. Give 100 to 150 mg PO tid at 8-hour intervals. Initial dose is 300 mg PO qd at 8-hour intervals with adjustments in dosage made after 2 weeks depending on free T_4 levels and symptoms. Continue therapy 6 to 18 months before tapering.
Iodine products	Lugol's Iodine	Give 2 to 6 drops solution tid. Used before surgery.
	Thryo-Block	Give 130 mg potassium iodine tablets.

creased blood pressure; tremor; warm, moist, smooth skin; and proximal muscle weakness. Weight loss and the signs of congestive heart failure may be the predominant manifestations of hyperthyroidism in the elderly.

Laboratory findings may show elevated free T_4 index, increased T_3, or decreased TSH.

The nurse should obtain a complete health history, including hypersensitivity to antithyroid drugs, other medications taken concurrently that could cause drug interactions, and pregnancy or breastfeeding.

▼ **Planning**

The patient's compliance to therapy should be encouraged to avoid hyperthyroidism. Antithyroid drugs have a high incidence of achieving remission if taken correctly for 1 to 2 years.

▼ **Implementation**

The therapeutic objective is to correct the hypermetabolic state with a minimum of side effects and with the smallest incidence of hypothyroidism. Clinical response to the antithyroid drugs usually takes 1 to 2 weeks, because the drugs do not affect the release of the thyroid hormone. Response depends on the inhibition of thyroid hormone synthesis, the amount of preformed hormone in the gland, and the peripheral rate of conversion of the thyroid hormones. Generally, therapy is maintained for 12 to 24 months and then reduced to see if a remission occurs. Titration of

dosage to gain maximal therapeutic response with the lowest dosage is the objective.

See Table 15-13 for a summary of antithyroid products.

▼ **Evaluation**

Laboratory blood tests should be done before initiating antithyroid therapy and done periodically once the patient is on a maintenance dosage. Before therapy is started, a white blood cell count with differential is done and is repeated with any sign of infection. Serum T_4 and TSH levels are monitored initially and after every 2 weeks of therapy until a euthyroid state is achieved, usually in 3 to 5 months. Once the patient has been euthyroid (normal) for 6 to 12 months, a decision may be made to reduce the dosage and ascertain whether a remission has occurred. If remission is achieved, therapy is discontinued.

▼ **Patient and family teaching**

The nurse should provide the patient and family with the following instructions:
1. The patient should take this medication exactly as directed by the physician.
2. Because clinical response usually takes from 1 to 2 weeks to achieve, the dosage should not be increased until each dosage level can be individually evaluated.
3. Some patients experience side effects from this

drug, such as fever, sore throat, malaise, unusual bleeding or bruising, headache, skin rash, and enlargement of cervical lymph nodes (in the neck); these symptoms should be reported to the physician.

4. Bed rest, adequate diet, and avoidance of occupational and domestic stress are also useful modalities of therapy.

SUMMARY

A variety of hormones and steroids are used in medical therapy. Unlike many other medications, hormones and steroids are natural or manufactured preparations that replace, increase, or decrease the effects of substances produced in the body. Hormones and steroids are part of a complex message system linking together various organs and biologic systems. Important hormones or steroids covered in this chapter are insulins, oral hypoglycemics, agents that act on the uterus, pituitary and adrenocortical hormones, sex hormones, oral contraceptives, and thyroid preparations. It is important for the nurse to have a basic understanding of how these preparations work in the body, a familiarity with the major adverse effects that can occur, and a lesson plan with the important points to cover when teaching the patient and family.

 CRITICAL THINKING QUESTIONS

1. Identify characteristics of the two major types of diabetes mellitus, including overall differences in their treatment.

2. Seven-year-old Jessica has just been found to have type I juvenile diabetes (IDDM). Her mother has brought her in to the clinic. Draw up a patient and family teaching plan that includes not only an explanation of insulin therapy but also meal planning. Also, describe adverse reactions to insulin and applicable nursing actions to be taken. Include the Somogyi effect.

3. Describe the preparation and administration of several insulin products. Why do these vary? Which preparation(s) is Jessica most likely to be started on?

4. Identify the different roles and actions of each of the three types of drugs used for the uterus.

5. Mrs. Kline has been in labor for a number of hours since her water broke, and the physician has started infusing oxytocin. Why is it important to monitor Mrs. Kline very carefully? Don't forget to explain the delicate margin between therapeutic and adverse effects.

6. Draw up a chart to help you sort out the various uses, adverse effects, drug interactions, and associated nursing actions for the major pituitary and adrenocortical hormones.

7. Develop a generic teaching plan for the patient receiving long-term hormone therapy.

8. Describe the most important aspects of the nursing process for the patient receiving androgen therapy, paying particular attention to the adverse reactions and drug interactions.

9. During her hospital stay, Ms. James has begun estrogen therapy. She will continue to take estrogen after she is discharged. What would you include in a teaching plan for Ms. James regarding risks and possible adverse effects?

10. Ms. Marra, a young woman, comes to your clinic to begin taking oral contraceptives for the first time. Write a list of points to make in instructing her, particularly on the importance of sticking to a strict regimen and obtaining regular checkups once she is taking this drug.

11. Explain the difference between hypothyroidism and hyperthyroidism.

12. Mr. Moore is starting a thyroid replacement regimen. As you are preparing to instruct him on its use and effects, he makes the comment that "replacement therapy" sounds to him like he will experience immediate results. What points will you want to be sure to make about sensitivity, therapeutic response, and follow-up? Be sure to include the signs of myxedema.

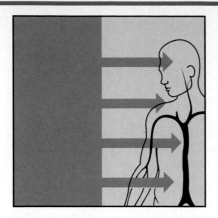

CHAPTER 16

Immunologic Agents

OBJECTIVES

At the conclusion of this chapter you should be able to:

1. Define common terms used in immunology.
2. Explain the differences among the three different types of immunity.
3. Outline typical immunization plans for children and adults.
4. List the major adverse effects of common immunologic drugs.
5. Identify at least three drugs used in in vivo testing.

KEY TERMS

antigen-antibody response, p. 345
antiserums, p. 346
artificially acquired active immunity, p. 345
immunity, p. 345
naturally acquired active immunity, p. 345
passive immunity, p. 346
toxoid, p. 345
vaccines, p. 345

OVERVIEW

Immunologic agents are biologic preparations such as vaccines, toxoids, and other serologic agents used primarily to prevent or modify disease in an otherwise healthy individual. Depending on the composition of the biologic agents, they provide active or passive immunity to specific diseases. These different mechanisms are discussed in general, with specific product information summarized in Table 16-2.

Immune System

The immune system is part of the lymphatic system, which is composed of the lymph vessels, lymph nodes, and other lymph organs (Fig. 16-1). This system removes foreign substances from the blood and lymph, combats disease, maintains tissue fluid balance, and absorbs fats. It moves lymph from its source, the body tissues, to the point where it reenters the bloodstream. The structures of the lymphatic system are of two kinds: those that are concerned with the transport of lymph, and those that are composed principally of lymphatic tissue but serve other specific functions. The former comprise lymph capillaries, lymph vessels, and lymph ducts. The latter include the lymph nodes, spleen, tonsils, and thymus, collectively called lymph organs.

The lymphatic system provides transport as well as having organs producing the T cells that help provide immunity.

ACTION

A bacterium, a virus, or a foreign protein that invades the body is called an antigen. The body responds to the antigen by forming antibodies, which are special proteins manufactured by the lymphatic tissue and the reticuloendothelial system that are designed to help neutralize or resist the invading proteins and provide **immunity** in the patient. In this **antigen-antibody response,** a specific antigen provokes a specific antibody to be produced. This is called **naturally acquired active immunity.** Some antibodies remain circulating for the life of the person, providing constant immunity to that antigen. An example is when a child develops chickenpox, and the body develops antibodies to the chickenpox virus. These antibodies circulate for the rest of the person's lifetime, providing constant immunity. Other antibodies are active for only a short period of time.

The lymphoid tissue and the reticuloendothelial system tissues produce antibodies whether the invading protein is a live antigen capable of producing disease, a weakened or attenuated antigen, or an antigen that has been killed. Thus laboratories can produce **vaccines** that contain either weakened or dead antigens, so that individuals can develop immunity to some diseases. This is called **artificially acquired active immunity.** Whether a weakened or dead antigen is given depends on the disease and the research that has demonstrated how best to protect patients. Rubeola vaccine is an example of a weakened antigen. When a person who is vaccinated for measles (rubeola) with live, attenuated measles virus develops a very mild case of measles, the body produces antibodies that protect the individual. Some diseases may require periodic booster injections to keep the antibody level high enough to protect the patient from disease (Table 16-1).

Some disease-causing proteins come from invading bacteria and are called toxins. Toxins act like antigens to stimulate the antibody-producing system to pro-

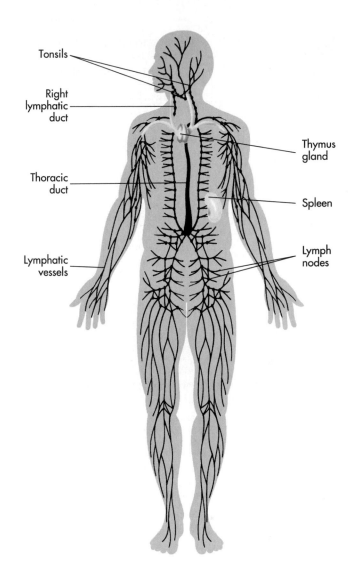

Fig. 16-1   The lymphatic system.

duce antitoxins, which act to neutralize the toxins in the same way that antibodies neutralize antigens. When a toxin is attenuated, or weakened, it is called a **toxoid.** A toxoid produces immunity because the body cannot distinguish between the toxin and the toxoid. The most common example is the use of tetanus toxoid to protect patients from *Clostridium tetani.*

Once a person has had an antigen-antibody response, the antibodies are stored in the body. Globulins are special collections of protein antibodies stored in blood serum and plasma that may be taken from the blood of one person and given to another individual who has not had the antigen-antibody response. These antibodies then circulate to immediately protect the new individual, but the protection lasts for only a short time. A common example is the hepatitis B immune globulin. This form of protection

Table 16-1 Recommended primary immunization series

Agent	Preferred ages and intervals	Dose/route	Booster
DPT*	2, 4, 6, and 15 months 4- to 6-week intervals	0.5 ml IM	4 to 6 years
TOPV†	2, 4, 6‡, and 15 months 6- to 8-week intervals	Oral drops	4 to 6 years
Measles	15 months	0.5 ml SQ	None
Mumps	15 months	0.5 ml SQ	None
Rubella	15 months	0.5 ml SQ	None
Td§	Used after 6 years of age for primary series; three doses at 4- to 6-week intervals	0.5 ml IM	Fourth dose 1 year after third, then every 10 years throughout adulthood
Haemophilus b	If 2 to 6 months; 3 doses at 2-month intervals	0.5 ml IM	15 months
	—7 to 11 months; 2 doses 2 months apart	0.5 ml IM	15 months
	—12 to 14 months, 1 dose	0.5 ml IM	15 months
	—15 to 59 months, 1 dose	0.5 ml IM	No booster

*Combined diphtheria, pertussis, tetanus toxoids.
† Live oral polio vaccine, trivalent.
‡ Sixth month dose optional, depending on prevalence and epidemiology of disease in community.
§ Combined tetanus and diphtheria toxoids, adsorbed adult.

is called **passive immunity.** Concentrated antibody injections may also be called **antiserums,** and the antibodies may be from human or animal sources.

USES

Vaccines and toxoids constitute the biologic agents used in the routine schedule of active immunizations for adults and children. Specific biologic agents are reserved for use in individuals in special circumstances where disease is endemic in nature and presents a high risk of infection (e.g., yellow fever, cholera, typhoid).

Other vaccines are recommended for individuals with increased susceptibility to specific disease states (e.g., pneumococcal vaccine, influenza vaccine).

An additional group of biologic agents is used in screening procedures to identify individuals exposed to a specific disease state or with a potentially active disease process (e.g., PPD, histoplasmin, coccidioidin).

In special circumstances, certain biologic agents may be useful to modify a disease process in the previously unimmunized individual (e.g., gamma globulins).

ADVERSE EFFECTS

In general, mild adverse effects are common and include localized pain and swelling that are mild and of short duration. There are rare instances of more serious problems. The risk of complications from the disease outweighs the risk of adverse effects for all biologic products. Adverse effects occasionally seen include altered levels of consciousness, headaches, lethargy, rash, urticaria, vesiculation, diarrhea, increased respiratory rate, shortness of breath, arthralgia, fever, lymphadenopathy, and malaise.

Most states have laws requiring infants and children to be properly immunized before starting school. A special fund has been established by the federal government that pays for the medical costs incurred if a patient has a serious adverse effect from the required immunization. A certain percentage of the fee paid by the patient for each immunization goes toward this fund.

DRUG INTERACTIONS

Theoretically there is an increase in adverse effects when several vaccines are given at the same time that have known potent side effects (e.g., cholera, plague, and typhoid). The recent recipient of passive antibodies (from a maternal or a vaccine source, or through blood products) may not demonstrate adequate active antibody response to live, attenuated vaccine administration.

 ## NURSING IMPLICATIONS AND PATIENT TEACHING

▼ Assessment

The nurse should obtain a complete health history, including the patient's previous immunization status and reaction to biologic agents; history of allergy, especially to eggs or feathers; results of any known allergy testing; the presence of underlying disease or concurrent infections; the use of immunosuppressant drugs, immune serums, blood, or blood products; or the possibility of pregnancy.

The patient may have a history of exposure to a specific organism, or plans to travel to areas where disease may be endemic. Whether the individual is at risk for infection needs to be assessed, as well as if there are children requiring primary immunizations.

▼ Planning

Immunizations should not be given to patients with active infectious processes, severe febrile illness, or a history of previous serious side effects. Live, attenuated vaccine is usually contraindicated in pregnancy.

Many biologic agents are prepared with animal serum or in chick embryos. Thus individuals with known allergies may have sensitivity reactions to these preparations. Live, attenuated virus vaccine should not be given if there is a recent history of acquired passive antibodies (immune serum globulin).

Patients should be screened for concurrent or incubating illness. There is an increased risk in using immunologic agents in any individual with a compromised immune status (e.g., neonates, the elderly, patients on immunosuppressive therapy, AIDS patients, or patients with chronic disease).

All vaccines should be used with caution in breast-feeding and pregnant individuals.

▼ Implementation

It is important to follow specific protocols and schedules for administration. There are usually specialized storage instructions, modes of administration, sites, and site preparation techniques. It is also important to consult the package insert for each manufacturer's product.

The dosage schedule recommended for primary immunization of infants, children, and adults can be found in Table 16-1.

Uncomfortable reactions to active vaccines are frequent and generally range from localized irritation and soreness to a systemic response with fever, malaise, and anorexia. Specific biologic agents may predispose the recipient to a variety of hypersensitivity reactions. These range from a localized rash, pruritus, or urticaria to an anaphylactic response.

A record of the patient's immunizations should be kept, and the patient should be provided with a record to take home for his or her personal file.

Occasionally antibody blood titers are helpful before vaccine administration to assess antibody development. This is particularly true for rubella.

▼ Evaluation

Patients receiving immune serums should be evaluated for suppression or modification of the disease. Other patients should be monitored for adverse effects. Adverse effects may occur immediately or be delayed for some time after the preparation has been administered. On all visits, patients should be asked whether or not their immunizations are current. There has been a decrease in the extent of pediatric immunizations over the past few years, and few adults obtain needed booster immunizations.

▼ Patient and family teaching

The nurse should provide the patient and family with the following instructions:

1. Localized discomfort may often be relieved by symptomatic measures, such as the use of warm compresses to the area, acetaminophen, rest, and sometimes antihistamines.
2. The patient should record the immunization in a personal health file.
3. The patient should notify the physician immediately if fever, rash, itching, or difficulty breathing develops.
4. The patient or family should periodically discuss immunizations with the physician to make certain that they have adequate immunity.

See Table 16-2 for a summary of agents used for immunity.

Table 16-2 Agents for immunity

Generic name	Comments and dosage
AGENTS FOR ACTIVE IMMUNITY **Toxoids**	
Diphtheria, tetanus toxoid, whole cell pertussis, *Haemophilus influenzae* type b	Immunization for infants and children under 6 years. Produces local reactions, fever, malaise, generalized aches, and pain. *Primary immunizations:* 2 doses of 0.5 ml IM, 6 to 8 weeks apart and third dose 1 year later.
Diphtheria, tetanus toxoid, acellular pertussis	*Booster:* 0.5 ml IM at 5- to 10-year intervals. Vaccine different for children and adults.
Diphtheria toxoid, adsorbed	
Diphtheria and tetanus toxoids; combined	
Diphtheria and tetanus toxoids and pertussis vaccine, adsorbed	
Tetanus toxoid	Immunization in adults and children. May produce local reactions, fever, chills, malaise, and myalgia. *Tetanus toxoid adsorbed:* 2 doses of 0.5 ml IM, 4 to 6 weeks apart, then third dose 6 to 12 months later. *Booster:* q 10 years. *Tetanus toxoid, fluid:* 3 doses of 0.5 ml IM or SQ at 4- to 8-week intervals and fourth dose 6 to 12 months after third dose. *Booster:* 5 to 10 years, depending on risk of wound.
Bacterial vaccines	
BCG	For TB protection in international travelers in high-risk areas, high-risk infants and children. 0.2 to 0.3 ml on skin. Use multiple-puncture disk.
Cholera vaccine	Required on travel to certain areas. May produce transitory local reactions, fever, headache, and malaise. Give 2 doses of 0.5 ml SQ or IM 1 week to 1 month apart.
Haemophilus b conjugate	Routine immunization. Give 3 doses 2 months apart for adults.
Meningitis vaccine Group A, Group C Groups A and C Groups A, C, Y, and W-135	Induces formation of antibodies, leading to immunity to specific organisms. Does not provide immunity against all varieties. Give 0.5 ml SQ.
Plague vaccine	Reduces incidence and severity of disease. Give 2 doses 1 month apart, follow with third dose 1 to 3 months later. See dosage schedule in package insert.
Pneumococcal vaccine, polyvalent	Produces immunity against a variety of pneumococcal infections. Give 0.5 ml IM or SQ. Revaccinations necessary in 3 or more years.
Typhoid vaccine	Give when there has been exposure to known carrier or foreign travel to area where typhoid is endemic. May produce local reactions, fever, chills, malaise, and myalgia. *Primary immunization:* 2 doses of 0.5 ml SQ 4 or more weeks apart, 0.25 ml for children. *Booster:* 0.3 ml SQ or 0.1 ml intradermal q 3 years; for children under age 10, the dose is 0.25 ml SQ or 0.1 ml intradermal.
Viral vaccines	
Hepatitis B vaccine (Hepavax-B)	For immunization against all known subtypes of hepatitis B virus. May produce local reactions, malaise, fatigue, nausea, myalgia, and headache. *Adults:* 1 ml IM, repeat in 1 and 6 months. *Children under 10:* 0.5 ml; repeat with second dose in 1 month, third dose in 6 months.
Influenza virus vaccine	Annual vaccination of high-risk persons. May produce localized reactions, fever, malaise, and myalgia. Dosage schedule varies from year to year.

Table 16-2   Agents for immunity—cont'd

Generic name	Comments and dosage
Measles virus vaccine, live attenuated	Give before or immediately after exposure to measles or as immunization for children 15 months or older. May develop fever and rash between 5th and 12th day after injection. Give 1 ampule SQ.
Measles, mumps, and rubella virus vaccine, live	Same as above.
Measles and rubella virus vaccine, live	Immunization for children 15 months to puberty. Give 1 ampule SQ.
Mumps virus vaccine, live	Give to children 15 months or older and adults. May develop fever or parotitis. Give 1 ampule SQ.
Pertussis vaccine (in combination)	See Diphtheria (above).
Poliovirus vaccine, live, oral, trivalent TOPV, Sabin	Prevention of polio in infants and children up to 18 years. May provoke rare vaccine-related paralysis. Give 3 doses of 0.5 ml PO started at 6 to 12 weeks of age, second dose 6 to 8 weeks later, third dose 8 to 12 months after second dose. *Booster:* On entering school.
Poliomyelitis vaccine, inactivated IPV, Salk	Immunization for those with compromised immune systems. May provoke allergic reactions. Give 3 doses of 1 ml each SQ at 4- to 6-week intervals, then 1 dose of 1 ml 6 to 12 months after the third dose. *Booster:* 1 ml SQ every 2 to 3 years.
Rubella virus vaccine, live	Immunization for children 15 months to puberty. May produce rash, sore throat, fever, headache, and urticaria. Give 1 ampule SQ.
Rubella and mumps virus vaccine, live	Immunization for children 15 months to puberty. Give 1 ampule SQ.
Yellow fever vaccine	Given only at approved World Health Organization centers for people traveling abroad. Give 0.5 ml SQ with revaccination in 10 years as needed.

AGENTS FOR PASSIVE IMMUNITY
Antitoxins and antivenins

Diphtheria antitoxin	For prevention and treatment of diphtheria. Give 20,000 to 120,000 units IM, IV as therapy; 10,000 units IM prophylaxis.
Tetanus antitoxin (equine)	For prevention and treatment of tetanus; give 1500 to 5000 units IM, SQ for prophylaxis; 50,000 to 100,000 units IM and IV for treatment.
Black widow spider species antivenin	*Adults and children:* Inject 1 vial IM, preferably in the region of the anterolateral thigh so that a tourniquet may be applied in the event of a systemic reaction. Symptoms usually subside in 1 to 3 hours.

Immune serums

Immune globulin IV (IGIV)	For the maintenance treatment of patients who are unable to produce sufficient amounts of IgG antibodies. Used in immunodeficiency syndrome, idiopathic thrombocytopenic purpura, and beta cell chronic lymphocytic leukemia. Usually give 200 mg/kg IV once a month.
Cytomegalovirus immune globulin (CMV-IGIV)	For the attenuation of primary CMV disease associated with kidney transplantation. Usually give 15 mg/kg/hr IV.
RH$_O$(D) immune globulin	Effectively suppresses the immune response of nonsensitized Rh-negative mothers after delivery of an Rh-positive infant. Give 1 vial IM.
Lymphocyte immune globulin, antithymocyte globulin	Used in management of allograft rejection in renal transplant patients. Give 5 to 30 mg/kg/day IV.
Hepatitis B immune globulin (human)	For postexposure or high-risk patient prophylaxis. Produces local reactions, urticaria, and fever. Give 0.06 mg/kg IM as soon as possible and repeat 28 to 30 days after exposure.
Immune serum globulin, human (HISG)	Hepatitis A, rubeola prophylaxis; immunoglobulin deficiency; passive immunization for varicella in immunosuppressed patients. Give 0.02 to 1.2 ml/kg IM, depending on reason for use.

Continued.

Table 16-2 Agents for immunity—cont'd	
Generic name	**Comments and dosage**
Tetanus immune globulin, human (HTIG)	For temporary postexposure prophylaxis. Give 4 units/kg IM.
Varicella-zoster immune globulin, human (VZIG)	For temporary passive immunity to varicella. Give deep IM, according to dosage schedule on package insert.
Rabies prophylaxis products	
Antirabies serum, equine origin (ARS)	Give on suspected exposure to rabies. May produce serum sickness, urticaria, local pain, and erythema. See package insert for dosage schedule.
Rabies immune globulin, human (RIG)	Immunization for those suspected of exposure to rabies. May produce fever and soreness at injection site. Give 20 IU/kg IM; half the dose may be used to infiltrate the wound.
Rabies vaccine, human diploid cell cultures (HDCV)	For prophylaxis and postexposure treatment. May produce nausea, headache, muscle aches, abdominal pain, and local reactions. See package insert for dosage schedule.
In vivo diagnostic biologic agents	
Candida and trichophyton	Give 0.1 ml shallow SQ to detect sensitivity.
Coccidioidin	Used to identify people with active disease or exposure to the fungal infection coccidioidomycosis. Give lowest possible dosage intradermally, evaluate 24 to 48 hours later. Positive reaction is area of erythema and induration 5 mm or greater in size.
Histoplasmin	Used to identify people with active disease or exposure to histoplasmin. Give 0.1 ml per intradermal injection and evaluate 24 to 48 hours later. Positive reaction is area of erythema and induration 5 mm or greater in size.
Mumps skin test antigen	Demonstrates cutaneous hypersensitivity to mumps virus. Give 0.1 ml antigen intradermally and evaluate 24 to 48 hours later. Positive reaction is area of erythema and induration 5 mm or greater in size.
Tuberculin purified protein derivative (Mantoux)	Designed to identify persons with active tuberculosis, exposure to tuberculosis, or needing further testing. Give 0.1 ml of intermediate strength PPD intradermally and evaluate in 24 to 48 hours. Positive reaction must have erythema and induration 9 mm or more in size; areas 5 to 9 mm are questionable; areas under 5 mm are negative.
Tuberculin PPD multiple puncture device	Used to identify persons with active tuberculosis, exposure to tuberculosis, or needing further testing.
Tuberculin Old, multiple puncture device	Same as above.

SUMMARY

Immunologic agents provide active or passive immunity to specific disease states. Types of immunologic agents are vaccines, toxoids, and other serologic agents used to prevent or modify disease. Immunity can either be naturally acquired or artificially acquired. It is important to follow specific protocols and schedules for administering these products.

 ## CRITICAL THINKING QUESTIONS

1. Outline the differences in the three different types of immunity and their individual effects.
2. There has been considerable debate about the benefits of immunization versus the relatively rare but serious adverse effects. In a two-column format, outline the benefits versus the risks. Where do you stand? Did the outline put things in a different perspective for you?

3. You are asked to give immunizations to four children, of various ages, who are visiting your clinic this afternoon. Draw up a fairly generic list of assessment, planning, and implementation strategies.

4. Identify drug interactions and hypersensitivity or allergic reactions commonly seen with immunologic agents. Suggest appropriate actions the nurse and patient can take in response to these.

5. Mr. Alexander has come into your office because he has a "cold." He seems to be getting better, he says, but needs to put in some late hours at work this week. He wonders whether the doctor can give him a medication to "speed up the recovery." However, the physician explains that in response to his illness, his body has developed its own antibodies. What kind of immune response has taken place?

6. Give examples of the process or development of each of the following types of immunity: (a) artificially acquired active immunity; (b) artificially acquired passive immunity; (c) naturally acquired active immunity; and (d) naturally acquired passive immunity.

7. Identify and suggest ways to counteract the most common side effects of immunologic agents.

8. After giving him an immunization, you explain to Mr. Stavros that he will need a booster later. Mr. Stavros has never heard of a booster. Explain what this is, along with the rationale for getting one.

9. When might a patient exhibit extra sensitivity to an immunologic agent?

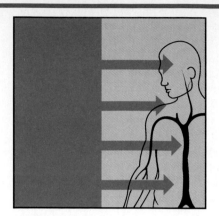

CHAPTER 17
Musculoskeletal and Antiarthritis Medications

OVERVIEW

This chapter summarizes the medications helpful in treating problems affecting the bones, joints, muscles, and ligaments. There are a variety of musculoskeletal disorders that produce varying degrees of pain, disability, and deformity. The drugs used to treat these problems are selected on the basis of the severity of the problem and the pathologic mechanisms underlying the disorder. Many acute problems, such as sprains, fractures, or tears, require only short-term therapy. Some disorders, such as arthritis, may require long-term therapy with a variety of medications, with more powerful drugs required as the disability progresses. Many of these products are associated with significant adverse reactions, and the patient requires close monitoring of response to therapy.

This chapter is divided into four sections. Section One deals with antiinflammatory and analgesic medications, the salicylates and nonsteroidal antiinflammatory drugs (NSAIDs), used to treat common orthopedic problems. Section Two presents skeletal muscle relaxants. Section Three introduces a variety of medications used to treat arthritis: the slow-acting antirheumatic drugs (SAARDs). The agents used to treat high uric acid levels found in gout are presented in Section Four.

Muscular and Skeletal Systems

The muscular and skeletal systems work together to provide support and movement for the body (Figs. 17-1 and 17-2). The skeletal system is composed of the bones, associated cartilage, and joints, while the muscular system involves those muscles attached to the skeleton.

The skeleton protects, supports, and allows body movement, produces blood cells in the long bones, and stores minerals. The muscular system provides movement of body parts, maintains posture, and produces body heat.

Pathologic conditions may arise within the body itself, or in the muscular or ligament attachments. Often injuries are due to trauma or to long-term wear or overuse. While some traumatic skeletal injuries heal well and the patient has no residual problems, some injuries may form the site for continuing arthritis pain and deformity.

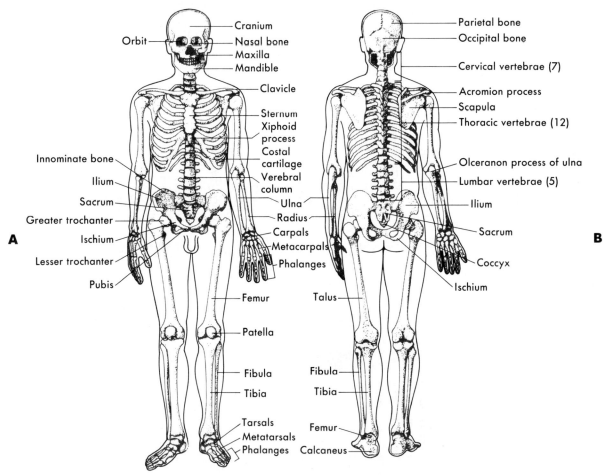

Fig. 17-1   The skeletal system.

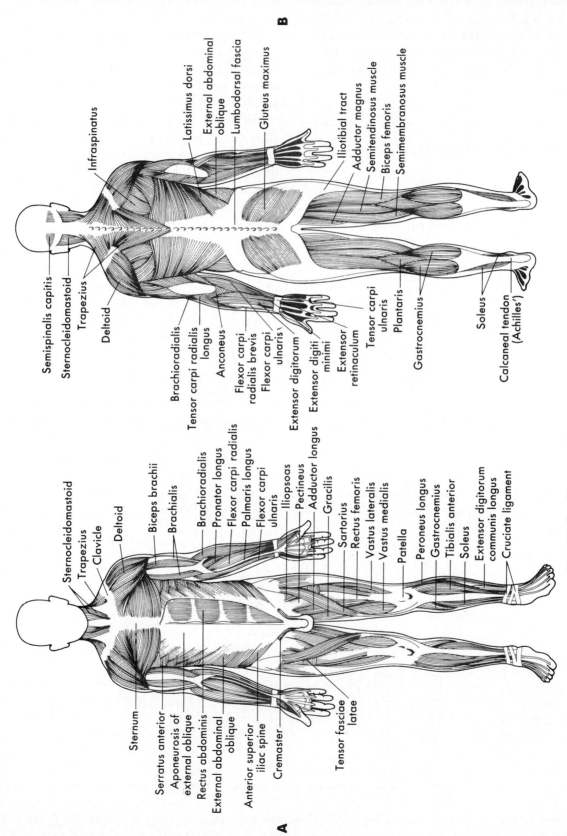

Fig. 17-2 The muscular system.

A

Sternocleidomastoid
Trapezius
Clavicle
Deltoid
Biceps brachii
Brachialis
Brachioradialis
Pronator longus
Flexor carpi radialis
Palmaris longus
Flexor carpi ulnaris
Iliopsoas
Pectineus
Adductor longus
Gracilis
Sartorius
Rectus femoris
Vastus lateralis
Vastus medialis
Patella
Peroneus longus
Gastrocnemius
Tibialis anterior
Soleus
Extensor digitorum communis longus
Cruciate ligament

Sternum
Serratus anterior
Aponeurosis of external oblique
Rectus abdominis
External abdominal oblique
Anterior superior iliac spine
Cremaster
Tensor fasciae latae

B

Semispinalis capitis
Sternocleidomastoid
Trapezius
Deltoid
Infraspinatus
Brachioradialis
Tensor carpi radialis longus
Anconeus
Flexor carpi radialis brevis
Flexor carpi ulnaris
Extensor digitorum
Extensor digiti minimi
Extensor retinaculum
Tensor carpi ulnaris
Plantaris
Gastrocnemius
Soleus
Calcaneal tendon (Achilles')

Latissimus dorsi
External abdominal oblique
Lumbodorsal fascia
Gluteus maximus
Illiotibial tract
Adductor magnus
Semitendinosus muscle
Biceps femoris
Semimembranosus muscle

SECTION ONE: ANTIINFLAMMATORY ANALGESIC AGENTS

Objectives

At the conclusion of this section you should be able to:

1. List the indications for use of salicylates and NSAIDs preparations.
2. Explain the mechanism of action for salicylates and NSAIDs.
3. Identify common adverse reactions associated with the use of these products.
4. Use the nursing process in administering these medications to patients with musculoskeletal disorders.
5. Develop a teaching plan for patients taking salicylates or NSAIDs.

OVERVIEW

Aspirin is one of the most commonly taken medications. The ease with which it can be purchased and the high percentage of self-administration does not diminish the importance of this drug in treating common and significant musculoskeletal problems. Aspirin has greater antiinflammatory action than other salicylates and is preferred in the treatment of many problems. The NSAIDs are relative newcomers on the market but are powerful agents to help decrease pain and inflammation. Interest in and research on NSAIDs are expanding. Both salicylates and NSAIDs are thought to inhibit the production of prostaglandins, a substance believed to cause greater sensitivity of peripheral pain receptors to painful stimuli.

SALICYLATES

ACTION

Salicylates are used to treat mild to moderate pain and reduce fever. They have analgesic, antipyretic, and antiinflammatory effects. The exact mechanism of action for these agents is not understood. It is known that they reduce fever partially by vasodilation; they also inhibit prostaglandin synthesis, which affects the pain stimulation and inflammatory process. They have a depressant effect on the central and peripheral pain receptors. They also interfere with factor III of the clotting mechanism. Aspirin is the most potent prostaglandin inhibitor of this group and therefore has the greatest antiinflammatory effect of the salicylates.

USES

Salicylates are used to treat various forms of arthritis (e.g., rheumatoid, osteoarthritis, degenerative joint disease). They are used to treat systemic fever produced by viral illnesses or in therapy for pain arising from trauma to soft tissue or muscle. Myalgias, neuralgias, arthralgias, headache, and dysmenorrhea are also indications for salicylates. The antiinflammatory effects are useful in treating systemic lupus erythematosus, acute rheumatic fever, and similar conditions. They are also used to decrease platelet aggregation as a prophylactic measure in patients with coronary artery disease.

ADVERSE REACTIONS

Adverse reactions to antiinflammatory analgesics include tinnitus, visual disturbances, edema, hives, rashes, anorexia, epigastric discomfort, and nausea. In overdosage, symptoms may progress from mild to severe with hyperventilation, sweating, thirst, headache, drowsiness, skin eruptions, and electrolyte imbalance progressing to CNS depression, stupor, convulsions and coma, tachycardia, and respiratory insufficiency. Respiratory and metabolic acidosis are most often seen in children.

DRUG INTERACTIONS

Antiinflammatory analgesics increase the chance of gastrointestinal bleeding when used with alcohol. An increased paraaminosalicylic acid (PAS) effect may be caused by decreased excretion by the kidneys or decreased protein binding. There is an increased effect on anticoagulants, sulfonylureas, and sulfonamides if they are used concomitantly with salicylates. Ascorbic acid increases the effect of salicylates by increasing renal tubular reabsorption. Salicylates interact with NSAIDs to increase effects, side effects, and toxicities. Salicylates also potentiate the effects of phenytoin and inhibit hyperuricemia produced by pyrazinamide. Salicylates can affect many laboratory test results.

NURSING IMPLICATIONS AND PATIENT TEACHING

▼ Assessment

The nurse should obtain a complete health history to check for the presence of hypersensitivity to aspirin or other nonsteroidal antiinflammatory preparations, history of asthma or nasal polyps, gastrointestinal problems or ulcer disease, concurrent use of other drugs that may cause interactions, or other underlying hepatic or renal disease. These conditions are precautions or contraindications to the use of salicylates.

The physician may ask the nurse to check for occult blood in the patient's stool before beginning medication. This will help determine whether or not stool specimens positive for blood in the future are a chance event.

Antiinflammatory analgesics are effective for mild to moderate pain of a musculoskeletal nature and in conditions causing mild fever. They are useful for many of the same conditions in which nonsteroidal antiinflammatory drugs are used.

▼ Planning

Antiinflammatory analgesics should not be used in patients with hepatic disease. Patients on anticoagulant therapy or with abnormalities of clotting must be very careful when they use these products. They also should not be used before surgery, because of the platelet effect, or before labor, because bleeding may increase. They should be used with caution in patients with symptoms suggesting transient ischemic attacks. In patients with musculoskeletal pain that persists for more than 10 days, further evaluation is needed.

Antiinflammatory analgesics should not be used during pregnancy, especially during the third trimester, because they may have adverse effects on the fetus. Salicylates are excreted in breast milk.

These drugs should be used cautiously to determine the presence of gastric irritation, especially in patients with a past history of upper gastrointestinal problems. Also use them with caution in patients with blood dyscrasias or impaired renal function.

Hydration should be monitored carefully in children, because they seem to be more prone to salicylate intoxication.

Reye's syndrome, an acute, life-threatening problem, is characterized by vomiting and lethargy that may proceed to delirium and coma with permanent

CRITICAL DECISION
Reye's Syndrome

Children with recurrent upper respiratory tract infection symptoms within a short time span or with disorientation should not be given salicylates because of the positive association with Reye's syndrome.

brain damage and possible death. Use of aspirin after influenza or chickenpox also seems more highly correlated with the development of Reye's syndrome.

Many salicylate products are not recommended for use in children under 12 years of age. The nurse should check the individual agent when ordered for children.

▼ Implementation

The administration and dosage vary for each of the salicylate products. There are tablets, capsules, drops, chewable preparations, suppositories, and injectable forms of these products. Aspirin is the most active agent and has the greatest amount of salicylate per unit. Individual products should be checked for specifics.

Patients with diabetes who are testing their urine with Benedict's Clinitest may get incorrect readings. They may need to switch to another form of urine testing while using salicylate products. Salicylates also potentiate oral hypoglycemic agents, and diabetic patients should be alert to signs of hypoglycemia.

▼ Evaluation

The dosage should be reduced or the drug discontinued if tinnitus develops. The patient should be monitored for the therapeutic effect: subjective relief of pain and reduction in temperature to 101° F or below. The nurse should also observe for fever that does not resolve and progression of the disease.

For arthritis, higher dosages are usually needed to control the symptoms. The dosage should be gradually increased while the patient is monitored for subjective improvement, increased strength of grip, increased mobility, and improved ability to carry on normal activities. Patients taking medication over a long time should be monitored for signs of occult bleeding with regular blood counts and stool checks. The nurse should check for signs of toxicity, especially tinnitus. Periodic checks of serum salicylate levels may be beneficial if the dosage is approaching maximum levels, or if there is a question of patient compliance.

▼ Patient and family teaching

The nurse should provide the patient and family with the following instructions:

1. These drugs may cause gastric upset because they are so strong. This symptom may be reduced by taking medicine with food, milk, or a full glass of water.
2. The patient should notify the physician if he or she notices any ringing in the ears, any abnormal bleeding, bruising, or bloody or black, tarry stools.
3. Chronic problems may require taking the medicine for more than a week before the patient notices any decrease in symptoms.
4. The medicine should be taken regularly to reduce inflammation. If the medicine is taken irregularly, a high level of medicine in the blood is not maintained, and symptoms cannot be reduced as successfully as with regular use.
5. The patient should not take any other medications without the knowledge of the physician. This includes drugs that the patient may purchase over the counter.
6. The physician should be contacted if the fever does not decrease in 24 to 48 hours, or if the patient becomes lethargic or hard to awaken.
7. This medicine should be kept out of the reach of children and all others for whom it is not prescribed.
8. If the patient is unable to take the medicine in the form prescribed, the physician should be called so that another form may be ordered. Medicine is available in chewable tablets and in suppositories to aid in administration.

NONSTEROIDAL ANTIINFLAMMATORY DRUGS

ACTION

Nonsteroidal antiinflammatory drugs (NSAIDs) have analgesic, antiinflammatory, and antipyretic effects and are used to treat rheumatic diseases, degenerative joint disease, osteoarthritis, and acute musculoskeletal problems. The exact mode of action of NSAIDs is not known, although it is believed that they work by inhibiting the synthesis of prostaglandins. These agents are also associated with the inhibition of platelet aggregation, but this effect appears to be dose re-

lated. Ibuprofen has been approved for use in dysmenorrhea because of its prostaglandin inhibition.

USES

When the patient's history and physical examination have documented a disease process that significantly affects the person's normal pattern of living (because of changes in mobility or pain), the use of NSAIDs is indicated. They are specifically indicated in the treatment of moderate to severe musculoskeletal pain, rheumatoid arthritis, osteoarthritis, ankylosing spondylitis, degenerative joint disease, and acute or chronic problems involving the bursa or tendons.

ADVERSE REACTIONS

Adverse reactions to NSAIDs include asthma, fluid retention, hypertension, confusion, dizziness, blurred or decreased vision, malaise, somnolence, tinnitus, pruritus, skin irritation or rash related to sun exposure, abdominal pain, anorexia, bloating, constipation, diarrhea, dyspepsia, flatulence, GI bleeding (upper or lower), heartburn, nausea, vomiting, hematuria (with some agents or worsened renal failure), and many forms of blood cell changes (see box on p. 360).

DRUG INTERACTIONS

Because the various NSAIDs are structurally somewhat different, their specific drug interactions vary; therefore the specific generic agents should be checked for drug interactions that should be monitored. Most products have significant drug interactions.

 NURSING IMPLICATIONS AND PATIENT TEACHING

▼ Assessment

The patient may complain of musculoskeletal pain or tenderness of involved areas, inflammation, stiffness, and an alteration in the normal activities of life. The onset may be insidious, with the patient showing only tiredness, or it may be sudden, or after a change in activity or minor trauma, depending on the particular type of arthritic problem. The specific history of onset, duration, and location are important factors in determining which arthritic condition exists. The

Table 17-1 Antiinflammatory analgesics

Generic name	Trade name	Comments and dosage
SALICYLATES		
Acetylsalicylic acid (ASA, aspirin)	Aspergum Ecotrin Empirin Bayer	The most commonly used antiinflammatory agent. It is the standard against which all other agents are compared. Hypersensitivity often exists. ■ *Mild to moderate pain:* 325 to 650 mg PO initially, then repeat q4h. ■ *Arthritis:* 2.6 to 5.2 gm/day PO in divided doses. ■ *Acute rheumatic fever:* up to 7.8 gm/day in divided doses. *Children:* 65 mg/kg/day in divided doses.
Diflusinal	Dolobid	A salicylic acid nonsteroidal derivative. Give 1 gm PO, then 500 mg q8 to 12h.
Acetylsalicylic acid (ASA) buffered choline salicylate	Alka-Seltzer Ascriptin Bufferin	Aspirin-antacid combinations are used with patients who experience gastrointestinal distress from plain aspirin. Give 325 to 850 mg q4h prn. Dosage and administration are the same as for plain aspirin (above).
Choline salicylate	Arthropan	This is a liquid form of salicylate with fewer gastrointestinal side effects than aspirin. Used if a sodium restriction is necessary. It has a nasty aftertaste that may be reduced by giving it in water. *Adults and children over 12 years:* 870 mg PO initially; repeat q3 to 4h; give no more than 6 times daily.
Salsalate	Amigesic Salsitab	*Adults:* 3000 mg/day in divided doses.
Magnesium salicylate	Doan's pills Mobidin Magan	A sodium-free salicylate with a lower incidence of GI problems than ASA. *Adults and children over 12 years:* 600 mg PO tid to qid. May be increased to 3.6 or 4.8 gm PO qd at 3- to 6-hour intervals.
Sodium salicylate	Sodium salicylate	Give 325 to 650 mg enteric coated tablet q4h.
Sodium thiosalicylate	Asproject Tusal Rexolate Arthrinol ♣	■ *Acute gout:* 100 mg q3 to 4h IM for 2 days, then 100 mg qd. ■ *Rheumatic fever:* 100 to 150 mg IM q4 to 6h for 3 days, then 100 mg tid until patient is without symptoms.
NONSTEROIDAL ANTIINFLAMMATORY AGENTS		
Fenamates		
Meclofenamate	Meclomen	Has the ability to block the action of prostaglandins as well as inhibit their synthesis, as opposed to the other NSAIDs that only inhibit prostaglandin synthesis. *Adults:* 200 to 400 mg PO qd in 3 to 4 divided doses. Maximum dose 400 mg/day.
Mefenamic acid	Ponstel Ponstan ♣	Recommended for the treatment of dysmenorrhea rather than arthritis or other acute musculoskeletal problems. Give 500 mg, then 250 mg q6h.
Acetic acids		
Diclofenac	Voltaren	Give 100 to 150 mg/day in divided doses.
Etodolac	Lodine	Give 800 to 1200 mg/day in divided doses.
Indomethacin	Indocin Indocid ♣	A *potent* prostaglandin synthesis inhibitor with significant toxic side effects; many adverse reactions (including blood dyscrasias) and drug interactions. ■ *Acute gouty arthritis:* 50 mg tid for 3 to 5 days, then reduce to 25 mg tid. Gradually wean patient off medication as soon as possible.
Ketorolac	Toradol	Use IM for short-term management of pain. Use orally also for short duration. Give 10 mg q4 to 6h. IM may give 30 to 60 mg IM as loading dose, followed by half the loading dose q6h prn.
Nabumetone	Relafin	Give 1000 mg as single daily dose with or without food.

Table 17-1   Antiinflammatory analgesics—cont'd

Generic name	Trade name	Comments and dosage
Sulindac	Clinoril	■ *Arthritis and ankylosing spondylitis:* 150 to 200 mg bid with food. Maximum dose 400 mg/day. ■ *Acute painful shoulder or gout:* 200 mg bid with food. Use for 7 days in gout, 7 to 14 days for painful shoulder.
Tolmetin	Tolectin	One of the few NSAIDs approved for the treatment of juvenile rheumatoid arthritis in children over the age of 2. ■ *Osteoarthritis:* 400 mg PO tid with meals. ■ *Rheumatoid arthritis:* 600 to 1600 mg/day in 3 to 4 divided doses with meals; maximum of 2 gm/day PO. *Children over 2 years:* 15 to 20 mg/kg/day in 3 to 4 divided doses with meals; dosages higher than 30 mg/kg/day not recommended.

Propionic acid derivatives

Fenoprofen	Nalfon	Administer medication 30 minutes before meals or 2 hours after meals because food interferes with absorption. ■ *Mild to moderate pain:* 200 mg PO q4 to 6h on empty stomach. ■ *Chronic pain:* 300 to 600 mg q6 to 8h on empty stomach; maximum dose 3200 mg/24 hours.
Flurbiprofen	Ansaid	Used in rheumatoid and osteoarthritis. Give 100 mg bid or tid.
Ibuprofen	Motrin Nuprin Advil	Approved for use in the treatment of dysmenorrhea. ■ *Mild to moderate pain:* 400 mg PO q4 to 6h. ■ *Chronic pain and acute exacerbations:* 300 to 600 mg PO q6 to 8h. ■ *Antiinflammatory response:* 800 mg q6 to 8h.
Ketoprofen	Orudis	Give 25 to 50 mg q6 to 8h for primary dysmenorrhea; higher doses in arthritis.
Naproxen	Anaprox Naprosyn	■ *Mild to moderate pain:* 500 mg initially, followed by 250 mg q6 to 8h, or 550 mg naproxen sodium followed by 275 mg naproxen sodium q6 to 8h. ■ *Rheumatoid arthritis, osteoarthritis, ankylosing spondylitis:* 250 mg to 375 mg PO q12h. Doses do not have to be equal. Long-term therapy may require the higher dosage range. If there is no symptomatic effect in 2 weeks, continue trial for 2 more weeks before discontinuing the agent. ■ *Acute gout:* 750 mg (825 mg naproxen sodium) followed by 250 mg (275 mg naproxen sodium) q8h until attack ends.
Oxaprozin	Daypro	Give 1200 mg PO once a day.

Pyrazole derivatives

Phenylbutazone Oxyphenbutazone	Azolid Butazolidin	These drugs have significant side effects and should be used only in short-term therapy and for exacerbations of acute problems. Medication should be taken with meals or milk, or use products that include antacids. ■ *Acute gout:* 400 mg initially, followed by 100 mg qid for 7 days. ■ *Other problems:* 300 to 600 mg in equal divided doses.

Oxicans

Piroxicam	Feldene	Indicated in the treatment of acute exacerbations and long-term management of rheumatoid and osteoarthritis. Give 20 mg qd. No therapeutic effects may be seen for 2 weeks.

nurse should evaluate the patient for signs of inflammation: tenderness, erythema, increased warmth, and swelling; joint stiffness, decreased range of motion, or crepitus may also be present. Distribution, location, pattern (i.e., monoarticular, asymmetric, symmetric), and number of involved joints must be determined.

NSAIDs are contraindicated in patients with past sensitivity to the drug. They are also not to be used in patients displaying hypersensitivity to aspirin, because all of the specific agents are closely related to aspirin and there is a potential for cross-sensitivity. Alternate agents in this category should not be given to patients who have manifested symptoms of bronchospasm, asthma, rhinitis, urticaria, nasal polyps, or angioedema after using any agents within this group.

The nurse should obtain a complete health history, including the presence of sensitivity to aspirin or any of the products within this group, gastrointestinal problems, renal dysfunction, history of asthma or allergic respiratory problems, anticoagulant therapy, bleeding problems, other drugs taken concurrently that may cause drug interactions, and the possibility of pregnancy or breastfeeding.

▼ Planning

Because the chemical structure varies among these agents, the specific drug should be checked before it is given.

Some agents should be used only for short-term therapy because of their toxic side effects. The duration of therapy should be considered when a particular agent is selected for chronic arthritic problems.

In uniarticular problems, it should be certain that all infective processes are ruled out. NSAIDs may relieve symptoms but not affect the invasive agent, allowing more extensive damage to take place if used inappropriately.

▼ Implementation

NSAIDs are first-line drugs in the treatment and control of the various forms of arthritis and in many of the uniarticular inflammatory processes. The chemical structure of these agents varies somewhat, and therefore failure to symptomatically improve with the use of one agent does not mean there will be no improvement with another. Salicylates are the most commonly used antiinflammatory agents. Because of the low cost, efficacy, and low toxicity of salicylates, all NSAIDs are compared with them in terms of their therapeutic benefits and side effects (Table 17-1).

▼ Evaluation

The full therapeutic effect of an agent may not be seen in many chronic problems for 1 to 2 weeks; therefore this delay should be considered before changing therapy.

The nurse should monitor the patient for therapeutic effects: reduction of symptoms and ability of the patient to return to previous activities without pain. The patient should be evaluated 3 to 4 weeks after starting the medication for the first signs of improvement. If there is no reduction in symptoms or if side effects develop, an alternative in this group can be tried.

The patient should be monitored for adverse effects, particularly for GI and CNS symptoms. Periodic laboratory analysis should also be carried out while the patient is taking this medicine. Stool specimens should be obtained to check for occult bleeding; complete blood cell counts with indices for anemia, hematologic problems, and ability to fight infection should be evaluated at least biannually.

▼ Patient and family teaching

The nurse should provide the patient and family with the following instructions:

1. These medications should be taken exactly as ordered. The dosage should not be increased or decreased unless recommended by the physician. Evaluation of the action of these drugs will require returning to the physician periodically for checkups.
2. These medications should be taken with meals or with milk to minimize gastric irritation. The patient may use an antacid with the medicine, unless specifically prohibited.
3. Patients who have chronic arthritic problems may need to take the medicine for 1 to 2 weeks before noting any improvement. The medicine should be taken regularly during this time to evaluate fairly whether or not it will be effective.

CRITICAL DECISION:
Gastrointestinal Upset

Gastrointestinal upset is the most common complication and should be reported to the physician. Bowel movements should also be checked for the presence of blood or tarry stools, which result from excessive irritation.

4. A certain level of medicine must be maintained within the body at all times to maintain the antiinflammatory effect of the drug. If the patient does not take the medicine regularly, the drug level may be too low to be effective.
5. If a dose is missed, it should be taken as soon as possible after the missed dose was due. If the next dose is due shortly, the missed dose should not be taken, but instead the regular dosage schedule should be resumed. An increased amount of medicine should not be taken to make up for a missed dose.
6. Blurred vision or any other eye problems, ringing in the ears, and rashes should be reported immediately to the physician.
7. Some patients experience drowsiness, lightheadedness, or decreased alertness from this medicine. Patients should not drive or perform tasks requiring alertness until they evaluate their reaction to this drug.
8. The patient should be cautioned not to take aspirin or any other antiinflammatory drug while using this product.

SECTION TWO: SKELETAL MUSCLE RELAXANTS

Objectives

At the conclusion of this section you should be able to:

1. Identify the primary indications for skeletal muscle relaxants.
2. Describe adverse effects associated with skeletal muscle relaxants.
3. Compare and contrast the actions of skeletal muscle relaxants.
4. Develop a teaching plan for patients taking skeletal muscle relaxants on a short-term basis.

ACTION

The main action of **skeletal muscle relaxants** is to decrease muscle tone and involuntary movement without loss of voluntary motor function. These drugs inhibit the transmission of impulses in the motor pathways at the level of the spinal cord and the brainstem (centrally acting), or they interfere with the contractile mechanism of the skeletal muscle fibers (direct myotrophic blocking). Other actions include mild sedation, reduction of anxiety and tension, and alteration of pain perception.

USES

Skeletal muscle relaxants are used to relieve pain in musculoskeletal and neurologic disorders involving peripheral injury and inflammation, such as muscle strain or sprain, arthritis, bursitis, low back syndrome, cervical syndrome, tension headaches, cerebral palsy, and multiple sclerosis.

ADVERSE REACTIONS

Adverse reactions to skeletal muscle relaxants include flushing, hypotension, syncope, tachycardia, ataxia, blurred vision, confusion, drowsiness, headache, insomnia, irritability, abdominal pain, anorexia, bleeding, diarrhea, hiccups, nausea, many blood cell disorders, anaphylactic reactions, asthmalike reaction, dermatoses, erythema, fever, pruritus, rash, dysuria, enuresis, urinary retention, dyspnea, nasal congestion, shortness of breath, wheezing, dyspepsia, euphoria, metallic taste, pain or sloughing at injection site, and tremors.

DRUG INTERACTIONS

Skeletal muscle relaxants are known to interact additively with CNS depressants, including sedatives, narcotic analgesics, antianxiety agents, hypnotics, and alcohol; general anesthetics; MAO inhibitors; tricyclic antidepressants; and anticholinergic drugs such as cyclobenzaprine and orphenadrine. Cyclobenzaprine may interfere with the antihypertensive activity of the alpha-adrenergic blockers.

 NURSING IMPLICATIONS AND PATIENT TEACHING

▼ Assessment

The patient may have a history of pain caused by acute muscular trauma or inflammation (sprains or strains), low back syndrome, arthritis, multiple sclerosis, muscular tension with or without intermittent relief, headache, and muscle rigidity.

The nurse should obtain a complete health history, including the presence of hypersensitivity, concurrent drug use that would produce drug interactions, and history of respiratory, renal, hepatic, or cardiac dysfunction. These drugs also should not be dispensed to women who are pregnant or breastfeeding or to persons with a history of drug dependency.

▼ Planning

Skeletal muscle relaxants used with other CNS drugs, including alcohol, will potentiate the sedative actions of this drug. Therefore, these drugs are not recommended for persons with a history of alcoholism or alcohol abuse.

The efficacy and safe use of these drugs have not been established in children.

▼ Implementation

Skeletal muscle relaxants are available in tablet and injectable forms. When given orally, these drugs are purported to be of questionable benefit. The oral dose would have to be 5 to 10 times greater than the parenteral dose to obtain true muscle relaxation. For this reason the parenteral form of these drugs is recommended over the oral form. The parenteral form of the drug can cause local tissue irritation.

In rare instances the first dose of skeletal muscle relaxants produces an idiosyncratic reaction within minutes or hours. Symptoms include extreme weakness, transient quadriplegia, dizziness, ataxia, temporary loss of vision, diplopia, mydriasis, dysarthria, agitation, euphoria, confusion, and disorientation. See Table 17-2 for a summary of skeletal muscle relaxants.

▼ Evaluation

Incidences of hepatotoxicity, nephrotoxicity, and blood dyscrasias have been reported with the use of skeletal muscle relaxants. Signs of hepatotoxicity include abdominal pain, high fever, nausea, and diarrhea. Signs of blood dyscrasias include fever, sore throat, mucosal irritation, malaise, and petechiae. Side effects that occur most commonly include drowsiness, diplopia, dizziness, weakness, mild muscular incoordination, anorexia, nausea, vomiting, syncope, and hypotension.

The drug should be discontinued if no improvement occurs after 45 days, because the risk of hepatotoxicity increases with long-term use of these drugs.

The lowest dosage possible should be used, and the patient should be monitored for signs and symptoms of hepatotoxicity, blood dyscrasias, dependence, and adverse drug reactions.

The acuteness of the musculoskeletal disorder or type of neurologic impairment dictates the duration of drug use. Abrupt termination of these drugs can cause withdrawal symptoms after long-term use, so the dosage should be gradually reduced before termination.

Table 17-2   Skeletal muscle relaxants

Generic name	Trade name	Comments and dosage
Baclofen	Lioresal	■ *Muscle relaxant, antispastic:* Begin dosage regimen with 5 mg tid for 3 days. Thereafter, increase the dosage in increments of 5 mg per dose q 3 days until the desired response is obtained. The dosage is adjusted according to the reversal of spasticity symptoms. The maximum daily dose is 80 mg.
Carisoprodol	Soma	■ *Muscle relaxant:* 350 mg PO tid and at bedtime. Administration with meals will help reduce gastric distress.
Chlorphenesin carbamate	Maolate Mycil ♣	■ *Muscle relaxation:* 800 mg tid until a therapeutic effect is achieved; then give maintenance dose of 400 mg tid. Treatment should not exceed 8 weeks.
Chlorzoxazone	Paraflex Parafon Forte DSC	*Adults:* 250 to 750 mg tid. Initial dose for painful musculoskeletal conditions should be 500 mg tid. If adequate response is not obtained, the dosage may be increased to 750 mg tid to qid and then gradually reduced to a maintenance dose of 250 mg tid once the therapeutic effect is achieved. Administration with meals may help avoid GI irritation. *Children:* Give 20 mg/kg not to exceed 125 mg to 500 mg tid. The tablets may be crushed and mixed with food.
Cyclobenzaprine	Flexeril	Relieves acute skeletal muscle spasm of local origin without interfering with muscle function. ■ *Local muscle spasm:* 10 mg tid to qid. Do not administer for longer than 2 to 3 weeks.
Dantrolene	Dantrium	■ *Spasticity* *Adults:* Begin therapy with 25 mg qd; increase to 25 mg bid to qid; and then by increments up to as high as 100 mg bid to qid if necessary. Doses higher than 400 mg per day are not recommended. Each dosage should be maintained for 4 to 7 days to determine the patient's response. *Children:* Begin with 1 mg/kg daily and increase by 0.5 mg/kg increments to a maximum of 3 mg/kg bid to qid.
Diazepam	Valium Valrelease	*Adults:* 2 to 10 mg PO bid to qid. Give sustained-release capsules 15 to 30 mg qd. *Geriatric or debilitated patients:* 2 to 2.5 mg PO qd or bid. Gradually increase dose as needed. ■ *Parenteral therapy:* Inject IV medication slowly only into large veins, 1 minute for each 5 mg. *Adults:* 5 to 10 mg IV initially, repeated prn at 10- to 15-minute intervals. Maximum IV dose is 30 mg. Therapy may be repeated in 2 to 4 hours as needed.
Metaxalone	Skelaxin	■ *Muscle relaxation*
Methocarbamol	Robaxin	*Adults:* 800 mg tid to qid. The drug may change the color of standing urine to green or black. ■ *Relief of muscle spasm:* 1.5 gm PO qid as initial loading dose for the first 3 to 4 days of treatment. The maintenance dose is 750 to 1000 mg qd in 4 divided doses. Intravenous and intramuscular dosage should not exceed 30 mg (3 vials) per day for more than 3 days, except in the treatment of tetanus. Specifically for intravenous dosage, do not exceed a rate of 3 ml (300 mg) per minute.
Orphenadrine citrate	Norflex	■ *Muscle spasm:* Administer 100 mg tablet in the morning and evening; or give 60 mg IM or IV q12h.
Quinine sulfate	Quinamm Legatrin	■ *Relief of leg muscle cramps:* 1 tablet at bedtime; increase the dose to add 1 tablet at the evening meal when necessary.

Continued.

Table 17-2	Skeletal muscle relaxants—cont'd	
Generic name	**Trade name**	**Comments and dosage**
COMBINATION PRODUCTS		
Chlorzoxazone and acetaminophen	Chlorzone Forte	Centrally acting skeletal muscle relaxant and analgesic. Its use is indicated in acute musculoskeletal conditions that require symptomatic relief from muscle spasms and pain. ■ *Relief of muscle spasm and pain:* 2 tablets qid.
Methocarbamol and aspirin	Robaxisal	A centrally acting skeletal muscle relaxant. ■ *Relief of muscle spasm and for analgesia:* 2 tablets tid to qid; or in severe conditions, 3 tablets tid to qid for 1 to 3 days.
Carisoprodol and aspirin (also comes with codeine)	Soma Compound	Combination centrally acting skeletal muscle relaxant. Used to treat acute muscle spasms and to relieve pain associated with musculoskeletal conditions. Has CNS depressant effects, and physical and psychologic addictive effects, and withdrawal effects occur with abrupt cessation of the drug. ■ *Relief of muscle spasm and pain:* 1 to 2 tablets tid to qid.
Orphedrine citrate, aspirin, and caffeine	Norgesic	Combination centrally acting skeletal muscle relaxants indicated for the relief of mild to moderate pain and muscle spasms of acute musculoskeletal conditions. ■ *Relief from pain and muscle spasms:* 1 to 2 tablets tid to qid.

The patient should be observed for signs and symptoms of therapeutic effect, such as increased range of motion, relief from muscle spasm, and pain relief.

▼ Patient and family teaching

The nurse should provide the patient and family with the following instructions:

1. The patient should take this medication as advised, and not stop taking it suddenly or increase the dosage without supervision.
2. The patient should avoid driving, operating heavy machinery, or doing tasks requiring alertness while taking skeletal muscle relaxants.
3. The patient should avoid taking medicines that depress CNS functions, for example, antihistamines, allergy or cold medications, sedatives, tranquilizers, sleeping medications, anticonvulsants, narcotic analgesics, or tricyclic antidepressants.
4. If a dose of medication is missed, it may be taken within the hour it was scheduled. If it is close to the next scheduled dose, only the regular dose should be taken and the missed dose should be omitted.
5. The physician should be contacted immediately if the following side effects occur: dizziness or fainting, mental depression, unusually fast heartbeat, wheezing, shortness of breath, difficult breathing, abdominal pain, high fever, nausea, diarrhea, sore throat, malaise, mucosal ulceration, or petechiae.
6. The patient should take the last dose at bedtime so that drowsiness will assist in producing sleep.
7. This medicine must be kept out of the reach of children and all others for whom it is not prescribed.

CRITICAL DECISION:
Skeletal Muscle Relaxants

Skeletal muscle relaxants, like other CNS depressants, can become habit forming. Their long-term use is not recommended.

SECTION THREE: ANTIARTHRITIS MEDICATIONS

Objectives

At the conclusion of this section you should be able to:

1. List at least three medications used to treat arthritis.
2. Describe the probable mechanisms of action for various antiarthritic medications.
3. Indicate why these medications are generally reserved for more serious forms of arthritis.
4. Identify adverse reactions commonly associated with these preparations.
5. Describe specific things for which the nurse should monitor in a patient receiving these medications.
6. Develop a teaching plan to help a patient on long-term therapy take the medications appropriately.

OVERVIEW

The term **arthritis** covers more than 100 different types of joint disease in which inflammation of a joint is present. The most common types are **rheumatoid arthritis** (a systemic disease that involves an autoimmune response caused by failure of the body to recognize its own tissue, resulting in destruction of the joint) and **osteoarthritis** (the commonly seen joint destruction, particularly in weight-bearing joints or stressed joints, gradually resulting from overuse and age).

Symptoms of arthritis include involvement of one or more joints, with swollen, painful, and inflamed joints developing. In rheumatoid arthritis, as the disease progresses, there is degeneration of the joint with permanent changes that produce deformities and immobility.

Most medications used in arthritis are designed to reduce pain, swelling, and inflammation. Gold compounds and penicillamine are the only products that are used to help slow or halt joint destruction.

Salicylates and NSAIDs are first-line drugs for the treatment of arthritis. The following products are used only in documented rheumatoid arthritis that has been progressive or without remission despite other methods of therapy, including high doses of nonsteroidal antiinflammatory drugs. None of these agents is without significant risk and toxic effects. Patients on these drugs need constant follow-up and regular evaluation.

The slow-acting antirheumatic drugs (SAARDs) useful in treating significant disease include hydroxychloroquine sulfate, penicillamine, methotrexate, and gold compounds. Each will be briefly described.

HYDROXYCHLOROQUINE SULFATE

ACTION

Hydroxychloroquine sulfate's mechanism of action is not understood. This is an antimalarial drug that in some way suppresses the formation of antigens in the body. These antigens produce the hypersensitivity reactions leading to the physiologic changes of rheumatoid arthritis and systemic lupus erythematosus.

USES

Hydroxychloroquine sulfate is used in documented cases of rheumatoid arthritis that have been progressive or without remission despite other methods of therapy, including high doses of NSAIDs. This agent is not without significant risk and toxic effects. Patients on this drug need constant follow-up and regular evaluation. This drug may also be used in confirmed diagnosis of systemic or discoid lupus erythematosus.

ADVERSE REACTIONS

The retinopathy does appear to be dose related, so patients should have an expert ophthalmologic evaluation before initiation of the drug and periodic checks every 3 to 6 months throughout therapy. The drug should be discontinued if there are any visual complaints or symptoms, such as seeing flashing lights or light streaks, because the retinal damage may progress even after the drug is discontinued.

This product must not be used with other slow-acting antirheumatic drugs, especially gold, because concurrent use will greatly increase the chance of dermatologic reactions.

CRITICAL DECISION:
Hydroxychloroquine Sulfate

The most serious side effect of hydroxychloroquine sulfate is damage to the eyes, which usually appears in two forms: (1) retinopathy with irreversible visual loss, and (2) corneal infiltration that may be somewhat reversible when the medication is stopped.

CRITICAL DECISION:
Adverse Reactions

About 50% of patients taking penicillamine have adverse reactions, some of which are fatal.

This medication requires 4 to 12 weeks of therapy before improvement is seen. If there is no improvement after 6 months, the drug should be discontinued.

If the drug is stopped while the patient is feeling relief from the symptoms, the agent can be reintroduced if the disease becomes exacerbated. Corticosteroids or NSAIDs may be used with this drug until the effects of this slow-acting drug become apparent.

PENICILLAMINE

ACTION AND USES

Penicillamine is a degradation of penicillin. It is a chelating agent used as a heavy metal antagonist and is helpful in conditions such as lead and copper poisoning. Its mode of action in the treatment of rheumatoid arthritis is not understood. It is known to be effective in relieving the symptoms of arthritis and in some way suppressing the disease progression.

Patients with a history of renal impairment or active renal impairment should not receive this drug, because of its potentially toxic effects on the kidneys. Penicillamine is contraindicated in combination with other drugs that could potentiate blood dyscrasias, such as gold compounds, cytotoxic drugs, or pyrazoline derivatives, such as phenylbutazone or oxyphenbutazone.

Blood dyscrasias and skin reactions are particularly dangerous. This drug has many toxic side effects, and as with gold, only about 30% of patients who are prescribed this agent obtain benefit from its use. The patient should be warned of this before starting the agent. This drug requires excellent patient compliance, because it is an oral preparation that patients must administer themselves.

The special dosage schedule enclosed as a package insert should be followed. Maintenance dosage is that dose at which clinical improvement begins to occur. When a maintenance dosage is reached, the blood

and urine follow-up should continue every 2 weeks for 6 months and then monthly thereafter for as long as the patient receives the medicine. If an exacerbation occurs during therapy, the use of NSAIDs is indicated rather than a rapid increase in the penicillamine dosage. No therapeutic effect may be seen for 3 to 6 months.

GOLD COMPOUNDS

ACTION AND USES

Gold compound therapy is also called chrysotherapy. The exact mechanism of action of gold is not known. Gold is a heavy metal that interferes with a wide range of biochemical reactions on a cellular level. It is felt that it may inhibit lysosomal enzyme activity in macrophages and decrease their phagocytic activity. It is also believed that it in some way affects the antigen formation in the autoimmune response of patients with rheumatoid arthritis. It appears to suppress the synovitis of active rheumatoid disease and therefore reduce the amount of damage done.

This drug has many contraindications and precautions to its use. It also has many toxic effects, and only 30% to 35% of patients gain benefit from its use. The patient should be warned of this before starting on this agent.

The most common side effects are mucocutaneous, which occur in about 15% of all patients. Gold dermatitis has a variety of appearances, but is always pruritic (often this pruritus occurs before the rash presents itself, and is seen most commonly periorbitally and on the palms and dorsum of the hands). Stomatitis may be seen with painful ulcers on the buccal mucosa, tongue, palate, or pharynx. These may be preceded by a metallic taste.

A number of patients experience what is known as the "nitritoid reaction" with the use of Myochrysine. This is a benign reaction caused by the aqueous medium of the gold. It results in the patient feeling flushed and lightheaded, and occasionally leads to fainting. These symptoms occur immediately after the injection, and for this reason it is advised that patients receiving Myochrysine lie down and remain recumbent for 10 to 15 minutes after the injection. This problem is self-limited and requires no other intervention.

The dosage regimen includes three phases in the administration and use of gold: (1) a 2- or 3-week period of injections that increase gradually to test for severe reactions or unusual problems; (2) a "loading period" of weekly injections, until a total dose of 1 gm of injected gold is reached; and (3) a decreasing frequency of dosage sequencing until a maintenance dosage is achieved. Follow the very specific dosage schedule included in the package insert.

Gold is a heavy metal and comes in two solution forms for injection: one in an oil medium and the other in an aqueous medium. They are both painful injections and should be given only in the gluteus maximus muscle. There is an oral form of gold that has been introduced only in the last few years.

METHOTREXATE

ACTION AND USES

Methotrexate (amethopterin) is a medication that has been used for years to treat various neoplastic and psoriatic conditions. The mechanism of action in rheumatoid arthritis is unknown. It may affect immune function. It reduces articular swelling and tenderness in 3 to 6 weeks, but there is no evidence that it induces remission or limits bone erosions.

Methotrexate is used in cases of severe rheumatoid arthritis that are unresponsive to other treatment. This product has a high possibility of severe adverse reactions, including death. It is most toxic to the bone marrow, liver, kidney, and lungs. It has many contraindications to use, drug interactions, and dosage precautions. The package insert should be consulted for specific information.

 NURSING IMPLICATIONS AND PATIENT TEACHING

▼ Assessment

After reading specific information from the package insert about the medication, the nurse should obtain a complete health history, including the complete diagnostic and therapeutic history of the patient's arthritis, presence of drug sensitivities, underlying

diseases such as renal, liver, cardiovascular, or hematopoietic diseases that would contraindicate any of these products, the possibility of pregnancy, or other drugs taken concurrently that might cause drug interactions.

▼ Planning

Only 30% to 35% of patients may benefit from these drugs. The patient should be counseled not to develop unrealistic hopes and should be made aware of the potential risk of many serious adverse reactions associated with these products.

▼ Implementation

Gold compounds are very painful on injection and must be given in the gluteus maximus muscle. Patients receiving Myochrysine injections should remain lying down for 15 minutes after the injection, and should then be helped carefully to their feet. They should be monitored for any symptoms of nitritoid reaction. The vial should be shaken well before administering the injection, and the concentration of the medication should be checked. The color of the medication should be checked; if it is darker than pale yellow, it should not be used.

See Table 17-3 for a summary of dosage information concerning antiarthritis medications.

▼ Evaluation

The nurse should observe for the therapeutic effect and monitor closely for the numerous and serious adverse effects that may develop.

▼ Patient and family teaching

The nurse should provide the patient and family with the following instructions:

1. These drugs are very potent and slow acting. They may be helpful in some patients in reducing symptoms or actually halting joint destruction caused by arthritis. They do not help all patients, and a thorough trial will take 12 to 20 weeks before response to the drug can be determined.

2. There are serious toxic effects that can occur with this drug. The patient must work closely with physician, keep appointments, and have laboratory work performed.

3. The patient and the physician should be alert for problems that may develop in the kidneys, lungs, liver, skin, or blood.

4. This medication requires frequent response and dosage monitoring.

5. Some patients experience a brief increase in pain and joint achiness for 1 to 2 days after receiving the injection, but it usually disappears. The patient should contact the physician if he or she is still having great discomfort after 2 days.

6. The most common adverse effects are skin rashes, itching, ulcers or sores in the mouth, and easy bruising or bleeding.

7. The physician should be notified if the patient notes a metallic taste in the mouth, purple blotches, bruising, or problems with bleeding.

 Table 17-3 Antiarthritis medications

Generic name	Trade name	Comments and dosage
SLOW-ACTING ANTIRHEUMATIC DRUGS (SAARDs)		
Hydroxychloroquine	Plaquenil	■ *Rheumatoid arthritis:* 400 to 600 mg PO qd with meals or food to prevent GI upset. *Maintenance dose:* Continue 400 to 600 mg PO qd for 4 to 12 weeks, until patient has symptomatic improvement. Then reduce dosage by 50% to 200 to 400 mg PO daily, and maintain that dosage.
Penicillamine	Cuprimine Depen	This product has a very specific dosage schedule that covers three specific phases. The format should be followed as closely as possible. See the package insert for details.
Methotrexate	Rheumatrex Amethopterin ♣	Therapy generally begins with 7.5 mg/week. An initial test dose is usually given before beginning a regular dosage schedule to detect any extreme sensitivity reactions. See the package insert for specific guidelines. Therapeutic response is generally seen in 3 to 6 weeks, and the patient may continue to improve for another 12 weeks. Optimal duration of therapy is unknown. Arthritis may worsen within 3 to 5 weeks of therapy ending.
GOLD COMPOUNDS		
Auranofin	Ridaura	Give 6 mg daily, either as 3 mg bid or 6 mg qd. If response is inadequate after 6 months, increase dosage to 9 mg/day. If no response after 3 more months, discontinue the drug. Comes as a capsule to be taken PO. Contains 29% gold.
Aurothioglucose	Solganal	There appear to be fewer skin eruptions and a greater incidence of stomatitis and albuminuria with this preparation. Oil and aqueous preparations may be alternated. This injection is painful and should be given deep into the gluteus maximus muscle. Contains 50% gold.
Gold sodium thiomalate	Myochrysine	This injection is painful and should be given only in the gluteus maximus muscle. This preparation is also responsible for producing a "nitritoid-like response" in some patients, and patient must remain lying down for 10 to 15 minutes after injection to decrease possibility of fainting. Shake vial well before injection, and make certain proper concentration of medication is used. Contains 50% gold.

SECTION FOUR: ANTIGOUT AGENTS

Objectives

At the conclusion of this section you should be able to:

1. Explain the action of uricosuric agents.
2. Identify indications for the use of uricosuric agents.
3. List common agents used in treatment or prophylaxis of gout.
4. Identify common adverse effects from uricosuric agents.
5. Develop a teaching plan for the patient taking uricosuric agents on a long-term basis.

OVERVIEW

Uric acid, a metabolite of protein, is present in the blood of individuals within very specific ranges. Several pathologic processes, metabolic changes, or drug interactions may be responsible for increasing the uric acid level of the blood.

Gout is a form of arthritis caused by overproduction or underexcretion of uric acid. The drugs used to treat gout vary in their method of action. Those used to treat acute attacks primarily relieve pain and inflammation; others alter the body's response to, production of, or distribution of uric acid.

High uric acid levels cause the uric acid to precipitate into crystals, usually in the kidney and in joint spaces. These crystals have very long, sharp, and jagged edges. When the crystals precipitate in the body, they tear and bruise the areas with which they come in contact. The result is swelling, heat, inflammation, and pain, the syndrome called gout.

ACTION

Uricosuric agents increase the elimination of urate salts by blocking renal tubular reabsorption. They also decrease the amount of circulating urate and urate deposition and promote reabsorption of urate deposits. Sulfinpyrazone also has platelet inhibitory and antithrombotic effects. Uricosuric agents do not have significant antiinflammatory or analgesic properties, and therefore are of little help during an acute episode of gout.

The mechanism of action of colchicine in relieving gouty attacks is not completely known. It is believed to be involved in the inhibition of leukocyte migration and phagocytosis that causes the inflammatory response in gout. It also decreases uric acid deposition. Colchicine is not an antiinflammatory, analgesic, or uricosuric agent. It is used to treat acute gouty attacks, or prophylactically with allopurinol or other uricosuric agents to prevent an acute attack when therapy with these agents is initiated.

Probenecid inhibits tubular reabsorption of urate, increasing uric acid excretion.

Allopurinol inhibits the production of uric acid by decreasing the production of xanthine oxidase, an enzyme that metabolizes purine hypoxanthine to xanthine and xanthine to uric acid. This drug has no analgesic or antiinflammatory properties, and is therefore not beneficial in the treatment of acute gout, but rather is used in prophylactic therapy for recurrent or chronic gout, and in patients with renal failure significant enough to increase their uric acid levels to a point where they may develop gouty attacks.

USES

Uricosuric agents are primarily used to reduce uric acid levels in patients who are underexcreters. The diagnosis of gout is confirmed by serum uric acid levels greater than 7 mg/100 ml and a 24-hour urine test for uric acid of less than 800 mg/day. The patient has usually had more than one acute episode before being started on these agents.

The patient should not be started on uricosuric agents during an acute episode of gout, because these agents may induce an attack or worsen the severity of an existing attack. Colchicine is often given concurrently when initiating treatment with these agents to prevent the precipitation of an acute episode of gout brought on by a shift in the miscible urate pool. Sulfinpyrazone is used only in patients refractory to all other modalities.

Colchicine is used when the diagnosis of gout is either confirmed or suspected by the patient's history and physical examination and when examination of joint fluid is not possible. It relieves the pain of acute attacks. It is also used in conjunction with allopurinol or other uricosuric agents to avoid precipitating a gouty attack until the serum uric acid level is reduced to normal and stabilized. It has no effect on uric acid levels itself. It may be used prophylactically to prevent recurrent attacks, but only in combination with a uricosuric agent.

Allopurinol usually is used when objective findings demonstrate any of the following conditions:

1. On a general diet, the patient overproduces uric acid (24-hour urine test shows uric acid excretion greater than 700 mg/day).
2. A uric acid nephropathy with impaired renal function (creatinine clearance less than 80 ml/min).
3. Tophi, or small masses of crystals on bony prominences.
4. Documentation of kidney stones by flat plate of the abdomen.
5. Primary or secondary hyperuricemia associated with blood dyscrasias and their treatment.
6. Gout not controlled by uricosuric drugs alone, caused by the patient's intolerance of the drug, or ineffectiveness of drug.
7. Drug is for prophylactic therapy in patients with lymphomas, leukemias, or other malignancies requiring chemotherapy or radiation therapy that results in an increase in the serum uric acid level.

Probenecid is often used to treat venereal diseases with penicillin preparations, because of its ability to increase the plasma level of penicillin. Levels may increase two to four times normal, irrespective of the route of penicillin administration.

ADVERSE REACTIONS

Uricosuric agents may produce drug fever, dizziness, pruritus, rashes, anorexia, constipation, diarrhea, nausea, vomiting, exacerbation of acute attacks of gout; rarely anaphylaxis, nephrotic syndrome, hepatic necrosis, and aplastic anemia are seen.

Colchicine may cause abdominal pain, severe diarrhea, nausea, and vomiting; prolonged use may cause bone marrow depression, peripheral neuritis, purpura, myopathy, and hair loss. There is usually a latent period between overdosage and onset of symptoms. Deaths have been reported with as little as 7 mg.

Allopurinol may produce drowsiness, alopecia, rash (even up to several months after therapy is started), purpuric lesions, diarrhea, abdominal pain, nausea, vomiting, and blood dyscrasias. It may also produce idiosyncratic drug reactions with fever, chills, arthralgias, skin rash, pruritus, nausea, vomiting, interstitial nephritis, occasional development of cataracts, and vasculitis that may lead to hepatotoxicity and death.

DRUG INTERACTIONS

Salicylates antagonize the uricosuric action of these drugs. Uricosurics potentiate the effects of the following drugs by decreasing renal tubular excretion: sulfonamides, sulfonylureas, naproxen, indomethacin, rifampin, dapsone, pantothenic acid, aminosalicylic acid, and methotrexate. Additionally, sulfinpyrazone affects anticoagulants by potentiating their platelet aggregation effects.

Colchicine is inhibited by acidifying agents and potentiated by alkalinizing agents. Patients taking this drug may have an increased sensitivity to CNS depressants. Colchicine also decreases gut absorption of vitamin B_{12}. Sympathomimetics are enhanced by colchicine.

Hypersensitivity may occur in patients with renal compromise who are taking thiazides and allopurinol concurrently. Concomitant use with ampicillin may increase the chance for skin rashes. Allopurinol will increase the half-life of anticoagulants and many other drugs.

 NURSING IMPLICATIONS AND PATIENT TEACHING

▼ Assessment

The patient may complain of an initial or recurrent attack of inflammation, erythema, swelling, extreme tenderness, and pain, usually in a single or asymmetric joint pattern. At least 50% of initial attacks occur in the great toe at the metatarsal phalangeal joint (podagra). This disease usually manifests itself in the lower extremities. Joints affected may be in the instep, ankles, heels, or knees, although some patients are also bothered in wrists, fingers, and elbows. In patients with a severe or progressive form of the disease, additional joints may be involved. These symptoms are sudden in onset, and the patient may complain of being unable to tolerate clothing, shoes, or even bed coverings on the site of inflammation. There may be a historical association of minor trauma to the involved joint, obesity, alcohol ingestion, use of a new drug such as hydrochlorothiazide, or low-dose aspirin consumption.

The nurse should obtain a complete health history, including the presence of hypersensitivity, concurrent drug administration that could cause drug interactions, history of underlying disease, or the possibility of pregnancy. These conditions are precautions or contraindications to the use of antigout medications. The frequency and severity of the attacks should be assessed to determine whether therapy with colchicine is indicated.

▼ Planning

The nurse can assist in obtaining a 24-hour urine test for uric acid level and creatinine clearance and baseline laboratory tests as ordered by the physician.

Uricosuric agents are to be started only after the acute attack has subsided. Prophylactic therapy is recommended in patients having more than one acute attack per year. If affected less often than that, the patient should try to control attacks by having colchicine on hand.

Initiation of therapy with uricosuric agents may precipitate an acute attack of gout, and concomitant use of colchicine is often given to prevent such an attack.

The use of salicylates in small or large doses is contraindicated in patients taking probenecid, because salicylates antagonize the uricosuric action of this drug. Patients needing mild analgesia should be instructed to use only acetaminophen products.

Allopurinol may precipitate a gouty attack during the initial treatment phase. This is easily preventable by oral prophylactic use of colchicine 0.5 mg twice daily for 2 weeks to 1 month. Good fluid intake and neutral or alkaline pH of urine are important to prevent the possibility of xanthine calculi. Patients with impaired renal function require decreased dosage, and renal function should be carefully monitored.

In transferring patients from uricosuric agents to allopurinol, a gradual increase of allopurinol with a gradual decrease of the other agent should be made over a period of several weeks. The patient should be monitored to maintain a normal serum uric acid level.

▼ Implementation

The patient's urine should be alkalinized to prevent hematuria or formation of urate stones, especially during the initial stages of therapy. Injectable doses of colchicine are not to be given intramuscularly or subcutaneously, but must be given only intravenously.

See Table 17-4 for a summary of dosage and information concerning some common antigout medications.

▼ Evaluation

The nurse should evaluate the therapeutic effects (decrease in frequency and severity of gouty attacks) and monitor for progression of the arthritis process (joint deformity, destruction, or tophus formation).

With colchicine, the nurse should observe for therapeutic effects and adverse reactions. The patient treating acute attacks with a loading dose can usually reach a maximum dose level before the onset of GI side effects. The patient should be checked frequently for weakness, anorexia, nausea, vomiting, or diarrhea, because these are the first indications of toxicity, and if these appear the dosage should be reduced. The nurse should watch for symptoms of vitamin B_{12} deficiency.

The potential effect of allopurinol is seen 5 to 10 days after therapy is started. The dosage should be adjusted to maintain a serum uric acid level of less than 7 mg/100 ml. Levels as low as 2 to 3 mg/100 ml are not harmful. Adverse reactions such as rash, appearance of tophi, and change in joint deformities should be monitored.

If a maculopapular rash develops in the patient taking allopurinol anytime during therapy, the drug should be stopped immediately and it should not be restarted.

▼ Patient and family teaching

The nurse should provide the patient and family with the following instructions:

1. The uricosuric drugs will not alter acute gouty attacks, but they help prevent attacks if they are taken regularly. During the initial dose, an acute attack may be precipitated, but this will decrease future chances of severe attacks. The drugs do not cure gout, but they should help control it.
2. Uricosuric medication should be taken as outlined by the physician. It should be taken with meals to help decrease gastrointestinal upset.
3. The patient should drink at least 8 glasses of fluid (especially water or citrus juices) every day while taking uricosuric medication to prevent the development of kidney stones.
4. The patient should observe stools and urine for blood.

Table 17-4   Antigout medications

Generic name	Trade name	Comments and dosage
URICOSURIC AGENTS		
Probenecid	Benemid Probalan Probenecid	Increases urate excretion. Often used with penicillin to treat venereal disease. There is cross-sensitivity to phenylbutazone and other pyrazoles. *Initial dosage:* 250 mg bid for 1 week. *Maintenance:* 500 mg bid.
Sulfinpyrazone	Anturane	This drug is reserved for patients who are refractory to all other modalities of therapy. *Initial dose:* 200 to 400 mg/day in two divided doses; take with meals. *Maintenance dose:* 400 mg/day in divided doses; may be increased to 800 mg/day or reduced to as low as 200 mg/day as long as serum uric acid level remains normal. Therapy should be continued even during acute episodes and patient may be switched from other uricosuric agents to this drug at full maintenance dose.
ANTIGOUT ANALGESIC PREPARATIONS		
Colchicine	Colchicine	*Acute attack of gout:* Begin therapy at first warning of an acute attack. The delay of only a few hours greatly reduces the therapeutic effectiveness. *PO:* 1 to 1.2 mg initially, followed by 1 tablet q1 to 2h until pain is relieved, or nausea, vomiting, or diarrhea develops. Total dose is 4 to 8 mg. Pain is usually relieved in 12 hours and gone in 24 to 48 hours. *IV:* 1 to 2 mg initially, then 0.5 mg q3 to 6h until pain is relieved; total dose is 4 mg. *Prophylactic therapy:* 0.5 to 1 mg/day in single or divided doses, usually in combination with a uricosuric agent.
Allopurinol	Zyloprim	Gastrointestinal side effects are usually reduced if taken with meals. The dosage to control gout and hyperuricemia is variable. The average is 200 to 300 mg for patients with mild gout; 400 to 600 mg for those with moderately severe or tophaceous gout. Dosages over 300 mg should be given in divided doses; less than that can be given once daily.
Combination products:	ColBenemid Proben-C Probenecid with Colchicine Pro-Biosan ✦ Verban ✦	Therapy may be increased by 500 mg/day q 4 weeks with a maximum dose of 2 gm or until urine urate excretion is less than 700 mg/day. If an acute attack occurs, continue regimen and add colchicine 0.25 mg bid for 1 week, then 0.5 mg bid until uric acid levels are within normal range. Colchicine can then be discontinued until there is another attack. If attacks occur frequently, then the two agents should be used together indefinitely. Once normal uric acid levels have been maintained for 6 months, daily dosage may be decreased by 500 mg every 6 months until there is a slight rise in the uric acid level. Drug is maintained at that level.

5. The physician should be contacted if any rash, stomach problems, or any new or troublesome symptoms develop.

6. This medication must be kept out of the reach of children and all others for whom it is not prescribed.

7. Colchicine should be kept on hand in case the patient develops an attack of gout. At the first sign of difficulty, the patient should take 2 tablets, and then 1 tablet every hour or every 2 hours until the symptoms are relieved or until the patient develops nausea, diarrhea, or vomiting. The patient should not take more than 12 tablets.

8. If the patient is taking colchicine regularly with other drugs, it should be taken with meals to reduce gastrointestinal upset.

9. Colchicine must be taken regularly as ordered if it is to help prevent gouty attacks.

10. While the patient is taking the drug on a daily basis, the drug should be stopped if the patient notices symptoms of nausea, vomiting, or diarrhea, and the physician should be notified. The patient should also report any skin rash, fever, sore throat, unusual bleeding, or bruising.

11. The patient should not take any other medications without the knowledge of the physician; some drugs interact adversely with this product.

SUMMARY

This chapter discussed musculoskeletal and antiarthritis medications, which are used to treat problems affecting bones, joints, muscles, and ligaments. Drugs used to treat these disorders are selected on the basis of the severity of the problem and the pathologic mechanisms underlying the disorder. Many acute problems require only short-term therapy. Some disorders, such as arthritis, may require long-term therapy with a variety of medications, including more powerful medications as the disease progresses. Many of these products are associated with significant side effects, and therefore require close monitoring.

 CRITICAL THINKING QUESTIONS

1. Mr. Lionhart has started taking a salicylate for his arthritis. He says he has a sister with lupus who is also taking salicylates. Mr. Lionhart wonders about the discrepancy in their dosages, despite the fact that he and his sister are similar in body weight and size. Explain the importance of different dosages depending on the problem.

2. What kinds of adverse reactions should you advise Mr. Lionhart to watch out for?

3. In assessing Mr. Lionhart, his physician asks you to test for "occult blood." What is that and how do you test for it?

4. Generate a teaching plan for guiding Mr. Lionhart in when and how to take his medication for the best possible antiinflammatory response.

5. Ms. French is receiving an NSAID for her rheumatoid arthritis. Why might this drug be preferred over ASA or salicylate therapy? What adverse reactions should Ms. French be told to watch out for?

6. Mr. Henson has been prescribed an oral skeletal muscle relaxant. Mr. Henson asks, "Wouldn't an injection or something be more helpful?" What is a possible rationale for the oral form? Explain to Mr. Henson (a) proper dosage adherence and (b) how to monitor for adverse reactions.

7. Create a table to compare and contrast the four major antiarthritis medications in the following area: (a) uses, (b) adverse reactions, (c) precautions, and (d) appropriate nursing interventions. Are the nursing implications the same for all four drugs? Explain.

8. Because these drugs are some of the most dangerous on the market, carefully prepare a teaching plan that includes a discussion of the high incidence of serious and potentially fatal adverse effects. Naturally, this plan should stress the requirement of excellent patient compliance.

9. Discuss the two etiologies of high uric acid levels in light of common signs and symptoms of each.

10. Develop a patient teaching plan for helping patients identify the signs and symptoms of gout and the difference between prophylactic and acute treatment. Be sure to include a warning against taking prophylactic drugs during an acute attack.

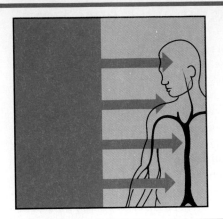

CHAPTER 18
Topical Preparations

OBJECTIVES

At the conclusion of this chapter you should be able to:

1. Identify major categories of medications used topically.
2. List at least three preparations used to treat eye, ear, and skin problems.
3. Indicate major adverse effects that might be expected from topical products.

KEY TERMS

anorectal preparations, p. 375

antiglaucoma agents, p. 376

antipsoriatics, p. 376

antiseptics, p. 375

mydriasis, p. 376

pediculocides, p. 376

scabicides, p. 376

vasoconstrictors, p. 376

OVERVIEW

This chapter presents a brief overview of the many products that may be used topically. Many of these products are purchased over the counter. The nurse plays a major role in teaching the patient the proper administration of these medications. Side effects are usually localized unless systemic sensitization develops.

Integumentary System

The integumentary system comprises the skin, hair, nails, and sweat glands (Fig. 18-1). The skin provides the most important barrier to infection and protects the body, regulates temperature, prevents water loss, and produces vitamin D precursors.

The skin, the mucous membranes, and the surfaces of the eye, ear, nose, mouth, and vagina are often the site of minor infections. Medications are frequently required to treat disease in these areas. Special prepa-

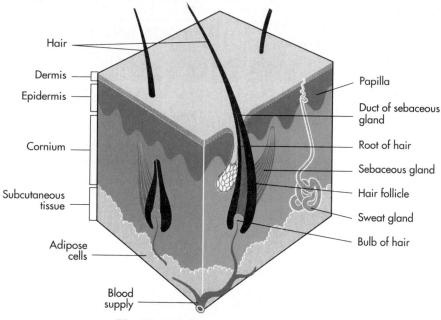

Fig. 18-1   The integumentary system.

rations and procedures are often required in order to allow medication to penetrate deep within these tissues.

ANORECTAL PREPARATIONS

ACTION AND USES

Anorectal preparations include over-the-counter preparations for topical anesthesia or healing of the rectal area. They are used for symptomatic relief of discomfort associated with hemorrhoids. They may be used on a long-term basis, or for hemorrhoids associated with pregnancy, prolonged sitting, or other temporary problems.

ADVERSE REACTIONS

The patient may have sensitization to the product.

MOUTH AND THROAT PREPARATIONS

ACTION AND USES

These miscellaneous products are used to soothe minor oral inflammation. Some release oxygen to provide cleansing while others contain an anesthetic property to reduce pain. These preparations are indicated for minor oral inflammation, such as canker sores, dental irritation, irritation after dental procedures, relief of dryness of mouth and throat, or to treat minor sore throat discomfort and control of coughs caused by colds.

Products are available in mouthwashes, sprays, solutions, troches, lozenges, and disks. The patient should be taught the appropriate administration technique for the relevant drug. Administration should not exceed 3 or 4 days for normal therapy.

OPHTHALMIC DRUGS

ACTION AND USES

There are a wide variety of preparations used for eye problems. Local anesthetics are useful in procedures such as tonometry, gonioscopy, cataract surgery, and removal of foreign bodies from the cornea. **Antiseptics** are used for the prevention of gonorrheal ophthalmia neonatorum when babies are born and if germicidal or astringent action is needed. Antiinfectives are used to treat common eye infections caused by bacteria, fungi, or viruses. Artificial tears provide tearlike lubrication to relieve dry eyes, eye irritation secondary to wearing contact lenses, or deficient tear production caused by a wide variety of disorders. Diagnostic products include topical fluorescein stains, used to detect foreign bodies or scratches.

Antiglaucoma agents make up a large class of medications, with a variety of actions. Carbonic anhydrase inhibitors, such as acetazolamide, are sulfonamide diuretics that reduce the secretion of aqueous humor in the eye. Mydriatic-cyclopegics block the action of acetylcholine. The sphincter of the iris is paralyzed, causing **mydriasis,** or abnormal dilation of the pupil, and the ciliary muscles are paralyzed, blocking accommodation, or adjustment of the focus of the eye. Atropine and scopolamine are long-acting agents that produce complete cycloplegia, or paralysis. Homatropine, cyclopentolate, and tropicamide have shorter durations of action and are most useful for diagnostic procedures. Long-acting cholinesterase inhibitors include miotic-antiglaucoma agents that inactivate acetylcholinesterase. This provides iris sphincter contraction, leading to miosis and ciliary muscle constriction, which leads to increased aqueous humor outflow. Parasympathomimetic or miotic drugs, such as carbachol, act as cholinergic agonists to reduce intraocular pressure through miosis as a result of iris sphincter contraction. This leads to an increased outflow of aqueous humor by opening up the anterior chamber angle. Cholinesterase inhibitors, such as physostigmine salicylate, temporarily inactivate acetylcholinesterase to allow increased parasympathetic tone from accumulation of endogenous acetylcholine. This causes iris sphincter contraction, resulting in miosis and increased ciliary muscle constriction and reduction of aqueous humor outflow. Timolol is a beta-blocker that reduces intraocular pressure, probably by reducing the production of aqueous humor. Sympathomimetic agents, such as epinephrine, produce vasoconstriction and decreased intraocular pressure in open-angle glaucoma, probably as a result of decreased aqueous humor production. Phenylephrine acts as a mydriatic, causing constriction of the dilator muscles of the pupil, leading to mydriasis and vasoconstriction of the arterioles of the conjunctiva. **Vasoconstrictors,** such as naphazoline, cause direct stimulation of the alpha receptors of vascular smooth muscle, leading to vasoconstriction. This action lasts for several hours. It is especially important for the nurse to avoid dilating the eyes of a patient who may have glaucoma, because angle closure could be provoked, leading to a surgical emergency.

Each of these preparations has numerous precautions, contraindications, and minor adverse effects. See the package inserts for more detailed information and Table 18-1 for a summary.

OTIC PREPARATIONS

ACTION AND USES

Topical antibiotics are used to control superficial infections of the ear through bactericidal or bacteriostatic mechanisms. Other products may be used in prophylaxis of infections for swimmers, and for removing ceruminous (ear wax) accumulations. There are also some steroid products available for ear problems. See individual products for precautions, contraindications, and adverse effects.

TOPICAL SKIN PREPARATIONS

ACTION AND USES

Topical preparations for the skin may include medicated bar soaps and foams, sulfur preparations, topical antibiotics, and medications used for acne. A wide variety of steroids are also available for topical use in a variety of dermatologic disorders. These preparations come in mild, intermediate, and strong concentrations. Fluorinated products should not be used on the face, because they may cause thinning and may leave scars. **Antipsoriatics** accelerate scaling and healing of dry lesions in chronic psoriasis. Antiseborrheic shampoos promote shedding and softening of the horny cell layer and inhibit the growth of microorganisms in seborrhea and dandruff. Acyclovir is a relatively new antiviral agent used to treat herpes simplex. This agent helps reduce the severity of symptoms and lengthen the time between outbreaks. **Scabicides** and **pediculocides** are used to treat scabies and pediculosis. There are also a variety of burn preparations, cauterizing agents, emollients, keratolytics, and wet dressings and soaks on the market. These agents all have their own specific precautions, adverse reactions, and drug interactions. The specific product information should be consulted. These preparations are summarized in Table 18-1.

SUMMARY

This chapter presented a brief overview of the wide variety of topical preparations available, many of which are over-the-counter products. The nurse's role in these medications often is one of teaching the patient how to apply or administer the products. Side effects are usually localized unless systemic sensitization develops.

Table 18-1	Topical preparations	
Generic name	**Trade name**	**Comments and dosage**

ANORECTAL PREPARATIONS

	Anusol Nupercainal	Apply ointment morning and night and after each bowel movement. For suppositories, insert one after each bowel movement.
	Anusol-HC Anugard-HC	Contains hydrocortisone. Insert suppository morning and bedtime for 3 to 6 days, or until inflammation subsides. Apply cream to anal area and gently rub in tid to qid for 3 to 6 days.
Hydrocortisone foam	Cortifoam	Contains hydrocortisone. Insert one applicatorful PR qd or bid for 2 to 3 weeks, then qod. Decrease therapy gradually. Steroid used for antiinflammatory treatment of ulcerative proctitis and distal ulcerative colitis.

MOUTH AND THROAT PREPARATIONS
Oral preparations

Carbamide peroxide	Cankaid Proxigel	Do not dilute. Apply directly to affected area qid, expectorate after 2 to 3 minutes.

Lozenges and troches

	Cepacol Cepastat Chloraseptic Sucrets	Dissolve 1 lozenge in mouth up to qh if needed. Take no more than 12 lozenges daily.

Gargles, gels, mouthwashes, and sprays

	Cepacol Chloraseptic	Follow directions on bottle or package. Wide variation among products.
Nystatin	Mycostatin Nilstat	Antifungal. Take 400,000 to 600,000 units qid. Take half of each dose, hold in one side of mouth for at least 2 minutes and then swallow. Repeat, using rest of medication on other side of mouth.

Saliva substitutes

	Orex	Used to relieve dry mouth and throat; spray into mouth as needed.

Throat disks

	Soretts Colrex Medikets Oracin	Allow lozenge to dissolve slowly; do not use more than 4 lozenges per hour.

OPHTHALMIC DRUGS
Local anesthetics

Benoxinate Fluorescein	Fluress Novesin ♣	Often used when suturing of eye is required. Instill 1 to 2 drops before procedure.
Proparacaine	Alcaine	Use 1 to 2 drops immediately before tonometry, 2 to 3 minutes before suture removal or removal of foreign body.
Tetracaine	Pontocaine	Instill 1 or 2 drops or ½ to 1 inch of ointment to lower conjunctival area.

Antiseptic ointments

Silver protein	Argyrol	Instill 1 to 3 drops in eyes q3 to 4h for several days for minor eye infections or before eye surgery. Stains hands and clothing.

Continued.

Table 18-1 Topical preparations—cont'd

Generic name	Trade name	Comments and dosage
OPHTHALMIC ANTIINFECTIVES (preparations must be labeled "ophthalmic")		
Antibiotics		
Bacitracin	AK-Tracin	Apply sparingly into conjunctival sac bid to tid.
Chloramphenicol	Chloroptic	Apply small amount of ointment to the lower conjunctival sac, or instill 2 drops of solution q3h for the first 48 hours, then prn. Continue for at least 48 hours after the eye appears to be normal.
Tetracycline	Achromycin	Apply ointment to affected eye q2h prn; 1 to 2 drops bid to qid.
Erythromycin	Ilotycin	Apply to affected eye qd or more often, depending on severity of infection.
Gentamicin	Garamycin Genoptic Gentacidin	Instill 1 to 2 drops into affected eye q4h. In severe infections, dosage may be increased to as much as 2 drops hourly. Apply ointment sparingly bid to tid.
Polymyxin B	Aerosporin	Instill 1 to 2 drops of 0.1% to 0.25% qh; increase prn.
Sulfacetamide sodium	AK-Sulf Sodium sulamyd	Instill 1 to 2 drops q2 to 3h during day, less at night. May also apply ½- to 1-inch ribbon of ointment in lower conjunctival sac at night.
Tobramycin	Tobrex	Instill 1 to 2 drops 4 to 6 times daily.
Antiviral agents		
Idoxuridine	Herplex Stoxil ♣	Saturate tissue for best results. Instill 1 drop in infected eye qh during day. At night, instill 1 drop qoh.
Trifluridine	Viroptic	Instill 1 drop onto the cornea of eye with corneal ulcers q2h while awake for a maximum of 9 drops/day. Continue until reepithelialization, then for 7 days give 1 drop q4h while awake.
Vidarabine	Vira-A	Apply ½ inch of ointment to the lower conjunctival sac 5 times daily at 3-hour intervals.
Artificial tears		
	Isopto alkaline Liquifilm Forte Tears Plus Tearisol	1 to 3 drops may be instilled in the eyes tid to qid or prn. Some of these preparations, such as Tearisol, are not to be used with soft contact lenses. Keep the solution free from contamination.
ANTIGLAUCOMA AGENTS		
Sympathomimetics		
Apraclonidine	Iopidine	Instill 1 drop 1% solution before laser surgery.
Epinephrine	Epifrin Eppy/N	Instill 1 to 2 drops into affected eyes qd to bid.
Dipivefrin	Propine	Instill 1 drop 0.1% solution into eyes q12h.
Beta-blockers		
Betaxolol	Betoptic	Instill 1 drop bid.
Carteolol	Ocupress	Instill 1 drop 1% solution bid.
Levobunolol	Betagan	Instill 1 drop 0.25% solution qd.
Metipranolol	OptiPranolol	Instill 1 drop 0.3% solution bid.
Timolol	Timoptic	Instill 1 drop 0.25% solution bid.

Table 18-1   Topical preparations—cont'd

Generic name	Trade name	Comments and dosage
Miotics, direct-acting		
Carbachol	Isopto-carbachol	Instill 1 or 2 drops up to 3 times daily.
Pilocarpine	Pilocar	Instill 1 or 2 drops up to 6 times daily.
	Pilostat	
Pilocarpine ocular therapeutic system	Ocusert	The system is placed in and removed from the eye by the patient, according to instructions in the package. Releases 20 or 40 μg pilocarpine per hour for 1 week.
Miotics, cholinesterase inhibitors		
Demecarium	Humorsol	Instill 1 or 2 drops into eyes qd.
Echothiophate	Phospholine Iodide	Instill 1 to 2 drops qd.
Isoflurophate	Floropryl	Apply 0.25-inch strip ointment in conjunctival sac.
Physostigmine	Eserine	Instill 2 drops into the eyes up to 4 times daily.
Carbonic anhydrase inhibitors		
Acetazolamide	Diamox	Give 250 mg to 1 gm PO qd in divided doses for chronic open-angle glaucoma.
Dichlorphenamide	Daranide	Give priming dose of 100 to 200 mg PO; follow with 100 mg q12h until the desired response is achieved. Maintenance dosage is 25 to 50 mg bid to qid.
Methazolamide	Neptazane	Give 50 to 100 mg PO bid to qid.
Cholinergic blocking agents		
Mydriatic-cycloplegics		
Atropine	Atropisol	1 drop of 0.5% or 1% solution qd to tid, or 0.3 gm to 0.5 gm of 1% ointment qd to tid.
Cyclopentolate	Cyclogyl	Give 1 drop of 1% or 2% solution; repeat in 5 minutes. Refraction can occur in 40 to 50 minutes.
Homatropine	AK-Homatropine	Give 1 drop of 2% or 5% solution; repeat 2 to 5 times until desired results occur.
Scopolamine	IsoptoHyoscine	Give 1 drop of 0.25% solution qd to tid.
Tropicamide	Mydriacyl	Give 1 drop of 1% solution; repeat in 5 minutes.
Mydriatics		
Phenylephrine	Isopto-Frin	■ *Mydriasis:* 1 drop of 2.5% to 10% solution topically on conjunctiva. Repeat in 5 minutes prn. ■ *Vasoconstriction:* 1 drop of 0.02% to 0.15% solution topically to conjunctiva tid to qid prn. ■ *Conjunctivitis:* 1 to 2 drops qh until condition improves, and then 1 drop tid to qid.

OTHER OPHTHALMIC PREPARATIONS
Alpha-adrenergic blocking agents

Dapiprazole	Rev-Eyes	Instill 2 drops followed 5 minutes later by an additional 2 drops.

VASOCONSTRICTORS

Naphazoline	Allerest	Use 1 to 2 drops bid to tid prn to relieve irritation or redness. Mydriasis occurs within 1 hour, recedes within 6 hours of administration. Do not give to patients with angle-closure glaucoma or narrow anterior angle.
	Degest 2	
	Vasocon	
Oxymetazoline	OcuClear	Instill 1 or 2 drops q6h.
Tetrahydrozoline	Murine Plus	Use 1 to 2 drops in each eye bid to tid prn. Mydriasis occurs in 1 hour, recedes within 6 hours. Do not give to patients with narrow-angle glaucoma.
	Visine	

Continued.

Table 18-1   Topical preparations—cont'd

Generic name	Trade name	Comments and dosage
EYE DIAGNOSTIC PRODUCTS		
Fluorescein	Fluor-I-Strip	For examination of corneal and conjunctival epithelium, pour 1 drop sterile water on strip, touch to cornea, and close lid for 60 seconds. Use Wood's lamp to visualize.
OTIC PREPARATIONS (preparations must be labeled "otic")		
Acetic acid	Domeboro	Used for external ear infections and prophylaxis of swimmer's ear. Instill 2 drops in ear, morning and evening for prophylaxis; insert saturated wick into ear and keep moist for 24 hours by occasionally adding a few drops of solution for external ear infection. Remove wick after 24 hours and instill 5 drops tid to qid.
Benzocaine	Americaine Auralgan	Swab ear with solution; instill 4 to 5 drops of warmed solution. Insert cotton pledget in meatus. Patient should remain on side for a few minutes.
Carbamide peroxide	Debrox	To remove ear wax, instill 5 to 10 drops, keeping head tilted so that solution stays in. Maintain position for a few minutes. Repeat bid for 3 to 4 days. May use before irrigation with bulb syringe.
Chloramphenicol	Chloromycetin	*Adults and children:* Instill 2 to 3 drops into the ear tid. Effective against many gram-positive and gram-negative organisms.
Desonide, acetic acid	Tridesilon	Useful in superficial infections of the external canal. Instill 3 to 4 drops into affected ear tid to qid.
Polymyxin B sulfate	Aerosporin	Used in acute and chronic otitis externa, otitis media. Give 2 to 4 drops, tid to qid prn.
Triethanolamine polypeptide oleate-condensate	Cerumenex	To remove cerumen. May be given as drops to loosen cerumen. Use patch test to check for sensitivity 24 hours before use. Tilt patient's head to 45-degree angle and fill ear canal with solution. Insert cotton plug for 30 minutes. Gently flush ear with warm water using a soft, rubber syringe.
TOPICAL SKIN PRODUCTS **Acne products**		
Benzoyl peroxide bars and soaps	Desquam-X Xerac BP5 Clearasil	Apply qd to affected areas after cleansing skin. After 3 to 4 days, if redness, dryness, and peeling do not occur, increase application to bid. Use instead of soap. These products promote drying of skin and provide a gently abrasive action when applied. If undue skin irritation develops, discontinue and consult physician. Available over the counter.
Sulfur preparations	Xerac Fostex Transact	Thin film of medication should be applied qd or bid to clean skin. Used to treat oily skin and mild acne.
Tretinoin	Retin-A	Apply to affected area, clean skin only, qd at bedtime. Start with low doses; may irritate skin initially. Makes individuals more sensitive to the sun and they must wear sunscreen. Also evidence that this product restores skin collagen and turgor, reversing fine wrinkles. Do not use in pregnant women.
Isotretinoin	Accutane	This product must not be taken by women who are pregnant, because severe fetal abnormalities may be produced. Women in childbearing years should be protected by adequate contraception methods during the course of therapy. ■ *Cystic acne:* 1 to 2 mg/kg/day divided into 2 doses for 2 weeks. Dosage may then be adjusted for individual weight and severity of disease.

Table 18-1   Topical preparations—cont'd

Generic name	Trade name	Comments and dosage
TOPICAL ANTIINFECTIVES		
Bacitracin	Baciguent	Apply small amount to infected area tid; comes as cream.
Chlortetracycline	Aureomycin	Apply small amount to infected area tid; comes as cream.
Chloramphenicol	Chloromycetin	Apply small amount to infected area tid; comes as cream.
Clindamycin	Cleocin T	Apply small amount to infected area bid.
Erythromycin	Akne-mycin	Apply small amount to infected area tid; comes as cream.
Gentamicin	Garamycin	Apply small amount to infected area tid; comes as cream.
Mupirocin	Bactroban	New topical antibiotic. Used to treat impetigo. May produce superinfection. Apply small amount to affected area tid. May cover with gauze. Must be reevaluated by physician within 3 days.
Neomycin sulfate	Myciguent	Apply small amount to infected area tid; comes as cream.
Combinations	Neosporin	Combination polymyxin B, neomycin, and bacitracin. Apply small amount to infected area tid; comes as cream.
	Polysporin	Apply small amount to infected area tid; comes as cream. Combination polymyxin B and bacitracin. Apply small amount to infected area tid; comes as cream.
TOPICAL CORTICOSTEROIDS		
Betamethasone dipropionate	Diprosone	Fluorinated product, relatively expensive. Comes as cream, lotion, ointment, or topical aerosol. Use sparingly for dermatoses needing antiinflammatory medication.
Betamethasone valerate	Beta-Val Valisone	Fluorinated product that may be used with occlusive dressings; comes as cream, lotion, or ointment. Apply sparingly qd to tid for adults.
Desonide	Tridesilon	Gently rub in medication bid to qid.
Desoximetasone	Topicort	Do not use near eyes; apply sparingly qd to bid.
Fluocinolone acetonide	Flurosyn Synalar	Rub cream in gently, bid to qid. Apply very sparingly; use less frequent applications for children.
Fluocinonide	Lidex	Comes as cream, gel, or ointment; apply tid to qid.
Flurandrenolide	Cordran Drenison ♣	Shake lotion well; protect from light, heat, and freezing. Also comes as a film tape. Apply sparingly bid to tid.
Halcinonide	Halog	Ointment, cream, solution; protect ointment from light. Apply sparingly bid to tid.
Hydrocortisone	Hycort Cortizone	One of the few steroids that can be used safely on the face, axilla, groin, and under the breasts; comes as ointment, cream, or lotion. Apply thin coat qd to qid; increase strength as indicated by condition.
Hydrocortisone acetate	Cortaid Lanacort	This form is more expensive. Apply thin coat of ointment or apply the cream gently and sparingly. Apply qd to qid as needed by condition. The lowest doses are available without a prescription.
Methylprednisolone	Medrol	Very expensive; apply ointment qd to qid.
Triamcinolone acetonide	Aristocort Kenalog	Fluorinated steroid, highest potency; has many precautions to use. Apply to affected area bid to qid. Do not use on face.
Hydrocortisone plus antibiotics	Cortisporin Neo-Cortef	Comes with neomycin sulfate and polymyxin B. Apply to affected area bid to tid; withdraw gradually if medication has been used for a long time.
Triamcinolone plus antifungals	Mycolog	Many precautions and warnings. Apply ointment to affected areas bid to tid. Ototoxicity and nephrotoxicity have been reported if preparation is overused.

Continued.

Table 18-1 Topical preparations—cont'd

Generic name	Trade name	Comments and dosage
ANESTHETICS FOR MUCOUS MEMBRANES AND SKIN		
Benzocaine	Anbesol Teething syrup ♣	Used for toothaches, wounds, ulcers, and lesions of oral mucosa. Apply 20% aerosol or gel to affected areas bid to tid.
Butamben picrate	Butesin Picrate	Temporary relief of pain caused by minor burns. Apply sparingly to small areas as needed.
Dibucaine	Nupercainal	For abrasions, minor burns, sunburn, and hemorrhoids. Apply ointment or cream sparingly to affected area bid to tid.
Dyclonine	Dyclone	Used as topical anesthetic in anesthetizing of wounds, lesions, and ulcers of the oral mucosa.
Lidocaine	Unguentine Plus	Ointment and jelly used as dental anesthetics.
Tetracaine	Pontocaine	Used in hemorrhoids and minor skin disorders. Apply sparingly tid to qid.
ANTIPSORIATICS		
Ammoniated mercury	Emersal	Apply qd to bid to treat psoriasis.
Anthralin	Anthra-Derm Anthra Forte ♣	Apply thin layer of 0.1% ointment qd to bid for 2 weeks.
ANTISEBORRHEIC PRODUCTS		
Shampoos	Danex Sebulon	Massage into wet scalp for 5 min; rinse and repeat; rinse thoroughly. May use daily. Decrease to 1 to 2 times weekly as symptoms disappear. Tolerance often develops after a short time. It may be necessary to switch from one type of shampoo to another to control symptoms.
Povidone-iodine	Betadine	Shampoo with 2 tsp to hair and scalp. Lather with warm water and rinse. Repeat application and allow to remain on scalp 5 min; rinse thoroughly. Use twice a week until improvement, then once weekly.
Selenium	Selsun Selsun Blue	Massage 1 to 2 tsp into wet scalp. Allow medicated shampoo to remain on scalp for 2 to 3 min; rinse thoroughly; repeat application and rinse. Use twice a week for 2 weeks, then weekly for 2 weeks.
Sulfacetamide	Sebizon	Shampoo hair and rinse. Then apply medication at bedtime and allow it to remain on scalp overnight.
ANTIVIRAL AGENTS		
Acyclovir	Zovirax	For treatment of herpes simplex. Cover all lesions q3h, 6 times a day for 6 days. Approximately ½-inch ribbon of ointment per 4 square inches of surface area should be used. Oral forms are available for treatment of herpes simplex labialis (cold sores).
BURN PREPARATIONS		
Mafenide	Sulfamylon	Apply qd or bid to a thickness of approximately ¹⁄₁₆ inch. No dressing is required.
Nitrofurazone	Furacin Novofuran ♣	Soluble dressing: apply directly to lesions daily; topical cream: apply directly to lesion once daily or every few days.
Silver nitrate	Silver Nitrate	Saturate dressing with warmed solution and apply to burn wound. Mold dressing to body surface and cover with dry dressing. Reapply solution q2h. Change dressing at least once daily.
Silver sulfadiazine	Silvadene	Apply qd or bid to a thickness of approximately ¹⁄₁₆ inch. Dressing not required.

Table 18-1   Topical preparations—cont'd

Generic name	Trade name	Comments and dosage
SCABICIDES/PEDICULOCIDES		
Crotamiton	Eurax	Used in scabies and very pruritic skin conditions. Massage into skin of the whole body; 24 hours later, apply a second coat. Clothing and bed linen should be changed after 24 hours. Bath should be taken 48 hours after the last application.
Gamma benzene hexachloride	Kwell Lindane	Creams or lotions should be applied in a thin layer over skin and left for 24 hours. May repeat in 2 weeks. May use shampoo for pediculosis capitis.
MISCELLANEOUS SKIN PREPARATIONS **Cauterizing agents**		
Dichloroacetic acid	Bichloracetic Acid	Apply petrolatum to tissue surrounding area to be treated. Solution should then be carefully applied to lesion. A kit is provided with detailed instructions.
Monochloroacetic acid	Monocete	Used for removing verrucae or warts. Do not drip solution on normal tissue or mucous membranes. Apply solution with cotton tip applicator or capillary tube. Cover with bandage and allow to remain in place for 4 to 6 days. May require more than one application.
Silver nitrate	Solution or sticks	Apply to local area as needed.
Emollients		
Dexpanthenol	Panthoderm	Stimulates epithelization and granulation. Aids in the healing of skin lesions and relieves pruritus. Apply directly to clean skin qd to bid.
Urea	Aquacare	Hydrates skin and aids in removing scales and crusts. Apply directly to clean skin bid to tid, affected area only.
Colloidal baths	Alpha Keri Aveeno	Bath additives for treating widespread eruptions. Limit bath time to 30 minutes and patient should be aware preparations often make tub slippery. Follow directions on packet or bottle.
Keratolytics		
Salicylic acid	Mediplast Salacid Wart-Off	Use creams for corns and calluses. Apply directly to area qd for 2 weeks. Cut out piece of plaster to fit callus, or apply gels to well-hydrated skin. Check callus q24h; discontinue if irritation develops.
Transdermal nicotine patches	ProStep Habitrol Nicoderm Nicotrol	Used to decrease withdrawal symptoms as part of smoking cessation program. Do not have serious side effects. In association with behavior-modification programs, use patch daily. ProStep: Use 3 weeks at higher strength, then 3 weeks at lower strength. Habitrol/Nicotrol/Nicoderm: 2 weeks at each of three strengths in decreasing order of strength.
Wet dressings and soaks		
Burow's solution	Domeboro	Used for open wet dressings. They cool and dry through evaporation, which causes local vasoconstriction. Used in inflammatory conditions of skin. Moisten dressing and apply multiple layers to prevent rapid drying and cooling. Reapply q15 to 30 min as indicated, for 4 to 8 hours.

CRITICAL THINKING QUESTIONS

1. Define each of the following terms: antiglaucoma agent, antipsoriatic, antiseptic, mydriasis, pediculocide, scabicide, and vasoconstrictor.

2. Mr. Samms comes to the clinic for an eye examination. His pupils must be dilated first. Describe the precautions you must take in dilating his pupils.

3. Mr. Samms' physician has recommended an OTC ophthalmic product for control of mild glaucoma. Explain glaucoma to Mr. Samms, along with the actions and effects of the antiglaucoma agents.

4. While waiting for his prescription, Mr. Samms asks you what exactly his new medicine is called. What are at least three types of medications he might take for glaucoma?

5. Mr. Samms also has to take medication in the form of eye drops for 1 week for a separate, minor disorder. He has never needed eye drops until now. He tells you that he is nervous about being able to self-administer these. Develop a teaching plan for describing or demonstrating this process to Mr. Samms.

6. What are the differences in administering eye ointment instead of drops?

7. Mrs. Johnson and her 4-year-old son both come into the clinic needing treatment for swimmer's ear. Review the process of administering ear drops for each.

8. The physician also discovers that Mrs. Johnson's ears are filled with wax. What medication is the doctor most likely to order for this?

9. Conduct an informal investigation at your nearest pharmacy or drug store: Compare administration instructions on the labels or (if you can get access to them!) the package inserts of several OTC skin products. Are some more specific in their instructions than others? Why might that be?

10. List at least six different types of topical medications and the uses associated with each.

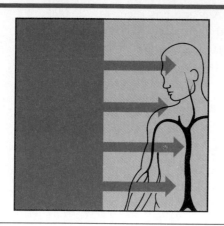

CHAPTER 19
Vitamins, Minerals, and Electrolytes

OBJECTIVES

At the conclusion of this chapter you should be able to:

1. Identify the actions and indications for vitamins and minerals.
2. List at least six products used to treat vitamin or mineral deficiencies.
3. Identify indications for electrolyte replacement.
4. Present a teaching plan for patients who require vitamin or mineral supplements.

KEY TERMS

ascorbic acid, p. 389
dehydration, p. 401
fluid and electrolyte mixtures, p. 401
minerals, p. 392
niacin, p. 387
riboflavin, p. 387
thiamine, p. 386
vitamin A, p. 386
vitamins, p. 385

OVERVIEW

This chapter discusses the clinical uses of vitamins, minerals, and electrolytes. An overview of the action, the indications for use, and common adverse effects and drug interactions is presented. Brief comments are included about the information of clinical importance to the nurse. Summaries of medications available on the market are included in tables at the ends of each major discussion.

VITAMINS

OVERVIEW

Vitamins are chemical compounds found naturally in plant and animal tissues but not synthesized in the human body. They are necessary for life and essential to normal metabolism. They can act as coenzymes to regulate the synthesis of compounds. Vitamins are classified into two types: fat-soluble (which are stored in the body), and water-soluble (which are excreted in the urine). Usually, vitamins may be obtained in sufficient amounts from a well-balanced nutritious diet, except when certain conditions prevent their ingestion (such as intravenous therapy when a patient is taking nothing by mouth) or prevent their metabolism (as in disorders that inhibit fat metabolism). Such conditions may require vitamin supplementation until a normal diet can be resumed or the underlying problem corrected.

A deficiency of one vitamin in a diet that is otherwise adequate is rare. Deficiency signs and symptoms in a patient may point to a lack of one vitamin, but usually a deficiency of several vitamins will be found. With the vast number of multiple vitamin preparations that are easily available to consumers and the active media advertising, hypervitaminosis of several vitamins is more likely to occur than deficiencies.

Although debates occur over natural versus synthetic vitamin preparations, vitamins are vitamins and the cheapest preparation is as therapeutic as a more expensive preparation. There are still many mysteries about the action of vitamins in the body, and needless overconsumption of vitamins should be avoided.

VITAMIN A

ACTION AND USES

Vitamin A is a fat-soluble long-chain alcohol that comes in several isometric forms: retinol, retinene, carotene, and retinoic acid. Its best understood action is aiding visual adaptation in changes from light to darkness. Less understood actions include aiding in the stabilization and maintenance of cell membrane structure, especially epithelial cell membranes, therefore helping the body to resist infection; affecting the synthesis of protein, which affects growth of skeletal and soft tissue; and playing an essential role in reproduction. A quantity sufficient to meet a 2-year requirement is stored in the normal adult Kupffer cells of the liver.

Vitamin A is used to treat deficiency that may be provoked by sprue, colitis, regional enteritis, biliary tract or pancreatic disease, or partial gastrectomy. It is used for the treatment of specific eye diseases and night blindness.

ADVERSE REACTIONS

If vitamin A is given in high doses over a long period, the treatment should be interrupted at times to avoid hypervitaminosis. Any patient receiving 25,000 USP IU or over should be closely supervised. Pregnant women should not receive more than 6000 IU daily, or they may risk fetal abnormalities.

DRUG INTERACTIONS

Women taking oral contraceptives often show significant elevation in plasma vitamin A levels and should be closely monitored for hypervitaminosis. Mineral oil interferes with the absorption of fat-soluble vitamins. Certain antihyperlipidemic agents may also affect absorption of this product.

 NURSING IMPLICATIONS AND PATIENT TEACHING

One IU or USP unit of vitamin A is equivalent to 0.6 µg of beta-carotene or 0.3 µg retinol. This medication may be given PO, IV, or IM, depending on the rapidity of needed replacement.

Recommended daily intake (RDA) includes:

Children 0 to 9 years: 300 to 450 µg/day
Children 9 to 18 years: 575 to 750 µg/day
Adults 18 to 75 years and older: 750 µg/day
Pregnant women (second and third trimester): 750 µg/day
Lactation: 1200 µg/day

Some foods rich in vitamin A include animal products, such as dairy products, eggs, organ meats (all contain preformed vitamin A); and deep orange, yellow, and green fruits and vegetables (contain carotene). In addition, some fortified sources of vitamin A include infant formula, skim milk, margarine, and some cereals.

VITAMIN B₁

ACTION AND USES

Vitamin B₁, or **thiamine,** is water soluble and functions as a coenzyme closely involved with carbohydrate metabolism. Thiamine participates in 24 different reactions, including the citric acid cycle. It also has been thought to have a role in neurophysiology. Thiamine is excreted in the urine.

Vitamin B₁ is used to treat beriberi, which is rare in the United States but does sometimes occur. It is usually found in conjunction with alcoholism, gastric lesions, or hyperemesis of pregnancy. Symptoms include anorexia, vomiting, fatigability, aching muscles, ataxia of gait, and emotional disturbances, such as moodiness or depression.

ADVERSE REACTIONS

Adverse reactions to thiamine include sensitivity reactions, particularly after parenteral administration, that can be of a severe allergic type, including anaphylaxis. Fatalities may occur. Sensitivity tests should be done before the therapeutic dose is given. IV doses should be administered very slowly. Also seen are feelings of warmth, pruritus, urticaria, nausea, angioneurotic edema, pulmonary edema, sweating, tightness of the throat, weakness, and cyanosis.

DRUG INTERACTIONS

Neutral or alkaline solutions will produce poor stability of thiamine preparations.

NURSING IMPLICATIONS AND PATIENT TEACHING

Thiamine is easily leached out of food and is destroyed when food is heated over 100° C, fried in hot pans, or cooked for a long time under pressure. There is some loss of thiamine during dehydration of vegetables. The product is also sensitive to ultraviolet light. Foods rich in thiamine include pork, whole grains, enriched breads, cereals, and legumes. Satisfactory sources include green vegetables, fish, meats, fruit, and milk.

VITAMIN B₂

ACTION AND USES

Vitamin B₂, or **riboflavin**, is water soluble and functions as a precursor of two essential enzymes that deal with intermediary metabolism of proteins, fats, and carbohydrates. It is related to the release of energy to the cells and is active in tissue respiratory systems. It is used for the prophylaxis or treatment of riboflavin deficiency. Early symptoms include soreness and burning of the tongue, lips, and mouth, discomfort in eating and swallowing, photophobia, lacrimation, burning and itching of the eyes, visual fatigue, and the loss of visual acuity.

DRUG INTERACTIONS

Riboflavin is only slightly soluble in water. Riboflavin can be depleted by oral contraceptives, even in low doses. This depletion has been shown through studies to be greater when patients have been taking oral contraceptives over a period of at least 3 years.

NURSING IMPLICATIONS AND PATIENT TEACHING

This product should be protected from light by keeping it in a tightly closed, light-resistant container. This medication turns the urine a yellow color. Food sources naturally rich in riboflavin include milk, eggs, liver, kidneys, heart, green leafy vegetables, and enriched breads and cereals.

VITAMIN B₃

ACTION AND USES

Vitamin B₃, or **niacin,** is water soluble and an essential component of two coenzymes (nicotinamide adenine dinucleotide [NAD] and nicotinamide adenine dinucleotide phosphate [NADP]), which transfer hydrogen in intracellular respiration. These coenzymes convert lactic acid to pyruvic acid and function in energy release and in amino acid metabolism.

Niacin is used to prevent or treat deficiency states. Deficiency can be caused by a limited dietary intake of niacin, excessive dietary intake of leucine (which increases the daily need for niacin), generalized anorexia related to disease or other problems, or malabsorptive syndrome. The deficiency disease is pellagra, which is rare but may be more prevalent where corn is the major staple food. It is usually found in conjunction with other vitamin deficiencies.

Deficiency symptoms are characterized by mucous membrane, cutaneous, gastrointestinal, and CNS manifestations. Anorexia, irritability, anxiety, and mental changes such as hallucinations, lassitude, apprehension, and depression may be especially prominent.

Gastrointestinal symptoms include glossitis, or swollen, beefy, red tongue; stomatitis; and diarrhea. Dermatitis of different body parts exposed to sun or trauma may develop, as well as lesions on the skin from sun, fire, or heat. Mental changes that are subjective early in deficiency may progress to disorientation, loss of memory, confusion, hysteria, and sometimes maniacal outbursts.

ADVERSE REACTIONS

Adverse reactions to niacin include dry skin, pruritus, skin rash, gastrointestinal disorders, allergies, feelings of warmth, headache, tingling of the skin, and transient flushing.

DRUG INTERACTIONS

Sympathetic blocking agents (antihypertensives) may increase the vasodilatory effect of niacin, leading to postural hypotension.

 NURSING IMPLICATIONS AND PATIENT TEACHING

Flushing is a frequent side effect of niacin. If patients feel weak or dizzy, they should lie down until they feel better. Usually this reaction does not require discontinuing the drug.

The recommended intake is 8 mg/1000 Kcal for infants and 6.6 mg/1000 Kcal for children and adolescents. Not less than 8 mg/day should be given. The recommended intake for adults is 13 mg/day for women and 18 mg/day for men.

Foods rich in niacin are lean meats, peanuts, yeast, and cereal (especially bran and germ). Other good sources include eggs, liver, red meat, whole grain, and enriched bread.

VITAMIN B₅

ACTION AND USES

Vitamin B₅, or pantothenic acid, is essential for the synthesis of coenzyme A, which has a role in the release of energy in fats, proteins, and carbohydrates. This vitamin has been used to treat paralytic ileus after surgery, possibly acting to stimulate gastrointestinal motility. Deficiency states are produced only in the laboratory.

 NURSING IMPLICATIONS AND PATIENT TEACHING

When food is cooked above the boiling point, considerable loss of pantothenic acid occurs. The loss is smaller when food is moderately cooked or baked. Much of the original vitamin content is lost from frozen meat in the liquid that drips off during thaw-

ing. This vitamin is available naturally in all plant and animal tissues. Rich sources include yeast, liver, kidney, egg yolk, wheat bran, and fresh vegetables. Human milk contains 2.2 mg/L and cow's milk 3.4 mg/L.

VITAMIN B₆

ACTION AND USES

Vitamin B₆, or pyridoxine hydrochloride, is water soluble and functions as a coenzyme in the metabolism of protein, carbohydrates, and fat.

Pyridoxine is used to treat pyridoxine deficiency seen in inborn errors of metabolism, such as vitamin B₆ dependency; vitamin B₆–responsive chronic anemia; and other rare vitamin problems.

Pyridoxine deficiency is most likely to develop in the elderly and in women of childbearing age, especially those who are pregnant or breastfeeding. Women taking oral contraceptives, alcoholics, and those whose diets are of poor quality and quantity, or whose diets are rich in refined foods are also at risk.

Symptoms of deficiency include weakness, nervousness, irritability, and difficulty in walking. There may also be personality changes in adults, such as depression and a loss of sense of responsibility.

ADVERSE REACTIONS

No adverse effects are usually seen in patients taking pyridoxine. Pyridoxine dependency may develop in adults taking doses exceeding 200 mg/day for a month.

DRUG INTERACTIONS

Oral contraceptives may induce pyridoxine deficiency. Concurrent use with levodopa will neutralize CNS effects. Pyridoxine may prevent chloramphenicol-induced optic neuritis. Some drugs interfere enough to produce symptoms of deficiency.

 NURSING IMPLICATIONS AND PATIENT TEACHING

Pyridoxine should be kept in a tightly sealed, light-resistant container. Good food sources of vitamin B₆ include yeast, wheat, corn, egg yolk, liver, kidney, and muscle meats; limited amounts are available from milk and vegetables. Appropriate food preparation is important in preserving this vitamin. Freezing of vegetables results in a 20% loss of pyridoxine, and the milling of wheat results in a 90% loss.

VITAMIN B$_{12}$

ACTION AND USES

Vitamin B$_{12}$ is water soluble and contains cobalt. It is produced by the bacterium *Streptomyces griseus*. It functions in many metabolic processes in protein, fat, and carbohydrate metabolism. The coenzymes of B$_{12}$ are also part of the erythrocyte-maturing factor of the liver and are required in the synthesis of DNA. Vitamin B$_{12}$ has a hemopoietic activity identical to the antianemia factor of the liver, and it is essential for growth, cell reproduction, and nucleoprotein and myelin synthesis. Vitamin B$_{12}$ interacts with folate in metabolic functions, and a deficiency in B$_{12}$ renders folate useless in the body.

Vitamin B$_{12}$ is used to treat all B$_{12}$ deficiency conditions, including pernicious anemia (with or without neurologic manifestations); malabsorption syndromes; certain other anemias; hemorrhage; blind loop syndrome; pregnancy; and chronic liver disease complicated by deficiency of vitamin B$_{12}$; malignancy; thyrotoxicosis; and renal disorders. Vitamin B$_{12}$ is also used as the flushing dose in Schilling's test. Symptoms of deficiency are rare, occurring mainly in persons on strict vegetarian diets, because vitamin B$_{12}$ is found only in animal products. Symptoms include dyspepsia, sore tongue, breathlessness, and a characteristic stiff back, often dubbed a "poker" or "vegan" back.

ADVERSE REACTIONS

Allergy to vitamin B$_{12}$ is rare. The patient may report itching, feeling of swelling of the entire body, or a severe anaphylactic reaction. A few patients may experience mild pain, localized skin irritation, or mild transient diarrhea after an injection of cyanocobalamin.

DRUG INTERACTIONS

Alcohol, colchicine, and paraaminosalicylic acid lower the absorption of vitamin B$_{12}$. Some antibiotics lower the response to vitamin B$_{12}$ therapy.

 NURSING IMPLICATIONS AND PATIENT TEACHING

Irreparable neurologic damage may occur if a deficiency state continues longer than 3 months or when treatment for pernicious anemia includes only folic acid. If colchicine, paraaminosalicylic acid, or excessive alcohol intake occurs for more than 2 weeks, malabsorption of vitamin B$_{12}$ may occur.

Recommended daily intake of cyanocobalamin for adults is 3 μg. The best food sources of B$_{12}$ include organ meats; bivalves, such as clams and oysters; nonfat dry milk; seafoods, such as lobster, scallops, flounder, haddock, swordfish, and tuna; and fermented cheese such as Camembert and limburger.

VITAMIN C

ACTION AND USES

Vitamin C, or **ascorbic acid,** has multiple functions, some of which are understood more than others. Vitamin C functions in a number of enzyme systems and is involved in intracellular oxidation-reduction potentials. It aids in the conversion of folic acid and the metabolism of certain amino acids, facilitates the absorption of iron and calcium, and inhibits the absorption of copper in the gastrointestinal tract. Ascorbic acid protects vitamins A and E and polyunsaturated fatty acids. It is also necessary for the formation of the ground substance of bones, teeth, connective tissue, and capillaries and for the synthesis of collagen. Ascorbic acid aids in wound healing and may be involved in blood clotting.

Ascorbic acid is used to treat debilitated patients, especially postoperatively in elderly patients with fractures and as a supplement for burn victims or patients undergoing severe stress. Infection, smoking, chronic illness, and febrile states may increase the need for vitamin C. It is used adjunctly with iron therapy and in patients on prolonged intravenous therapy. Premature infants require relatively large doses. It is also used for the prophylaxis and treatment of scurvy, the deficiency syndrome.

With modern refrigeration and processing methods of citrus fruits, scurvy is rarely seen in the United States but may be found when other vitamin deficiencies are present. Symptoms include tender, painful muscles, joints, and bones; muscle cramps; loss of appetite; fatigue; weakness; and sore gums. Wound healing is impaired, and hemorrhagic manifestations are demonstrated by subperiosteal bleeding and petechial hemorrhages. Vasomotor instability, bruising, faulty bone and tooth development, loosened teeth, and gingivitis also may develop.

ADVERSE REACTIONS

The patient may experience mild, transient soreness at injection sites if the medication is given intramuscularly or subcutaneously. Patients may also experience temporary episodes of faintness or dizziness when intravenous injections are given too rapidly. Excessive doses are usually rapidly excreted into the urine. Doses in excess of 1 to 3 gm daily may result in gastrointestinal complaints, glycosuria, oxaluria, and development of renal stones, especially in patients prone to these problems. Patients who chronically overuse vitamins may develop a state of conditioned need.

DRUG INTERACTIONS

Ascorbic acid may have varying effects on anticoagulants, inhibiting the action of some and prolonging the intensity and duration of others. Ascorbic acid increases the effect of salicylates through elevated renal tubular reabsorption. There is also an increased chance of crystallization of sulfonamides in urine when ascorbic acid is administered concurrently. Ascorbic acid decreases the effect of tricyclic antidepressants by decreasing renal tubular reabsorption. Calcium ascorbate may cause cardiac dysrhythmias in patients receiving digitalis. Ascorbic acid is chemically incompatible with potassium penicillin G and should not be mixed in the same syringe. Smoking may lead to increased vitamin C requirements by decreasing ascorbic acid serum levels. Intermittent use of ascorbic acid in patients taking ethinyl estradiol may increase the risk of contraceptive failure. Large doses of vitamin C may interfere with urine testing of some diabetic testing methods.

 NURSING IMPLICATIONS AND PATIENT TEACHING

Vitamin C comes in three major forms that may be given orally or parenterally: ascorbic acid, sodium ascorbate, and calcium ascorbate. The recommended daily intake is 60 mg for adults.

Vitamin C is easily destroyed by air, heat, and light. This medication should be kept tightly capped in its own container. Foods high in vitamin C should not be boiled for long periods of time or left uncovered in the refrigerator.

Good food sources of vitamin C include green, leafy vegetables; oranges; grapefruit; strawberries; cauliflower; cantaloupe; beef liver; asparagus; and potatoes.

VITAMIN D

ACTION AND USES

Vitamin D is a term applied to a group of fat-soluble, chemically similar sterols. The three main categories within this group include (1) ergocalciferol (vitamin D_2), which is very limited in nature in both distribution and concentration but can be artificially manufactured by ultraviolet irradiation on ergot and yeasts; (2) cholecalciferol (vitamin D_3), which occurs naturally in fish liver oils and can be formed in animals and humans by ultraviolet irradiation on the skin; and (3) other lesser compounds (D_4, D_5, D_6, D_7), which are formed by irradiation of sterols. The term "vitamin D" has therefore become a rather ambiguous term.

The main action of this group of sterols is the movement of calcium and phosphorus ions into three main sites: small intestine (to promote absorption of calcium and phosphorus from the gut); kidney (to effect phosphate reabsorption in the proximal convoluted tubules and, to a lesser extent, to stimulate calcium and sodium reabsorption); and bone (to facilitate the mineralization of newly formed bone).

These preparations are used to treat childhood rickets and adult osteomalacia, hypoparathyroidism, and familial hypophosphatemia. In childhood, rickets may be demonstrated by complaints of excessive sweating and gastrointestinal disturbances. These may be the first symptoms, preceding any objective findings. In adult cases of osteomalacia, patients may complain of skeletal pain and progressive muscular weakness.

ADVERSE REACTIONS

Symptoms of vitamin D toxicity include anorexia, nausea, weakness, weight loss, vague aches and stiffness, constipation, diarrhea, convulsions, anemia, mild acidosis, and impairment of renal function. The renal effects are usually reversible. A variety of more serious system effects may all be seen in adults. Dwarfism may be present in infants and children. Most toxic effects persist for several months for adults at doses of 100,000 IU or more daily or for children at doses of 20,000 IU or more daily. Reactions gradually disappear if treatment is discontinued at the first sign of symptoms.

DRUG INTERACTIONS

Mineral oil and some of the antihyperlipidemic agents may interfere with the absorption of fat-soluble vitamins. Thiazide diuretics and vitamin D together contribute to hypercalcemia. There is a possible connection between dilantin and phenobarbital use leading to hypocalcemia, which in turn may contribute to rickets or osteomalacia.

 NURSING IMPLICATIONS AND PATIENT TEACHING

The dosage of vitamin D must be individualized and given under close supervision, because the margin between the therapeutic and the toxic levels is narrow. Calcium intake should be sufficient to achieve a serum calcium level between 9 and 10 mg/dl. In rickets, up to 12,000 to 500,000 IU/day can be taken. In hypoparathyroidism, initially give 50,000 to 200,000 IU/day with a maintenance dosage of 50,000 to 400,000 IU/day.

Most people obtain all the vitamin D they need from the food in their diet. Natural sources of vitamin D are few, and the majority of vitamin D must be obtained from fortified sources. Fortified foods high in this vitamin are milk, evaporated milk, infant formula, powdered skim milk, and human milk. Cereals, margarine, and diet foods also contain vitamin D supplements. Vitamin D should be protected from light in a light-resistant container.

VITAMIN E

ACTION AND USES

Vitamin E is fat soluble and consists of naturally occurring tocopherols. Vitamin E is considered an essential nutrient for humans even though its specific functions are not yet understood. Vitamin E may

function as an antioxidant, preventing damage to cellular membranes. It stabilizes red blood cell walls and protects them from hemolysis. It may also enhance vitamin A use and suppress platelet aggregation.

Many purported uses of vitamin E are controversial and unproven. The only established use is to prevent or treat vitamin E deficiency, though evidence suggests men and women can significantly lower their risk of coronary heart disease by taking vitamin E supplements.

ADVERSE REACTIONS AND DRUG INTERACTIONS

Vitamin E appears to be the least toxic of the fat-soluble vitamins. No signs and symptoms of toxicity or hypervitaminosis have been identified as yet in humans.

 NURSING IMPLICATIONS AND PATIENT TEACHING

Food sources of vitamin E are primarily from plants. The highest amounts are found in vegetable oils such as soybean or corn, with meat and dairy products providing less. An accurate assessment of tocopherol levels in food is difficult to obtain. The amount in the body depends on the initial concentration of vitamin E and the processing, storage, and preparation of the food. Vitamin E products should be stored in tightly closed, light-resistant containers.

VITAMIN K

ACTION AND USES

Vitamin K enhances hepatic formation of active prothrombin (factor II), proconvertin (factor VII), plasma thromboplastin component (factor IX), and the Stuart factor (factor X), which are essential for normal blood clotting. The exact mechanism is unknown. Menadione (K_3) and phytonadione (K_1) are synthetic lipid-soluble forms of vitamin K. Menadiol sodium diphosphate (K_4) is changed in the body to menadione (K_3). Menadione is not commonly available now.

Vitamin K is used to treat or prevent various coagulation disorders that result in impaired formation of factors II, VII, IX, and X. The American

Academy of Pediatrics recommends routine phytonadione (K_1) administration at birth to prevent hemorrhagic disease of the newborn. Vitamin K will not counteract the anticoagulant activity of heparin.

ADVERSE REACTIONS

Specific adverse reactions to menadione (K_3)/menadiol sodium diphosphate (K_4) include headache, rash, urticaria, gastric upset, redness, and pain or swelling at injection site. Specific adverse reactions to phytonadione (K_1) include brief hypotension, rapid and weak pulse, dizziness, flushing, sweating, unusual taste sensations, redness, and pain or swelling at injection site.

Severe reactions, including fatalities, have occurred with the use of intravenous phytonadione, even when precautions have been taken (dilution of drug, slow infusion).

DRUG INTERACTIONS

Concurrent use of vitamin K with oral anticoagulants may decrease the effects of the anticoagulant. Mineral oil and cholestyramine inhibit gastrointestinal absorption of oral vitamin K.

 NURSING IMPLICATIONS AND PATIENT TEACHING

The preferred routes of administration of vitamin K are subcutaneous or intramuscular. Intravenous administration is not recommended because of the risk of anaphylaxis.

A summary of selected vitamin preparations on the market is included in Table 19-1.

MINERALS
OVERVIEW

There are 19 nonorganic homogeneous substances called **minerals** present in the body, at least 13 of which are essential to good health. These minerals carry positive or negative charges, leading to the formation of salts. Minerals are obtained from a diet varied in animal and vegetable products that meets the energy and protein needs of the body. The Food and Nutrition Board of the National Research Council has established recommended daily intakes for calcium and iron. Calcium, iron, and iodine are the three elements most frequently missing in the diet. Zinc, iron, copper, magnesium, and potassium are the five minerals most frequently involved in disturbances of metabolism. As electrolytes, these preparations are commonly infused to critically ill patients unable to take food orally.

CALCIUM
ACTION AND USES

Calcium is a major mineral in the body and is essential for muscular and neurologic activity, especially in the cardiac system. Calcium functions in the formation and repair of skeletal tissues (bones and teeth); activates several enzymes that influence cell membrane permeability and muscle contraction; aids in blood clotting by stimulating the release of thromboplastin and the conversion of fibrinogen to fibrin; activates pancreatic lipase; influences the intestinal absorption of cobalamin; and in extracellular fluids is involved in the transmission of neurotransmitters, and in metabolic processes. Calcium is also involved in the regulation of lymphocyte and phagocyte function through interaction with calmodulin.

Calcium is used as a supplement when dietary levels of calcium are inadequate. Calcium requirements may be increased during pregnancy, breast-feeding, adolescence, and for postmenopausal women. Calcium is also used to treat neonatal hypocalcemia and to prevent and treat postmenopausal and senile osteoporosis. It may also be used as a supplement to parenterally administered vitamin D in cases of hypoparathyroidism, pseudohypoparathyroidism, rickets, and osteomalacia.

ADVERSE REACTIONS

The nurse should watch for symptoms of hypercalcemia such as polyuria, constipation, abdominal pain, dryness of mouth, anorexia, nausea, and vomiting.

DRUG INTERACTIONS

Vitamin D is essential for the absorption of calcium in the body. Calcium status is affected by the calcium/phosphorus ratio in the body and by the level of protein in the diet. Phytic acid (found in bran and whole grain cereals) and oxalic acid (found in spin-

Table 19-1   Vitamins

Generic name	Trade name	Comments and dosage
Vitamin A	Aquasol A Del-Vi-A	Give 50,000 to 100,000 IU/day for 3 days for 2 weeks; follow with 10,000 to 20,000 IU/day for 2 months.
Vitamin B₁ (thiamine)	Biamine Thiamilate	Medication may be given PO, IM, or IV. Daily average dose is 0.5 mg/1000 Kcal intake, or usually 1 to 1.4 mg/day. Usual dosage is 50 mg IM for deficiency states, and 5 to 10 mg daily as dietary supplement for adults and children over 12 years of age.
Vitamin B₂ (riboflavin)	Riboflavin	Give 0.4 mg to 0.6 mg for infants; 0.8 to 1.2 mg for children; 1.4 to 1.6 mg for males, and 1.1 mg to 1.3 mg for females. For deficiency states, usually give 50 mg IM and 5 to 10 mg daily as dietary supplements for adults and children over 12.
Vitamin B₃ (nicotinic acid, niacin)	Niacor Nicobid Novonacin ♣	May be given IM, SQ, or IV; the IV route with slow drip is preferred when parenteral medication is necessary. ■ *Deficiency states:* 50 to 100 mg qd. ■ *Pellagra:* Up to 500 mg/day. ■ *Hyperlipidemia:* 1 to 2 gm tid; maximum dosage is 6 gm/day.
Niacinamide	Nicotinamide	500 mg PO qd, or may give 100 to 200 mg 1 to 5 times daily parenterally, depending on the severity of the symptoms.
Vitamin B₅ (calcium pantothenate)	Calcium Pantothenate	A daily intake of 5 to 10 mg is thought to be adequate, with the lower level suggested for children and the upper level suggested for pregnant and breastfeeding women. A dosage of 2 mg/day has been suggested for infants and 4 to 7 mg/day for adolescents. Usual dosage is 10 mg/day.
Vitamin B₆ (pyridoxine)	Beesix Hexa-Betalin ♣ Nestrex	Recommended daily allowances range from 2 to 2.2 mg. Preparation may be given PO, IM, or IV. ■ *Dietary deficiency:* 10 to 20 mg/day for 3 weeks, then 2 to 5 mg/day for several weeks. ■ *Vitamin B₆ dependency states:* May give up to 600 mg/day initially, dropping to 50 mg/day for life.
Vitamin B₁₂ (cyanocobalamin)	Ener-B Bedoz ♣ Rubion ♣	■ *Nutritional deficiency:* Give 25 to 250 μg/day PO. ■ *Vitamin B₁₂ deficiency:* 1000 μg/day PO. If patients have normal gastrointestinal absorption, give 15 μg/day along with other multiple vitamins. In other cases, give 30 μg IM or SQ daily for 5 to 10 days, and then 100 to 200 μg monthly. ■ *Schilling's test:* 1000 μg IM as a flushing dose.
Vitamin C Ascorbic acid	Ascorbicap Cetane Cevalin	■ *Prophylactically:* 50 to 100 mg as indicated. ■ *Therapeutically:* 100 mg or more as needed.
Calcium ascorbate	Apo-C ♣	■ *Parenterally:* 100 to 250 mg given slowly qd to bid up to a maximum of 1 to 2 gm daily.
Sodium ascorbate	Cenolate	■ *Parenterally:* 100 to 250 mg given slowly qd to bid up to a maximum of 1 to 2 gm daily.

Continued.

Table 19-1 Vitamins—cont'd

Generic name	Trade name	Comments and dosage
Vitamin D		
Calcifediol	Calderol Calcifedrol ✦	Give 300 to 350 µg/week administered qd or qod. Usually can give 20 to 50 µg/day or 100 to 200 µg qod.
Calcitriol	Rocaltrol D-Tabs ✦ Calcijex	Initially give 0.25 µg/day. May increase by 0.25 µg/day at 2 to 4 week intervals until satisfactory response is obtained. Some patients may respond to doses of 0.25 µg qod. Patients undergoing hemodialysis may require doses of 0.5 to 1 µg/day.
Dihydrotachysterol	Hytakerol DHT	*Initial:* 0.75 to 2.5 mg daily for several days. *Maintenance:* 0.2 to 1 mg daily, titrated by serum calcium levels. Average dose is 0.6 mg.
Ergocalciferol (D$_2$)	Calciferol	■ *Vitamin D–resistant rickets:* 50,000 to 500,000 IU daily. ■ *Hypoparathyroidism:* 50,000 to 400,000 IU of vitamin D daily plus 4 gm of calcium lactate, administered 6 times daily.
Vitamin E	Aquasol E	A range of 10 to 20 IU of vitamin E should provide adequate levels for an adult diet. For premenstrual syndrome (PMS), 300 IU of an alcohol-free product is taken PO qd.
Vitamin K		
Phytonadione	Aquamephyton Konakion Mephyton	■ *Anticoagulant-induced prothrombin deficiency:* 2.5 to 10 mg or up to 25 mg initially. Frequency and dosage of subsequent therapy are determined by prothrombin time response. See package insert for other uses.
Paraaminobenzoic acid	Potaba	Accessory food factor. *Adults:* 12 gm daily in divided doses.

ach and rhubarb) may interfere with calcium absorption by combining with it to form insoluble salts in the intestine. Calcium compounds and calcium-rich substances, such as milk, interfere with the absorption of oral tetracyclines, and use together should be avoided. Administration of corticosteroids may also decrease the absorption of calcium.

NURSING IMPLICATIONS AND PATIENT TEACHING

In patients with low calcium levels, carpal spasm may be elicited by compressing the upper arm with a blood pressure cuff, causing ischemia to the distal nerves. The patient may report a tingling sensation and may inadvertently flex his or her arm.

Excessive amounts of calcium may lead to hypercalcemia and hypercalciuria, especially in hyperthyroid patients. Serum and renal calcium levels should be monitored to detect the development of renal stones; calcium should not be given to patients who already have renal stones.

Calcium products come in combination with various other chemicals, with a concentration of between 6% and 40%. Preparations come in both parenteral and oral forms.

Recommended daily intake is 800 mg/day for adults, 1200 mg/day for adolescents, 800 mg/day for children, 360 to 540 mg/day for infants from birth to 1 year, and 1500 mg/day for nursing mothers.

Milk and dairy products are the richest sources of calcium. Egg yolks and most dark green, leafy vegetables are also good sources.

FLUORIDE

ACTION AND USES

Fluoride is concentrated in bones and teeth and is present in soft tissues only in minute amounts. It is an essential trace element, but has not been proven to be essential to life. Fluoride is incorporated into the surface enamel of teeth in higher concentrations than in deeper layers. This strengthening of the enamel provides greater resistance to the dissolution or demineralization by acids produced in dental plaque. It has therefore been found useful in reducing dental caries.

Fluoride is recommended for the prevention of dental caries. It may be used topically or systemically. It is primarily administered in localities with unfluoridated water supplies or to individuals having a genetic tendency for dental caries.

ADVERSE REACTIONS

Gastric distress, headache, urticaria, and weakness may be seen in hypersensitive individuals. Excessive salivation, mottling of teeth, gastrointestinal disturbances, and nausea are seen in acute overdosage.

DRUG INTERACTIONS

Fluoride in the water supply may produce calcium fluoride, a poorly absorbed product, when taken with dairy foods.

 NURSING IMPLICATIONS AND PATIENT TEACHING

Fluoride is available in gels, pastes, drops, tablets, capsules, and mouth rinses. The preparation and quantity chosen should be adjusted to the fluoride level of the local water supply. The county water commissioner should be contacted for this information.

Fluoride products should be taken as ordered: tablets and drops may be dissolved in water used for making infant formula or added to food or juices. Tablets may also be swallowed, chewed, or allowed to dissolve slowly in the mouth. Products are best taken following meals. For rinses and gels, teeth should be brushed thoroughly and then the coating should be applied to clean teeth. The fluoride coating should

not be swallowed. The patient should not rinse the mouth, eat, or drink for 30 minutes after treatment. Plastic containers should be used for diluting fluoride drops or rinses, and glass should be avoided. Milk may decrease absorption of oral fluoride products, so the patient should avoid taking fluoride with milk or dairy products.

IRON

ACTION AND USES

Iron is an essential mineral for the synthesis of myoglobin and hemoglobin. It stimulates the hematopoietic system and increases hemoglobin in the correction of iron deficiency states.

It is used to treat symptomatic iron deficiency anemia only after the cause of the anemia has been identified, and it is used to prevent hypochromic anemia during infancy, childhood, pregnancy, and breastfeeding, in patients recovering from other anemias, and after some gastrointestinal surgeries.

ADVERSE REACTIONS

Adverse reactions to iron supplements include constipation, cramping, diarrhea, epigastric or abdominal pain, gastrointestinal irritation, and allergic-type reactions to any component of the iron preparation. Symptoms of overdosage may occur after 30 minutes to several hours and include lethargy, nausea, vomiting, abdominal pain, diarrhea, melena, and dyspnea. Coma and metabolic acidosis may occur as well as symptoms of systemic absorption.

DRUG INTERACTIONS

Large iron doses may cause false-positive test result for occult blood using the toluidine test (Hematest, Occultest, Clinistix). Absorption of oral iron is inhibited by antacids (particularly magnesium trisilicate–containing antacids), milk, and eggs. Patients receiving chloramphenicol concurrently with iron may show a delayed response to iron therapy. Absorption of iron increases with concurrent administration of ascorbic acid in doses of 200 mg per 30 mg of iron. Iron interferes with absorption of oral tetracyclines. Vitamin E decreases the response to iron therapy. Many other isolated medications may have interactions.

NURSING IMPLICATIONS AND PATIENT TEACHING

The cause of the anemia must be identified and treated. The nurse should obtain stools for occult blood tests after the patient has been on a red meat–free diet for at least 3 days. Although dietary inadequacies may contribute to iron deficiency, especially in those over age 75, blood loss is the primary cause. Heavy menstrual periods and multiple pregnancies in women may produce anemia.

Hematologic laboratory values may be normally decreased in the elderly, leading to overprescribing of iron for geriatric patients. Liquid preparations can discolor teeth and should be taken through a straw after dilution with liquid.

Replacement of iron in iron deficiency anemia should be 90 mg to 300 mg of elemental iron daily in divided doses (6 mg/kg/day.) Remission of symptoms should be apparent within 2 weeks and laboratory studies normal within 2 months if diagnosis and treatment are adequate. Therapy for 4 to 6 months after the anemia has been corrected is advised to replenish iron stores. Absorption is enhanced if the iron is taken on an empty stomach with water or in an acid environment, although stomach irritation can be minimized by taking after meals. Taking iron preparations after a meal can reduce their absorption by 40% to 50%. Different oral preparations vary in cost and percentage of elemental iron. Product selection must be based on how well it is absorbed, how well it is tolerated, and the individual needs of the patient. All simple oral iron preparations are available over the counter.

The recommended daily intake of elemental iron is adult males, 10 mg; adult females, 18 mg (with an additional 10 mg during pregnancy or lactation); children, 10 to 15 mg. A diet high in natural iron should be encouraged to meet these requirements. Fish, meat, and dried fruits are the best sources of dietary iron.

Iron can cause dark green or black stools. The patient should report constipation, diarrhea, nausea, or abdominal pain to the physician.

MAGNESIUM

ACTION AND USES

Magnesium is an electrolyte essential to several enzyme systems. It is important in maintaining osmotic pressure, ion balance, bone structure, muscular contraction, and nerve conduction.

ADVERSE REACTIONS

Excessive magnesium intake may produce diarrhea.

NURSING IMPLICATIONS AND PATIENT TEACHING

Magnesium deficiencies are seen primarily when malabsorption syndromes are present. Magnesium is usually used with other vitamins as a general dietary supplement when multiple deficiencies are suspected. Deficiency states have been associated with convulsions, retarded growth, digestive disturbances, spasticity of muscles and nerves, accelerated heart beat, dysrhythmias, nervous conditions, and vasodilation.

Magnesium is available in adequate quantities in meat, milk, fruits, and vegetables and special dietary planning is unnecessary.

MANGANESE

ACTION AND USES

Manganese activates many enzymes, assists in normal skeletal and connective tissue development, helps in the initiation of protein synthesis, and plays a part in the synthesis of cholesterol and fatty acids. It is distributed throughout the body tissues and fluids. No precise recommended daily allowances have been established.

Manganese is used in dietary supplementation. Usually it is used with other vitamins when multiple deficiencies are suspected. Research subjects with manganese deficiency experience weight loss, changes in beard and hair growth (usually slowed growth), and occasional nausea and vomiting. There are no known adverse effects or drug interactions.

Nuts, whole wheat cereals, and grains are the foods richest in manganese. Tea and cloves are exceptionally rich. Meat, fish, and dairy products have low amounts of manganese.

POTASSIUM

ACTION AND USES

Potassium is the principal intracellular cation of most body tissues, participating in the maintenance of normal renal function, contraction of muscle, and transmission of nerve impulses.

Prophylactic administration of potassium may be used in the therapy of nephrotic syndrome, in hepatic cirrhosis accompanied by ascites, and in patients with hyperaldosteronism who maintain normal renal function. Potassium products are used prophylactically or to replace potassium that may be lost as a result of long-term diuretic therapy, digitalis intoxication, or low dietary intake of potassium; or for depletion resulting from vomiting and diarrhea, diabetic acidosis, metabolic alkalosis, or corticosteroid therapy; or to counteract increased renal excretion of potassium because of acidosis, certain renal tubular disorders, or diseases that produce increased secretion of glucocorticoids or aldosterone.

ADVERSE REACTIONS

Adverse reactions to potassium supplements include nausea, vomiting, diarrhea, abdominal discomfort, and gastrointestinal bleeding. Potassium intoxication or hyperkalemia may result from overdosage of potassium or from a change in the patient's underlying condition, which makes an accumulation of potassium possible. Signs and symptoms of potassium intoxication include flaccid paralysis, paresthesias of the hands and feet, mental confusion, restlessness, listlessness, weakness, and heaviness of the legs. Hypotension and cardiac dysrhythmias leading to heart block may also develop. Potentially fatal dysrhythmias may develop if potassium cannot be excreted (or if it is administered too rapidly intravenously). Detection of hyperkalemia mandates immediate treatment because lethal levels may be reached in a few hours in untreated patients.

DRUG INTERACTIONS

Potassium should not be used in patients receiving potassium-sparing agents, such as aldosterone antagonists or triamterene.

 ## NURSING IMPLICATIONS AND PATIENT TEACHING

All potassium supplements must be diluted properly or taken with plenty of liquid to avoid development of gastrointestinal ulcerations.

The usual adult dietary intake of potassium ranges between 40 and 60 mEq/day. The loss of 200 or more mEq of potassium from the total body store is sufficient to produce hypokalemia.

The dosage must be titrated to the individual's needs and the patient should be closely monitored during therapy, especially in the initial stages of therapy. For patients on concurrent diuretic therapy, 20 mEq per day is usually adequate for the prevention of hypokalemia. In cases of potassium depletion, 40 to 100 mEq/day or more may be required for replacement.

Potassium comes in various salt combinations, with potassium chloride being the form most frequently prescribed. It may be ordered either by percentage of potassium chloride or in milliequivalents of potassium chloride, with 10 mEq KCl per 15 ml equivalent to 5% KCl.

Potassium also comes as potassium gluconate, potassium citrate, potassium acetate, and potassium bicarbonate; in combinations; and with additions of vitamin C, ammonium chloride, citric acid, betaine HCl, and L-lysine monohydrochloride.

Many health care providers advocate eating a potassium-rich diet as well as taking this type of supplement. If a potassium-rich diet is ordered, the foods that might be included are bananas, citrus fruits (especially tomatoes and oranges), apricots, and dried fruits such as raisins, prunes, and dates. Cantaloupe and watermelon (in season), nuts, dried beans, beef, and fowl also contain ample quantities of potassium.

ZINC

ACTION AND USES

Zinc is a constituent of many enzymes and is essential for normal growth and tissue repair. Zinc functions in the mineralization of bone and in the detoxification and oxidation of methanol and ethylene glycol, and it plays a role in the synthesis of DNA and the synthesis of protein from amino acids. It is important in wound healing and functions in the mobilization of vitamin A from liver stores.

Zinc is used to prevent zinc deficiency and to treat delayed wound healing. It has been used experimentally in rheumatoid arthritis and acne.

Patients may complain of abnormalities of taste and smell, rough skin, and anorexia with profound disinterest in food. Patients may demonstrate sexual immaturity, delayed wound healing, and decreased absorption of dietary folate.

ADVERSE REACTIONS

Adverse reactions to zinc supplements include gastric ulceration, nausea, and vomiting. Doses in excess of 2 gm produce emesis. Acute zinc intoxication produces drowsiness, lethargy, lightheadedness, staggering gait, restlessness, and vomiting leading to dehydration.

DRUG INTERACTIONS

Calcium competes with zinc for absorption. Phytates form insoluble complexes with zinc and interfere with its absorption. Zinc impairs the absorption of tetracycline derivatives.

 ## NURSING IMPLICATIONS AND PATIENT TEACHING

The minimum daily requirements of zinc include: infants to 1 year, 3 to 5 mg/day; children 1 to 10 years, 10 mg/day; adolescents 11 to 18 years, 15 mg/day; adults, 15 mg/day; pregnant women, 20 mg/day; lactating women, 25 mg/day.

Seafoods and meats are rich sources of natural zinc; cereals and legumes also have significant amounts of this mineral.

See Table 19-2 for a summary of minerals.

 ## NURSING IMPLICATIONS AND PATIENT TEACHING

▼ Assessment

The nurse should obtain a complete health history, including the presence of hypersensitivity, pregnancy, breastfeeding, underlying systemic disease, hereditary disorders, and concurrent use of medications. The patient should be assessed for symptoms of multiple deficiency or disease states.

▼ Planning

Many medications require baseline laboratory assessment before initiating therapy so that progress may be monitored.

The nurse should make certain that the medication is stored in the proper manner: protected from light and heat to avoid destruction of the medication.

▼ Implementation

The nurse should make certain that the route of administration is appropriate before attempting to give the medication. Many products must be given very slowly or by certain routes.

▼ Evaluation

The nurse should monitor for the therapeutic effect or the development of adverse effects and obtain a follow-up laboratory report to document the therapeutic results.

▼ Patient and family teaching

The nurse should provide the patient and family with the following instructions:

1. The patient should take the medication exactly as ordered. If a dose is missed, the patient should take it as soon as he or she remembers, but should not take it if it is almost time for the next dose. The doses should not be doubled. The physician should be informed if doses of vitamin K are missed.

2. The patient will need to make regular return visits to see the physician while taking some vitamins. The patient should inform all physicians and dentists that he or she is taking specific products.

3. The patient must not take other medications, including over-the-counter drugs, without first discussing them with the physician.

4. Some forms of the drugs may cause unusual taste sensations, and must be protected from light and heat, or have special storage instructions. The patient must be taught the specific care of the medications.

5. The patient should avoid overdosage of the medication; too many vitamins are not helpful and lead to dependency on them.

6. The patient should eat well-balanced meals. The physician or nurse should teach the patient about the foods to eat that contain the naturally occurring vitamins.

7. Vitamin and mineral preparations should be kept out of the reach of children and all others for whom they are not prescribed.

8. Vitamins and minerals sold as special products in health food stores may have no nutritional superiority over cheaper products.

Table 19-2   Minerals

Generic name	Trade name	Comments and dosage
CALCIUM		
Calcium acetate	Phos-Ex	Has 25% calcium.
Calcium carbonate	Os-Cal 500	Has 40% concentration of calcium, the largest of any calcium product. Give 1 to 1.5 gm PO tid with meals.
Calcium citrate	Citracal	Has 21% calcium.
Calcium gluconate	Calcium Gluconate	Comes in both oral and parenteral forms. IV infusion is preferred over IM injection and is used frequently in emergency situations. Check equivalency of all oral products, because they vary from preparation to preparation. In parenteral forms, 10 ml contains 90 mg (4.5 mEq) calcium. *Oral:* Give 1 to 2 gm several times daily. *Parenterally:* 1 to 15 gm daily intravenously for adults; 500 mg/kg/day in divided doses for children.
Calcium glubionate	Neo-Calglucon	Oral preparation contains 6% calcium. Administer before meals to increase absorption. *Adults (including pregnant and breastfeeding women) and children 4 years or older:* 15 ml tid. *Children under 4 years:* 5 to 10 ml tid.
Tricalcium phosphate	Posture	Has 39% calcium.
Calcium lactate	Calcium Lactate	Contains 13% calcium and is given orally. It is available without prescription. Give 325 mg to 1.3 gm PO tid with meals.
FLUORIDE		
Fluoride (oral)	Fluoritab Flura	Adjust dosage according to local water fluoride level. ■ *General oral dosages:* 1 mg daily. *Children 3 years old and under:* 0.5 mg daily.
Fluoride (topical)	Fluorigard Dermalar ♣ Fluorinse Fluonicle ♣ Prevident	Products used between professional dental fluoride treatments for patients who have excessive problems with tooth decay. After brushing, hold preparation in mouth for at least 1 minute, then spit out. Do not swallow; do not eat, drink, smoke, or rinse mouth for at least 15 to 30 minutes after treatment to obtain maximum benefit. *Adults and children over 12 years:* 10 ml qd. *Children 6 to 12 years:* 5 to 10 ml qd.
IRON-CONTAINING PRODUCTS		
Ferrous fumarate	Feostat Femiron	Few reported side effects with this product and better tolerated than sulfate or gluconate. Contains 33% elemental iron. *Adults:* 600 to 800 mg/day PO in divided doses. *Children under 5 years:* 100 to 300 mg/day PO in 3 to 4 divided doses.
Ferrous gluconate	Fergon Simron	Less corrosive than ferrous sulfate. It is indicated for those patients who cannot tolerate sulfate because of gastric irritation. It contains 11.6% elemental iron. *Adults:* 320 to 640 mg PO tid. *Children 6 to 12 years:* 100 to 300 mg PO tid. *Children under 6 years:* 120 to 300 mg PO qd.
Ferrous sulfate	Feratab Mol-Iron	Ferrous sulfate is the standard preparation against which all other iron salts are compared. Optimal compound because it is the least expensive and contains 20% elemental iron. Timed-release capsules are more expensive and less well absorbed but reportedly have fewer side effects. *Adults:* 300 to 1200 mg PO qd in divided doses. *Children:* 600 mg PO qd in divided doses.

Continued.

Table 19-2   Minerals—cont'd

Generic name	Trade name	Comments and dosage
Ferrous sulfate exsiccated	Fer-In-Sol Feosol Slow FE	This product contains more elemental iron per mg of compound than other products. It is more expensive than plain ferrous sulfate. The liquid preparation of Feosol cannot be mixed with juice. *Iron deficiency states:* 30 to 90 mg elemental iron qd.
Iron dextran	InFeD	Used in cases where oral iron administration is impossible or unsatisfactory. Parenteral iron has caused fatal anaphylactic-type reactions and must be used with care. *Test dose:* 0.5 ml IV or IM 1 hour before the therapeutic dose, to rule out hypersensitivity. Calculate the total dose required to return hemoglobin and iron stores to normal using the following formula: $$0.3 \times \text{Weight in lb} \times \left(100 - \frac{\text{hemoglobin g/dl} \times 100}{14.8}\right) = \text{mg iron}$$ For patients weighing less than 30 lb, reduce to 80% total calculated. The Z-track method should be used for injection into the gluteus maximus muscle only. Inject deeply using a 2- or 3-inch needle of 19 to 20 gauge.

MAGNESIUM

Magnesium	Magonate Maglucate ♣	RDA for adult males is 350 mg; adult females, 330 mg. As a dietary supplement give 27 to 133 mg qd to tid.

MANGANESE

Manganese	Chelated Manganese	No RDA has been determined. Suggested daily intake includes 0.5 to 0.7 mg PO for infants, 2.5 to 5.0 mg PO for adolescents, and 3 to 7 mg PO for adults.

PHOSPHORUS

Phosphorus	Neutra-Phos	*Adults:* 800 to 1200 mg. May have mild laxative efect.

POTASSIUM

Potassium chloride
  Liquids
  Powders
  Tablets
	Cena-K
	Kaon
	Klor-Con
	K-Lyte
	K-Lor
	Slow-K
		Wide variation in concentration, price, flavor. Make certain medication is diluted with water or juice or is taken with adequate quantities of liquid. Titrate to individual requirements. Usual dosage is 20 mEq/day for prophylaxis and 40 to 100 mEq/day for treatment of potassium depletion.

Combinations of potassium gluconate; potassium citrate; potassium acetate; potassium bicarbonate

Effervescent tablets Liquids Powders Tablets	Kaochlor-Eff K-Lyte Duo-K Kaon Kaylixir Kolyum Kaon	These products, most of which require prescriptions, are used primarily in patients in whom chloride is restricted. Because some of these products do contain chloride, it is important to carefully choose the potassium salt desired. There is wide variability in the cost of these products, with most tending to be more expensive than potassium chloride products. Effervescent tablets must be dissolved completely in water before administration. Dosage should be titrated to individual needs. Usual dosage is 20 mEq/day for prophylaxis and 40 to 100 mEq/day for treatment of potassium depletion.

SODIUM CHLORIDE

Sodium chloride	Slo-Salt	Supplementation on rare occasions.

ZINC

Zinc	Orazinc	Give 10 to 20 mg/day.

ELECTROLYTE SOLUTIONS

ACTION AND USES

Fluid and electrolyte mixtures are solutions of water and calories in the form of carbohydrates, with such minerals and electrolytes as sodium, potassium, chloride, calcium, and phosphorus. These are given in the event that oral food intake has been suspended, or for the prevention of dehydration and electrolyte loss, especially in diarrhea. Fluid deficits can result from inadequate intake, excessive loss, or both. Causes include vomiting, bowel obstruction (which causes a pooling of fluid and electrolytes), diarrhea, and fever (producing increased use of fluid and electrolytes). The body attempts to compensate for the reduced circulating volume by pulling in extracellular fluid first and then intracellular fluid. This contributes to an imbalance of both fluid and electrolytes that must be corrected.

Fluid and electrolytes may be given either orally or parenterally, to prevent dehydration when oral intake is temporarily halted and to replace moderate losses of fluids and electrolytes (see Table 19-3 and the box on p. 402). Electrolyte solutions are especially useful in managing dehydration from diarrhea in infants.

CRITICAL DECISION:
Symptoms of Dehydration

Symptoms of dehydration include fatigue and a general feeling of malaise coupled with thirst. The patient may have a history compatible with progressive or acute dehydration. Geriatric patients may appear asymptomatic, even with severe dehydration.

 NURSING IMPLICATIONS AND PATIENT TEACHING

Signs of **dehydration** include weight loss, dry skin, lack of sweat, dry mucous membranes, decreased urinary output, lowered blood pressure, rapid pulse, and increased respirations. In infants dehydration may also include sunken fontanelles and loss of skin turgor. Fluid and electrolytes are also required in the comatose or acutely ill patient who is unable to take oral substances for a prolonged period of time.

These solutions are contraindicated when the patient has severe or continuing diarrhea or other major fluid loss that requires intravenous replacement, or has intractable vomiting, intestinal obstruc-

 Table 19-3   Fluid and electrolytes for oral administration

ORAL ELECTROLYTE SOLUTIONS

Pedialyte	Dosage should be based on water requirements calculated on the basis of total body surface area for infants and young children. A general guide uses 1500 ml/m^2 for maintenance during illness and 2400 ml/m^2 for maintenance and replacement of mild to moderate losses (as in diarrhea or vomiting.) *Replacement in mild to moderate fluid losses: Children 5 to 10 years of age:* 1 to 2 quarts/day. *Older children and adults:* 2 to 3 quarts/day.

SALT SUBSTITUTES

Adolph's salt substitute Morton salt substitute NoSalt Neocurtasal Nu-Salt	Over-the-counter preparations that can be used in both cooked and uncooked foods to make food more palatable for patients with sodium restrictions. These potassium chloride preparations come in a salt shaker dispenser and are used in slightly less than normal amounts of NaCl. Contraindicated in patients with severe kidney disease or oliguria. Long-term use may require iodine supplements in some patients.

SODIUM BICARBONATE

Sodium bicarbonate	Used as gastric, systemic, and urinary alkalinizer. May relieve symptoms of occasional overeating and indigestion. Give 325 mg to 2 gm 2 to 4 times daily. Daily maximum intake should not exceed 16 gm.

Fluid and electrolytes for parenteral administration

Products available in a variety of concentrations, volumes, and combinations.
    See the physician's order and the package insert.

Amino acids

Amino acid substrates with electrolytes in a variety of combinations.

Carbohydrates

Dextrose in water with 2.5% to 70% concentrations.
5% or 10% alcohol in 5% dextrose infusions
10% fructose in water
10% invert sugar in water

Electrolytes

0.2% to 5% sodium chloride solutions
Potassium chloride or potassium acetate for injection

Calcium chloride for injection
Calcium gluconate for injection
Calcium gluceptate for injection
Calcium products—combined
Magnesium sulfate or magnesium chloride for injection
Sodium bicarbonate for injection
Sodium lactate for injection
Sodium acetate for injection
Tromethamine for slow infusion
Sodium phosphate for injection
Potassium phosphate for injection
Ammonium chloride for injection

Trace metals (for slow infusion)

Zinc, copper, manganese, molybdenum, chromium, selenium, and iodine

tion or bowel perforation, decreased renal function, or when the homeostatic mechanism of the body is impaired.

The prescribed amount should not be exceeded. If the patient is still thirsty after taking the recommended dose, additional fluids in the form of water or other nonelectrolyte fluids should be given.

SUMMARY

Vitamins and minerals are essential for the body to function properly. They are often taken as supplements when dietary levels are inadequate. There is much yet to be learned about the action of vitamins and minerals in the body. It is important to note that overconsumption can create as many problems as deficiency and should be avoided. Electrolytes are given in the event that oral food intake has been suspended or given to prevent dehydration and electrolyte loss.

 CRITICAL THINKING QUESTIONS

1. What are the two types of vitamins? How does each type react differently, overall, within the body?
2. What are two circumstances under which a patient may

be unable to obtain sufficient amounts of vitamins, despite the availability of a well-balanced, nutritious diet?
3. Explain the difference between vitamins and minerals; define *electrolytes*.
4. Mr. Baker leads a very athletic life and is proud of his strict diet and voluminous intake of vitamins, which he keeps, he says, on the kitchen counter so he won't forget them. He comes to the clinic feeling "a little under the weather." He is surprised and confused when he is told that he has hypervitaminosis. Explain what that is.
5. Mr. Baker is still confused, insisting that more is better when it comes to vitamins—"and minerals, too, as far as that goes." Discuss with Mr. Baker the narrow difference between therapeutic and toxic levels of vitamins, minerals, *and* electrolytes. Use potassium as an example.
6. Create a nutrition chart to show Mr. Baker how he can get adequate amounts of vitamins, minerals, and electrolytes by eating a well-balanced diet. Be prepared to counteract Mr. Baker's frequent protest: "A vitamin is a vitamin!"
7. What three minerals are most often missing from our diets? Why is that?
8. You are asked to monitor a new patient, Ms. Falk, for dehydration, among other things. What are some of the symptoms of dehydration?
9. Ms. Falk has been told she needs fluid and electrolyte supplementation. Explain to her the rationale for such therapy and its benefits.

Bibliography

Alfaro-LeFevrer J, et al: *Drug handbook: a nursing process approach*, Menlo Park, CA, 1992, Addison-Wesley.

American Pharmaceutical Association: *Handbook of nonprescription drugs*, ed 9, Washington, 1990, American Pharmaceutical Association.

American Medical Association: *AMA drug evaluations*, ed 7, Philadelphia, 1987, WB Saunders.

Arundt K: *Manual of dermatologic therapeutics*, ed 4, Boston, 1988, Little, Brown.

Asperheim MK: *The pharmacologic basis of patient care*, ed 5, Philadelphia, 1985, WB Saunders.

Baer CL, Williams BR: *Clinical pharmacology and nursing*, ed 2, Springhouse, Pa, 1991, Springhouse.

Beck RK: *Pharmacology for prehospital emergency care*, Philadelphia, 1992, FA Davis.

Benitz WE: *The pediatric drug handbook*, ed 2, St Louis, 1988, Mosby.

Billups NA: *American drug index*, ed 37, Philadelphia, 1993, JB Lippincott.

Clark, JB, Queener SF, Karb VB: *Pharmacologic basis of nursing practice*, ed 4, St Louis, 1992, Mosby.

Clayton BD: *Basic pharmacology for nurses*, St Louis, 1992, Mosby.

Dale MM, Dickenson AH: *Companion to pharmacology: a study guide for self assessment and revision*, New York, 1993, Churchill Livingstone.

DeWit SC, editor: *Keane's essentials of medical-surgical nursing*, ed 3, Philadelphia, 1992, WB Saunders.

Dison N: *Simplified drugs and solutions for nurses*, ed 10, St Louis, 1988, Mosby.

Dukes MN, Aronson JK: *Side effects of drugs annual 17*, Amsterdam, 1993, Elsevier Science.

Gerald MC, O'Bannon FV: *Nursing pharmacology and therapeutics*, ed 2, Norwalk, Conn, 1988, Appleton & Lange.

Gilman AG, Goodman LS, Gillman A: *Goodman & Gilman's pharmacological basis of therapeutics*, ed 8, New York, 1990, McGraw-Hill.

Grahame-Smith DG, Aronson JK: *Oxford textbook of clinical pharmacology & drug therapy*, ed 2, London, 1992, Oxford University Press.

Harkness RR: *Drug interactions handbook*, Englewood Cliffs, NJ, 1991, Prentice-Hall.

Henney D: *Drugs in nursing practice*, ed 4, New York, 1992, Churchill Livingstone.

Hitner H, Nagle BT: *Basic pharamacology for health occupations*, ed 3, Westerville, Oh, 1993, Glencoe.

Hodgson BB, Kizior RJ, Kingdon RT: *Nurse's drug handbook*, Philadelphia, 1993, WB Saunders.

Janney C, Timpke J: *Calculation of drug dosages*, ed 4, Penn Valley, Va, 1993, TJ Designs.

Katzung BG: *Basic and clinical pharmacology*, ed 5, Norwalk, Conn, 1992, Appleton & Lange.

Liska K: *Drugs and the human body*, ed 3, New York, 1990, Macmillan.

Long JW, Rybacki, JJ: *Essential guide to prescription drugs*, New York, 1994, Harper Collins.

Malik MA: *American drug reference*, New York, 1993, American Drug Reference.

Malseed RT: *Pharmacology, drug therapy and nursing considerations*, ed 3, Philadelphia, 1990, JB Lippincott.

Mann RE, Rawlins MD, Auty R: *A textbook of pharmaceutical medicine*, New York, 1993, Parthenon.

Mathewson MK: *Pharmacotherapeutics: a nursing process approach*, ed 2, Philadelphia, 1991, FA Davis.

McEvoy GK: *The American hospital formulary service*, Bethesda, Md, 1993, American Society of Hospital Pharmacists.

McKenry LM, Salerno E. *Mosby's pharmacology in nursing*, ed 18, St Louis, 1992, Mosby.

Medication teaching manual: a guide for patient counselling, ed 2, Bethesda, 1986, American Society of Hospital Pharmacists.

Melmon KL et al: *Melmon & Morrelli's clinical pharmacology: basic principles in therapeutics*, ed 3, New York, 1992, McGraw-Hill.

Modell W: *Drugs of choice*, New Rochelle, NY, 1993, The Medical Letter.

Neal MJ: *Medical pharmacology at a glance*, ed 2, Colchester, Vt, 1992, Blackwell Scientific.

Olin BR, ed: *Drug facts and comparisons*, Philadelphia, 1994, JB Lippincott.

Patterson HR, Gustafson EA, Sheridan ES: *Current drug handbook*, Philadelphia, 1988, WB Saunders.

Physicians' desk reference, ed 48, Oradell, NJ, 1994, Medical Economics Data.

Pirodsky DM, Cohn JS: *Clinical primer of psychopharmacology: a practical guide*, ed 2, New York, 1992, McGraw-Hill.

Radcliff RK, Ogden SJ: *Calculation of drug dosages*, ed 4, St Louis, 1990, Mosby.

Rall TW, editor: *Goodman and Gilman's essentials of pharmacology*, New York, 1993, McGraw-Hill.

Rees J, Ritter J, Spector R: *Aids to clinical pharmacology and therapeutics*, ed 3, New York, 1993, Churchill Livingstone.

403

Rice J, Skelley EG: *Medications and mathematics for the nurse,* ed 7, Albany, NY, 1993, Delmar.

Sacks S, Spector R: *Aids to pharmacology,* ed 3, New York, 1993, Churchill Livingstone.

Smeltzer SC, Bare BG, editors: *Brunner and Suddarth's textbook of medical-surgical nursing,* ed 7, Philadelphia, 1992, JB Lippincott.

Spencer RT: *Clinical pharmacology and nursing management,* ed 4, Philadelphia, 1992, JB Lippincott.

Spratto GR, Woods AL: *RN magazine's nurses' drug reference '93,* Albany, NY, 1993, Delmar.

Stockley IH: *Drug interactions,* ed 2, Colchester, Vt, 1992, Blackwell Scientific.

Taylor C, Lillis C, LeMone P: *Fundamentals of nursing,* ed 2, Philadelphia, 1993, JB Lippincott.

Trouce J: *Clinical pharmacology for nurses,* ed 14, New York, 1993, Churchill Livingstone.

USP DI United States Pharmacopeia Dispensing Information: vol 1, *Drug information for the health care provider;* vol 2, *Advice for the patient,* Rockville, Md, 1990, United States Pharmacopeial Convention Inc.

Wallace B: *Nursing pharmacology,* ed 2, Boston, 1992, Jones & Bartlett.

Wilson BA, Shannon MT: *Nurse's drug guide,* Norwalk, Conn, 1992, Appleton & Lange.

Index